VISUALIZING NUTRITION

EVERYDAY CHOICES

D0813505

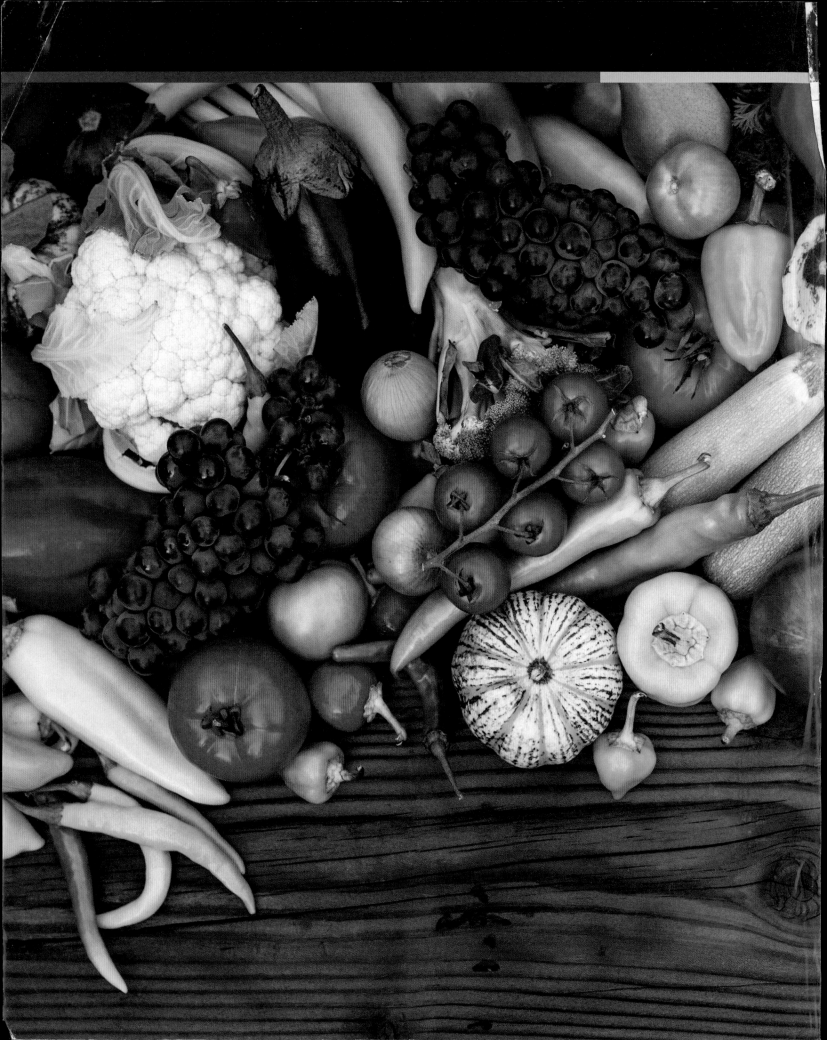

VISUALIZING NUTRITION
EVERYDAY CHOICES

CANADIAN EDITION

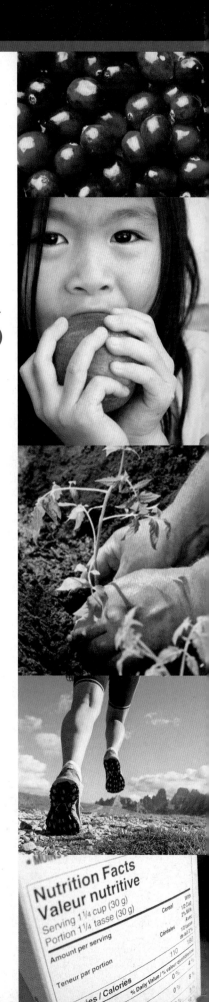

Mary B. Grosvenor, MS, RD

Lori A. Smolin, PhD,
University of Connecticut

Diana L. Bedoya, MSc,
Simon Fraser University

WILEY

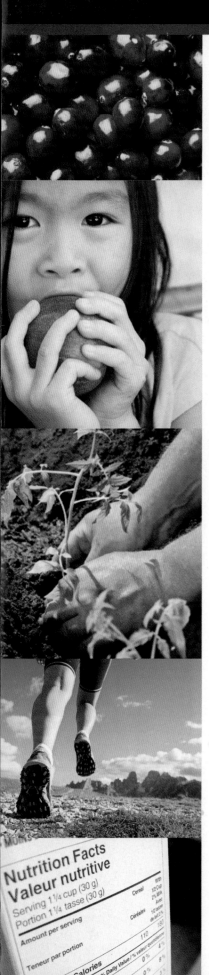

Vice President & Publisher: Veronica Visentin
Acquisitions Editor: Rodney Burke
Marketing Manager: Patty Maher
Editorial Manager: Karen Staudinger
Production Manager: Tegan Wallace
Developmental Editor: Joanne Sutherland
Production Editor: Andrea Grzybowski
Media Editor: Channade Fenandoe
Publishing Services Coordinator: Lynda Jess
Editorial Assistant: Luisa Begani
Layout: codeMantra
Cover Design: Harry Nolan

Title page credits: (facing page) ©iStockphoto.com/Jasmina007, title and copyright pages (top to bottom) ©iStockphoto.com/mphilllips007, ©iStockphoto.com/ktaylorg, ©iStockphoto.com/Sveta, ©iStockphoto.com/Gorfer, ©iStockphoto.com/timmy

Library and Archives Canada Cataloguing in Publication

Grosvenor, Mary B., author
    Visualizing nutrition / Mary B. Grosvenor, Lori A. Smolin,
Diana L. Bedoya.—Canadian edition.
Includes index.
ISBN 978-1-118-16174-6 (bound)
    1. Nutrition—Textbooks. I. Smolin, Lori A., author
II. Bedoya, Diana L., 1981-, author III. Title.
QP141.G76 2013   612.3
C2013-903972-4

Printing and binding: Quad Graphics
Printed and bound in the United States.
1 2 3 4 5 QG 18 17 16 15 14

John Wiley & Sons Canada, Ltd.
6045 Freemont Blvd.
Mississauga, Ontario L5R 4J3
Visit our website at: www.wiley.ca

How Is Wiley Visualizing Different?

Wiley Visualizing is based on decades of research on the use of visuals in learning.[1] The visuals teach key concepts and are pedagogically designed to **explain, present,** and **organize** new information. The figures are tightly integrated with accompanying text; the visuals are conceived with the text in ways that clarify and reinforce major concepts, while allowing students to understand the details. This commitment to distinctive and consistent visual pedagogy sets Wiley Visualizing apart from other textbooks.

The textbooks offer an array of remarkable photographs, maps, media, and film from photo collections around the world, including those of National Geographic. Wiley Visualizing's images are not decorative; such images can be distracting to students. Instead, they are purposeful and the primary driver of the content. These authentic materials immerse the student in real-life issues and experiences and support thinking, comprehension, and application.

Together these elements deliver a level of rigour in ways that maximize student learning and involvement. Wiley Visualizing has proven to increase student learning through its unique combination of text, photographs, and illustrations, with online video, animations, simulations, and assessments.

(1) Visual Pedagogy. Using the Cognitive Theory of Multimedia Learning, which is backed up by hundreds of empirical research studies, Wiley's authors create visualizations for their texts that specifically support students' thinking and learning—for example, the selection of relevant materials, the organization of the new information, or the integration of the new knowledge with prior knowledge.

(2) Authentic Situations and Problems. *Visualizing Nutrition: Everyday Choices, Canadian Edition* benefits from National Geographic's more than century-long recording of the world and offers an array of remarkable photographs, maps, media, and film. These authentic materials immerse the student in real-life issues in environmental science, thereby enhancing motivation, learning, and retention (Donovan & Bransford, 2005).[2]

(3) Designed with Interactive Multimedia. *Visualizing Nutrition: Everyday Choices, Canadian Edition* is tightly integrated with *WileyPLUS*, our online learning environment that provides interactive multimedia activities in which learners can actively engage with the materials. The combination of textbook and *WileyPLUS* provides learners with multiple entry points to the content, giving them greater opportunity to explore concepts and assess their understanding as they progress through the course. *WileyPLUS* is a key component of the Wiley Visualizing learning and problem-solving experience, setting it apart from other textbooks whose online component is mere drill-and-practice.

Wiley Visualizing and the WileyPLUS Learning Environment are designed as a natural extension of how we learn

To understand why the Visualizing approach is effective, it is first helpful to understand how we learn.

1. Our brain processes information using two main channels: visual and verbal. Our *working memory* holds information that our minds process as we learn. This "mental workbench" helps us with decisions, problem-solving, and making sense of words and pictures by building verbal and visual models of the information.

2. When the verbal and visual models of corresponding information are integrated in working memory, we form more comprehensive, lasting mental models.

3. When we link these integrated mental models to our prior knowledge, stored in our *long-term memory*, we build even stronger mental models. When an integrated (visual plus verbal) mental model is formed and stored in long-term memory, real learning begins.

The effort our brains put forth to make sense of instructional information is called *cognitive load*. There are two kinds of cognitive load: productive cognitive load, such as when we're engaged in learning or exert positive effort to create mental models; and unproductive cognitive load, which occurs when the brain is trying to make sense of needlessly complex content or when information is not presented well. The learning process can be impaired when the information to be processed exceeds the capacity of working memory. Well-designed visuals and text work with effective pedagogical guidance to reduce the unproductive cognitive load in our working memory.

---

[1] Mayer, R.E. (Ed.) *The Cambridge Handbook of Multimedia Learning.* New York: Cambridge University Press, 2005.
[2] Donovan, M.S., and Bransford, J. (Eds.) *How Students Learn: Science in the Classroom.* Washington, DC: The National Academy Press, 2005. Available at http://www.nap.edu/openbook.php?record_id=11102&page=1. Accessed June 9, 2013.

Wiley Visualizing is designed for engaging and effective learning

The visuals and text in *Visualizing Nutrition: Everyday Choices, Canadian Edition* are specially integrated to present complex processes in clear steps and with clear representations, organize related pieces of information, and integrate related information with one another. This approach, along with the use of interactive multimedia, minimizes unproductive cognitive load and helps students engage with the content. When students are engaged, they're reading and learning, which can lead to greater knowledge and academic success.

Research shows that well-designed visuals, integrated with comprehensive text, can improve the efficiency with which a learner processes information. In this regard, SEG Research, an independent research firm, conducted a national, multi-site study evaluating the effectiveness of Wiley Visualizing. Its findings indicate that students using Wiley Visualizing products (both print and multimedia) were more engaged in the course, exhibited greater retention throughout the course, and made significantly greater gains in content area knowledge and skills, compared with students in similar classes that did not use Wiley Visualizing.[3]

The use of *WileyPLUS* can also increase learning. According to a white paper titled "Leveraging Blended Learning for More Effective Course Management and Enhanced Student Outcomes" by Peggy Wyllie of Evince Market Research & Communications, studies show that effective use of online resources can increase learning outcomes. Pairing supportive online resources with face-to-face instruction can help students to learn and reflect on material, and deploying multimodal learning methods can help students to engage with the material and retain their acquired knowledge.

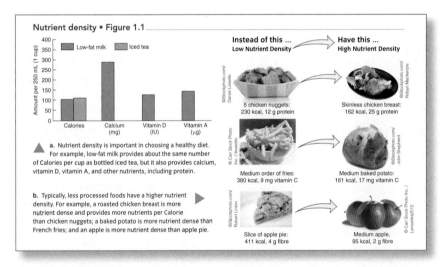

Nutrient density (Figure 1.1) To augment the definition of nutrient density, which appears in the text, this two-part figure integrates a graphic depiction of the concept of nutrient density with a photographic illustration. The arrows visually guide students to the more nutrient-dense choice, while captions add specific information on the nutrient density of each food.

---

[3]SEG Research. *Improving Student-Learning with Graphically-Enhanced Textbooks: A study of the Effectiveness of the Wiley Visualizing Series*, 2009. Available at http://www.wiley.com/college/visualizing/doc/Wiley_Visualizing_Effectiveness_Report.pdf. Accessed June 9, 2013.

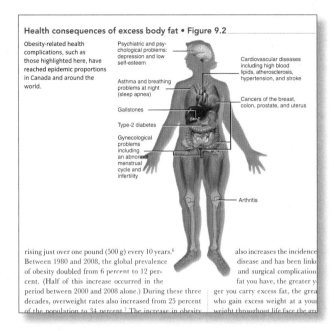

Health consequences of excess body fat • Figure 9.2

Obesity-related health complications, such as those highlighted here, have reached epidemic proportions in Canada and around the world.

Psychiatric and psychological problems: depression and low self-esteem

Cardiovascular diseases including high blood lipids, atherosclerosis, hypertension, and stroke

Asthma and breathing problems at night (sleep apnea)

Cancers of the breast, colon, prostate, and uterus

Gallstones

Type-2 diabetes

Gynecological problems including an abnormal menstrual cycle and infertility

Arthritis

rising just over one pound (500 g) every 10 years.[6] Between 1980 and 2008, the global prevalence of obesity doubled from 6 percent to 12 percent. (Half of this increase occurred in the period between 2000 and 2008 alone.) During these three decades, overweight rates also increased from 25 percent of the population to 34 percent.[7] The increase in obesity

also increases the incidence disease and has been linke and surgical complication fat you have, the greater y ger you carry excess fat, the grea who gain excess weight at a you weight throughout life face the gr

Health consequences of excess body fat (Figure 9.2)

This visual overview enhances learning by visually relating the health conditions associated with obesity to the area of the body affected. Organizing the list of health conditions and their effects reduces cognitive load.

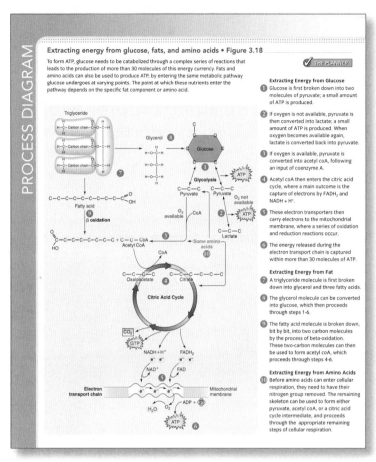

PROCESS DIAGRAM

Extracting energy from glucose, fats, and amino acids • Figure 3.18

To form ATP, glucose needs to be catabolized through a complex series of reactions that leads to the production of more than 30 molecules of this energy currency. Fats and amino acids can also be used to produce ATP, by entering the same metabolic pathway glucose undergoes at varying points. The point at which these nutrients enter the pathway depends on the specific fat component or amino acid.

THE PLANNER

Extracting Energy from Glucose

1. Glucose is first broken down into two molecules of pyruvate; a small amount of ATP is produced.

2. If oxygen is not available, pyruvate is then converted into lactate; a small amount of ATP is produced. When oxygen becomes available again, lactate is converted back into pyruvate.

3. If oxygen is available, pyruvate is converted into acetyl coA, following an input of coenzyme A.

4. Acetyl coA then enters the citric acid cycle, where a main outcome is the capture of electrons by $FADH_2$ and $NADH + H^+$.

5. These electron transporters then carry electrons to the mitochondrial membrane, where a series of oxidation and reduction reactions occur.

6. The energy released during the electron transport chain is captured within more than 30 molecules of ATP.

Extracting Energy from Fat

7. A triglyceride molecule is first broken down into glycerol and three fatty acids.

8. The glycerol molecule can be converted into glucose, which then proceeds through steps 1-6.

9. The fatty acid molecule is broken down, bit by bit, into two carbon molecules by the process of beta-oxidation. These two-carbon molecules can then be used to form acetyl coA, which proceeds through steps 4-6.

Extracting Energy from Amino Acids

10. Before amino acids can enter cellular respiration, they need to have their nitrogen group removed. The remaining skeleton can be used to form either pyruvate, acetyl coA, or a citric acid cycle intermediate, and proceeds through the appropriate remaining steps of cellular respiration.

Cellular respiration (Figure 3.18) Visually ordering the steps in this process diagram makes metabolism easier to understand. Various process illustrations appear throughout the book to review, reinforce, and build students' knowledge of how processes occur both inside and outside the body.

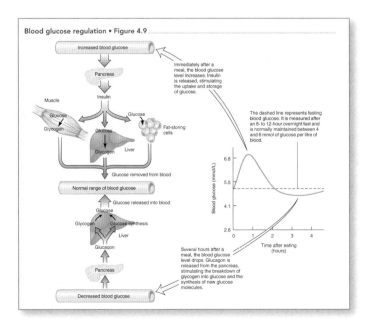

Blood glucose regulation • Figure 4.9

Immediately after a meal, the blood glucose level increases. Insulin is released, stimulating the uptake and storage of glucose.

The dashed line represents fasting blood glucose. It is measured after an 8- to 12-hour overnight fast and is normally maintained between 4 and 6 mmol of glucose per litre of blood.

Several hours after a meal, the blood glucose level drops. Glucagon is released from the pancreas, stimulating the breakdown of glycogen into glucose and the synthesis of new glucose molecules.

Blood glucose regulation (Figure 4.9)

Physically integrating textual elements with the visual elements, as shown here, eliminates split attention (when we divide our attention among several sources of different information).

Guided Chapter Tour

How Are the Wiley Visualizing Chapters Organized?

Student engagement is more than just exciting videos or interesting animations—engagement means keeping students motivated to keep going. It is easy to get bored or lose focus when presented with large amounts of information, and it is easy to lose motivation when the relevance of the information is unclear.

Each Wiley Visualizing chapter engages students from the start

Chapter opening text and visuals introduce the subject and connect the student with the material that follows.

Chapter Introductions illustrate key concepts with intriguing stories and striking images.

Chapter Outlines guide students through the chapter.

Lipids: Oils, Fats, Phospholipids, and Sterols

"Sausages taste good. Pork chops taste good," wrote filmmaker Quentin Tarantino in the original screenplay of *Pulp Fiction*. Fat makes foods taste good, smell good, and feel good to our palate. Tarantino understands the appeal of fat. As for its function, we have to rely on study, not entertainment.

The word *fat* has come to be associated with unhealthiness, unfitness, and obesity. Fitness gurus and enthusiastic celebrities declare that "fat is bad," whether you are considering which fast-food meal to choose or trying to remove it from your waist. Their 30-second commercial or half-hour program for a new diet regimen or exercise contraption—or both—gives little consideration to the vital role that fats play in healthy nutrition. There is, in reality, nothing intrinsically "bad" about dietary fats. The body uses fats as building blocks for other molecules, for vitamin absorption and storage, as a source of energy, and for energy storage. Fats are as important to a well-balanced diet as carbohydrates, proteins, and vitamins; without fats, the body cannot function.

Unfortunately, the amount of dietary fat we require and the amount we desire are often two very different things. In the case of the body's requirements for these substances, moderation is key. Whatever our bodies don't use remains in reserves of stored fat. Depending on our lifestyle choices, these abundant unused reserves may become not only unnecessary but harmful to our health.

CHAPTER OUTLINE

Fats in Our Food   130
- Sources of Fat in Our Food
- Canada's Changing Fat Intake

Types of Lipids   131
- Triglycerides and Fatty Acids
- Phospholipids
- Sterols

Absorbing and Transporting Lipids   138
- Digestion and Absorption of Fat
- Transporting Lipids in the Blood

Lipid Functions   142
- Fat as a Source of Energy

Lipids in Health and Disease   145
- Heart Disease
- Cancer
- Obesity

Meeting Lipid Needs   153
- Fat and Cholesterol Recommendations
- Choosing Fats Wisely
- ■ Thinking It Through: Improving Heart Health

CHAPTER PLANNER ✓

☐ Stimulate your interest by reading the introduction and looking at the visual.

☐ Scan the Learning Objectives in each section: p. 130 ☐ p. 131 ☐ p. 138 ☐ p. 142 ☐ p. 145 ☐ p. 153 ☐

☐ Read the text and study all figures and visuals. Answer any questions.

Analyze key features

☐ Nutrition InSight, p. 132

☐ Process Diagram, p. 139 ☐ p. 141 ☐ p. 143 ☐ p. 146 ☐

☐ Debate, p. 151

☐ Thinking It Through, p. 154

☐ What Should I Eat?, p. 157

☐ Stop: Answer the Concept Checks before you go on: p. 130 ☐ p. 138 ☐ p. 141 ☐ p. 145 ☐ p. 152 ☐ p. 157 ☐

End of chapter

☐ Review the Summary and Key Terms.

☐ Answer the Critical and Creative Thinking Questions.

☐ Answer What is happening in this picture?

The **Chapter Planner** gives students a path through the learning aids in the chapter. Throughout the chapter, The Planner icon prompts students to use the learning aids and to set priorities as they study.

Wiley Visualizing guides students through the chapter

The content of Wiley Visualizing gives students a variety of approaches—visuals, words, interactions, video, and assessments—that work together to provide a guided path through the content.

Process Diagrams enable students to grasp important topics with less effort by guiding them with clear step-by-step narrative.

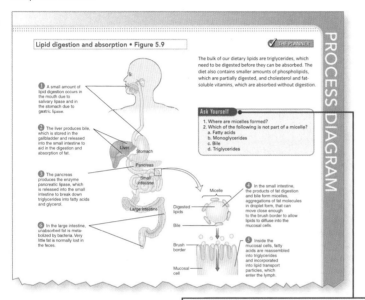

Ask Yourself, Think Critically, or Interpreting Data questions appear with many figures throughout the text. Ask Yourself questions require students to focus on the visual itself, making sure students understand the concept presented in the visual.

WileyPLUS

WileyPLUS **Interactive Process Diagrams** provide additional visual examples and descriptive narration of a difficult concept, process, or theory, allowing the students to interact and engage with the content. Many of these diagrams are built around a specific feature such as a Process Diagram.

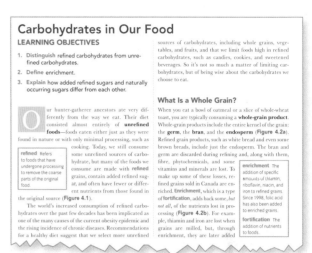

Learning Objectives at the start of each section indicate in behavioural terms the concepts that students are expected to master while reading the section.

Nutrition InSight features are multipart visual features that focus on a key concept or topic in the chapter, exploring it in detail or in broader context using a combination of photos, diagrams, maps, figures, and data.

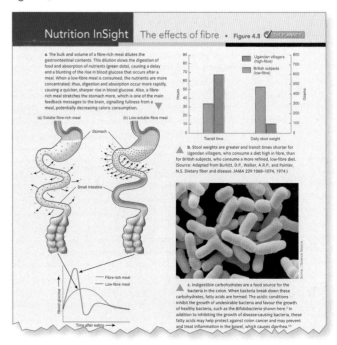

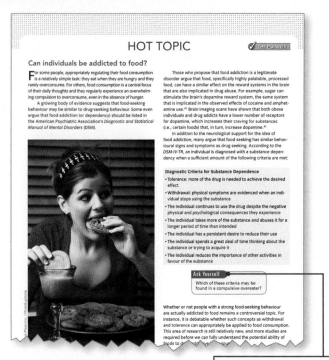

Hot Topic boxes highlight the latest research on a concept or phenomenon that is topical in the media or among nutrition scientists. Photos and figures are used to improve students' understanding of the subject.

Ask Yourself questions challenge students to think beyond what they have learned in the text and images.

What Should I Eat? provides simple, usable tips that help students translate the nutrition recommendations discussed in each chapter into healthy food choices.

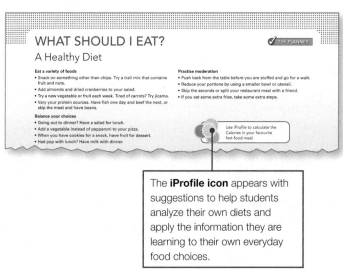

The **iProfile icon** appears with suggestions to help students analyze their own diets and apply the information they are learning to their own everyday food choices.

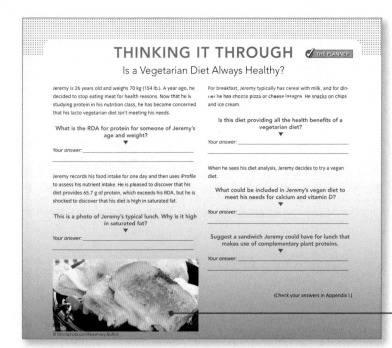

Thinking It Through exercises use a critical thinking approach to walk students through the thought processes needed to make nutritional decisions and solve related problems. These exercises appear in each chapter of the book to help students apply their developing nutrition knowledge to everyday situations. They present a nutrition-related case study and then guide the students through the logical progression of thought needed to collect the appropriate information and solve the case.

Each Thinking it Through includes a photo, graph, or table that must be used to answer one of the questions.

Debate explores both sides of a controversial nutrition topic. Students synthesize the material for greater understanding.

Each debate raises a relevant issue related to the chapter.

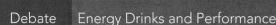

Debate Energy Drinks and Performance ✓ THE PLANNER

The Issue: Energy drinks are sold alongside sports drinks, and manufacturers of these beverages often sponsor athletes and athletic events. Should they be used as ergogenic aids? Is drinking them a safe way to improve your game?

© Tony Cenicola/The New York Times/ReduxStock

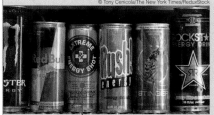

Energy drinks have been available for purchase in Canada only since 2004, but the popularity of such drinks as Red Bull, Monster, and Full Throttle has soared over the past decade. They promise to keep you alert to study, work, drive, party all night, and perhaps excel at your next athletic competition. The main ingredients in these drinks are sugar and caffeine. Glucose is an important fuel for exercise, and caffeine is known to enhance endurance, so these drinks may seem like an ideal ergogenic aid.

A traditional sports drink, like Gatorade, contains about 28 g of sugar in 500 mL; a typical energy drink provides twice this much (55 to 60 g). Since carbohydrate fuels activity, it may seem that the additional sugar would provide energy for prolonged exercise. But more is not always better during activity. The double load of sugar cannot be absorbed quickly, and unabsorbed sugar in the stomach can cause gastrointestinal distress and slow fluid absorption.

The caffeine content of energy drinks ranges from 50 to 500 mg per can or bottle. Caffeine is an effective ergogenic aid that enhances endurance when consumed before or during exercise.[46] But too much caffeine, referred to as caffeine intoxication, causes nervousness, anxiety, restlessness, insomnia, gastrointestinal upset, tremors, increased blood pressure, and rapid heartbeat. Numerous cases of caffeine-associated death, seizure, and car-

diac arrest have occurred after consumption of energy drinks.[47–49] Even if the caffeine in an energy drink increases endurance, depending on when it is consumed, it can also affect timing and coordination and hurt overall performance. These effects are of particular concern because a recent *Consumer Reports* analysis found that approximately one-third of reviewed energy drinks contained caffeine levels significantly higher than were declared on their labels.[50] Caffeine is also a diuretic; at the levels contained in these drinks, it may contribute to dehydration, particularly in first-time users. Because of caffeine's potential for toxicity at high doses, Health Canada is currently considering limiting the amount of caffeine in these beverages to a maximum level of 180 mg per container, regardless of size.[51]

Energy drinks often contain other ingredients that promise to improve performance, such as B vitamins, taurine, guarana, and ginseng. B vitamins are needed to produce ATP, so they are marketed to enhance energy production from sugar. But unless you are deficient in these vitamins, drinking them in an energy drink will not enhance your ATP production. Taurine is an amino acid that may reduce the amount of muscle damage and improve exercise performance and capacity, but not all research supports these claims.[52] Guarana is an herbal ingredient that contains caffeine and small amounts of the stimulants theobromine and theophylline. The extra caffeine from guarana (which is not included in the caffeine content listed for these beverages) may contribute to caffeine toxicity. Ginseng is also claimed to have performance-enhancing effects, but these effects have not been demonstrated scientifically.[52] In general, the amounts of these ingredients are too small to have much effect, and the safety of consuming them in combination with caffeine prior to or during exercise has yet to be established.[52]

Ask Yourself

a. So should you down an energy drink before your next competition? They do provide a caffeine boost, but is it so much caffeine that you also risk dehydration, high blood pressure, and heart problems?

b. Energy drinks provide sugar to fuel activity, but will they upset your stomach? What about the herbal ingredients—do they offer a benefit you are looking for?

Ask Yourself questions at the end of each debate ask students to integrate and evaluate the information presented.

Tables, graphs, and photos focus student attention and add information and are often the focus of Think Critically questions.

---

proteins that have complementary amino acid patterns can meet an individual's essential amino acid requirements without consuming any animal proteins.

Canada's Food Guide recommendations

Choose a diet that includes a variety of foods, which will provide enough protein and enough of each of the essential amino acids to meet the body's needs. If you follow the food guide recommendations, your diet will include both animal and plant sources of protein (**Figure 6.17**). A 250-mL glass of milk provides about 8 g of protein, and a serving of meats and alternatives can add another 7 to 10 g of protein. These two food groups contain the foods that are the highest in protein. Each serving from the grains group and a serving of vegetables provides 1 to 3 g, but because we eat a larger number of servings from these groups, they make an important contribution to our protein intake. However, just getting enough protein does not ensure a healthy diet. The sources of your dietary proteins also affect the healthfulness of your diet, particularly how well it meets the recommendations for fat and fibre intake (see *What Should I Eat?*).

Vegetarian Diets

In many parts of the world, diets based on plant proteins, called vegetarian diets, have evolved mostly out of necessity because people are living in areas where animal sources of protein are limited, either physically or economically. Compared with raising plants, raising animals requires more land and resources, and purchasing animals is more expensive than purchasing plants. The developing world relies on plant foods to meet protein needs. For example, in rural Mexico, most dietary protein comes from beans, rice, and tortillas (corn); in India, most dietary protein comes from lentils and rice. As a population's economic prosperity rises, the proportion of animal foods in its diet typically increases, but in developed countries, vegetarian diets are often followed for reasons other than economics, such as health, religion, personal ethics, or environmental awareness. Vegan diets eliminate all animal

vegetarian diets Diets that include plant-based foods and eliminate some or all foods of animal origin.

vegan diets Plant-based diets that eliminate all animal products.

Margin Glossary Terms (in **green boldface**) define important terms in each chapter. Other important terms appear in **black boldface** and are defined in the text.

Student understanding is assessed at different levels

Wiley Visualizing with *WileyPLUS* offers students lots of practice material for assessing their understanding of each study objective. Students know exactly what they are getting out of each study session through immediate feedback and coaching.

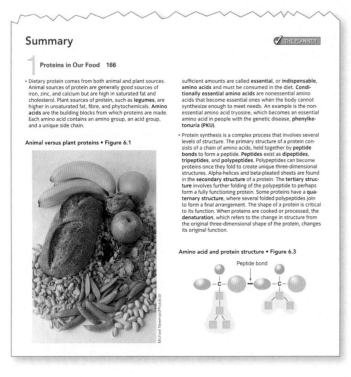

Summary

✓ THE PLANNER

1 Proteins in Our Food 166

• Dietary protein comes from both animal and plant sources. Animal sources of protein are generally good sources of iron, zinc, and calcium but are high in saturated fat and cholesterol. Plant sources of protein, such as **legumes**, are higher in unsaturated fat, fibre, and phytochemicals. **Amino acids** are the building blocks from which proteins are made. Each amino acid contains an amino group, an acid group, and a unique side chain.

Animal versus plant proteins • Figure 6.1

sufficient amounts are called **essential**, or **indispensable**, **amino acids** and must be consumed in the diet. **Conditionally essential amino acids** are nonessential amino acids that become essential ones when the body cannot synthesize enough to meet needs. An example is the nonessential amino acid tryosine, which becomes an essential amino acid in people with the genetic disease, **phenylketonuria (PKU)**.

• Protein synthesis is a complex process that involves several levels of structure. The primary structure of a protein consists of a chain of amino acids, held together by **peptide bonds** to form a peptide. **Peptides** exist as **dipeptides**, **tripeptides**, and **polypeptides**. Polypeptides can become proteins once they fold to create unique three-dimensional structures. Alpha-helices and beta-pleated sheets are found in the **secondary structure** of a protein. The **tertiary structure** involves further folding of the polypeptide to perhaps form a fully functioning protein. Some proteins have a **quaternary structure**, where several folded polypeptides join to form a final arrangement. The shape of a protein is critical to its function. When proteins are cooked or processed, the **denaturation**, which refers to the change in structure from the original three-dimensional shape of the protein, changes its original function.

Amino acid and protein structure • Figure 6.3

Peptide bond

The **Summary** revisits each major section, with informative images taken from the chapter. These visuals reinforce important concepts.

CONCEPT CHECK STOP

1. **How** is *Eating Well with Canada's Food Guide* related to the DRIs?

2. **What** is the significance of the specific rainbow design of Canada's Food Guide?

3. **How** many servings of grain product do you require each day? How many would be recommended if you were of the opposite gender?

Concept Check questions at the end of each section allow students to test their comprehension of the learning objectives.

Critical and Creative Thinking Questions

1. Keep a three-day diet record. Use iProfile to analyze the nutrient composition of your diet. Would your diet meet the energy, protein, and micronutrient needs of a 25-year-old pregnant woman who is 165 cm (5'5") tall, weighed 59 kg (130 lb.) at the start of her pregnancy, and is now in her second trimester? If not, what foods or supplements should need to be added to meet these needs?

2. Many people object to infant formula manufacturers advertising their products in developing nations. Do you feel it is appropriate to promote the use of formula in developing nations? Why or why not?

3. HIV, the virus that causes AIDS, passes via breastfeeding to one out of seven infants born to HIV-infected mothers; yet, in developing countries, some HIV-positive women are advised to breastfeed. Explain this recommendation, considering what you have learned about the benefits of breastfeeding.

4. If an infant is born weighing 2.7 kg (6 lb.), what might the baby weigh at 4 months of age and at 12 months? Why?

5. Sia, a vegan woman, has just learned she is pregnant. What nutrient deficiencies are common for vegans? For pregnant women? What supplements would you recommend Sia take during her pregnancy?

6. Marina, a 16-year-old, is four months pregnant. She is 163 cm (5'4") tall and weighed 50 kg (110 lb.) before she became pregnant. Her typical diet, which provided 1,800 kilocalories, 60 g of protein, and 15 mg of iron, met her needs before she became pregnant. What changes in the amounts of energy, protein, and iron would you recommend now that Marina is in her second trimester?

Critical and Creative Thinking Questions challenge students to think more broadly about chapter concepts. The level of these questions ranges from simple to advanced; they encourage students to think critically and develop an analytical understanding of the nutrition concepts discussed in the chapter. Some exercises feature clinical applications, which help reinforce the importance of nutrition in both health promotion and disease prevention. Some exercises can be assigned as collaborative learning exercises to encourage students to work together and learn from each other to solve a problem.

Self-Test

(Check your answers in Appendix K.)

1. Which DRI standards can be used as goals for individual intake?
   a. AIs
   b. RDAs
   c. EARs
   d. A and B only

2. Based on the following graph, which shows one day's intake of selected nutrients, which of these statements about this person's nutrient intake is true?

Nutrient	Percent of recommendation 0% 50% 100%
Vitamin A	75%
Vitamin C	115%
Iron	54%
Calcium	75%
Saturated fat	134%

   a. She has an iron deficiency.
   b. She consumes the recommended amount of vitamin A.
   c. If she consumes this amount of iron every day, she is at risk for iron deficiency.
   d. She has osteoporosis.

3. Which DRI standard can help you determine whether a supplement contains a toxic level of a nutrient?
   a. RDA
   b. AI
   c. EAR
   d. UL

4. Which letter labels the DRI standard that represents the average needs of the population?

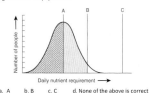

   a. A b. B c. C d. None of the above is correct.

5. Which of the following statements is false?
   a. An EER value gives the amount of energy needed to maintain body weight.
   b. Your EER stays the same when you gain weight.
   c. If you consume more calories than your EER, you will gain weight.
   d. Your EER depends on your age, gender, weight, height, and activity level.

6. Which of the following is *not* a food group in *Eating Well with Canada's Food Guide*?
   a. milk
   b. meat and alternatives
   c. vegetables and fruit
   d. fats and sweets

7. *Eating Well with Canada's Food Guide* recommends that _____ consume a daily supplement of vitamin D
   a. men and women over the age of 50
   b. women of childbearing age
   c. vegetarians
   d. people with osteoporosis

8. Which of the following is not a recommendation in the "Make each Food Guide Serving Count" section of *Eating Well with Canada's Food Guide*?
   a. Make at least half of each day's grain products whole grain.
   b. Consume at least two food guide servings of fish each week.
   c. Choose fresh vegetables and fruit over frozen.
   d. Select lower-fat milk alternatives.

9. Use the following label to determine which of the following statements about the amount of saturated fat in this product is true.

Nutrition Facts Valeur nutritive		
Per 1 cup (220 g)/par 1 tasse (225 g)		
Amount Teneur		% Daily Value % valeur quotidienne
Calories / Calories 250		
Fat / Lipides 12 g		18 %
Saturated / saturés 3 g		15 %
+ Trans / trans 1.5 g		
Cholesterol / Cholestérol 30 mg		10 %
Sodium / Sodium 470 mg		20 %
Carbohydrate / Glucides 31 g		10 %
Fibre / Fibres 0 g		0 %
Sugars / Sucres 5 g		
Protein / Protéines 5 g		
Vitamin A / Vitamine A		4 %
Vitamin C / Vitamine C		2 %
Calcium / Calcium		20 %
Iron / Fer		4 %

Visual end-of-chapter **Self-Tests** pose questions to test students' understanding of key concepts. Graphs, diagrams, and other images from the chapter encourage students to actively and visually engage with the material.

What is happening in this picture?

Clara Hughes is shown after receiving her sixth Olympic medal at the Vancouver Olympics in 2010. At age 38, which we consider middle age, she was twice the age of many of her competitors. Clara is one of the only athletes to have won multiple medals at both the summer and winter Olympics.

Think Critically

1. How does Clara's physiological age compare with her chronological age?
2. How do you think Clara's lean body mass compares with that of the average 38-year-old woman?

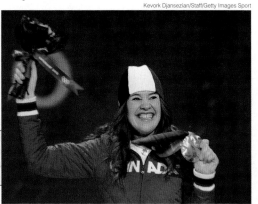

What is happening in this picture? presents a photograph that illustrates the practical application of chapter concepts. The photograph is paired with Think Critically questions that ask students to apply what they have learned in the chapter to analyze and interpret what they observe in the photo.

Preface

Why *Visualizing Nutrition?*

Visualizing Nutrition: Everyday Choices, Canadian Edition provides the rigour needed in the study of science while integrating photography and illustrations into the learning process. Information that would be buried in the text of other books is presented within the context of colourful illustrations and vibrant photographs. The images grab students' attention and, along with the text, tell the absorbing story of nutrition. The text captures the interest of students from every background and engages them by demonstrating the applications of the science of nutrition to everyday choices.

This book is intended to serve as an introductory textbook for undergraduate students. The accessible format of *Visualizing Nutrition: Everyday Choices, Canadian Edition* assumes that readers have little prior knowledge of nutrition and allows students to easily relate their individual experiences with food to nutrition concepts and the science of nutrition. The text uses a critical thinking approach to teaching human nutrition, bringing nutrition out of the classroom by asking students to apply the logic of science to their own nutrition concerns. *Visualizing Nutrition: Everyday Choices, Canadian Edition* educates students about the functions and sources of individual nutrients and focuses on the total diet. As a result, students understand that no one food choice determines the healthfulness of their overall dietary pattern. The examples and exercises throughout the book allow students to think critically while exploring the similarities and differences in the diets and health concerns of the diverse ethnic and cultural mix of the Canadian population and the rest of the world. The text presents information using a clear, concise writing style and addresses the most recent advances in nutrition science. Each chapter extensively references the most current literature

Visualizing Nutrition: Everyday Choices, Canadian Edition is unique in its integrated approach to the presentation of nutrition science. While the chapter organization follows the traditional format of nutrition books, this book also integrates practical knowledge and health and disease information. To set a strong foundation on which to build an understanding of nutrition, Chapter 3 features a detailed overview of digestion and metabolism. The concepts outlined in Chapter 3 are then used in future chapters as the basis for a more specific discussion of digestion and metabolism and how these processes relate to different nutrients and concepts. Throughout the textbook, discussions of nutrition, health, and disease are integrated to consistently engage student interest. Students can incorporate the digestion and metabolism information of Chapter 3 into what they learn about carbohydrates, lipids, and protein in Chapters 4, 5, and 6 to gain a fuller picture of how a nutrient's function in metabolism relates to its role in health and disease. This integration continuously reinforces the application of nutrition science to students' lives and increases their appreciation of how and why our food choices affect our health.

What is the organization of this book?

- The first two chapters of this book introduce nutrition science. **Chapter 1**, "**Nutrition: Everyday Choices**," begins by discussing the Canadian diet—how it has changed and how healthy it is—and by emphasizing that food choices affect both our current and future health. This chapter provides an overview of the nutrients and their roles in the body and defines the basic principles of balance, variety, and moderation that are key to a healthy diet. It also introduces the scientific method and the steps students need to follow to distinguish accurate nutrition information from inaccurate hearsay. **Chapter 2**, "**Guidelines for a Healthy Diet**," begins with a brief history of nutrition recommendations in Canada and a discussion of the value of these recommendations for assessing the nutritional health of populations and individuals. This chapter then takes the science out of the laboratory to show how advances in nutrition knowledge have been used to develop the Dietary Reference Intakes (DRIs), *Eating Well with Canada's Food Guide*, and Canadian food labels.

- **Chapter 3**, "**Digestion: From Meals to Molecules**," provides students with the background they need to understand how nutrients are used by their bodies. This chapter discusses how food is digested, how nutrients from foods are absorbed into the body and transported to the cells where metabolism occurs, and how wastes are removed. This chapter provides an overview of metabolism that outlines how food energy is converted into the cellular energy required to fuel the chemical reactions essential for body function.

- Chapters 4, 5, and 6 feature the energy-yielding nutrients of carbohydrates, lipids, and proteins. Each of these chapters begins with a discussion of the respective macronutrient in the food we eat. The body of each chapter then illustrates the digestion and absorption of these nutrients, their functions, and the impact of each on health and particular disease states. Each chapter ends with a discussion of how to choose foods to meet current dietary recommendations, emphasizing the types and proportions of these nutrients needed to optimize health. **Chapter 4**, "**Carbohydrates:**

Sugars, Starches, and Fibres," compares the health impacts of refined grains and added sugar with whole grains and foods that naturally contain sugars. **Chapter 5, "Lipids: Oils, Fats, Phospholipids, and Sterols,"** points out that, relative to their caloric intake, Canadians are not consuming too much fat but are often choosing the wrong types of fat for a healthy diet. **Chapter 6, "Proteins and Amino Acids,"** discusses animal and plant sources of protein. This chapter discusses how to meet protein needs and how to plan a healthy vegetarian diet.

- The next two chapters present the micronutrients and water. **Chapter 7, "Vitamins,"** begins with a general overview of vitamins: where vitamins are found in the diet, factors affecting their bioavailability, and how they function. The chapter then discusses each vitamin individually, providing information on sources in the diet, functions in the body, impact on health, recommended intakes, and potential for toxicity. The chapter ends with a discussion of dietary supplements. **Chapter 8, "Water and Minerals,"** addresses water, a nutrient that is often overlooked, and the major and trace minerals. The chapter presents the sources of these nutrients in the diet and discusses their functions in the body, their relationships to health and disease, and their recommended intakes. A discussion of hypertension illustrates the importance of certain minerals in blood pressure regulation and the impact of the total diet on healthy blood pressure. A discussion of nutrients and bone health includes a section on the relationship between nutrition and the development of osteoporosis. Sections on trace minerals discuss health concerns related to both deficiencies and excesses.

- **Chapter 9, "Energy Balance and Weight Management,"** begins with a discussion of the obesity epidemic and the effect of excess body fat on health. It then presents the various causes of obesity from a complex systems perspective and reinforces the multifactorial nature of the disease. The chapter illustrates the impact of small changes in diet and behaviour on long-term weight management and presents up-to-date information on how body weight is regulated and the role of genetic, psychological, environmental, and lifestyle factors in determining body fatness. The chapter includes recommendations for healthy body weight and composition and equations for determining energy needs. It also discusses weight-loss options. The chapter ends with a comprehensive discussion of eating disorders and their causes, consequences, and treatment.

- **Chapter 10, "Nutrition, Fitness, and Physical Activity,"** discusses the relationships among physical activity, nutrition, and health and includes the most up-to-date activity recommendations from the Canadian Society for Exercise Physiology. It emphasizes both the importance of exercise for health maintenance and the impact nutrition can have on exercise performance. Because nutrients fuel activity, this chapter serves as a review of metabolism. This chapter discusses the macronutrients and micronutrients needed for the production of adenosine triphosphate (ATP). A discussion of ergogenic aids for competitive athletes directs students to conduct a risk-benefit analysis of these products before deciding whether to use them.

- **Chapter 11, "Nutrition during Pregnancy and Infancy,"** addresses the role of nutrition in human development, including the nutritional needs of women during pregnancy and lactation as well as the nutritional needs of infants. The chapter also discusses the benefits and risks of breastfeeding versus bottle feeding.

- **Chapter 12, "Nutrition from 1 to 100,"** travels through the life cycle, discussing the energy and nutrient needs of growing children, adolescents, adults, and older adults. The chapter discusses the importance of learning healthy eating habits early in life. The chapter addresses how nutrition affects aging and how aging affects nutrition. It presents the interrelationships between aging and nutritional status and the impact of medications and chronic disease on nutritional status. The chapter ends with a discussion of alcohol's effects on metabolism and its impact on health at all stages of life.

- **Chapter 13, "How Safe Is Our Food Supply?"** discusses the risks and benefits associated with the Canadian food supply and includes information on the impact of microbial hazards, chemical toxins, food additives, irradiation, and food packaging. It details the use of HACCP (Hazard Analysis Critical Control Point) system to ensure safe food and the advances in technology that help identify the sources of food-borne illness. The chapter ends with a discussion of biotechnology, including an explanation of how plants are genetically modified and the potential benefits and risks.

- **Chapter 14, "Feeding the World,"** discusses the coexistence of hunger and malnutrition with obesity in both developed and developing nations. It examines the causes of world hunger and potential solutions that can affect the amounts and types of food that are available.

Features of the Canadian Edition

Visualizing Nutrition: Everyday Choices, Canadian Edition includes the most recent nutrition recommendations, captivating features, clear illustrations, and critical thinking pedagogy.

- A focus on the recommendations found in *Eating Well with Canada's Food Guide* are first discussed in Chapter 2 and addressed in all applicable subsequent chapters.

- Detailed information is presented on Canadian menu labelling regulations, including a focus on the labelling of natural health products. The 2011 Canadian Physical Activity Guidelines and the Canadian Sedentary Behaviour Guidelines are presented in Chapter 10.

- Hot Topic: This feature summarizes nutrition topics that are current and topical in the media or among nutrition scientists. The hot topics cover such issues as food addiction, menu labelling, the health value of soy protein, and school breakfast programs.

- Canadian statistics, research, and examples are used throughout the textbook to promote the study of nutrition from a Canadian perspective. This textbook also contains images that convey the diversity of the Canadian population.

- A detailed complex systems approach is applied to the study of obesity.

- Metabolism is covered in detail in Chapter 3, including specifics on the various stages of cellular respiration.

- Current topics of interest are discussed, including weight bias, nutrition and acne, medium-chain fatty acids, and food insecurity in Canada.

- An appendix on motivational interviewing lists specific questions that can be used to motivate behaviour change.

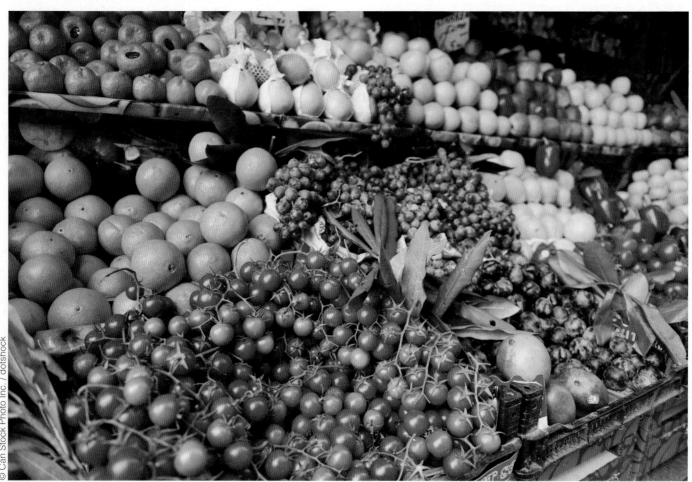

© Can Stock Photo Inc. / dotshock

How Does Wiley Visualizing Support Instructors?

Wiley Visualizing Site

The Wiley Visualizing site hosts a wealth of information for instructors using Wiley Visualizing, including ways to maximize the visual approach in the classroom and a white paper titled "How Well-Designed and Well-Used Visuals Can Help Students Learn," by Matt Leavitt, instructional design consultant. Visit Wiley Visualizing at www.wiley.com/college/visualizing.

Wiley Custom Select

Wiley Custom Select gives you the freedom to build your course materials exactly the way you want them, offering your students a cost-efficient alternative to traditional texts. In a simple three-step process you can create a solution containing the content you want, in the sequence you want, delivered how you want. Visit Wiley Custom Select at customselect.wiley.com.

Book Companion Site

www.wiley.com/go/grosvenorcanada

All instructor resources are housed on the book companion site (www.wiley.com/go/grosvenorcanada).

PowerPoint Presentations

(Available in *WileyPLUS* and on the book companion site.)

A complete set of highly visual PowerPoint presentations—one per chapter—is available online and in *WileyPLUS* to enhance classroom presentations. Tailored to the textbook's topical coverage and learning objectives, these presentations are designed to convey key text concepts, illustrated by embedded text art.

Test Bank

(Available in *WileyPLUS* and on the book companion site.)

The Test Bank has approximately 80 test items per chapter, many of which incorporate visuals from the book. The test items include true/false, multiple-choice, and essay questions testing a variety of comprehension levels. The test bank is available online in MS Word files, as a Computerized Test Bank, and in *WileyPLUS*. The easy-to-use test-generation program fully supports graphics, print tests, student answer sheets, and answer keys. The software's advanced features allow you to produce an exam to your exact specifications.

Instructor's Manual

(Available in *WileyPLUS* and on the book companion site.)

The Instructor's Manual includes a one-page summary of each chapter as well as creative ideas for in-class activities. Guidance is also provided on how to maximize the effectiveness of visuals in the classroom.

1. **Use visuals during class discussions or presentations.** Point out important information as the students look at the visuals, to help them integrate separate visual and verbal mental models.
2. **Use visuals for assignments and to assess learning.** For example, learners can be asked to identify samples of concepts portrayed in visuals.
3. **Use visuals to encourage group activities.** Students can study together, make sense of, discuss, hypothesize, or make decisions about the content. Students can work together to interpret and describe a visual or use the visual to solve problems and conduct related research.
4. **Use visuals during reviews.** Students can review key vocabulary, concepts, principles, processes, and relationships displayed visually. This recall helps link prior knowledge to new information in working memory, building integrated mental models.
5. **Use visuals for assignments and to assess learning.** For example, learners can be asked to identify samples of concepts portrayed in visuals.
6. **Use visuals to apply facts or concepts to realistic situations or examples.** For example, a familiar image, such as a hungry child with a bloated belly, can illustrate key information about the nutritional impact of famine, linking this new concept to prior knowledge.

Nutrition Visual Library

All photographs, figures, maps, and other visuals from the text are online and in *WileyPLUS* and can be used as you wish in the classroom. These online electronic files allow you to easily incorporate images into your PowerPoint presentations as you choose, or to create your own handouts.

Wiley Faculty Network

The Wiley Faculty Network (WFN) is a global community of faculty, connected by a passion for teaching and a drive to learn, share, and collaborate. Their mission is to promote the effective use of technology and enrich the teaching experience. Connect with the Wiley Faculty Network to collaborate with your colleagues, find a mentor, attend virtual and live events, and view a wealth of resources all designed to help you grow as an educator. Visit the Wiley Faculty Network at www.wherefacultyconnect.com.

Acknowledgements

Throughout the process of writing and developing this text, we benefited from the comments and constructive criticism provided by the instructors listed below. We offer our sincere appreciation to these individuals for their helpful review.

Nooshin Alizadeh-Pasdar, *University of British Columbia*
Nick Bellisimo, *Mount Saint Vincent University*
Tristaca Caldwell, *Acadia University*
Bob Demers, *Niagara College*
Barbara Dunlop, *George Brown College*
Catherine Field, *University of Alberta*
Debra Fingold, *Seneca College*
Kristin Hildahl, *University of Manitoba*
Dragan Jovanovic, *Concordia University*
Kathy Keiver, *University of the Fraser Valley*

Lynne Lafave, *Mount Royal University*
Paul Leblanc, *Brock University*
Karen McLaren, *Canadore College*
Donna Pegg, *Durham College*
Raylene Reimer, *University of Calgary*
Susan Somerville, *Humber College*
Sally Stewart, *University of British Columbia Okanagan*
Norman Temple, *Athabasca University*
Christine Wellington, *University of Windsor*
Ami Whitlock, *Centennial College*

Thank you as well to those who worked on the supplements that accompany the textbook: Joanna Komorowski, University of Ottawa; Caroline Mullins, Brandon University; and Andrea Olynyk, University of Guelph-Humber. A big thank you as well to Deanna Durnford for coordinating them all.

Special Thanks

I am extremely grateful for the various members of the editorial and production teams at John Wiley and Sons Canada that guided me through the various challenging steps involved in this process. The staff was always a pleasure to work with and worked tirelessly to help me stay on track throughout the development of this edition. I would like to especially thank our developmental editor, Joanne Sutherland, who was there from the beginning, guiding the process and providing the right amount of motivational, technical, and emotional support needed. My production editor, Andrea Grzybowski, was also a critical component in helping me complete the countless specifics involved in finalizing and producing the textbook in a timely fashion; I could have never finished it without her. My acquisitions editor, Rodney Burke, was the person responsible for "getting the ball rolling" with this Canadian edition and organizing the excellent team responsible for producing each separate element of the text. This supportive team also included the good eyes and excellent suggestions of copyedi-tor Mariko Obokata and proofreader Laurel Hyatt, who helped me Canadianize the language and avoid silly grammatical errors. Photo researcher Kristiina Paul also lent her good eye to help find a diverse range of images that helped visualize nutrition concepts from a Canadian perspective. Her diligent work as a permissions coordinator was another essential component necessary for producing the final book. I would also like to thank Kia Vance and Sarah Frood, my research assistants, for their hard work and excellent results. I am further grateful to Luisa Begani, my editorial assistant, Belle Wong, my indexer, and the talented group of figure artists for helping to bring this project to fruition. I would lastly like to thank my marketing manager, Patty Maher, for helping me to communicate the unique features of this book to those who will find them most useful.

Diana Bedoya

About the Authors

Mary B. Grosvenor holds a bachelor of arts in English and a master of science in Nutrition Science, affording her an ideal background for nutrition writing. She is a registered dietitian and has worked in clinical as well as research nutrition, in hospitals and communities large and small in the western United States. She teaches at the community college level and has published articles in peer-reviewed journals in nutritional assessment and nutrition and cancer. Her training and experience provide practical insights into the application and presentation of the science in this text.

Lori A. Smolin received a bachelor of science degree from Cornell University, where she studied human nutrition and food science. She received a doctorate from the University of Wisconsin at Madison, where her doctoral research focused on B vitamins, homocysteine accumulation, and genetic defects in homocysteine metabolism. She completed postdoctoral training both at the Harbor-UCLA Medical Center, where she studied human obesity, and at the University of California—San Diego, where she studied genetic defects in amino acid metabolism. She has published articles in these areas in peer-reviewed journals. Dr. Smolin is currently at the University of Connecticut, where she has taught both in the Department of Nutritional Science and in the Department of Molecular and Cell Biology. Courses she has taught include introductory nutrition, life cycle nutrition, food preparation, nutritional biochemistry, general biochemistry, and introductory biology.

Diana Bedoya earned her undergraduate degree at the University of Guelph, where she majored in biomedical science. She then earned her master's degree in biomedical physiology and kinesiology from Simon Fraser University. Her master's project focused on what is now a passion of hers, psychological and environmental approaches to promoting healthy eating and physical activity behaviours in overweight people. She is currently a lecturer at Simon Fraser University and Fraser International College, where she has taught nutrition and health courses to thousands of students. In both her professional and personal life, she is committed to encouraging individuals to make lifestyle choices that promote healthier, more enjoyable lives.

Dedication

To my sons, David and John, and my husband, Peter. In the beginning, their contribution was support and patience with my long hours but over the years it has grown to include editing and writing as well. Thanks for keeping my projects, and me, on track.

(from Mary Grosvenor)

To my sons, Zachary and Max, who have grown up along with my textbooks, helping me to keep a healthy perspective on the important things in life. To my husband, David, who has continuously provided his love and support and is always there to assist with the computer and technological issues that arise when writing in the electronic age.

(from Lori Smolin)

To Amparo, Fidel, and Diego for being sources of encouragement and strength throughout my life. To Carrie, Diane, and Penny for helping develop my interest and knowledge in nutrition. To my editor, Jo, for being so easy to work with and for giving me the right amount of push to help me complete this book. And to my sister, Vanessa, for being the very definition of best friend.

(from Diana Bedoya)

Contents in Brief

Contents

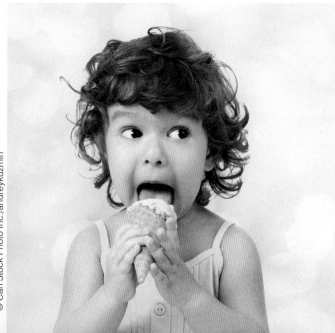

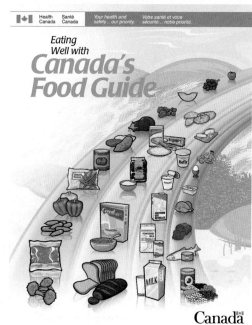

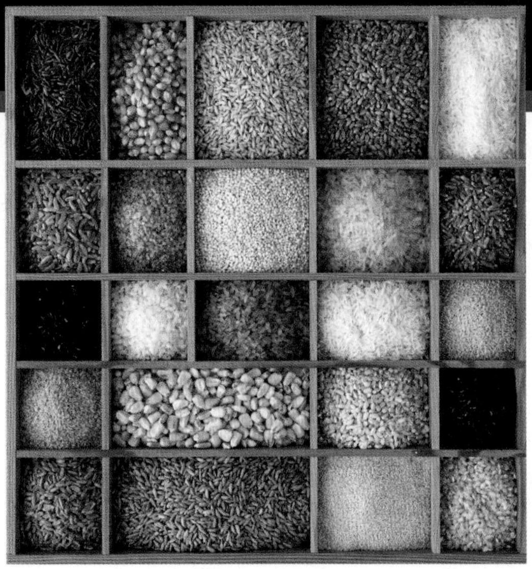

© Can Stock Photo Inc./Eschweitzer

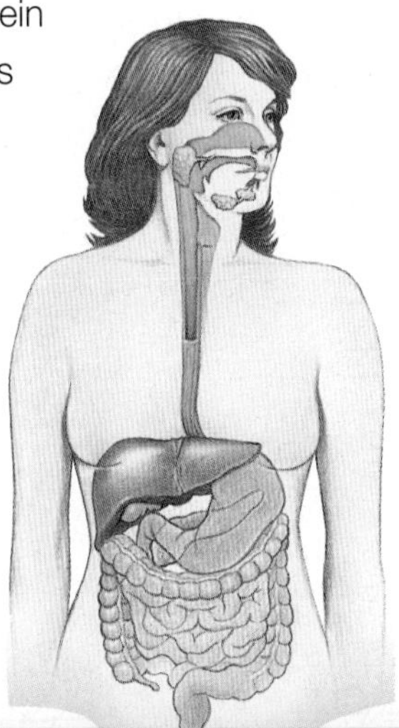

Contents **xxiii**

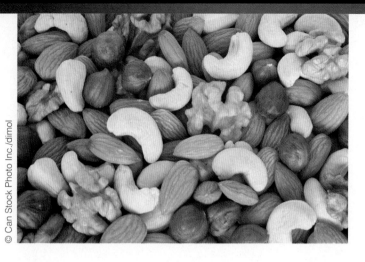
© Can Stock Photo Inc./dimol

Courtesy Diana Bedoya

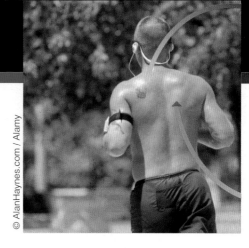

7 Vitamins 196

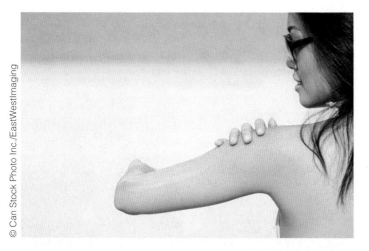

8 Water and Minerals 248

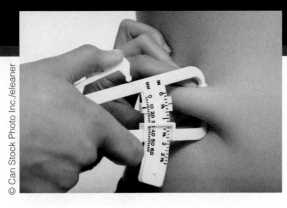

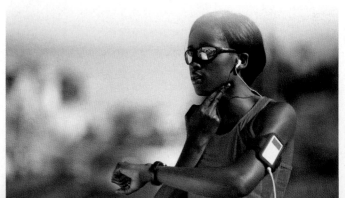

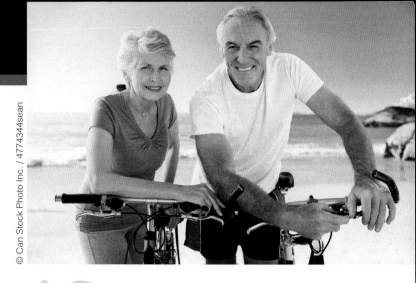

© Can Stock Photo Inc. / 4774344sean

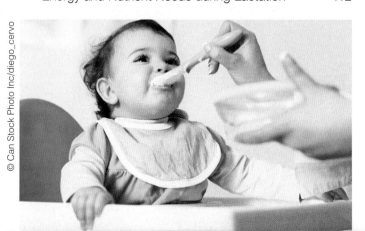

© Can Stock Photo Inc/diego_cervo

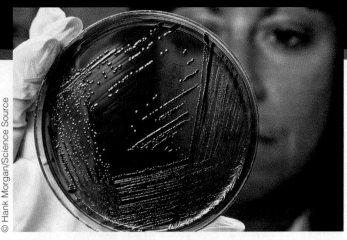

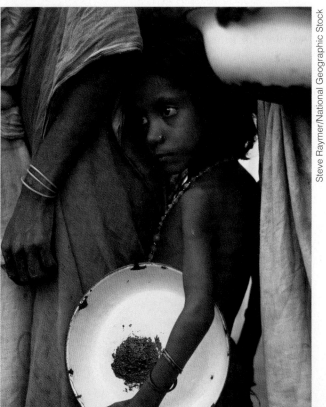

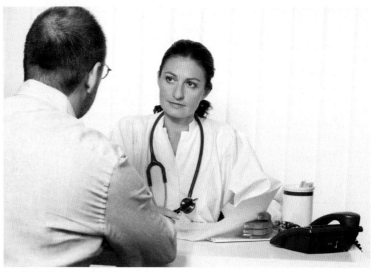

Can Stock Photo Inc./Gina Sanders

Nutrition InSight

Multipart visual presentations that focus on a key concept or topic in the chapter.

Process Diagrams

A series or combination of drawings and photos that describe and depict a complex process.

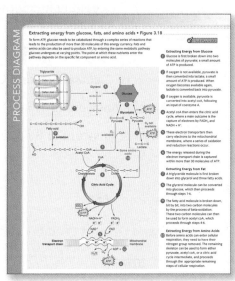

WileyPLUS

WileyPLUS is a research-based online environment for effective teaching and learning.

WileyPLUS builds students' confidence because it takes the guesswork out of studying by providing students with a clear roadmap:

- what to do
- how to do it
- if they did it right

It offers interactive resources along with a complete digital textbook that help students learn more. With *WileyPLUS*, students take more initiative so you'll have greater impact on their achievement in the classroom and beyond.

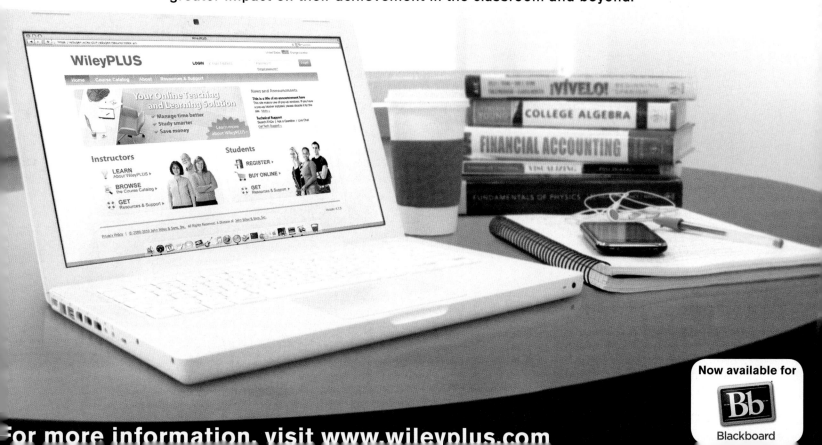

For more information, visit www.wileyplus.com

WileyPLUS

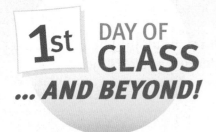
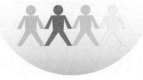
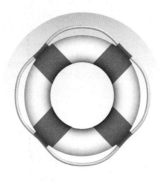
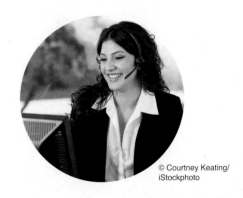

VISUALIZING NUTRITION

EVERYDAY CHOICES

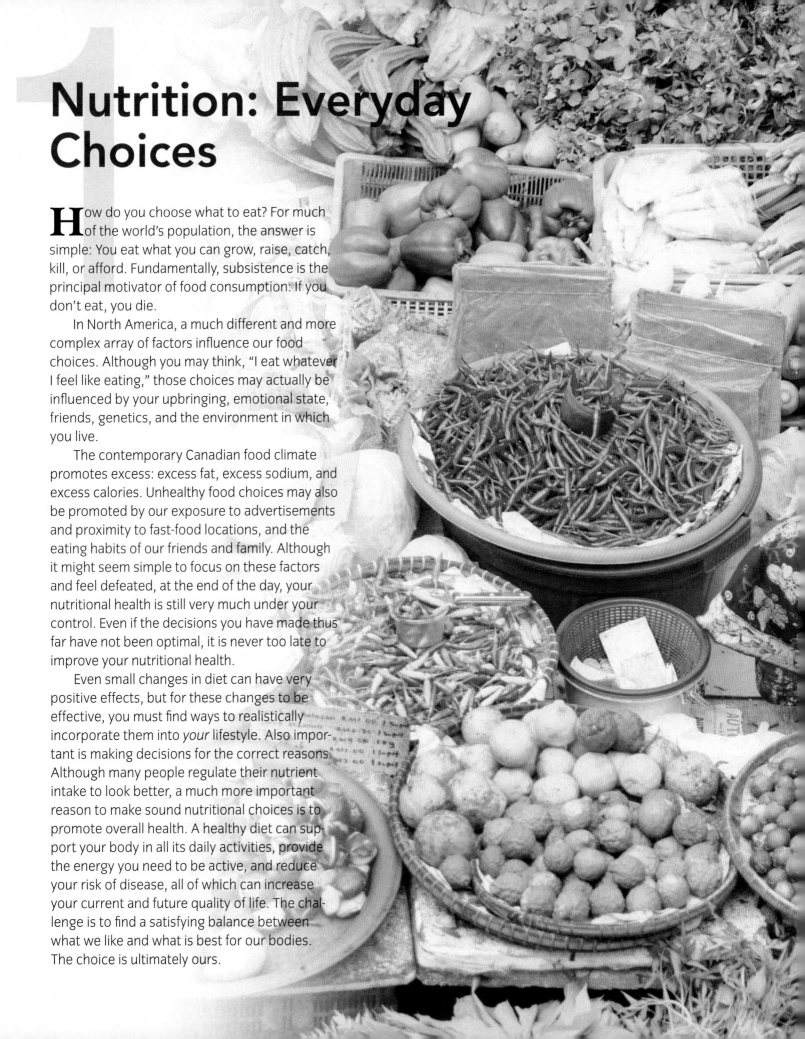

Nutrition: Everyday Choices

How do you choose what to eat? For much of the world's population, the answer is simple: You eat what you can grow, raise, catch, kill, or afford. Fundamentally, subsistence is the principal motivator of food consumption: If you don't eat, you die.

In North America, a much different and more complex array of factors influence our food choices. Although you may think, "I eat whatever I feel like eating," those choices may actually be influenced by your upbringing, emotional state, friends, genetics, and the environment in which you live.

The contemporary Canadian food climate promotes excess: excess fat, excess sodium, and excess calories. Unhealthy food choices may also be promoted by our exposure to advertisements and proximity to fast-food locations, and the eating habits of our friends and family. Although it might seem simple to focus on these factors and feel defeated, at the end of the day, your nutritional health is still very much under your control. Even if the decisions you have made thus far have not been optimal, it is never too late to improve your nutritional health.

Even small changes in diet can have very positive effects, but for these changes to be effective, you must find ways to realistically incorporate them into *your* lifestyle. Also important is making decisions for the correct reasons. Although many people regulate their nutrient intake to look better, a much more important reason to make sound nutritional choices is to promote overall health. A healthy diet can support your body in all its daily activities, provide the energy you need to be active, and reduce your risk of disease, all of which can increase your current and future quality of life. The challenge is to find a satisfying balance between what we like and what is best for our bodies. The choice is ultimately ours.

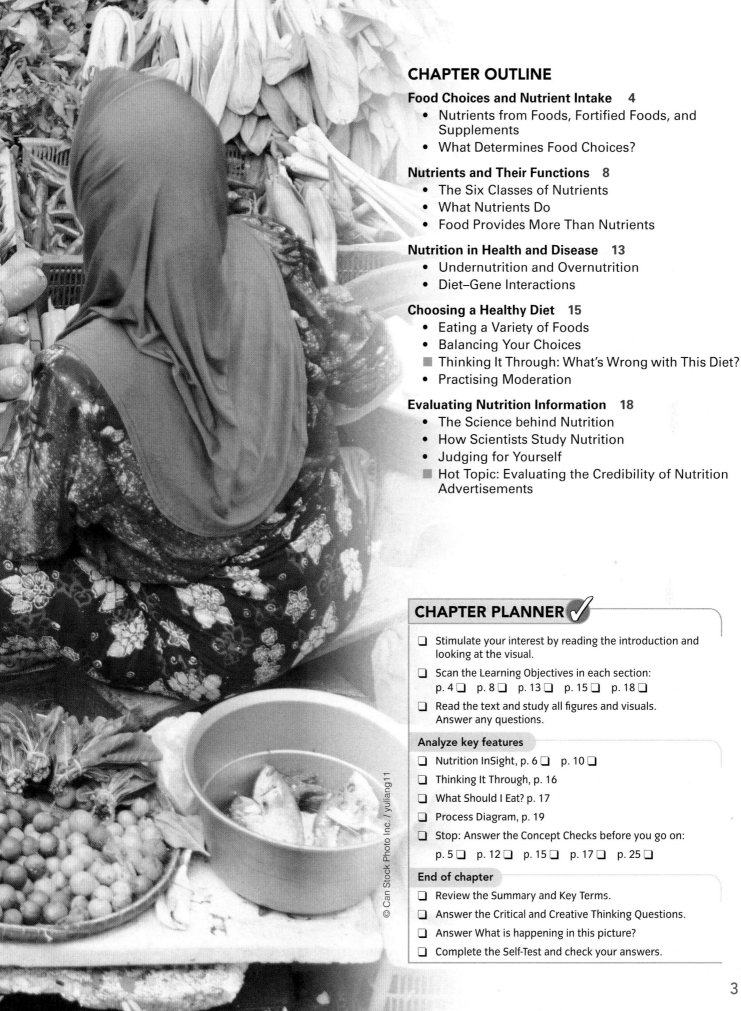

CHAPTER OUTLINE

CHAPTER PLANNER ✓

- ❑ Stimulate your interest by reading the introduction and looking at the visual.
- ❑ Scan the Learning Objectives in each section:
  p. 4 ❑   p. 8 ❑   p. 13 ❑   p. 15 ❑   p. 18 ❑
- ❑ Read the text and study all figures and visuals. Answer any questions.

Analyze key features

- ❑ Nutrition InSight, p. 6 ❑   p. 10 ❑
- ❑ Thinking It Through, p. 16
- ❑ What Should I Eat? p. 17
- ❑ Process Diagram, p. 19
- ❑ Stop: Answer the Concept Checks before you go on:
  p. 5 ❑   p. 12 ❑   p. 15 ❑   p. 17 ❑   p. 25 ❑

End of chapter

- ❑ Review the Summary and Key Terms.
- ❑ Answer the Critical and Creative Thinking Questions.
- ❑ Answer What is happening in this picture?
- ❑ Complete the Self-Test and check your answers.

© Can Stock Photo Inc. / yuliang11

Food Choices and Nutrient Intake

LEARNING OBJECTIVES

1. **Define** nutrient density.

2. **Compare** fortified foods and dietary supplements.

3. **Distinguish** essential nutrients from phytochemicals.

4. **Identify** the factors that determine food choices.

Have you ever thought about why you eat the way you do? Why did you choose that bowl of cereal with skim milk for breakfast over the bacon and eggs, or vice versa? And for lunch will you be seeking out a burger and fries, or do you feel like some pad thai today? On average, we make over 200 food-based decisions a day, from what to eat, to when, how much, where, and with whom.[1] These decisions regarding the foods we eat and the environments we choose to eat them in help determine the amounts and types of meals and, accordingly, the **nutrients** we consume. For example, when you are out with your friends, you are probably more likely to choose what your friends are having—perhaps a burger, fries, and a pint of beer. If you had instead prepared one of your favourite meals at home, it would probably be lower in calories, fat, and salt, and higher in health-promoting vitamins, minerals, and, potentially, fibre. To stay healthy, humans need more than 40 **essential nutrients**. Because our decisions, and thus the foods we eat, vary from day to day, so do the amounts and types of nutrients and the number of **calories** we consume. The amount of calories we consume is the fundamental dietary predictor of a healthy body weight, which reduces the risk of heart disease, cancer, type-2 diabetes, and numerous other **chronic diseases**.

> **nutrients** Substances in food that humans need to live and grow. They provide energy and structure to the body and regulate body processes.
>
> **essential nutrients** Nutrients that the body cannot make itself and, as a result, humans must consume to maintain health.
>
> **calorie** A unit of measure used to express the amount of energy provided by food. 1 kilocalorie = 1 Calorie = 1,000 calories.
>
> **chronic diseases** Long-term diseases such as heart disease or obesity that often negatively affect physical and mental health and increase risk of early mortality.

Nutrients from Foods, Fortified Foods, and Supplements

Any food you eat adds nutrients to your diet, but to make your overall diet healthy, it is important to choose nutrient-dense foods. Foods with a high **nutrient density** contain more nutrients per kilocalorie than do foods with a lower nutrient density (**Figure 1.1**), giving you more bang for your caloric buck! If a large proportion of your diet consists of foods that are low in nutrient density, such as soft drinks, chips, and candy, you will have a difficult time meeting your nutrient needs without exceeding your calorie needs, and you are less likely to feel full after your meal. By choosing nutrient-dense foods, you can meet all your nutrient needs and have calories left over for occasional treats that are lower in nutrients and higher in calories.

> **nutrient density** A measure of the nutrients provided by a food relative to its calorie content.

In addition to nutrients that occur naturally in foods, we obtain nutrients from **fortified foods**. The fortification of foods, which is mandated by the federal government, has helped to eliminate nutrient deficiencies in Canada. Examples of this mandated fortification that have been part of the food supply for decades include foods such as milk with added vitamin D and grain products with added B vitamins and iron.

> **fortified foods** Foods to which one or more nutrients have been added.

Today, grocery store aisles are lined with products that have been voluntarily fortified by manufacturers. Vitamins and minerals are routinely added to breakfast cereals and a variety of snack foods at the discretion of the manufacturer. These added nutrients contribute to the diet but do not necessarily eliminate deficiencies and may

Nutrient density • Figure 1.1

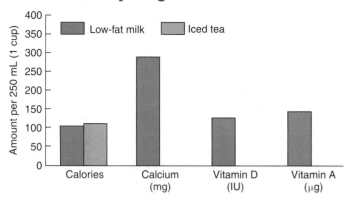

Amount per 250 mL (1 cup)

Legend: Low-fat milk | Iced tea

Categories: Calories, Calcium (mg), Vitamin D (IU), Vitamin A (µg)

Instead of this ...
Low Nutrient Density

Have this ...
High Nutrient Density

5 chicken nuggets:
230 kcal, 12 g protein

Skinless chicken breast:
162 kcal, 25 g protein

Medium order of fries:
380 kcal, 9 mg vitamin C

Medium baked potato:
161 kcal, 17 mg vitamin C

Slice of apple pie:
411 kcal, 4 g fibre

Medium apple,
95 kcal, 2 g fibre

a. Nutrient density is important in choosing a healthy diet. For example, low-fat milk provides about the same number of Calories per cup as bottled iced tea, but it also provides calcium, vitamin D, vitamin A, and other nutrients, including protein.

b. Typically, less processed foods have a higher nutrient density. For example, a roasted chicken breast is more nutrient dense and provides more nutrients per Calorie than chicken nuggets; a baked potato is more nutrient dense than French fries; and an apple is more nutrient dense than apple pie.

actually increase the likelihood of consuming nutrients in excess.

Dietary supplements are another source of nutrients, with numerous Canadian adults taking some sort of daily dietary supplement, such as multivitamins. Supplements provide nutrients but do not offer all the benefits of food and may provide a false sense of security regarding health. Furthermore, they increase the risk that an individual will consume toxic levels of a nutrient.

> **dietary supplements**
> Products sold to supplement the diet; may include nutrients (vitamins, minerals, amino acids, fatty acids), enzymes, herbs, or other substances.

personal convictions—such as environmental consciousness or vegetarianism. Tradition and values may dictate which foods we consider appropriate, but individual preferences for taste, smell, appearance, and texture affect which foods we actually consume. All these factors relate to our food choices because food does more than meet our physiological requirements. Food also provides sensory pleasure and helps meet our social and emotional needs (**Figure 1.2**).

What Determines Food Choices?

So how do you personally make your 200 daily food decisions? Do you eat oranges to boost your vitamin C intake or ice cream to add a little calcium to your diet? Probably not. We need these nutrients to survive, but we generally choose foods for reasons other than the nutrients they contain. Sometimes, we choose a food simply because it is put in front of us. Often, our choices depend on what and how we have learned to eat, the foods considered to be socially acceptable in our cultural heritage or religion, the food choices we think are healthy, or our

CONCEPT CHECK STOP

1. **Which** has a higher nutrient density, a can of pop or a glass of milk?

2. **Why** are foods fortified?

3. **Why** is it better to meet your vitamin C needs by eating an orange than by taking a dietary supplement?

4. **What** factors determine which foods you eat at a family picnic?

a. We use food as reward and punishment. A well-behaved child may be rewarded with an ice cream cone, while a child who misbehaves may be sent to bed without dessert. We also use food to commemorate milestones such as birthdays and anniversaries.

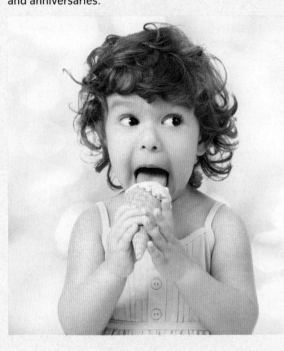

b. Food can provide comfort and security. "Comfort foods" such as hot tea, chicken soup, ice cream, and chocolate help us to feel better when we are sick, cold, tired, or lonely.

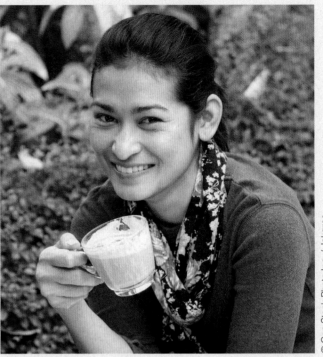

c. We can choose only from foods that are available to us. What is available is affected by season, geography, economics, health, and living conditions. In many parts of the world, food choices are limited to foods produced locally. In more developed regions, many non-native and seasonal foods, such as these pineapples, are available year-round because they can be stored and shipped from distant locations.

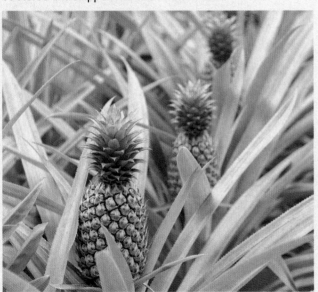

d. Food preferences and eating habits are learned as part of an individual's family, cultural, national, and social background. In many parts of the world, insects, such as these fried larvae, are considered a delicacy but in Canadian culture, insects are considered food contaminants, and most people would refuse to eat them.

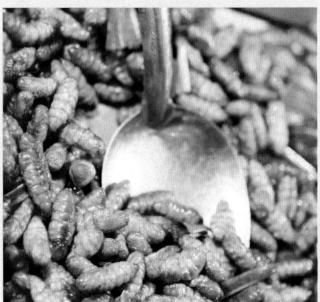

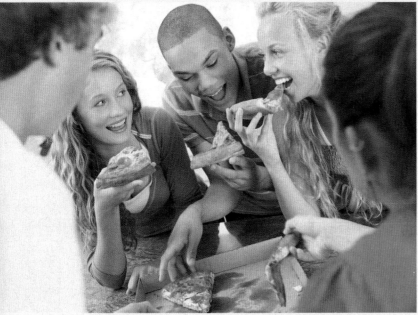

© Can Stock Photo Inc. / monkeybusiness

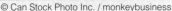

e. For an undergrad, stopping for pizza after class may be part of being accepted by his or her peers. Food is the centrepiece of everyday social interactions. We meet friends for dinner or coffee and celebrate most major occasions with food. The family dinner table is a focal point for communication, where experiences of the day are shared.

© iStockphoto.com/drbimages

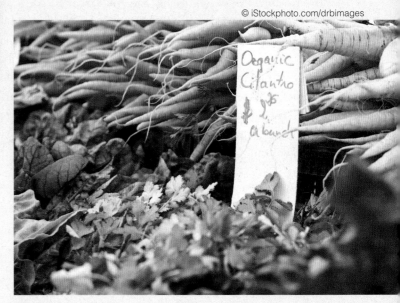

f. Often people's attitudes about what foods they think are good for them or good for the environment affect what they choose. For example, you may choose organic produce because you are concerned about exposure to pesticides, or green tea to increase your intake of antioxidants. You may also choose to buy local foods, those grown within 100 km of your home, because you are environmentally conscious and want to minimize the associated environmental harm of transporting foods to our stores.

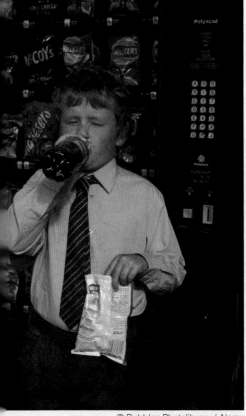

g. Food choices are often restricted by economic factors as well. Unfortunately, a fast food meal or packaged foods such as chips, pop, and TV dinners are often comparably cheaper than more nutrient-dense foods like fruits, vegetables, and lean meats. Being on a restricted income such as a "student budget" can limit which foods you can purchase without breaking the bank. Grocery shopping, cooking at home, and meal planning can help alleviate some of this budgetary burden.

© Bubbles Photolibrary / Alamy

Food Choices and Nutrient Intake **7**

Nutrients and Their Functions

LEARNING OBJECTIVES

1. **List** the six classes of nutrients.
2. **Discuss** the three functions of nutrients in the body.

There are six classes of nutrients: carbohydrates, lipids, proteins, water, vitamins, and minerals. Carbohydrates, lipids, proteins, and water are considered **macronutrients** because they are needed in large amounts. Vitamins and minerals are referred to as **micronutrients** because they are needed in small amounts. Together the macronutrients and micronutrients in our diet provide us with energy, contribute to the structure of our bodies, and regulate the biological processes that go on inside us. Each nutrient provides one or more of these functions, but all nutrients together are needed to provide for growth, maintain and repair the body, and support reproduction.

The Six Classes of Nutrients

Foods are often described in terms of their main nutrient composition. Words like "carbs" or "fatty foods" suggest that a food is high in a specific nutrient. Most foods, however, offer a combination of different nutrients, all with varying, similar, contrasting, or complementary functions. Nutrients are differentiated by their basic molecular structure. For example, carbohydrates, lipids, and proteins all provide energy to the body and are classified as **organic compounds** because they all contain carbon in their structure. Although we tend to think of each of them as being a single nutrient, there can actually be different types of molecules in these classes. **Carbohydrates** include starches, sugars, and fibre (**Figure 1.3a**). Several types

organic compounds Substances that contain carbon bonded to hydrogen in their molecular structure.

carbohydrates A class of nutrients that includes sugars, starches, and fibres. Chemically, they all contain carbon, hydrogen, and oxygen, in the same proportions as in water (H_2O).

fibre A type of carbohydrate that cannot be digested by human enzymes.

of **lipids** play important roles in nutrition (**Figure 1.3b**). The most familiar of these lipids are **cholesterol**, **saturated fats**, and **unsaturated fats**. The most common lipids in the Canadian diet are triglycerides, which are composed of a glycerol molecule attached to three fatty acids, which can be either saturated, unsaturated, or both. There are thousands of different **proteins** in our bodies and our diets. All proteins are made up of units called **amino acids** that link together in different combinations to form different proteins (**Figure 1.3c**).

Water, unlike the other classes of nutrients, is only a single substance. Water makes up about 60% of an adult's body weight. Because we can't store water, the water the body loses through sweat, urination, and respiratory functions must constantly be replaced by water obtained from the diet. In the body, water acts as a lubricant, a transport fluid, and a regulator of body temperature.

Vitamins are organic molecules that are needed in small amounts to maintain health. Thirteen vitamins perform a variety of unique functions in the body, such as regulating energy production, maintaining vision, protecting cell membranes, and helping blood to clot. **Minerals** are essential **elements** that can be found on the periodic table. They perform a variety of diverse functions in the body. For example, iron is an element needed for the transport of oxygen in the blood, and calcium

lipids A class of nutrients often referred to as fats. Chemically, they contain carbon, hydrogen, and oxygen, and most do not dissolve in water.

cholesterol A type of lipid that is found in the diet and in the blood. It is an essential component of every cell and can be used to form hormones, bile, and vitamin D. High blood levels of cholesterol can increase the risk of heart disease.

saturated fats Lipids that contain no double bonds in their structure. They are most abundant in solid animal fats and may be associated with an increased risk of heart disease.

unsaturated fats Lipids that contain one or more double bonds in their structure. They are most abundant in plant oils and may be associated with a reduced risk of heart disease.

proteins A class of nutrients that includes molecules made up of one or more intertwining chains of amino acids. They contain carbon, hydrogen, oxygen, and nitrogen. They promote the growth and development of the body.

Carbohydrates, lipids, and proteins • Figure 1.3

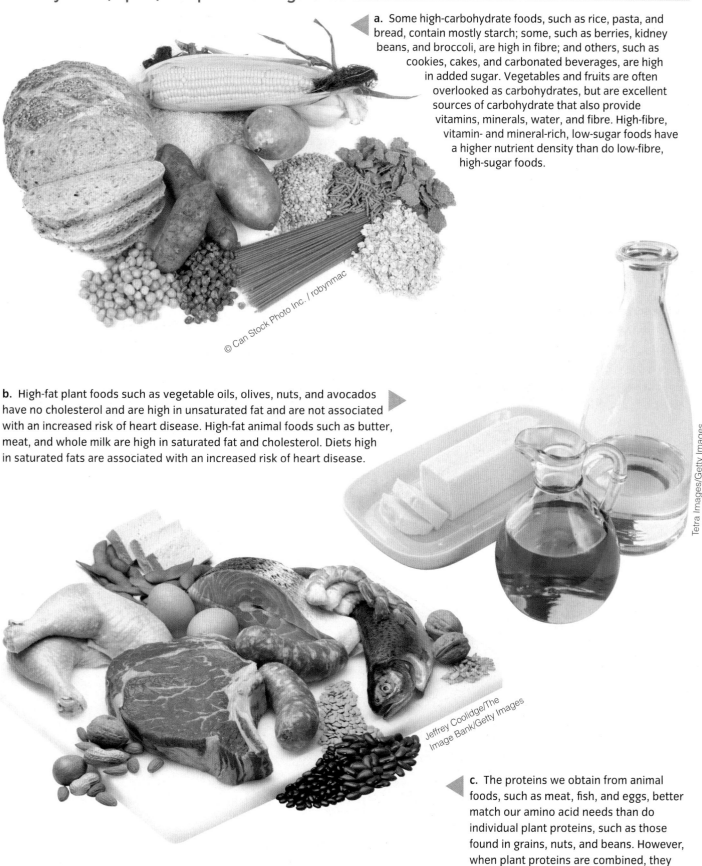

a. Some high-carbohydrate foods, such as rice, pasta, and bread, contain mostly starch; some, such as berries, kidney beans, and broccoli, are high in fibre; and others, such as cookies, cakes, and carbonated beverages, are high in added sugar. Vegetables and fruits are often overlooked as carbohydrates, but are excellent sources of carbohydrate that also provide vitamins, minerals, water, and fibre. High-fibre, vitamin- and mineral-rich, low-sugar foods have a higher nutrient density than do low-fibre, high-sugar foods.

© Can Stock Photo Inc. / robynmac

b. High-fat plant foods such as vegetable oils, olives, nuts, and avocados have no cholesterol and are high in unsaturated fat and are not associated with an increased risk of heart disease. High-fat animal foods such as butter, meat, and whole milk are high in saturated fat and cholesterol. Diets high in saturated fats are associated with an increased risk of heart disease.

Tetra Images/Getty Images

Jeffrey Coolidge/The Image Bank/Getty Images

c. The proteins we obtain from animal foods, such as meat, fish, and eggs, better match our amino acid needs than do individual plant proteins, such as those found in grains, nuts, and beans. However, when plant proteins are combined, they can provide all the amino acids we need.

is an element important in muscle contraction, nerve conduction, and keeping bones strong. We consume vitamins and minerals in almost all the foods we eat. Some are natural sources: Oranges contain vitamin C, milk provides calcium, and carrots give us vitamin A. Other foods are fortified with vitamins and minerals; fortified breakfast cereals often have 100% of the recommended intake of many vitamins and minerals. Dietary supplements are another source of vitamins and minerals for some people.

What Nutrients Do

Figure 1.4 illustrates some of the ways in which various nutrients are involved in providing energy, forming body structures, and regulating physiological processes. Carbohydrates, lipids, and proteins are often referred to as **energy-yielding nutrients** because they provide energy that can be measured in calories. This energy allows our body to perform the various activities it needs to do, such as carrying both the nerve signals that tell us to think, feel, and move and the muscle contractions that makes us move. Unfortunately, if the energy that you take in from meals is greater than the amount you burn fuelling basic body processes plus physical activity, that excess energy is stored as fat tissue for later use. It is therefore important to moderate the amount of calories consumed. The "calories" people talk about and see listed on food labels are actually **kilocalories**, units of

---

Nutrition InSight · Nutrient functions • Figure 1.4 ✓ THE PLANNER

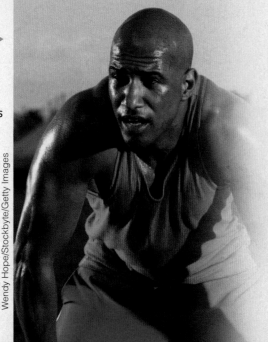

a. Physical activity, whether it consists of gardening, walking to the mailbox, or mountain biking through the Rockies, is fuelled by the energy in the carbohydrates, fats and, less often, proteins.

© Can Stock Photo Inc. / KAValles

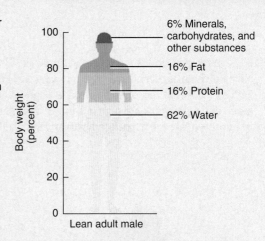

Body weight (percent) — 100, 80, 60, 40, 20, 0 — Lean adult male

6% Minerals, carbohydrates, and other substances
16% Fat
16% Protein
62% Water

b. The shape and structure of our bodies are formed and maintained by proteins, lipids, carbohydrates, minerals, and water.

c. Water helps regulate body temperature. When body temperature increases, sweat is produced, which cools the body as the heat evaporates from the skin.

Wendy Hope/Stockbyte/Getty Images

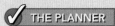

d. Lipids, such as the hormone testosterone, shown in the diagram, help regulate body processes. Testosterone is made from cholesterol. In men, it stimulates sperm production and the development of secondary sex characteristics such as body and facial hair, a deep voice, and increased muscle mass.

1,000 calories (abbreviated as kcalorie or kcal). When spelled with a capital *C*, Calorie means kilocalorie. Carbohydrates provide 4 kilocalories (kcal) per gram; they are the most immediate source of energy for the body. Lipids also help fuel our activities and are the major form of stored energy in the body. One gram of lipid provides 9 kcal. Protein can supply 4 kcal per gram but is not the body's first choice for meeting energy needs because protein's other vital roles take priority. Alcohol is not a nutrient because it is not needed for life; it nonetheless provides about 7 kcal per gram. Water, vitamins, and minerals do not provide energy (calories).

With the exception of vitamins, all the classes of nutrients are involved in forming and maintaining the body's structure. For example, fat deposited under the skin provides cushioning and insulation for the body, and proteins form the ligaments and tendons that hold our bones together and attach our muscles to our bones. Minerals harden bone. Protein and water make up the structure of the muscles, which helps define our body contours, and protein and carbohydrates form the connective tissue that holds us together. On a smaller scale, lipids, proteins, and water form the structure of individual cells. Lipids and proteins make up the membranes that surround each cell, and water and dissolved substances fill the cells and the spaces around them.

All six classes of nutrients play important roles in regulating body processes. Thousands of chemical reactions and physiological processes are needed to maintain relatively constant levels of hundreds of parameters, including body temperature, blood pressure, blood sugar level, and blood acidity. Proteins, vitamins, and minerals are regulatory nutrients that help control how quickly chemical reactions take place throughout the body. For example, lipids and proteins are needed to make regulatory molecules called **hormones** that stimulate or inhibit various body processes.

Food Provides More Than Nutrients

Food contains both nutrients, which are essential for normal body functioning, and other substances, which, although not essential to life, can be beneficial for health. In plants, these health-promoting substances are called phytochemicals (**Figure 1.5**). Although animal foods contain fewer phytochemicals, they do contain

phytochemicals
Substances found in plant foods that are not essential nutrients but may have health-promoting properties.

Foods that are high in phytochemicals • Figure 1.5

Fruits, vegetables, and whole grains provide a variety of phytochemicals, such as those highlighted here. Although a large number of individual phytochemicals are available as dietary supplements at grocery and health food stores, there is little evidence that they provide the same health benefits that can be obtained from natural food sources that are high in phytochemicals.[2] Foods provide mixtures of these chemicals, and we do not yet know which combinations provide the greatest health benefits.

Garlic, broccoli, and onions provide sulphur-containing phytochemicals that help protect us from some forms of cancer by inactivating carcinogens or stimulating the body's natural defenses.[3,4]

Yellow-orange fruits and vegetables, such as peaches, apricots, carrots, and cantaloupe, as well as leafy greens, are rich in carotenoids, which are phytochemicals that may prevent oxygen from damaging our cells.[8]

Soybeans are a source of phytoestrogens, hormone-like compounds found in plants that may reduce the risk of certain types of cancer and cause small reductions in blood cholesterol.[5,6,7]

Purple grapes, berries, and onions provide red, purple, and pale yellow pigments called flavonoids, which prevent oxygen damage and may reduce the risk of cancer and heart disease.[9,10]

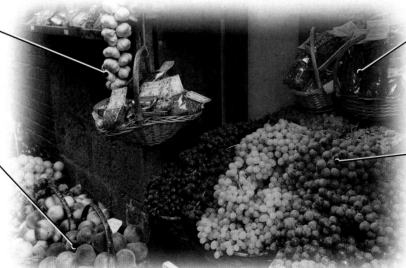

TODD GIPSTEIN/National Geographic Stock

Examples of functional foods   Table 1.1

Food	Potential health benefit
Blueberries	May reduce the risk of heart disease and cancer.[10, 11]
Breakfast cereal with added flaxseed	Helps reduce blood cholesterol levels and the overall risk of heart disease.[12]
Chocolate	May help reduce blood pressure and other risk factors for heart disease.[13]
Garlic	Helps reduce blood cholesterol levels and the overall risk of heart disease.[14]
Kale	May reduce the risk of age-related blindness (macular degeneration).[15]
Margarine with added plant sterols	Reduces blood cholesterol levels.[16]
Nuts	May reduce the risk of heart disease.[17]
Oatmeal	Helps reduce blood cholesterol.[18]
Orange juice with added calcium	Helps prevent osteoporosis.
Salmon	Reduces the risk of heart disease.[19]
Tea, green and black	May reduce the risk of certain types of cancer.[20]
Whole-grain bread	Helps reduce the risk of cancer, heart disease, obesity, and diabetes.[21]

substances called zoochemicals, which also have health-promoting properties.

In addition to providing basic nutrients such as carbohydrates, fats, and vitamins, some foods contain additional chemicals that may provide health benefits beyond basic nutrition. Such foods have been termed **functional foods**. The simplest functional foods are unmodified whole foods that naturally contain substances that promote health and protect against disease, such as broccoli and fish; but other foods that are fortified with nutrients or enhanced with phytochemicals or other substances are also classified as functional foods (**Table 1.1**). These modified foods, such as vitamin water, orange juice with added calcium, and eggs with added omega-3 fatty acids, have also been called **designer foods** or **neutraceuticals** and are ubiquitous in grocery store aisles. As food manufacturers cash in on the concept that "health sells," the line has blurred between what is a dietary supplement and what is a food (**Figure 1.6**).

> **functional foods** Foods that have health-promoting and/or disease-preventing properties beyond basic nutritional functions.

To further advance this growing field of study, the Richardson Centre for Functional Foods and Nutraceuticals opened at the University of Manitoba in 2006. It has been heralded as one of the most advanced bioprocessing and product development facilities in the nation and the world.

Are these foods or dietary supplements? • Figure 1.6

Energy bars fortified with 23 vitamins and minerals, bottled water enhanced with vitamin C, fruit juice with added phytochemicals, soft drinks with vitamins and amino acids—are these foods or are they dietary supplements? Before purchasing these highly fortified products, consider whether they provide the benefits they claim to provide and whether they are safe.

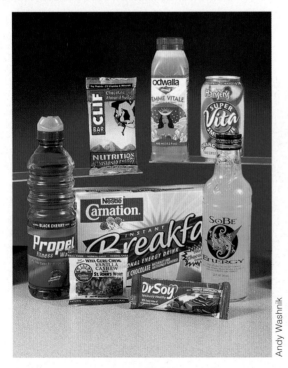

Andy Washnik

CONCEPT CHECK STOP

1. **Which** classes of nutrients provide energy?

2. **What** three nutrient functions help ensure normal growth, maintenance of body structure and functions, and reproduction?

Nutrition in Health and Disease

LEARNING OBJECTIVES

1. **Describe** the different types of malnutrition.

2. **Explain** ways in which nutrient intake can affect health in both the short term and the long term.

3. **Discuss** how the genes you inherit affect the amounts of nutrients and food components that optimize your health.

W hat we eat has an enormous impact on how healthy we are now and how likely we are to develop diseases in the future. Consuming either too much or too little of one or more nutrients or energy will result in **malnutrition**. Malnutrition can affect your health not just today but 20, 30, or 40 years from now. The impact of your diet on your health and quality of life is also affected by your genetic background.

> **malnutrition**
> A condition resulting from an energy or nutrient intake either above or below that which is optimal.

Undernutrition and Overnutrition

Undernutrition occurs when intake doesn't meet the body's needs (**Figure 1.7**). The more severe the deficiency, the more dramatic the symptoms. Some nutrient deficiencies occur quickly. Dehydration, which is a deficiency of water, can cause symptoms in a few hours. Drinking water can relieve the headache, fatigue, and dizziness caused by dehydration almost as rapidly as these symptoms appeared. Other nutritional deficiencies may take much longer to become evident. Symptoms of scurvy, a disease caused by a deficiency in vitamin C, appear after months of deficient intake; **osteoporosis**, a condition in which the bones become weak and break easily, occurs after years of consuming a calcium-deficient diet.

We typically think of malnutrition as undernutrition, but **overnutrition**, an excess intake of calories or nutrients, is also a concern. An overdose of iron can cause liver failure, for example, and too much vitamin B_6 can cause nerve damage. Because foods generally do not contain high enough concentrations of nutrients to be toxic, these nutrient toxicities usually result from taking large doses of vitamin and mineral supplements. However, health problems can result from chronic overconsumption of calories and certain nutrients from foods. The typical Canadian diet, which provides more calories than we need, has resulted in a frightening epidemic of obesity: The majority of Canadians (approximately 60%!)

Undernutrition • Figure 1.7

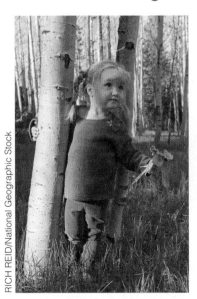

RICH REID/National Geographic Stock

a. Even though this child looks normal and healthy, she has low iron stores. If the iron content of her diet is not increased, she will eventually develop iron deficiency anemia. Mild nutrient deficiencies like hers may go unnoticed because the symptoms either are not immediately apparent or are nonspecific. Two common nonspecific symptoms of iron depletion are fatigue and a decreased ability to fight infection.

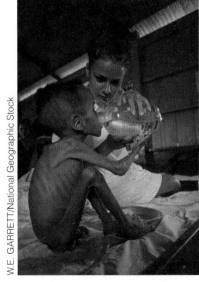

W.E. GARRETT/National Geographic Stock

b. The symptoms of starvation, the most obvious form of undernutrition, occur gradually over time when the energy provided by the diet is too low to meet the body's needs. Body tissues are broken down to provide the energy to support vital functions, resulting in loss of body fat and wasting of muscles.

Overnutrition • Figure 1.8

a. Obesity is a form of overnutrition that occurs when energy intake surpasses energy expenditure over a long period, causing the accumulation of an excessive amount of body fat. Adults are not the only ones who are getting larger. It is estimated that just over 30% of Canadian children and adolescents ages 2 to 17 years are overweight.[24]

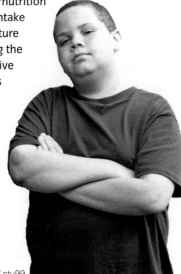

© Can Stock Photo Inc. / stu99

b. The top three causes of death in Canada are nutrition related.[25] They are all thought to be exacerbated by obesity.

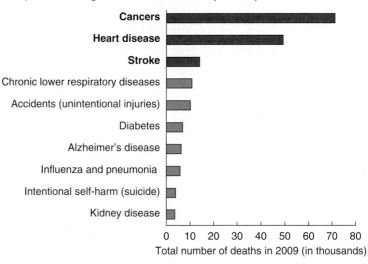

Total number of deaths in 2009 (in thousands)

are overweight or obese (**Figure 1.8a**).[22] Moreover, diets that are high in sodium may contribute to high blood pressure; an excess intake of fat may contribute to heart disease; and a dietary pattern that is high in red meat and saturated fat and low in fruits, vegetables, and fibre may increase the risk of colon cancer[23] (**Figure 1.8b**).

Diet–Gene Interactions

Diet affects your health, but diet alone does not determine whether you will develop a particular disease. Each of us inherits a unique combination of **genes**. Some genes can increase or decrease your risk of developing heart disease, cancer, high blood pressure, and type-2 diabetes (**Figure 1.9**). The strength and type of impact your genes make on health is affected by what you eat, and your genetic makeup determines how a certain nutrient will affect you. For example, some people inherit a combination of genes that results in a tendency to have high blood pressure. When these individuals consume even an average amount of sodium, their blood pressure increases (discussed further in Chapter 8). Others inherit genes that allow them to consume more sodium without much of a rise in blood pressure. Those whose genes dictate a significant rise in blood pressure with a high-sodium diet can reduce their blood pressure, and the complications associated with high blood pressure, by eating a diet that is low in sodium.

> **genes** Specific segments of DNA that are responsible for determining specific inherited traits.

Our increasing understanding of human genetics has given rise to the discipline of **nutritional genomics** or **nutrigenomics**, which explores the interaction between genetic variation and nutrition.[26] This research has led to the development of the concept of "personalized nutrition," the idea that a diet based on the genes an individual has inherited can be used to prevent, moderate, or cure chronic disease. Although today we do not yet know enough that we can take a sample of your DNA and use it to tell you what to eat to optimize your health, we do know that certain dietary patterns can reduce the risk of many chronic diseases.

> **nutritional genomics** or **nutrigenomics** The study of how diet affects our genes and how individual genetic variation can affect the impact of nutrients or other food components on health.

Nutritional genomics • Figure 1.9

Your actual risk of disease results from the interplay between the genes you inherit and the diet and lifestyle choices you make.

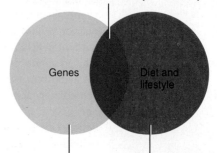

The genes you inherit may give you a greater or lesser tendency to develop conditions like obesity, heart disease, high blood pressure, or diabetes.

The nutrients and food components you consume and the amount of exercise you get can increase or decrease your risk of developing nutrition-related diseases.

1. **What** causes malnutrition?

2. **How** can your diet today affect your health 20 years from now?

3. **Why** might the diet that optimizes health be different for different people?

Choosing a Healthy Diet

LEARNING OBJECTIVES

1. **Explain** why it is important to eat a variety of foods.

2. **Describe** how you can eat your favourite foods that are low in nutrient density and still have a healthy diet.

3. **Discuss** how dietary moderation can reduce the risk of chronic disease.

 healthy diet is one that provides the right number of calories to keep your weight in the desirable range; the proper balance of carbohydrates, proteins, and fat; plenty of water; and sufficient but not excessive amounts of vitamins and minerals. Such a healthy diet is rich in whole grains, fruits, and vegetables; high in fibre; moderate in fat, sugar, and sodium; and low in unhealthy fats (*trans* fat and saturated fat). In short, a healthy diet is based on variety, balance, and moderation (see *Thinking It Through*).

Eating a Variety of Foods

In nutrition, choosing a variety of foods is important because no single food can provide all the nutrients the body needs for optimal health. *Variety* means choosing foods from different food groups—vegetables, grains, fruits, dairy products, and meats and beans. Some of these foods are rich in vitamins and phytochemicals, others are rich in protein and minerals, and all are important.

Variety also means choosing diverse foods from within each food group. Different vegetables provide different nutrients. Potatoes, for example, are the preferred vegetable for many Canadians. Potatoes provide vitamin C but are low in vitamin A. If potatoes are your only vegetable, it is unlikely that you will meet your nutrient needs. If instead you have a salad, potatoes, and broccoli,

you will be getting plenty of vitamins C and A as well as many other vitamins and minerals. Making varied choices both from the different food groups and from within each food group is also important because nutrients and other food components interact. Such interactions may be positive, enhancing nutrient utilization, or negative, inhibiting nutrient availability. Variety averages out these interactions.

Variety involves choosing different foods not only each day but also each week and throughout the year. If you had apples and grapes today, have blueberries and cantaloupe tomorrow. If you can't find good local tomatoes in the winter, replace them with a winter vegetable such as squash.

Balancing Your Choices

Choosing a healthy diet is a balancing act. Healthy eating doesn't mean giving up your favourite foods. There is no such thing as a good food or a bad food—only healthy diets and unhealthy diets. Any food can be part of a healthy diet—even the occasional slice of cheesecake—as long as your diet throughout the day or week provides enough of all the nutrients you need without excesses of any. If you consider your daily, weekly, and monthly food decisions as a whole, you want to make sure that *most* of your choices are healthy in nature. If, for example, your friend won't let you avoid "Sunday Funday," which includes Caesars, chicken wings, nachos, and fries, then the next day, or that night, you can consume a smaller meal of fruits, vegetables, and other fibre-rich foods. Making nutrient-dense choices can help balance out the fat- and protein-rich wings, the fat- and salt-rich nachos and fries, and the often empty calories found in alcoholic beverages.

THINKING IT THROUGH 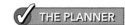 ✓ THE PLANNER

What's Wrong with This Diet?

For many undergrads, their first year at university is the first time they make their own decisions about what to eat. The choices they make aren't always the best, however, and many students' food choices lead to the "freshman 15"—the 15 or so pounds (7 kg) that are often gained in the first year away from home. Learning how to choose a healthy diet can both prevent this weight gain and maximize health status so that the first-year experience can be fully enjoyed.

Amad loves fast food. He grabs a doughnut for breakfast, a burger and fries for lunch, and either tacos or pizza for dinner.

What's wrong with Amad's diet?
▼

Amad's diet needs more balance. An occasional fast-food meal is fine, but eating these foods every day results in a diet that is high in calories and fat and low in some vitamins and minerals. Amad needs to balance his fast-food choices, which are low in nutrient density, with meals that are higher in nutrient density. For example, if he plans to eat a doughnut for breakfast, he can balance this fast-food choice with a nutritionally dense lunch—a sandwich on whole-grain bread with lettuce, tomatoes, and peppers. If his dinner is high in calories, he can balance these calories by snacking on low-calorie, nutrient-dense fruits and vegetables.

What about Brandi? She has cereal with milk for breakfast, a peanut butter sandwich for lunch, and meat with rice and a lettuce salad for dinner every day.

What's wrong with Brandi's diet?
▼

Your answer: _____

_____

Loretta takes advantage of the variety of foods offered at the cafeteria. She often has two types of whole-grain cereals each day for breakfast, selects eight or more ingredients at the salad bar, and includes two or three vegetables with her dinner. Despite these healthy choices, her diet has a problem.

Based on this photo, what might be wrong with Loretta's diet?
▼

Your answer: _____

_____

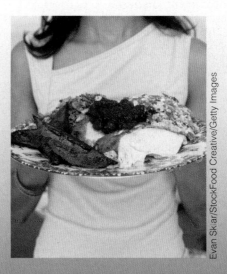

Evan Skar/StockFood Creative/Getty Images

(Check your answers in Appendix I.)

A balanced diet also balances the calories you take in with the calories you use up in your daily activities so that your body weight stays in the healthy range (**Figure 1.10**).

Practising Moderation

Moderation means not overdoing it—watching portion sizes and passing up the super sizes. Moderation means not having too many calories, too much fat, too much sugar, or too much sodium—and, conversely, not having too little of these. Choosing moderately will help you maintain a healthy weight and prevent some of the chronic diseases prevalent in the Canadian population (see *What Should I Eat?*).

The fact that more than 60% of adult Canadians are overweight demonstrates that we have not been practising moderation when it comes to calorie intake.[22] Moderation makes it easier to balance your diet and allows you to enjoy a greater variety of foods.

WHAT SHOULD I EAT?
A Healthy Diet

Eat a variety of foods

- Snack on something other than chips. Try a trail mix that contains fruit and nuts.
- Add almonds and dried cranberries to your salad.
- Try a new vegetable or fruit each week. Tired of carrots? Try jicama.
- Vary your protein sources. Have fish one day and beef the next, or skip the meat and have beans.

Balance your choices

- Going out to dinner? Have a salad for lunch.
- Add a vegetable instead of pepperoni to your pizza.
- When you have cookies for a snack, have fruit for dessert.
- Had pop with lunch? Have milk with dinner.

Practise moderation

- Push back from the table before you are stuffed and go for a walk.
- Reduce your portions by using a smaller bowl or utensil.
- Skip the seconds or split your restaurant meal with a friend.
- If you eat some extra fries, take some extra steps.

Use iProfile to calculate the Calories in your favourite fast-food meal.

Balance calories in with calories out • Figure 1.10

Extra calories you consume during the day can be balanced by increasing the calories you burn in physical activity.

If you have a Big Mac for lunch instead of a smaller plain burger, you will have to increase your energy expenditure by 300 kilocalories.

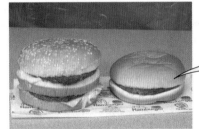

Andy Washnik

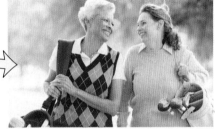

© Can Stock Photo Inc. / monkeybusiness

You could do this by playing golf for about an hour, carrying your own clubs.

If you have a grande Mocha Frappuccino instead of a regular iced coffee, you will have to increase your energy expenditure by 370 kilocalories.

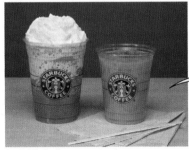

Andy Washnik

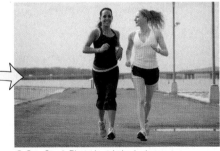

© Can Stock Photo Inc. / charlesknox

You could do this by running for about 40 minutes.

CONCEPT CHECK STOP

1. **Why** is variety in a diet important?

2. **How** might you balance the 600-kilocalorie cinnamon roll you had for a morning snack with your lunch choice?

3. **What** is the connection between obesity and moderation in a diet?

Evaluating Nutrition Information

LEARNING OBJECTIVES

1. **Explain** how the scientific method is used in nutrition.

2. **Discuss** three different types of experiments used to study nutrition.

3. **Describe** the components of a sound scientific experiment.

4. **Distinguish** between reliable and unreliable nutrition information.

We are bombarded with nutrition information almost every day. From the evening news and the morning papers, to the blogs, pop-ups, and pseudo health sites on the Internet, we are continually being offered tantalizing tidbits of nutrition advice that often sound so good we want to believe them. Food and nutrition information that used to take professionals years to disseminate now travels with lightning speed, reaching millions of people within hours or days. Much nutritional information is reliable, especially when it comes from a credible source, but some information can be misleading, especially when believing it means that someone stands to gain financially. To choose a healthy diet, we need to be able to sort out the useful material in this flood of information.

The Science behind Nutrition

Like all other sciences, the science of nutrition is constantly evolving. As new discoveries provide clues to the right combination of nutrients needed for optimal health, new nutritional principles and recommendations are developed. Sometimes, established beliefs and concepts give way to new information. For the average consumer, this information can often seem conflicting and frustrating. By first understanding how credible scientific studies are conducted, consumers can better understand and evaluate the nutrition information they encounter.

The **scientific method** refers to the systematic, unbiased approach that allows any science to acquire new knowledge and correct and update previous knowledge. The scientific method involves making observations of natural events, formulating **hypotheses**

hypotheses Proposed explanations for an observation or a scientific problem that can be tested through experimentation.

to explain these events, designing and performing experiments to test these hypotheses, and developing **theories** that explain the observed phenomenon based on the results (**Figure 1.11**). In nutrition, the scientific method is used to develop nutrient recommendations, understand the functions of nutrients, and learn about the role of nutrition in promoting health and preventing disease.

theories Formal explanations of an observed phenomenon made after a hypothesis has been repeatedly supported and tested through experimentation.

How Scientists Study Nutrition

When a scientist wants to learn how the diet affects health, he or she can use several methods to find the best evidence. **Epidemiology** seeks to understand the rates, distributions, and determinants of health and disease at the population level (**Figure 1.12**). For instance, nutritional epidemiologists might look at the significantly lower rates of heart disease found in Japan compared to those in North America and ask themselves whether the Japanese diet may provide protection against this disease. After comparing the food consumption patterns of the average Japanese citizen and the average North American, a nutritional epidemiologist might suggest that the high consumption of fish in Japan may provide protection against heart disease. Although epidemiology is effective establishing relationships amongst variables, it is critical to remember that association does not equal causation; that is, just because two factors are related, it does not prove that one causes the other. In this example, the Japanese population's lower body weight, physical activity patterns, or different genetic makeup may be responsible for their lower disease rates. Thus, not too many strict conclusions should be drawn from epidemiological evidence because of the difficulty of accounting for all the other various factors that could have produced similar results.

epidemiology The branch of science that studies health and disease trends and patterns in populations. In epidemiological studies, observations are made without the manipulation of variable.

Experimental evidence is better suited for drawing more specific conclusions as it can control for many of the confounding variables that can influence the results of epidemiological evidence. All experiments start with a hypothesis, typically a relationship that the scientist is trying

The scientific method • Figure 1.11

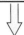 **THE PLANNER**

The scientific method is a process used to ask and answer scientific questions through observation and experimentation.

1 The first step of the scientific method is to make an observation and ask questions about that observation.

2 The next step is to propose an explanation for this observation. This proposed explanation is called a *hypothesis*.

3 Once a hypothesis has been proposed, experiments like this one are designed to test it. To generate reliable theories, the experiments done to test hypotheses must produce consistent, quantifiable results and must be interpreted accurately.

4 If the results from repeated experiments support the hypothesis, a scientific theory can be developed. A single experiment is not enough to develop a theory; rather, repeated experiments showing the same conclusion are needed to develop a sound theory. If experimental results do not support the hypothesis, a new hypothesis can be formulated. As new information becomes available, even a theory that has been accepted by the scientific community for years can be proved wrong.

Experimental Design

Observation

People who eat whole grains are less likely to develop type-2 diabetes.

Hypothesis

Whole grains regulate blood glucose levels.

Experiment

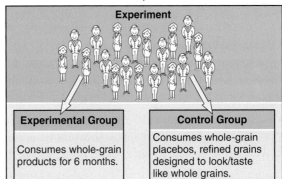

Experimental Group	Control Group
Consumes whole-grain products for 6 months.	Consumes whole-grain placebos, refined grains designed to look/taste like whole grains.

Results: Those who consumed whole grains had slower blood glucose increases after their meals.

Theory

Whole grains prevent the rapid post-meal glucose surges associated with type-2 diabetes.

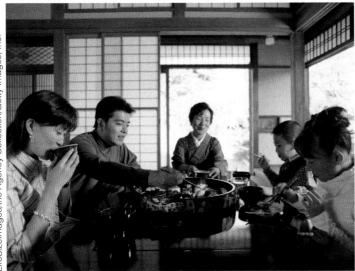

LifeSizeImages/the Agency Collection/Getty Images, Inc.

Epidemiological evidence • Figure 1.12

Epidemiology seeks to understand why health outcomes and disease rates differ among different populations. For instance, epidemiologists might look at the low levels of heart disease in Japan and try to determine the influencing factors. They might then look at the typical Japanese diet and notice that it contains more fish than the diets of populations with higher rates of heart disease. Although an association is evidenced, it doesn't mean that one factor is the sole cause of the other. In this example, it could be differences in saturated fat consumption, physical activity patterns and genetics, or a combination of these factors and others, that promote improved heart health in Japan.

to prove, which is phrased in a way that can be tested, such as "Eating whole grains helps regulate blood sugar levels" (see Figure 1.11). To test a hypothesis, you first need a **sample**, a group of people that are meant to represent the population being described. Ideally, if you wanted to study the effect of a specific dietary change on the health of all Canadians, you would randomly select a large number of people across the nation—people of all ages, ethnicities, and sizes; but making such a selection would be a very difficult task. Instead, scientists often need to use smaller samples of a specific group that is accessible to them, such as undergraduate students attending the university where the scientists work. The number of subjects needed depends on what is being studied. Fewer subjects are needed to demonstrate an effect that rarely occurs by chance. For example, if only one man in a million can increase his muscle mass by weight training for four weeks, then an experiment to test whether a supplement increases muscle mass in men who weight train for four weeks would require only a few subjects to demonstrate an effect. However, if many men can increase muscle mass by weight training for four weeks, then more experimental subjects would be needed to demonstrate that the increase in muscle mass was due to the supplement and not to the weight training alone.

In a scientific experiment, the individuals in the sample are assigned to one of two groups: the **experimental group**, who undergo the treatment to be tested, and the **control group**, who represent a similar demographic as the experimental group, but who don't receive the treatment being tested. Instead, the control group often receives a **placebo**, an artificial treatment that has no effect on the variable being measured. In the experiment described in Figure 1.11, our hypothesis is specifically tested by observing the effects of two different sets of grains. The experimental group receives whole grains, while the control group receives refined grains. To maximize the reliability of our study, both grains need to have an identical look, smell, and taste, but the experimental group's grains would be given whole grain, while the control group would receive refined grains that were coloured and flavoured with molasses to appear like whole grains. Since we would also not tell our subjects

experimental group In a scientific experiment, the group of participants who undergo the treatment being tested.

control group In a scientific experiment, the group of participants used as a basis of comparison. They are similar to the participants in the experimental group but do not receive the treatment being tested.

which groups they were in, our experiment is a **blind study**, which increases its credibility. Blind studies eliminate the potential for subjects to influence the results, even unknowingly, because they believe the study should lead to a specific result. Those who are conducting the studies also have the potential to influence the results, especially when money is at stake and a specific result is desired by those funding the study. Therefore, credibility is increased through the use of **double-blind experiments**, in which neither the experimenters nor the subjects in the experiment know which group each person belongs to.

Ideally, human subjects should be used to draw conclusions about diets in humans, but using humans is not always possible since some experiments are too costly, time-consuming, inconvenient for the subjects and, in some cases, using humans may be impossible for ethical reasons. In such situations, scientist may rely on **animal studies**, by using animals such as mice to act as models for human beings. Animal studies afford certain experimental advantages: It is easier to control their environment and behaviours, and their life cycles are typically shorter, meaning results can be observed in a shorter period of time. However, no animal is identical to a human except for a human. You should never completely trust a single animal study alone, because their bodies, although sometimes similar, function differently from the human body, and a completely different result may be observed in a human.

Biochemistry and molecular biology techniques are also used to study nutrient functions in the body. For example, biochemists can study the chemical reactions that generate energy and synthesize molecules, such as cholesterol, and molecular biology can be used to study how nutrients regulate our genes. Still another strategy for scientific study is computer modelling, which can be used to predict outcomes based on our current knowledge of a particular phenomenon. The specific serving size recommendations found in *Eating Well with Canada's Food Guide* were perfected using computer models that simulated different diets and modelled them for their ability to promote health.

After a study has run its course and results have been collected, the last crucial step is the interpretation of the results. Accurate interpretation is just as important as the careful conducting of a study, and the conclusions must accurately reflect the results of that specific study using that specific sample of the population. For example, if a study conducted on a large group of men indicates that a change in diet reduces cancer risk, the results of that study cannot be used to claim the same effect in women. Likewise, if the study looks only at the connection between a change in diet and colon cancer, the findings cannot be used to claim a reduced risk for other cancers. One way to ensure that the results of experiments are interpreted correctly is to have them reviewed by experts in the field who did not take part in the study being evaluated. This **peer-review process** is used to determine whether results should be published in scientific journals. The reviewing scientists must agree that the studies were conducted properly and that the results were interpreted fairly. Nutrition articles that have undergone peer review can be found in journals such as *The Canadian Journal of Clinical Nutrition*, *The American Journal of Clinical Nutrition*, *The Journal of Nutrition*, *The Canadian Medical Association Journal*, *Canadian Journal of Dietetic Practice and Research*, *The Canadian Journal of Public Health*, *Journal of the American Dietetic Association*, *The New England Journal of Medicine*, and *The International Journal of Sport Nutrition*. Newsletters from reputable institutions, such as the *Tufts Health & Nutrition Letter* and the *Harvard Health Letter*, are also reliable sources of nutrition and health information. The information in these newsletters comes from peer-reviewed articles but is written for a consumer audience.

Although experimental evidence is the most reliable type of nutritional evidence, much of the nutritional information available to consumers is in the form of **anecdotal evidence (Figure 1.13)**.

Judging for Yourself

Not everything you hear is accurate. Remember that much of the nutrition information we encounter is intended to sell products, which means that the information may have been embellished to make it more appealing. Understanding the principles scientists use to perform nutrition studies can help consumers judge the nutrition information they encounter in their daily lives (see *Hot Topic*). Some things that may tip you off to misinformation are claims that sound too good to be true, information from unreliable sources, information intended to sell a product, and information that is new or untested.

The following four questions can help you evaluate any piece of nutrition information you encounter:

1. **Does it make sense?** Some claims are too outrageous to be true. For example, if a product claims to increase your muscle size without any exercise or decrease your weight without a change in diet, common sense should tell you that the claim is too good to be true. In contrast, an article that tells you that adding exercise to your daily routine will help you lose weight and increase your stamina is not so outrageous. Always make sure that claims are in line with basic nutritional principles.

2. **What's the source?** If a claim seems reasonable, look to see where it came from. Personal testimonies are not a reliable source (see Figure 1.13), whereas more reliable sources are government

Anecdotal evidence is not proof • Figure 1.13

Anecdotal evidence is simply a story you may hear about someone else's experience with a specific nutritional concern. It often uses before and after pictures and "look at me now!" testimonials to convince consumers that the product being sold will improve health. Keep in mind that just because something worked for someone else, even your friend, it does not mean it will work for you. Also, some of these testimonials may be falsified because money is being exchanged. Only claims based on sound nutritional evidence and interpretation can be trusted.

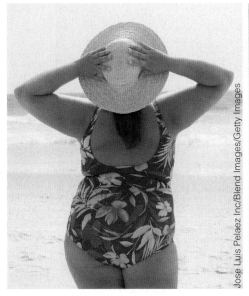
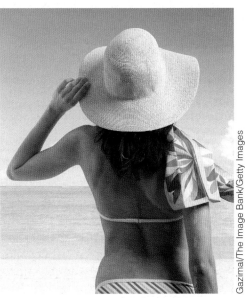

HOT TOPIC

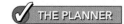

Evaluating the credibility of nutrition advertisements

This product must be amazing! It will increase your muscle strength, decrease your body fat, and boost your drive and motivation. These claims sound great to a consumer, but a scientist may have some concerns. Remembering what you have learned about credible nutritional information, look over the claim below and, before reading on, ask yourself:

Is this advertisement credible?

First of all, the claims about muscle strength and motivation are testimonials based on individuals' feelings and impressions; they are not objective measures.

A scientist would question whether the research evidence supports the claim that the product increases lean body mass and decreases body fat. The study measured the amount of lean tissue and fat tissue in weightlifters both before and then four weeks after they began consuming the Power Boost drink. The measures used provide quantifiable, repeatable data. The results report a gain of 5.2 kg of lean tissue and a loss of 4.5 kg of fat tissue in weightlifters taking Power Boost. These results sound convincing, but the results for the control group are not reported in the ad. When the results for the experimental group are compared with those for the control group, a different picture emerges. This comparison (see graph) shows that the control group gained almost as much lean mass and lost slightly more fat mass than those taking Power Boost.

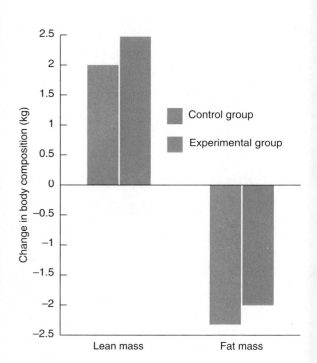

© Can Stock Photo Inc. / wacker

POWER BOOST

BOOST your STRENGTH • POWER up your DRIVE • MAXIMIZE your MASS

4 out of 5 users report:

"It increased my muscle strength."

"It pumped up my drive and motivation!"

Years of research have developed this special nutritional formulation. Just mix with water and drink one shake with every meal or snack.

University Study Shows: 25 experienced weightlifters added one POWER BOOST snacks 5 times a day for 4 weeks.

Lean body mass and fat mass were measured by underwater weighing before POWER BOOST was added and after 4 weeks of training with POWER BOOST.

RESULTS
The weightlifters gained an average of 2.4 kg (5.2 lb.) of lean muscle and lost 2 kg (4.5 lb.) of unwanted fat.

Think Critically Would you recommend this product? Why or why not?

recommendations regarding healthy dietary practices and information disseminated by universities. Government recommendations are developed by committees of scientists who interpret the latest well-conducted research studies and use their conclusions to develop recommendations for the population (see *Debate*). Information from universities is supported by research studies that are well scrutinized and published in peer-reviewed journals. Many universities also provide information that targets the general public. Nonprofit organizations such as the Canadian Dietetic Association and the Canadian Medical Association are also reliable sources of nutrition information.

If you are reading an article in a print medium or posted on a website, you can check the author's credentials to help evaluate the credibility of the information. Where does the author work? Does he or she have a degree in nutrition or medicine? Dietitians in Canada are credible because they have successfully completed a bachelor's degree focusing on nutrition and they have met established criteria for certification to provide nutrition education and counselling. Although nutritionists and nutrition counsellors may provide accurate information, the term *nutritionist* is not legally defined in most parts of Canada. Anyone can call themselves a nutritionist—from university professors with doctoral degrees from reputable universities to health food store clerks with no formal training, to your friend who once read an article about nutrition.

3. **What evidence is being presented?** In a criminal court, lawyers rely on evidence to support their arguments. The same is true in science: scientists believe only claims that can be supported by reliable, consistent evidence. Many blogs and advertisements make nutritional claims without any evidence or sources to back them up. On the other hand, any article found in a scientific journal will have ample evidence and other research results to support its conclusions. If a source makes outrageous claims without any evidence to support those claims, or if the evidence provided is anecdotal or attributes too much weight to a single, isolated study, more digging will be needed before you can establish whether that information is credible.

4. **Is it selling something?** If a person or company will profit from the information presented, be wary. Advertisements from such companies are designed to increase sales, and the company stands to profit if you believe the claims it makes. Even information presented in newspapers and magazines and on television may be biased or exaggerated because it is designed to help sell magazines or boost ratings, not necessarily to promote health and well-being. Even a well-designed, carefully executed study published in a peer-reviewed journal can be a source of misinformation if its results have been interpreted incorrectly or exaggerated (**Figure 1.14**).

Results may be misinterpreted to sell products • Figure 1.14

This rat, which was given large doses of vitamin E, lived longer than rats that consumed less vitamin E. So, will dietary supplements of vitamin E increase longevity in people? Not necessarily. The results of animal studies can't always be extrapolated to humans, but they are often the basis of claims in ads for dietary supplements.

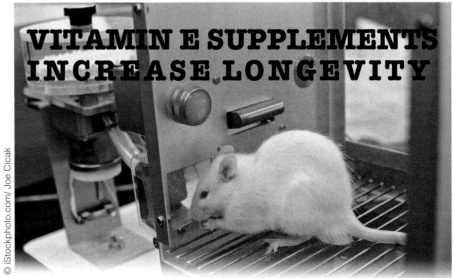

© iStockphoto.com/ Joe Cicak

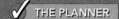

The Issue: The typical Canadian diet is not as healthy as it could be. These poor diets have contributed to our high rates of obesity, type-2 diabetes, and heart disease.[24,25] Should we as individuals take responsibility for our diet and health, or should the government intervene?

The economic burden of obesity is huge and affects health care spending and workplace productivity. Obesity has been estimated to cost Canadians $4 billion to $7 billion annually, both in direct and indirect costs.[27] So, who is responsible for the unhealthy diets we consume that promote obesity, and who should be responsible for changing what we eat?

Proponents of more government involvement in our food choices suggest that our food environment is the main cause of our unhealthy eating habits. They argue that the dramatic rise in obesity rates over the past four decades cannot be solely attributable to individual responsibility, but that our environment has changed in a way that makes eating healthfully a more difficult and expensive choice.

Obesity expert Kelly Brownell believes that environment plays a more powerful role in determining food choices than does personal irresponsibility.[28] Brownell and other proponents of government intervention argue that governments should treat toxic food environments like any other public threat and develop programs to keep us safe and healthy. Just as government regulations help to ensure that our food is not contaminated with harmful bacteria, laws can be used to ensure that food ordered at a restaurant will not contribute to heart disease or cancer. Unfortunately, unlike bacteria, individual foods are difficult to classify as healthy or unhealthy. Almost all food has some nutritional benefits, and the arguments are ongoing as to what constitutes "junk food" and what should be added or subtracted from our diets. However, many people believe certain actions can be taken to ensure healthier choices.

Proponents of government intervention suggest one option to encourage healthier choices is to tax junk food, making it more expensive, and to increase subsidies for fruits and vegetables, making them less expensive. Other suggestions include zoning restrictions to keep fast-food restaurants away from schools and child-care facilities and limitations on the types of foods that can be advertised on children's television. A good example of one such government intervention is the Quebec government's limitation on food advertising to children, which was implemented in 1980. While other factors may also have been at play, within the same period the bans have been in place, Quebec has seen a US$88 million annual drop in fast-food purchases,[29] leading many health professionals to argue that similar bans should be implemented across the country and the world.

All these ideas for promoting health through health-promoting public policies have pros and cons, and none will absolve individuals of their own responsibility for getting more exercise and making healthier food choices. Also, none of these solutions in isolation is enough to significantly improve the overall diets of Canadians. A disease such as obesity is a complex, multifaceted disorder that requires various interventions at various levels to see a significant effect on the weight of the nation.

Opponents of government involvement believe it is an infringement on personal freedom and suggest that individuals need to take responsibility for their own actions. They propose that the food industry work with the public to make healthier food more available and more affordable. Many food companies have already responded to the need for a better diet. For example, General Mills and Kellogg's offer whole-grain cereals. And the giant food retailer Walmart has announced a major campaign to make healthy food more affordable. But these are isolated cases and alone will not make a significant change on the health of Canadians.

Our current food environment makes unhealthy eating easy. Opportunities for high-calorie, fatty, salty, and sweet foods are available 24/7, and the portions offered are often massive. To preserve our public health and save health care dollars, Canadians need to change the way they eat. This change could be driven by government regulations and taxes, it could come from changes in the food industry, and/or it could come from individuals making healthier choices for their waistlines and health. A synergy of policy intervention, industry cooperation, and personal efforts is likely needed to solve this and other nutrition-related problems.

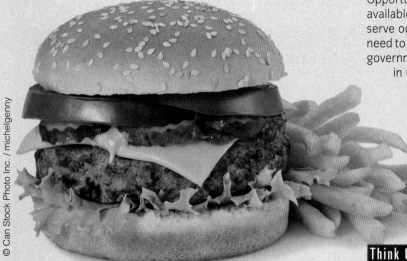

© Can Stock Photo Inc. / michelgenny

Think Critically If someone eats fast food daily and becomes obese, is that person to blame for eating the food, or is the restaurant to blame for not informing the person of the health risks?

5. Has it stood the test of time? Often the results of a new scientific study are on the morning news the same day they are presented at a meeting or published in a peer-reviewed journal. However, a single study cannot serve as a basis for a reliable theory. Results need to be reproduced and supported numerous times before they can be used as a basis for nutrition recommendations.

Headlines based on a single study should therefore be viewed skeptically. The information may be accurate, but not enough time has passed to repeat the work and reaffirm the conclusions. If, for example, someone has found the secret to easy weight loss, if the finding is valid, you will undoubtedly encounter this information again at some later time. If, however, the finding is not valid, it will fade away with all the other weight-loss concoctions that have come and gone.

CONCEPT CHECK

1. **What** is the difference between a hypothesis and a theory?
2. **How** is epidemiology used to study nutrition?
3. **Why** are control groups important in any scientific experiment?
4. **Why** is information in advertisements likely to be exaggerated or inaccurate?

Summary

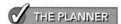

1   Food Choices and Nutrient Intake   4

- The foods you choose determine which **nutrients** you consume. The body requires more than 40 **essential nutrients** to function properly. Carbohydrates, fats, and proteins provide the body with energy, which is measured in **calories**. Although it is important to consume adequate amounts of the essential nutrients, the overconsumption of energy and of nutrients such as fats and sodium has promoted an increase in **chronic disease** in our population.

- Choosing foods that are high in **nutrient density** allows you to obtain more nutrients in fewer calories. **Fortified foods**, or foods to which nutrients have been added, and **dietary supplements** can also contribute nutrients to the diet.

- The food choices we make are affected by many factors other than nutrition, including food availability; what we learn to eat from family, culture, and traditions; personal tastes; and what we think we should eat to maintain health.

Food choices • Figure 1.2

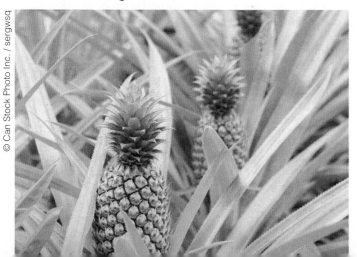

2   Nutrients and Their Functions   8

- Nutrients are grouped into six classes. Carbohydrates, lipids, proteins, and water are referred to as **macronutrients** because they are needed in large amounts. Vitamins and minerals are **micronutrients** because they are needed in small amounts to maintain health.

- **Carbohydrates, lipids**, and **proteins** are **organic compounds** that provide energy, typically measured in calories, more specifically kilocalories. Sugars, starches, and **fibre** are all carbohydrates; **saturated fats, unsaturated fats**, and **cholesterol** are the main lipids we consume; and the proteins we eat are made up of **amino acids**. Lipids, proteins, carbohydrates, **minerals**, and water perform structural roles, forming and maintaining the structure of our bodies. **Vitamins** are organic molecules that help put other nutrients to use, while minerals are non-organic **elements** that are involved in regulatory processes and help maintain body structure. All six classes of nutrients help regulate body processes. The energy, structure, and regulation provided by nutrients are needed for growth, maintenance and repair of the body, and reproduction.

- The **energy-yielding nutrients** provide energy to the body. Carbohydrates, fats, and proteins provide 4, 9, and 4 **kilocalories** per gram, respectively. Proteins and fats can also function as **hormones**, which are messengers that help regulate body processes.

- Food contains not only nutrients but also non-nutritive substances, such as **phytochemicals**, that may provide additional health benefits. Foods that provide health benefits beyond basic nutrition are called **functional foods**. Some foods are naturally functional and others are created through fortification. These foods that have been altered for the purpose of promoting health benefits are known as **designer foods** or **neutraceuticals**.

Nutrient functions • Figure 1.4

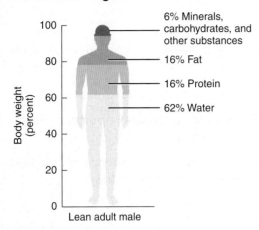

- 6% Minerals, carbohydrates, and other substances
- 16% Fat
- 16% Protein
- 62% Water

Body weight (percent)

Lean adult male

3 Nutrition in Health and Disease 13

- Your diet affects your health. The foods you choose contain the nutrients needed to keep you alive and healthy and prevent **malnutrition**.

- **Undernutrition** results from consuming too few calories and/or too few nutrients. For example, **osteoporosis** is a disease associated with the inadequate consumption of calcium. **Overnutrition** can result from a toxic dose of a nutrient or from a chronic excess of nutrients or calories, which over time contributes to chronic diseases.

- The diet you consume can affect your risk for developing a variety of chronic diseases, but your **genes** also play a large role in determining your disease susceptibility. The understanding of how genes and nutrition interact to affect health is explored in the discipline of **nutritional genomics** or **nutrigenomics**.

Undernutrition • Figure 1.7

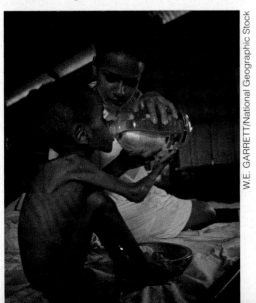

W.E. GARRETT/National Geographic Stock

4 Choosing a Healthy Diet 15

- A healthy diet includes a variety of nutrient-dense foods from the different food groups and a variety of foods from within each group. Variety is important because different foods provide different nutrients and health-promoting substances as well as a variety of tastes.

- Balance means mixing and matching foods and meals so you obtain enough of the nutrients you need and not too much of the ones that can potentially harm your health.

- Moderation means not ingesting too many or too few calories or too much or too little fat, sugar, and salt. Eating moderate portions helps you maintain a healthy weight and helps prevent chronic diseases such as heart disease and cancer.

Balance calories in with calories out • Figure 1.10

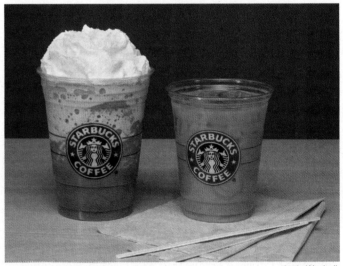

Andy Washnik

5 Evaluating Nutrition Information 18

- Nutrition uses the **scientific method** to study the relationships among food, nutrients, and health. The scientific method involves observing and questioning natural events, formulating **hypotheses** to explain these events, designing and performing experiments to test the hypotheses, and developing **theories** that explain the observed phenomena based on the experimental results.

- **Epidemiology** can help us learn more about how diets affect health by exploring relationships between different variables in different populations. Because causation cannot be established in an epidemiological study, **experimental evidence** is often used instead to establish a more direct link between variables. In an experiment, a **sample** of people is divided into an **experimental group**, which receives the experimental treatment, and a **control group**, which typically receives a **placebo**. In a well-designed study, neither group will know which treatment they are receiving, making it a **blind study**; when the researchers also do not know which group is which, it is a **double-blind study**, which further reduces potential bias. Experiments in humans are not always ethical or possible to perform, therefore, **animal studies** and **biochemistry and molecular biology techniques** are also often used to explore the science of nutrition. When a study has been completed, the results must be interpreted fairly and accurately. The **peer-review process** ensures that studies published in professional journals adhere to a high standard of experimental design and interpretation of results. On the other hand, **anecdotal evidence**, which is often used in advertising, does not adhere to this same process that ensures the quality and accuracy of information being presented.

• Not all the nutrition information we encounter is accurate. The first step in deciding whether a nutritional claim is valid is to ask whether the claim makes sense. If it sounds

too good to be true, it probably is. It is also important to determine whether the information came from a reliable source, whether it is trying to sell a product, and whether it has been confirmed by multiple studies.

Results may be misinterpreted to sell products
• Figure 1.14

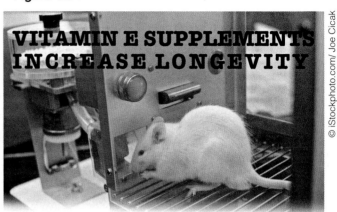

© iStockphoto.com/ Joe Cicak

Key Terms

- amino acids 8
- anecdotal evidence 21
- animal studies 20
- biochemistry and molecular biology technique 20
- blind study 20
- calorie 4
- carbohydrates 8
- cholesterol 8
- chronic diseases 4
- control group 20
- designer foods or neutraceuticals 12
- dietary supplements 5

- double-blind experiments 20
- elements 8
- energy-yielding nutrients 10
- epidemiology 18
- essential nutrients 4
- experimental evidence 18
- experimental group 20
- fibre 8
- fortified foods 4
- functional foods 12
- genes 14
- hormones 11

- hypotheses 18
- kilocalories 10
- lipids 8
- macronutrients 8
- malnutrition 13
- micronutrients 8
- minerals 8
- nutrient density 4
- nutrients 4
- nutritional genomics or nutrigenomics 14
- organic compounds 8
- osteoporosis 13
- overnutrition 13

- peer-review process 21
- placebo 20
- phytochemicals 11
- proteins 8
- sample 20
- saturated fats 8
- scientific method 18
- theories 18
- undernutrition 13
- unsaturated fats 8
- vitamins 8

Critical and Creative Thinking Questions

1. Which type of malnutrition—overnutrition or undernutrition—is most common in Canada today? Why? What are some potential consequences of this malnutrition?

2. Nutrients provide energy, structure, and regulation in our bodies. Based on the fact that about 50% of the calories we consume are from carbohydrates, yet less than 1% of our body weight is carbohydrates, which of these three functions do you think carbohydrates provide in the body? What is likely the function of a nutrient that is present in small amounts in the diet but in large amounts in the body?

3. A typical fast-food meal consists of a cheeseburger, fries, and pop. Use iProfile to calculate the kilocalories in this meal. For each food in this meal, suggest a more nutrient-dense alternative.

4. Emeryk is living in a university residence. Every day, he has a banana and a glass of orange juice for breakfast and potatoes or corn for dinner, but he doesn't eat any other fruits or vegetables. How can he improve his food choices? Why is such an improvement important?

5. Moderation and balance are important in choosing a healthy diet. Explain how these principles help a person maintain a healthy weight.

6. A scientist observes that colon cancer is rare in Japan but common in Canada. He hypothesizes that this difference is due to differences in diet. Propose an experiment that might be used to test this hypothesis.

7. Go to the Internet and locate an advertisement for a dietary supplement. What nutrients does the supplement contain? Does it contain substances that are not nutrients? Do you think this dietary supplement is worth the money? Why or why not?

What is happening in this picture?

A major benefit of Canada's multicultural nature is the diverse meal options that are available to us. Unlike countries like Japan, Thailand, and India, there is no similar dietary pattern that is common across the population. For some Canadians, a typical diet includes macaroni and cheese, pizza, hamburgers, and pop, while other Canadians enjoy eating foods of different ethnic origins, like this sushi dinner.

Lori Smolin

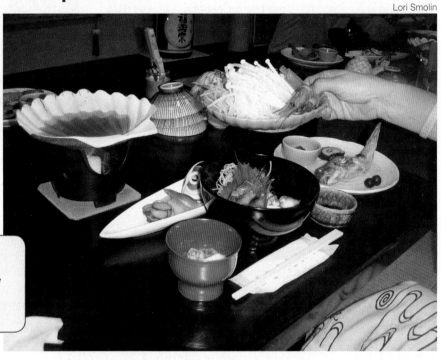

Think Critically

1. How does this meal fit into a healthy diet?
2. Why might some Canadians not choose these foods?
3. Does this meal illustrate variety, balance, and moderation? Why or why not?

Self-Test

(Check your answers in Appendix J.)

1. True or false: If you choose a high-fat, high-salt, fast-food lunch, your nutrient intake for the day cannot meet the recommendations for a healthy diet.

   a. True

   b. False

2. Which of these foods has the lowest nutrient density?

   a. an orange

   b. strawberry yogurt

   c. whole-wheat bread

   d. orange pop

3. Which group consists only of nutrients that are classified as energy-yielding nutrients?

   a. vitamins and minerals

   b. carbohydrates, lipids, and proteins

   c. lipids, carbohydrates, proteins, and water

   d. carbohydrates and vitamins

4. This graph indicates that _____.

   a. low-fat milk contains more calcium per kilocalorie than iced tea

   b. low-fat milk is more energy-dense than iced tea

   c. iced tea is more nutrient dense than milk

   d. low-fat milk has less vitamin D per kilocalorie than iced tea

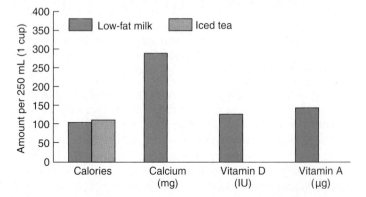

5. Which group consists only of nutrients that are considered micronutrients?

   a. protein and water

   b. carbohydrates, lipids, and proteins

   c. vitamins and minerals

   d. minerals and water

6. Which nutrient class provides the most kilocalories per gram?

   a. carbohydrates   c. lipids

   b. proteins   d. vitamins

7. Based on this illustration, which nutrient class makes up the greatest proportion of body weight?

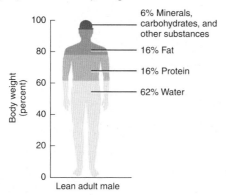

   a. protein   c. fat

   b. carbohydrate   d. water

8. Which of these statements about essential nutrients is false?

   a. If you do not get enough essential nutrients in your diet, your body will synthesize enough to meet its needs.

   b. If you do not get enough essential nutrients in your diet, deficiency symptoms will eventually appear.

   c. Some essential nutrients provide energy.

   d. Some essential nutrients provide structure.

9. Why is it better to obtain your nutrients from foods than from dietary supplements?

   a. Dietary supplements are more likely to contain toxic amounts of nutrients.

   b. Foods provide phytochemicals and zoochemicals.

   c. Foods provide pleasurable tastes and aromas.

   d. All of the above are correct.

10. Which of these factors can limit the availability of food?

   a. socioeconomic status   c. living conditions

   b. health status   d. All of the above are correct.

11. A diet that follows the principles of variety, balance, and moderation _____.

   a. can include all kinds of foods

   b. includes only foods that have high nutrient density

   c. includes exactly the right amount of each nutrient each day

   d. includes only unprocessed foods

12. Which of these sources would be most likely to exaggerate the beneficial effects of a dietary supplement?

   a. a government publication

   b. a dietitian's recommendations

   c. a pamphlet published by the manufacturer

   d. a peer-reviewed article in a scientific journal

13. When the scientific method is used, a hypothesis is first proposed and then tested through experimentation. Which of the following hypotheses can be tested by means of experiments that use a quantifiable measure?

   a. Iron supplements increase feelings of vitality.

   b. A high vitamin E intake makes you feel younger.

   c. Eating an apple a day will lower blood cholesterol.

   d. B vitamin supplements give you an energy boost.

14. Which of the following is a correct conclusion from an epidemiological study?

   a. A diet that is high in saturated fat causes heart disease.

   b. A higher incidence of coronary heart disease is associated with a higher intake of saturated fat.

   c. People who lower their intake of saturated fat will have fewer heart attacks.

   d. Moving to a country with less coronary heart disease will lower your intake of saturated fat.

15. In a scientific experiment, a group that is identical to the experimental group in every way except that its members do not receive the treatment being tested is called _____.

   a. a control group

   b. a placebo

   c. a variable

   d. an alternative group

THE PLANNER ✓

Review your Chapter Planner on the chapter opener and check off your completed work.

Guidelines for a Healthy Diet

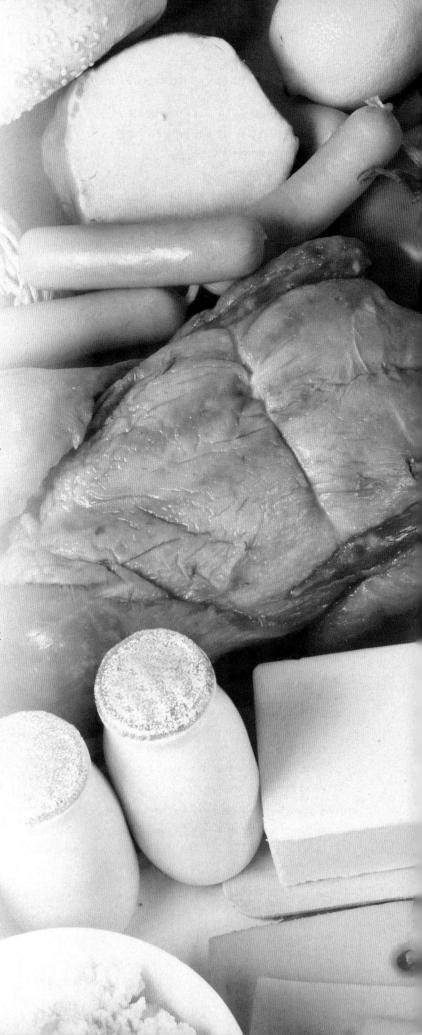

"**W**hat you don't know could kill you." Those words may have been the first nutrition recommendation in human history. Swallowing the wrong berry, gulping water from a suspect source, or tucking into a diseased organ from the most recent kill could have been fatal to early humans, who were hunter-gatherers. Such lessons would have served as anecdotal guideposts to survival. As societies developed, dietary cautions became taboos, sometimes laws, and ultimately, nutrition recommendations.

For the past 150 years, governments have been providing what we would call modern nutrition information. Today, this information is based on the results of thousands of studies examining the dietary factors associated with a population's highest level of health status. These results are then translated into an educational kit of dietary recommendations to inform the population which foods they should eat. The process of providing nutritional information to the population traces its roots to the Industrial Revolution that swept through Great Britain in the first half of the 19th century, when urban populations—and poverty and hunger—swelled. To ensure a healthy workforce, the British government developed minimum dietary guidelines utilizing the least expensive foods. It wasn't until World War I that the British Royal Society determined that a healthy workforce required not necessarily the least expensive diet but a healthy diet that included fruits, vegetables, and milk as elements of a solid nutritional foundation. Since then, virtually every national government, including the Canadian federal government, has sought, with varying degrees of success, to establish dietary standards for its citizens.

Today, modern public health agencies provide valuable information regarding nutritional choices. However, this information isn't always understood or used properly. As portion sizes grow, so do Canadian waistlines—and the attendant health concerns. "What you don't know could kill you" remains as vital an admonition today as it was 40,000 years ago.

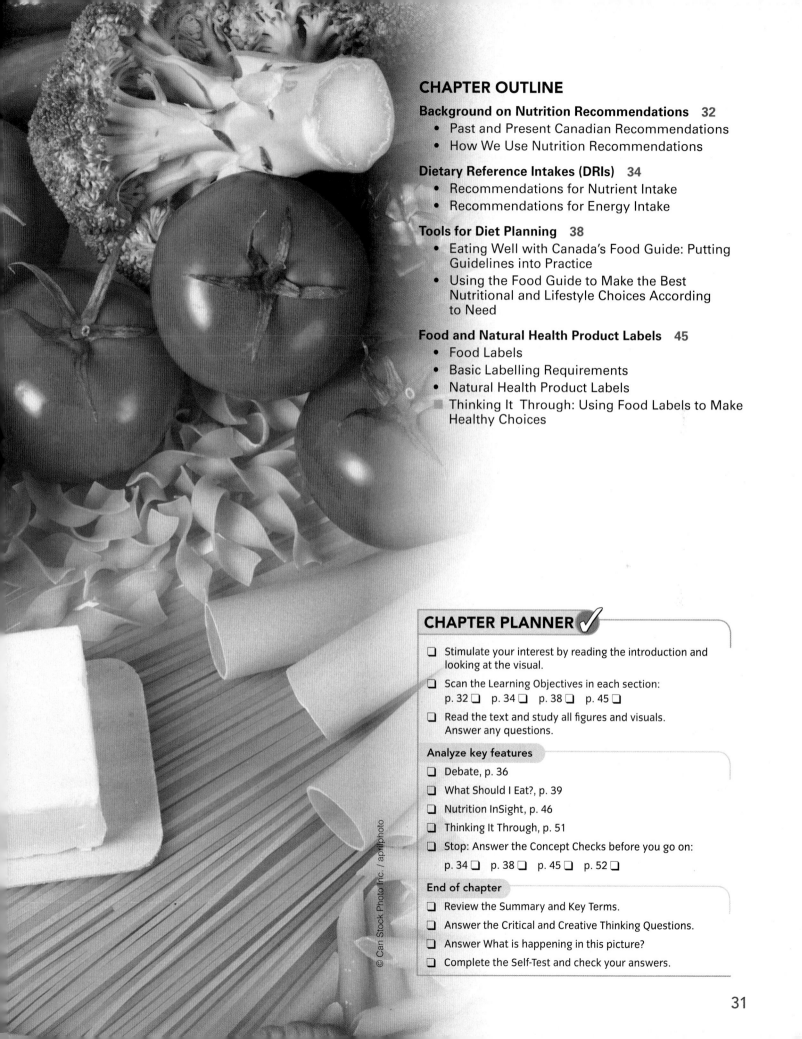

CHAPTER OUTLINE

CHAPTER PLANNER ✓

- ❑ Stimulate your interest by reading the introduction and looking at the visual.
- ❑ Scan the Learning Objectives in each section:
  p. 32 ❑   p. 34 ❑   p. 38 ❑   p. 45 ❑
- ❑ Read the text and study all figures and visuals. Answer any questions.

Analyze key features

- ❑ Debate, p. 36
- ❑ What Should I Eat?, p. 39
- ❑ Nutrition InSight, p. 46
- ❑ Thinking It Through, p. 51
- ❑ Stop: Answer the Concept Checks before you go on:
  p. 34 ❑   p. 38 ❑   p. 45 ❑   p. 52 ❑

End of chapter

- ❑ Review the Summary and Key Terms.
- ❑ Answer the Critical and Creative Thinking Questions.
- ❑ Answer What is happening in this picture?
- ❑ Complete the Self-Test and check your answers.

© Can Stock Photo Inc. / apriliphoto

Background on Nutrition Recommendations

LEARNING OBJECTIVES

1. **Explain** the purpose of government nutrition recommendations.

2. **Discuss** how Canadian nutrition recommendations have changed over the past 100 years.

3. **Describe** how nutrition recommendations are used to evaluate nutritional status and set public health policy.

W hat should we eat if we want to satisfy our nutrient needs, promote good health, and reduce the risk of disease? Our taste buds, food advertisers, and magazine and newspaper headlines can influence the numerous food consumption choices we make each day. But these choices may not always be healthy choices. Our taste buds respond to flavour and sensation, not necessarily to sensible nutrition; manufacturers want to sell products, and magazines want to sell advertising and subscriptions. Nutrition may not be the primary focus of the choices we are drawn to, and many alluring choices do not promote good health. Government recommendations, on the other hand, are based on credible nutritional evidence and are designed to enhance both individual health and public health. These recommendations can be used to plan diets and to evaluate what we are eating, both as individuals and as a population.

Past and Present Canadian Recommendations

The federal government recognizes that a population that eats well will be healthy and productive. Therefore, since 1938, Health Canada has helped to develop and review nutritional standards that are based on the most current scientific evidence available. The first food guidelines Canada ever released were the **Recommended Nutrient Intakes (RNIs)**, which provided information on the amount of essential nutrients needed to meet the needs of most Canadians. Canada's first food guide, *Canada's Official Food Rules* (**Figure 2.1**), was released in 1942 and drew many of its recommendations from the standards outlined in the RNIs. Today, as our scientific understanding of nutrition has evolved, so have the recommendations. Canadian guidelines have now merged with similar American guidelines to become the Dietary Reference Intakes (DRIs), which we will discuss in further detail later in this chapter.

CANADA'S OFFICIAL FOOD RULES
These are the Health-Protective Foods
Be sure you eat them every day in at least these amounts.
(Use more if you can)

MILK–Adults–½ pint. Children–more than 1 pint. And some CHEESE, as available.

FRUITS–One serving of tomatoes daily, or of a citrus fruit, or of tomato or citrus fruit juices, and one serving of other fruits, fresh, canned or dried.

VEGETABLES (In addition to potatoes of which you need one serving daily)–Two servings daily of vegetables, preferably leafy green, or yellow, and frequently raw.

CEREALS AND BREAD–One serving of a whole-grain cereal and 4 to 6 slices of Canada Approved Bread, brown or white.

MEAT, FISH, etc.–One serving a day of meat, fish, or meat substitutes. Liver, heart or Kidney once a week.

EGGS–At least 3 or 4 eggs weekly.

Eat these foods first, then add these and other foods you wish.

Some source of Vitamin D such as fish liver oils, is essential for children, and may be advisable for adults.

Canada's Official Food Rules (1942)[1] • Figure 2.1

Food guidelines distributed to the general Canadian public had humble beginnings. Canada's first food guide was *Canada's Official Food Rules*. It was much simpler than contemporary versions and included recommendations that were both similar and contrasting to today's guidelines. You will notice that the first food guide had six, not four, food groups: milk; fruits; vegetables; cereals and breads; meat, fish, or meat substitute; and eggs. It also recommended a weekly serving of liver, heart, or kidney, reflecting the food consumption patterns of a different time.

As our understanding of how nutrients affect health has evolved, so have the DRIs and the **food guides** that are based on those DRIs. Historical changes in the guides also reflect changes in Canadian lifestyles, health statuses, and dietary patterns. The latest version, entitled *Eating Well with Canada's Food Guide*, was released in 2007. Its changes include specific recommendations for various life stages and genders, as well as suggestions about the importance of incorporating physical activity in a healthy lifestyle.

How We Use Nutrition Recommendations

Nutrition recommendations are developed to address the nutritional concerns of the population and help individuals meet their nutrient needs. These recommendations can also be used to evaluate the nutrient intake of populations and of individuals within populations. Determining what people eat and how their nutrient intake compares with nutrition recommendations is important for assessing their **nutritional status**.

> **nutritional status**
> An individual's health, as it is influenced by the intake and utilization of nutrients.

Assessing nutritional status • Figure 2.2

THE PLANNER
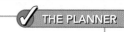

A complete assessment of an individual's nutritional status includes a diet analysis, a physical exam, a medical history, and an evaluation of nutrient levels in the body. An interpretation of this information can determine whether an individual is well nourished, malnourished, or at risk of malnutrition.

1 Determine typical food intake. Typical food intake can be evaluated by having people either record their food as they consume it or recall what they have eaten during the past day or so. Because food intake varies from day to day, an individual's intake should be monitored for more than one day to obtain a clearer view of overall consumption patterns. An accurate food record includes all food and beverages consumed, descriptions of cooking methods, and brand names of products. Obtaining an accurate record is often difficult because people may change what they are eating but not record it, or they may forget what they ate when recalling their consumption.

FOOD DIARY

Record all the food and beverages you eat. Include the food, how it was prepared, the amount you ate and the brand name. Don't forget to list all fats used in cooking and all spreads and sauces added.

Time	Food	Kind and how prepared	Amount
7:00 A.M.	Eggs	scrambled	2
	Butter	in eggs	5 mL
	toast	whole wheat	2 slices
	Butter	on toast	10 mL
	Milk	non-fat	250 ml
	Orange juice	from frozen concentrate	250 ml
12:00 P.M.	Big Mac	McDonalds	1

2 Analyze nutrient intake. A computer analysis of an individual's food intake can calculate nutrient intake and compare it with the appropriate nutrition recommendations. In this example, which shows only a few nutrients, the intakes of vitamin A, iron, and calcium are below the recommended amounts, and intakes of vitamin C and saturated fat are above the recommended amounts. Even though an individual may consume more or less than the recommended daily intake for a nutrient, keep in mind that the diet still may be acceptable if, over time, nutrient levels are greater than levels that could promote symptoms of deficiency and lower than levels that promote symptoms of toxicity.

Nutrient	Percent of recommendation 0% 50% 100%
Vitamin A	75%
Vitamin C	115%
Iron	54%
Calcium	75%
Saturated fat	134%

3 Evaluate physical health. A physical examination can detect signs of nutrient deficiencies or excesses. Measures of body dimensions such as height and weight can be monitored over time or compared with standards for a given population. Drastic changes in measurements or measurements that are significantly above or below the standards may indicate a nutritional deficiency or excess.

© Can Stock Photo Inc. / forestpath

4 Consider medical history. Personal and family medical histories are important because genetic risk factors affect an individual's risk of developing a nutrition-related disease. For example, if you have high cholesterol and your father died of a heart attack at age 50, you have a higher-than-average risk of developing heart disease and may need to modify your diet to reduce your risk.

Great-grand-parents

Grand-parents

Parents

● Affected by or at risk for heart disease

Kids

5 Assess with laboratory tests. Nutrient deficiencies and excesses can be detected by measuring nutrients, their by-products, or their functions in the blood, urine, and body cells (Appendix C). For instance, levels of iron and iron-carrying proteins in the blood can be used to determine whether a person has iron-deficiency anemia, and levels of blood cholesterol such as those shown here can provide information about an individual's risk of heart disease.

Blood Lipid Panel

Test	*Result (R)	Healthy range (HR)[2]
Cholesterol total	4.0 mmol/L	<4.5 mmol/L (6 to 19 years) < 5.2 mmol/L (20 to 79)
Triglycerides	1.5 mmol/L	<1.7 mmol/L
HDL ("good") cholesterol	1.4 mmol/L	>1.0 mmol/L men >1.3 mmol/L women
LDL ("bad") cholesterol	2.8 mmol/L	<3.4 mmol/L

To evaluate the nutritional status of a population, food intake can be assessed by having individuals track their food intake or by collecting information about the amounts and types of food available to the population to identify dietary trends.

Evaluating food intake data in conjunction with information about the health and nutritional status of individuals in the population (**Figure 2.2**) can help to identify relationships between dietary intake and health and disease. This evaluation is important for developing public health measures that address nutritional problems. For example, in 2004, the Canadian Community Health Survey helped public health officials recognize that 70% of males and 50% of females exceed their recommended daily caloric intake, and that magnesium and vitamin A were common nutrient deficiencies.[3] This finding led public health experts to develop programs and nutritional recommendations, such as the updated food guide, to improve both the diet and the fitness of Canadians.

CONCEPT CHECK STOP

1. **How** do nutrition recommendations benefit individual and public health?
2. **What** is the purpose of the RNIs?
3. **What** factors are considered in evaluating nutritional status?

Dietary Reference Intakes (DRIs)

LEARNING OBJECTIVES

1. **Summarize** the purpose of the DRIs.
2. **Describe** the four sets of DRI values used in recommending nutrient intake.
3. **List** the variables that affect energy needs (EERs).
4. **Define** the concept of the Acceptable Macronutrient Distribution Ranges (AMDRs).

The **Dietary Reference Intakes (DRIs)** are a set of scientifically based reference values for the amounts of energy, nutrients, and other food components in the diet that are recommended to be consumed to reduce chronic disease risk, promote general health, and minimize symptoms of deficiency.[4] When Health Canada designs a new food guide or a new set of dietary guidelines, it compares population data on what Canadians *do* consume with the DRIs, the amounts they *should* consume on a daily basis, and makes recommendations accordingly. For instance, when results of the 2004 Canadian Community Health Survey were compared with the Estimated Average Requirement (one of the DRIs) for vitamin A, it was found that more than 35% of Canadians were inadequate in vitamin A,[5] thereby increasing their risk for vision problems such as night blindness. The food guide now advises that Canadians consume at least one orange vegetable a day, as they are excellent sources of vitamin A.

The DRIs now replace both the Recommended Nutrient Intakes (RNIs) originally established in 1938 by Health Canada and the Recommended Dietary Allowances (RDAs) first established by the American Food and Nutrition Board in 1941. The DRIs include several types of recommendations that address both nutrient and energy intake and include values that are appropriate for people of different genders and stages of life (**Figure 2.3**).

DRIs for different groups • Figure 2.3

Because gender and life stage affect nutrient needs, Dietary Reference Intake values have been set for each gender and for various life-stage groups. These values take into account the physiological differences that affect the varying nutrient needs of men and women, infants, children, adolescents, adults, older adults, and pregnant and lactating women.

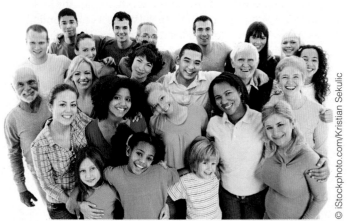

© iStockphoto.com/Kristian Sekulic

Understanding EARs, RDAs, and ULs • Figure 2.4

EARs and RDAs are determined by measuring the different amounts of nutrients required by different individuals in a population group and plotting the resulting values. Because a few individuals in the group need only a small amount, a few need a large amount, and most need an amount that falls between the extremes, the result is a bell-shaped curve like the one shown here.

The RDA is set by adding a safety factor to the EAR. About 97% of the population meets its needs by consuming this amount (shown as yellow shading). If nutrient intake meets the RDA, the risk of deficiency is very low. As intake falls, the risk of a deficiency increases.

An EAR is the average amount of a nutrient required for good health. If everyone in the population consumed this amount, only 50% would obtain enough of the nutrient to meet their requirements (shown as diagonal lines).

The UL is set well above the needs of everyone in the population and represents the highest amount of the nutrient that will not cause toxicity symptoms in the majority of healthy people. As intake rises above the UL, the likelihood of toxicity increases.

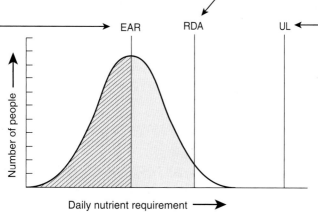

Recommendations for Nutrient Intake

DRIs for nutrient intake are an umbrella term for four sets of values. The **Estimated Average Requirements (EARs)** are the average amounts of nutrients or other dietary components required by healthy individuals within a specific gender and life-stage group (**Figure 2.4**). The EARs are determined from data on nutrient needs and are used to assess the adequacy of a population's food supply or typical intake. These requirements are not appropriate for evaluating an individual's intake but are used to calculate the **Recommended Dietary Allowances (RDAs)**. The RDAs recommend specific amounts of nutrients and other dietary components required to meet the needs of nearly all (97–98%) of the population and are typically set 20% above the EAR values. Most recommendations for adequate nutrient intake levels are based on the RDA for each specific nutrient (Figure 2.4).[6]

Sometimes, there is not enough data about nutrient requirements to establish EARs and RDAs. In these cases, **Adequate Intakes (AIs)** are set, based on the typical intake levels of people that are said to be healthy and show no symptoms of deficiency or toxicity. RDA or AI values can be used as goals for individual intake and to plan and evaluate individual diets (Appendix A and inside covers). These values are meant to represent the amounts that most healthy people should consume, on average, over several days or even weeks, not each and every day. Because these values are set high enough to meet the needs of almost all healthy people, intake below the RDA or AI does not necessarily mean that an individual is deficient, but the risk of deficiency is greater than would be the case if the recommended amount were consumed.[6]

The fourth set of values, **Tolerable Upper Intake Levels (ULs)**, specifies the maximum amount of a nutrient that most people can consume on a daily basis without some adverse effect (Figure 2.4). For most nutrients, it is difficult to exceed the UL by consuming food. Most foods do not contain enough of any one nutrient to cause toxicity; however, some dietary supplements (and fortified foods) may (see *Debate: Super-Fortified Foods*). For some nutrients, the UL is set for total intake from all sources, including food, fortified foods, and dietary supplements. For other nutrients, the UL refers to intake from

> **Estimated Average Requirements (EARs)** Nutrient intakes estimated to meet the needs of 50% of the healthy individuals in a given gender and life-stage group.

> **Recommended Dietary Allowances (RDAs)** Nutrient intakes that are sufficient to meet the needs of almost all healthy people in a specific gender and life-stage group.

> **Adequate Intakes (AIs)** Nutrient intakes that should be used as a goal when no RDA exists. AI values are an approximation of the nutrient intake that sustains health.

> **Tolerable Upper Intake Levels (ULs)** Maximum daily intake levels that are unlikely to pose risks of adverse health effects to almost all individuals in a given gender and life-stage group.

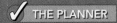

The Issue: Some foods, such as protein bars and energy drinks, are fortified with large amounts of nutrients. These foods add nutrients to the diet, but if eaten in large quantities or in combination with other highly fortified foods, they may pose a risk of toxicity. Are they a safe, healthy addition to your diet?

An orange, a tomato, a slice of bread, and a piece of grilled salmon—these foods are part of a healthy diet. But what about an energy drink with 23 added vitamins and minerals, a protein bar with 100% of your daily vitamin requirements, soft drinks with echinacea and green tea extract, fruit juice with added phytochemicals, and bottled water fortified with vitamin C? Are these products foods, or are they supplements?

Some may argue that fortified protein bars and juices are foods, not supplements, because they provide calories, just as traditional foods do, and the substances added to them, such as vitamin C, fish oil, or phytochemicals, also occur naturally in food. On the other hand, by definition, a supplement is a product intended to add nutrients or other substances to the diet, which these products certainly do. Does it matter whether these supplemental substances come in a food or in a pill? Opponents of these foods argue that it does matter because our decisions about eating foods differ from our decisions about supplements. Typically, we consider the dose when taking a supplement pill. But we eat to satisfy our sensory desires, fill our stomachs, and quench our thirsts. We don't think about whether the food or beverage might provide toxic amounts of nutrients.

In traditional foods, the amounts of nutrients are small, and the way they are combined limits absorption, making the risk of consuming a toxic amount of a nutrient almost nonexistent. In contrast, it is not difficult to swallow a very high dose of one or more nutrients from an excess of supplement pills or excessive servings of super-fortified foods. For example, if you drank 2 to 3 L of daily fluid as water fortified with vitamin C, niacin, vitamin E, and vitamins B6 and B12, you would exceed the UL for these vitamins. Then, if, in the same day, you also consumed 500 mL of fortified breakfast cereal and two protein bars, you would have an even greater risk of toxicity. The government labels these fortified products as foods, and we eat them like foods, but they may have the same toxicity risks as supplements.

Advocates of super-fortified foods point to the health-promoting substances these products add to our diet. But do super-fortified foods provide the same benefits that could have been sourced from the original food? In some cases they do. For example, if you get your calcium from orange juice, studies show that you are getting just about as much calcium as you would have consumed from milk.[7] On the other hand, fish oil consumed in capsules does not provide all the heart-health benefits of fish oil consumed in a piece of fish.[8]

So, are these products foods, or are they supplements? It is a fine line. Whether they are helpful or harmful depends on what is in them and how much you consume. Should the government regulate the amounts of nutrients that can be added to all foods? These answers depend on your view of the government's role in food regulation. Should we be gobbling these products without a thought? Probably not.

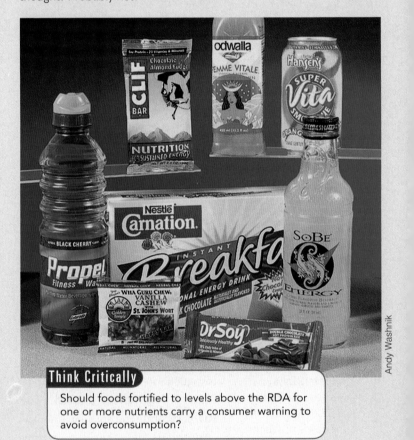

Think Critically

Should foods fortified to levels above the RDA for one or more nutrients carry a consumer warning to avoid overconsumption?

Andy Washnik

supplements alone or from supplements and fortified foods. Many nutrients have no UL because too little information is available to determine it.

Recommendations for Energy Intake

Instead of using an RDA value or UL for energy intake, there are two other types of recommendations for the amount of calories an individual should consume. The first, called **Estimated Energy Requirements (EERs)**, estimates the number of kilocalories needed to keep body weight stable. EER calculations take into account a person's age, gender, weight, height, and level of physical activity. A change in

Estimated Energy Requirements (EERs) Average energy intake values predicted to maintain body weight in healthy individuals.

The right amount of energy from the right sources
• Figure 2.5

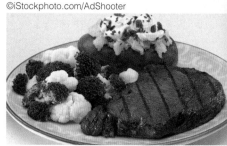

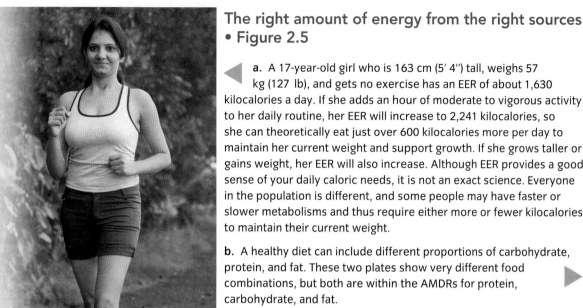

a. A 17-year-old girl who is 163 cm (5′ 4″) tall, weighs 57 kg (127 lb), and gets no exercise has an EER of about 1,630 kilocalories a day. If she adds an hour of moderate to vigorous activity to her daily routine, her EER will increase to 2,241 kilocalories, so she can theoretically eat just over 600 kilocalories more per day to maintain her current weight and support growth. If she grows taller or gains weight, her EER will also increase. Although EER provides a good sense of your daily caloric needs, it is not an exact science. Everyone in the population is different, and some people may have faster or slower metabolisms and thus require either more or fewer kilocalories to maintain their current weight.

b. A healthy diet can include different proportions of carbohydrate, protein, and fat. These two plates show very different food combinations, but both are within the AMDRs for protein, carbohydrate, and fat.

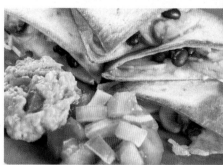

any of these variables will change the estimated energy needs (**Figure 2.5a**). To determine the most accurate value, Health Canada provides two sets of EER calculations for people 19 years of age or older, one for each gender.

Men

$$EER = 662 - (9.53 \times age\ [y]) + PA \times \{(15.91 \times weight\ [kg]) + (539.6 \times height\ [m])\}$$

Women

$$EER = 354 - (6.91 \times age\ [y]) + PA \times \{(9.36 \times weight\ [kg]) + (726 \times height\ [m])\}$$

Formulas for those in other age groups or for pregnant and lactating women can be found on the Health Canada website.

The value used to calculate the physical activity (PA) coefficient depends on the activity level of the individual and can be estimated using the values in **Table 2.1**.

The second type of energy recommendation, the **Acceptable Macronutrient Distribution Ranges (AMDRs)**, makes recommendations about the proportions of calories that should come from the energy-yielding nutrients: carbohydrates, fats, and protein. AMDRs are not exact values but ranges—20 to 35% of calories from protein, 45 to 65% of calories from carbohydrate, and 20 to 35% of calories from fat. These recommendations are intended to promote health while allowing flexibility in food intake patterns (**Figure 2.5b**).

> **Acceptable Macronutrient Distribution Ranges (AMDRs)** Healthy ranges of intake for carbohydrate, fat, and protein, expressed as percentages of total energy intake.

Physical activity coefficients (PA values) for use in EER equations	Table 2.1			
	Sedentary: Typical daily living activities (e.g., household tasks, walking to the bus)	**Low Active:** Typical daily living activities PLUS 30–60 minutes of moderate activity (e.g., walking at 5–7 km/h)	**Active:** Typical daily living activities PLUS at least 60 minutes of daily moderate activities	**Very Active:** Typical daily living activities PLUS at least 60 minutes of daily moderate activity PLUS an additional 60 minutes of vigorous activity or 120 minutes of moderate activity
Men age 19+	1.00	1.11	1.25	1.48
Women age 19+	1.00	1.12	1.27	1.45

Source: Health Canada. Dietary Reference Intakes Tables.[6]

CONCEPT CHECK **STOP**

1. **What** are RDAs and AIs used for?
2. **How** might you use ULs?

3. **What** are three variables that affect your energy needs?
4. **Why** are AMDR values given as ranges rather than as single numbers?

Tools for Diet Planning

LEARNING OBJECTIVES

1. **Outline** the recommendations found in *Eating Well with Canada's Food Guide*.
2. **Discuss** how chronic disease can be prevented by following *Eating Well with Canada's Food Guide*.
3. **Determine** your individualized food guide recommendations.

The DRIs show how much of each nutrient we need, but they do not help us to choose foods to meet these needs. Health Canada has accordingly used the DRIs to develop food guides to help Canadians make healthy nutritional choices: *Eating*

Well with Canada's Food Guide is Canada's most recent version of the guide. It divides foods into groups based on the main nutrients they supply and recommends appropriate amounts from each food group.

The food guide provides information and recommendations that are meant to improve knowledge about achieving health through appropriate nutrition and physical activity (**Figure 2.6**). As vital as these recommendations are, having this knowledge doesn't necessarily change the behaviour of every Canadian. Adopting a healthy diet or increasing physical activity levels are significant lifestyle changes that may take some time to fully implement. As you read the recommendations outlined over the next few

Recommendations for balancing food consumption with physical activity to achieve and maintain a healthy weight • Figure 2.6

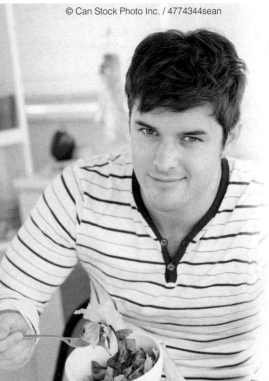

© Can Stock Photo Inc. / 4774344sean

a. To promote a healthy weight, Health Canada recommends moderating calorie intake, which can be achieved by limiting portion sizes and reducing consumption of added sugars, fats, and alcohol, which provide calories but few essential nutrients. The key to dietary-based weight management is consuming the appropriate number of calories rather than the relative proportions of carbohydrate, fat, and protein in the diet. The *What Should I Eat* section outlines some realistic changes that you may find useful.

b. To improve overall health, Health Canada recommends 150 minutes of moderate to vigorous physical activity per week, in accumulated intervals of at least 10 minutes at a time. Ideally, this activity should include aerobic exercise to strengthen the heart, stretching exercises for flexibility, and weightlifting to improve muscle strength and endurance. Greater health benefits can be obtained by engaging in more vigorous activity or by being active for longer periods.

The 150 minutes of weekly activity doesn't need to be exhaustive or achieved all at once. For example, this weekly activity can be accomplished with a 15-minute brisk walk to and from work each day. To maximize the powerful effects of physical activity on health, more daily physical activity and less sedentary activity is recommended. For those who are trying to lose weight or keep weight off, more activity is recommended.

© Can Stock Photo Inc. / monkeybusiness

WHAT SHOULD I EAT?
Following the Dietary Guidelines

Increase nutrient density
- Add more vegetables and less mayonnaise to your turkey sandwich.
- Choose to snack on fruit and nuts, in place of chips and cookies.
- Prepare a side dish made from whole grains, such as bulgur, quinoa, or brown rice, rather than packaged, flavoured white rice.
- Stir-fry a variety of vegetables.
- Serve strawberries rather than strawberry shortcake for dessert.

Balance intake with activity
- Don't skip breakfast; if you do, you may overeat later in the day.
- Pass on that second helping. When you eat out, split an entree with a friend.
- Walk an extra 1,000 steps; the more you exercise, the easier it is to keep your weight at a healthy level.
- Ride your bike to work or when running errands.
- Lift some weights or walk on a treadmill while watching the news.

Limit nutrients that increase health risks
- Read product labels and compare sodium levels and trans fat content before making a choice.
- Choose lean meat, fish, and low-fat dairy products to limit your consumption of fat.
- Drink water and skip the soft drink—it adds nothing but sugar to your diet.
- Pass on the salt; instead, try lemon juice or some basil and oregano.
- If you drink alcohol, stop after one drink.

 Use iProfile to look up the saturated fat and sugar content in your breakfast cereal.

pages, ask yourself, "Which recommendations apply to *my* lifestyle?" and, "Given my specific set of circumstances and environments, what realistic changes can *I* make to improve my health?" Nutrition-related behaviour change is a complex, yet critical process for improving overall health. We must first be *ready and willing* to change before any nutritional recommendations have a significant effect on our lives. This concept will be further discussed in Chapter 9.

Eating Well with Canada's Food Guide: Putting Guidelines into Practice

Since 1942, Canadians have relied on the advice offered in Canada's food guide. In fact, it is the second most frequently requested government document today.[7] *Eating Well with Canada's Food Guide* still focuses on the four food groups mentioned in previous versions, but now includes some important new information. The new food guide addresses the different needs of Canadians at different ages and life stages; includes culturally relevant foods; provides more alternatives to meat and dairy products; makes recommendations for different types of fats; addresses key nutrients, such as folate and vitamin D; and

makes recommendations about physical activity levels. **Figure 2.7** shows the messages and symbols contained in the new food guide. **Figure 2.8** provides further suggestions on how to estimate food servings.

Using the Food Guide to Make the Best Nutritional and Lifestyle Choices According to Need

In addition to providing the visual representation of Canada's Food Guide, Health Canada has also provided further recommendations to help you make wise choices from each group, shown in coloured boxes.

Vegetables and fruit Vegetables and fruits are excellent sources of vitamins, minerals, fibre, and phytochemicals, all of which promote health. The fibre and phytochemicals in vegetables and fruits can help improve body function and/or reduce the risk of diseases such as cancer, heart disease, and type-2 diabetes.

> **Eat at least one dark green and one orange vegetable each day.**
> Go for dark green vegetables such as broccoli, romaine lettuce and spinach.
> Go for orange vegetables such as carrots, sweet potatoes and winter squash.

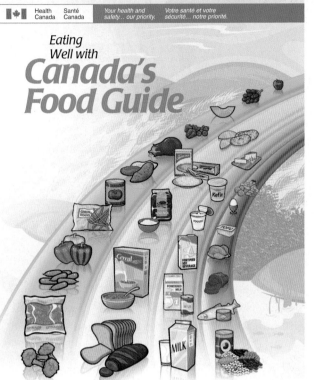

Eating Well with Canada's Food Guide

Canada

Eating Well with Canada's Food Guide: Messages and symbolism • Figure 2.7

a. New visual features in Canada's Food Guide:

1. The rainbow design is not merely aesthetic: Vegetables and fruits appear on the outer, larger arc of the rainbow, conveying that, compared with other foods, they should be consumed in the largest proportion. Meats and meat alternatives are featured in the inner, smaller arc, reflecting that, compared with other foods, they should be consumed in the smallest proportion.

2. For each food group, where a food lies in the arc demonstrates the recommended relative intake level for that nutrient with respect to the other foods featured in the same arc. For example, in the milk and milk alternatives category, pure milk is displayed as the most important dairy product to consume, while cheese is displayed as the least recommended, at the smaller end of the arc.

3. Many foods are featured in each group, reflecting the concept of variety.

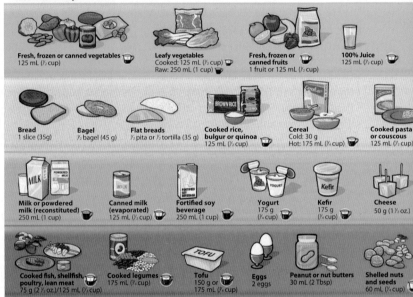

What is One Food Guide Serving?
Look at the examples below.

b. The new guide clarifies how many servings per food group each individual in the population should consume on a daily basis. This diet plan was tested using computer models and was found to be the most effective diet at preventing nutrient deficiencies and reducing the risk of chronic diseases.[9]

Recommended Number of Food Guide Servings per Day

	Children			Teens		Adults			
Age in Years	2-3	4-8	9-13	14-18		19-50		51+	
Sex	Girls and Boys			Females	Males	Females	Males	Females	Males
Vegetables and Fruit	4	5	6	7	8	7-8	8-10	7	7
Grain Products	3	4	6	6	7	6-7	8	6	7
Milk and Alternatives	2	2	3-4	3-4	3-4	2	2	3	3
Meat and Alternatives	1	1	1-2	2	3	2	3	2	3

The chart above shows how many Food Guide Servings you need from each of the four food groups every day.

Having the amount and type of food recommended and following the tips in *Canada's Food Guide* will help:
- Meet your needs for vitamins, minerals and other nutrients.
- Reduce your risk of obesity, type 2 diabetes, heart disease, certain types of cancer and osteoporosis.
- Contribute to your overall health and vitality.

Ask Yourself

Do your intake patterns fall within the recommended values?

c. Feedback from previous guides showed that Canadians were confused as to what comprised a food guide serving and often underestimated food serving sizes. The new guide provides more detailed instructions for estimating food servings, not only by size but also by weight, volume, or count. As you can see, both 125 mL (½ cup) of fresh vegetables and 125 mL (½ cup) of juice are considered a single food guide serving. A 50-g serving of cheese (about the size of a standard eraser) and 250 mL (1 cup) of milk each represent a single serving of milk or milk alternatives.

Oils and Fats
- Include a small amount – 30 to 45 mL (2 to 3 Tbsp) – of unsaturated fat each day. This includes oil used for cooking, salad dressings, margarine and mayonnaise.
- Use vegetable oils such as canola, olive and soybean.
- Choose soft margarines that are low in saturated and trans fats.
- Limit butter, hard margarine, lard and shortening.

d. Another new feature on the guide, which developed from consumer feedback, is the specific mention of how to include fats in a healthy diet. The Guide now specifically recommends choosing a small amount 30–45 mL (2–3 tablespoons) of unsaturated fats, while limiting trans and saturated fats.

Visual cues for estimating serving sizes
• Figure 2.8

If visual cues are more helpful to you for estimating serving sizes, you may find the following pictures helpful for understanding how many servings you are consuming.

Serving size	Example of Canada's Food Guide single serving of	Approximate visual equivalent
5 ml (1 tsp)	Not a CFG serving, but can be used to estimate use of margarine and other solid fats.	tip of thumb or die © Can Stock Photo Inc. / Gjermund
42 g (1.5 oz)	cheese	3 dominoes or 2 9-volt batteries © Can Stock Photo Inc. / toff955
30 mL (2 Tbsp)	Peanut or nut butters	golf ball or shot glass © Can Stock Photo Inc. / draghicich
75 g (2.5 oz)	Meat, fish	a deck of cards © Can Stock Photo Inc. / Violin
125 mL (1/2 cup)	Cooked vegetables Orange juice Cooked grain or pasta	1 tennis ball © Can Stock Photo Inc. / thesupe87
250 mL (1 cup)	Milk; fresh, frozen, or canned vegetables	a baseball © Can Stock Photo Inc. / Joe_Photo

Ask Yourself

Do you overestimate or underestimate the number of food guide servings in your meals?

The consumption of dark green vegetables is associated with decreased risk of heart disease and cancer. Orange vegetables tend to be rich in vitamin A, which is vital for proper eye function.

Choose vegetables and fruit prepared with little or no added fat, sugar or salt.
· Enjoy vegetables steamed, baked or stir-fried instead of deep-fried.

Try to eat vegetables in their most natural forms, which often contain the lowest amounts of disease-promoting nutrients and the highest amounts of vitamins, minerals, and phytochemicals

Have vegetables and fruit more often than juice.

Compared to its juice, the original vegetable or fruit often contains more fibre, vitamins, minerals, and phytochemicals. Also, juices can often contain added salts, sugars, and calories. The consumption of sugar-sweetened beverages, including soft drinks, juice drinks, sport drinks, and vitamin water, has been linked to the development of obesity, type-2 diabetes, and heart disease.[10] These beverages contain sucrose, high-fructose corn syrup, or fruit-juice concentrates that both sweeten the beverages and add extra calories.

Fresh, frozen, or canned vegetables options are all recommended as nutritious options. Frozen vegetables are often similar in nutritional content as their fresh counterparts (and sometimes better!), as long as they were frozen quickly. Canned vegetable options can also provide substantial nutrients, but try to pick those with the lowest sodium and preservative content.[11] Draining and rinsing canned vegetables can lower the sodium content substantially.

Be wary of products with "vegetable" or "fruit" in their names.[10] These products include candies, jams, ketchup, and vegetable or fruit drinks. Many of these products are composed mainly of sugar and fat and should not be included in the vegetable and fruit groups. Always check product labels to ensure you are getting the food you want.

Treat your tastebuds to a new vegetable or fruit.

Grain products Grain products, particularly whole grains, are a good source of dietary fibre and are typically low in fat.[11] Unfortunately, these carbohydrate-dense foods have received some negative attention in the media as a result of low-carbohydrate diets claiming that carbohydrates promote weight gain. Most scientists agree that *any* nutrients (including carbohydrates and fats) promote weight gain only when they are consumed in an amount that increases your overall energy intake beyond the required levels, leading to the storage of energy as fat tissue.

Make at least half of your grain products whole grain each day.
· Eat a variety of whole grains such as barley, brown rice, oats, quinoa and wild rice.
· Enjoy whole grain breads, oatmeal or whole wheat pasta.

Whole grains are associated with a decreased risk of heart disease and type-2 diabetes. The "white," "bleached," or "refined" grains you find in many baked goods do not provide these same benefits.

> **Choose grain products that are lower in fat, sugar or salt.**
> - Compare the Nutrition Facts table on labels to make wise choices.
> - Enjoy the true taste of grain products. When adding sauces or spreads, use small amounts.

Always check your labels! Even though a grain product may look brown, such as brown bread, it may just be its white counterpart that has been coloured with molasses. To be sure that you are buying whole grains, check that the first ingredients listed in your grain products include "whole wheat," "whole oats," "whole rye," "whole grain corn," "brown rice," "wild rice," or "oats." You will find a detailed description of how to read food labels later in this chapter.

Limit cookies, cakes, pastries, and pies to special occasions. A healthy diet has room for these foods—but not too much—as they are not nutrient-dense foods and tend to be filled with added calories and fat.

Milk and milk alternatives

Although some other food groups include a larger variety of foods, milk and milk alternatives have their own grouping because these foods are typically rich sources of two essential nutrients: calcium and vitamin D, which are vital for strong bones and teeth. Calcium is involved in numerous body processes, such as muscle contraction, hormone secretion, and nerve conduction, to name a few. Vitamin D helps promote strong bones and may have additional health benefits as well.

> **Drink skim, 1%, or 2% milk each day.**
> - Have 500 mL (2 cups) of milk every day for adequate vitamin D.
> - Drink fortified soy beverages if you do not drink milk.

If you do not drink milk, perhaps because you are lactose-intolerant, try the alternatives to dairy products, which still provide the essential nutrients provided by milk. For example, canned salmon with bones is another rich source of calcium. Many fortified foods, such as breakfast cereal and almond, soy, or rice milks, often have added calcium and vitamin D. However, if you are drinking a milk alternative such as soy milk that has been fortified with these nutrients, keep in mind that they often sink to the bottom of the container. To improve your nutrient content of these beverages, shake them vigorously before using.

> **Select lower fat milk alternatives.**
> - Compare the Nutrition Facts table on yogurts or cheeses to make wise choices.

Choose lower-fat yogurts and cheeses with less than 20% milk fats.[11] Use cream cheese, ice cream, coffee cream, whipping cream, and sour cream in moderation. These dairy products are often high in both fat and calories.

Meat and meat alternatives

Meat and meat alternatives are rich sources of protein, fats, and iron, and are a good source of many of the B vitamins that are essential for energy regulation. Many meat and meat alternative sources are dense in the above nutrients, so only a small amount of this food group is needed to satisfy your requirements. Another important reason not to over-consume meats is that their saturated fat content is high. A recent study found that as little as one daily serving of unprocessed meat was associated with a 13% increase in mortality risk, while processed meat, such as hot dogs and bacon, increased mortality risk by 20%. Conversely, replacing a serving of red meat with a meat alternative, such as nuts or leaner meats, reduced mortality risk significantly.[11]

> **Have meat alternatives such as beans, lentils and tofu often.**

These meat alternatives are often inexpensive, high in fibre, low in fat, and dense in nutrients.

> **Select lean meat and alternatives prepared with little or no added fat or salt.**
> - Trim the visible fat from meats. Remove the skin on poultry.
> - Use cooking methods such as roasting, baking or poaching that require little or no added fat.
> - If you eat luncheon meats, sausages or prepackaged meats, choose those lower in salt (sodium) and fat.

To moderate your fat consumption, choose baking, broiling, and barbecuing as low-fat alternatives to frying or sautéing. You can also use a spray bottle full of vegetable oil to grease your pan and minimize the use of fat.

As for sodium, a single serving of cold cuts can contain more than 1,000 mg, approximately half of the daily recommended amount! Make sure to always check product labels for sodium content.

Eat at least two Food Guide Servings of fish each week.
- Choose fish such as char, herring, mackerel, salmon, sardines and trout.

Most fish, especially cold-water fish, are significant sources of omega-3 fatty acids, which are associated with improved heart health. On the other hand, large fishes, such as tuna, tend to concentrate heavy metals such as mercury, which is known to be toxic. Luckily, Health Canada states that most Canadians do not need to worry about excessive mercury consumption from fish sources because the types of fish typical in the Canadian diet are relatively low in mercury, while still providing good sources of essential fatty acids,[12] These fish include pollock, salmon, smelt, rainbow trout, and many shellfish, such as clams and mussels. Conversely, *frozen and fresh* tuna, shark, swordfish, and orange roughy should be consumed less often because they provide the highest concentrations of mercury. Fortunately, most canned tuna uses younger tuna, which has had less time to concentrate heavy metals. The exception is albacore tuna, which has a higher potential for mercury intake. Canada's Food Guide advises that children and pregnant women should limit its intake.

Water Water is essential to many body processes. It is critical for maintaining appropriate blood pressure and helps regulate body temperature. Because of this latter role, drinking adequate amounts of water is especially important when exercising and during hot weather (**Figure 2.9**).

Age- and gender-specific recommendations In addition to the recommendations meant for the general population, further specific recommendations are provided for children, women of childbearing age, and men and women over age 50. For preschoolers and small children, Canada's Food Guide recommends respecting a child's ability to determine how much food to eat, offering children a variety of food, and supplementing good nutrition with fun physical activity. Women of childbearing age are advised to supplement their diet with a daily

Water recommendation for Canada's Food Guide • Figure 2.9

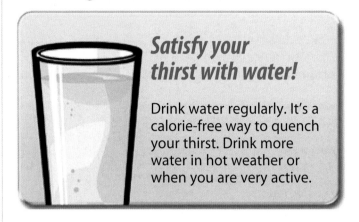

Satisfy your thirst with water!

Drink water regularly. It's a calorie-free way to quench your thirst. Drink more water in hot weather or when you are very active.

multivitamin containing supplemental iron to meet their higher needs and 400 micrograms of folic acid to decrease the risk of neural tube defects in their children. The food guide further recommends increasing food intake by *only* two or three food guide servings a day during pregnancy. Canadians over the age of 50 have an increased need for vitamin D, which will not be provided by following the food guide. Therefore, in addition to following the overall food guide recommendations, older adults should also supplement their diet with 400 international units (IU) of vitamin D per day.

Customizing your food guide The Health Canada website also provides the opportunity to customize your own food guide (**Figure 2.10**) by entering your gender and age group. After you learn your specific recommendations, you can then select healthy choices to satisfy those recommendations. Since the guide also focuses on physical activity, you can choose which activities to include to increase your daily energy expenditure. Another helpful resource can be found on the Dietitians of Canada website (www.dietitians.ca). The *Let's Make a Deal* feature allows consumers to select appropriate food choices for each meal from a selection of items that reflect the core values of Canada's Food Guide. You can track your food choices and see how each measures up in terms of food guide servings. The website also offer links to delicious recipes featured in the menu-selecting tool.

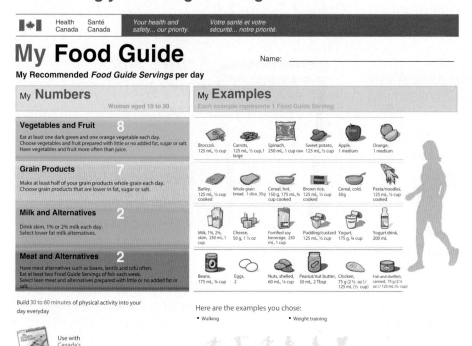

My **Food Guide**

Name: _____

My Recommended *Food Guide Servings* per day

My **Numbers**

Woman aged 19 to 30

Vegetables and Fruit   8

Eat at least one dark green and one orange vegetable each day.
Choose vegetables and fruit prepared with little or no added fat, sugar or salt.
Have vegetables and fruit more often than juice.

Grain Products   7

Make at least half of your grain products whole grain each day.
Choose grain products that are lower in fat, sugar or salt.

Milk and Alternatives   2

Drink skim, 1% or 2% milk each day.
Select lower fat milk alternatives.

Meat and Alternatives   2

Have meat alternatives such as beans, lentils and tofu often.
Eat at least two Food Guide Servings of fish each week.
Select lean meat and alternatives prepared with little or no added fat or salt.

Build 30 to 60 minutes of physical activity into your day everyday

Use with Canada's Food Guide

My **Examples**

Each example represents 1 Food Guide Serving

Here are the examples you chose:
- Walking
- Weight training

www.healthcanada.gc.ca/foodguide

Canadä

The interactive tool My Food Guide is found on Health Canada's website and allows you to customize your own guide based on your age, gender, and food preferences. It approximates how many servings from each group you require, and allows you to choose dietary options and various forms of physical activity that allow you to meet recommendations.

Eating Well with Canada's Food Guide— First Nations, Inuit, Métis • Figure 2.11

The First Nations, Inuit, and Metis version of *Eating Well with Canada's Food Guide* is similar to the main version of the guide in the types of foods found in each group, as well as the amount of servings required for different age and gender groups. The main difference is that the way the guide is presented better reflects Aboriginal dietary patterns and culture. For instance, the images contained within the inner circle reflect the importance of food as a connection with the family, community, and nature and as an element of spirituality. The outer circle shows the types of store-bought foods that are more typical and affordable in the remote communities where many Aboriginals live.

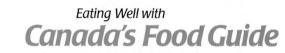

Eating Well with

Canada's Food Guide

First Nations, Inuit and Métis

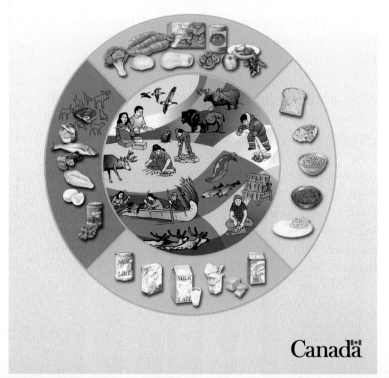

Canadä

Eating Well with Canada's Food Guide—First Nations, Inuit, and Métis Many different food guides have been produced over the years, and slightly different versions have been used in different parts of Canada, reflecting the specific food consumption patterns and nutritional needs particular to different regions. For the first time ever, a national guide specifically speaks to First Nations, Inuit, and Métis (**Figure 2.11**). This specifically tailored guide is meant to more accurately reflect the customs, traditions, and food choices that are relevant to Canada's Aboriginal populations and their tendency to consume store-bought foods, often because these foods are more readily available in the remote areas where many Aboriginal people live. Also, the graphics and content are specifically tailored to appeal to these populations. This version of Canada's Food Guide is available in Cree, Ojibwe, and Inuktitut.

CONCEPT CHECK

1. **How** is *Eating Well with Canada's Food Guide* related to the DRIs?

2. **What** is the significance of the specific rainbow design of Canada's Food Guide?

3. **How** many servings of grain product do you require each day? How many would be recommended if you were of the opposite gender?

Food and Natural Health Product Labels

LEARNING OBJECTIVES

1. **Discuss** how the information on food labels can help you choose a healthy diet.

2. **Determine** whether a food is high or low in fibre, trans fat, and kilocalories.

3. **Explain** how the order of ingredients on a food label is determined.

How do you know whether your frozen entree is a good source of vitamin C, how much fibre your breakfast cereal provides, or the amount of calcium in your daily vitamin/mineral supplement? You can find this information on food and supplement labels.

Food Labels

Food labels are designed to help consumers make healthy food choices by providing information about the nutrient composition of a food and how that food fits into the overall diet (**Figure 2.12**). Federal regulations control what can and cannot appear on a food label and what *must* appear on it. As of December 2007, Canadian manufacturers of prepackaged foods are required to conform to a set of new and very strict labelling rules—some of the strictest in the world. These regulations are designed to help consumers compare the nutritional quality of different products; shop for special diets, such as those required for people who have diabetes; and regulate intake of specific nutrients.[13] Knowing how to interpret the information on these labels can help you choose a healthy diet. Another major aim

a. Food labels must appear on all packaged foods except those produced by small businesses and those in packages too small to accommodate the information. This label from a macaroni-and-cheese product illustrates how the Nutrition Facts panel and the ingredient list can help you to evaluate the nutritional contribution this food will make to your diet.

Standard serving sizes are required to allow consumers to compare products. For example, the number of kilocalories in one serving of macaroni and cheese can be compared with the number of kilocalories in one serving of packaged rice because the values for both are for a standard 225-g (1-cup) serving.

Food labels must list the "% Daily Value" for total fat, saturated fat, cholesterol, sodium, carbohydrate, dietary fibre, vitamins A and C, calcium, and iron. A % Daily Value of 5% or less is considered low, and a value of 20% or more is considered high.

The label provides information about the amounts of nutrients whose intake should be moderated or minimized—total fat, saturated fat, trans fat, cholesterol, and sodium.

The label provides information about the amounts of nutrients that tend to be low in the Canadian diet—fibre, vitamins A and C, calcium, and iron.

The ingredients are listed in descending order by weight, from the most abundant to the least abundant. The wheat flour in the macaroni is the most abundant ingredient in this product.

Nutrition Facts
Valeur nutritive

Per 1 cup (220 g)/par 1 tasse (225 g)

Amount / Teneur	% Daily Value / % valeur quotidienne
Calories / Calories 250	
Fat / Lipides 12 g	18%
Saturated / saturés 3 g + Trans / trans 1.5 g	15%
Cholesterol / Cholestérol 30 mg	10 %
Sodium / Sodium 470 mg	20 %
Carbohydrate / Glucides 31 g	10%
Fibre / Fibres 0 g	0 %
Sugars / Sucres 5 g	
Protein / Protéines 5 g	
Vitamin A / Vitamine A	4 %
Vitamin C / Vitamine C	2 %
Calcium / Calcium	20 %
Iron / Fer	4 %

Ingredients
Enriched macaroni product (wheat flour, niacin, ferrous sulfate [iron], thiamine mononitrate, riboflavin, folic acid); cheese sauce mix (whey, modified food starch, milk fat, salt, milk protein concentrate, contains less than 2% of sodium tripolyphosphate, cellulose gel, cellulose gum, citric acid, sodium phosphate, lactic acid, calcium phosphate, milk, yellow 5, yellow 6, enzymes, cheese culture)

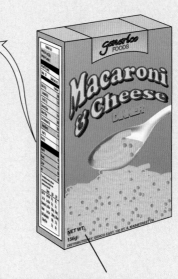

Labels must contain basic product information, such as the name of the product, the weight or volume of the contents, and the name and place of business of the manufacturer, packager, or distributor.

of standardization is to increase consumer knowledge of the associations between diet and health. Health Canada hopes that by implementing this mandatory labelling system, it may save approximately $5 billion in health-related costs over 20 years.[14]

Currently, labelling is required only on prepackaged foods. Some argue that food labelling should also extend to restaurants, which currently are not required to provide any nutritional information on their menus (see *Hot Topic*).

Basic Labelling Requirements

In most areas of Canada, food labels must provide nutritional information in both English and French and contain certain mandatory features. The **common name** of the food refers to the term generally used to refer to the product and must typically be approved by Canada's Food and Drug Regulations (FDR) to ensure that it accurately describes the product. For instance, a beverage made of water, sugar, and food colouring cannot call itself "juice."

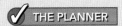

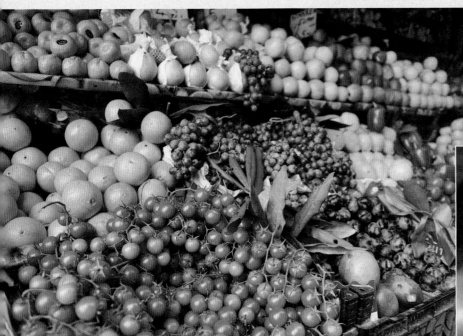

© Can Stock Photo Inc. / dotshock

b. Raw fruits, vegetables, fish, meat, and poultry are not required to carry individual labels.

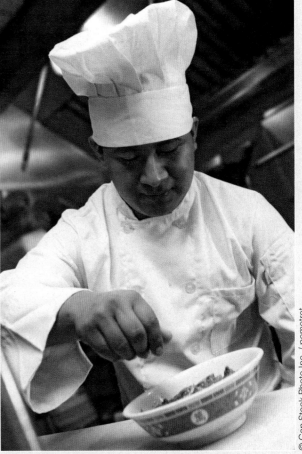

© Can Stock Photo Inc. / pemotret

c. Food served in restaurants and other eating establishments, such as delicatessens and bakeries, does not require labelling. However, if a claim is made about a food's nutritional content or health benefits, such as being "low-fat" or "heart-healthy," the eating establishment must provide nutritional information about that food, if requested.

The **net quantity declaration** must accurately reflect the weight, volume, measure, or numerical count of the product, and it must now be expressed in metric units. Previous labels were often expressed in different measures, leading to confusion. The label must also include the name and address of the company that has either produced or manufactured the prepackaged food so consumers can contact the company if they have any concerns or questions about the product.

The **durable life date** of the product is the amount of time that a product is anticipated to retain its freshness, taste, quality, and nutritional content.

Nutrition facts All food labels must contain a **Nutrition Facts** panel (**Figure 2.12**). This section of the label shows the type and quantity of nutrients in a standard serving. The serving size on the label is followed by the number of servings per container and the total kilocalories. This is an

Food and Natural Health Product Labels **47**

HOT TOPIC

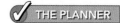

Should menu labelling be mandatory at Canadian restaurants?

Presently, in Canada, the inclusion of nutrition information on restaurant menus is completely voluntary. Some establishments choose to include this information to highlight the healthier nature of certain menu items or their entire menu. Other food providers post their nutrition information online or in brochures or posters in store. While this information may be available, very few people actually access it,[15] and many have no idea about the nutritional content of their meal. Accordingly, some people believe that menu labels should be more transparent about the nutritional content of the food they are providing to their customers.

Those in favour of labelling believe that including nutrition information on labels would help customers make more informed decisions since the calorie, salt, and fat content of menu items can often be underestimated by consumers.[16,17] Also, numerous surveys have shown that the majority of respondents are in favour of menu labelling.[17] Another argument in favour of menu labelling suggests that when restaurants are marketed as healthier options (e.g., Subway), patrons may underestimate the high caloric content of some of their options.[16]

Those opposed to menu labelling argue that it is difficult to accurately predict nutrition information because food is prepared in a slightly different manner each time, and many people modify the menu options. Others believe that it is not the government's role to legislate how restaurants conduct their business. Another opposing argument is that menu labelling alone will not solve the current obesity crisis, which is true since obesity is a complex problem, and multiple interventions at various levels and across multiple sectors are necessary to make a difference at the population level. Menu labelling could, however, be one of those interventions.

Menu labelling remains a controversial topic in nutrition research. While some evidence suggests that menu labelling can positively influence nutritional choices, the results are modest at best, and much more research is required to gain an accurate understanding of its potential impact.

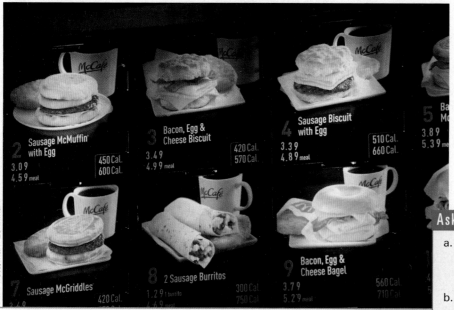

AP Photo/Mark Lennihan

Ask Yourself

a. Do you think restaurant chains should be required to include nutrition information on their menus? If so, should this legislation also apply to smaller restaurants?

b. What other arguments exist for and against menu labelling?

---

important area to check since you need to ensure the nutritional information accurately reflects the amount of food you are eating. If a person eats twice the standard serving, he or she is consuming twice the number of kilocalories, fat, and sodium listed. You should accordingly always compare your serving size against the net quantity declaration.

The next section of the Nutrition Facts panel lists the amounts of nutrients contained in a serving and, for most nutrients, the amount they provide as a percentage of the **Daily Value**. The % Daily Value is the amount of a nutrient in a food as a percentage of the Daily Value recommended for a

> **Daily Value**
> A reference value for the intake of nutrients used on food labels to help consumers see how a given food fits into their overall diet.

2,000-kilocalorie diet. For example, if a food provides 10% of the Daily Value for vitamin C, it provides 10% of the recommended daily intake for vitamin C in a 2,000-kilocalorie diet. This format is much more helpful than simply stating the amount of that nutrient in grams or milligrams, as most Canadians do not know how much of each specific nutrient they require. Because a Daily Value is a single standard for all consumers, it may overestimate the amount of a nutrient needed for some population groups, but it does not underestimate the requirement for any group except pregnant and lactating women.

Ingredient list Do you want to know exactly what goes into your food? The ingredient list is the place to look. The ingredient list presents the contents of the product in the order of their prominence by weight. A good rule of thumb is to check the first three ingredients, which are the most abundant ingredients in the product. If the first three ingredients are sugar, glucose, fructose, high-fructose corn syrup, honey, molasses, or the like, you know that the product contains mostly simple sugars. The ingredient list can also be very helpful to consumers who are allergic to nuts, who want to avoid animal products, or who are simply curious about the composition of the food they eat.

An ingredient list is required on all products containing more than one ingredient and is optional on products that contain a single ingredient. Food additives, including food colours and flavourings, must be listed among the ingredients.

Nutrient content and health claims Looking for low-fat or high-fibre foods (see *Thinking It Through*)? You may not even need to look at the Nutrition Facts. Food labels often contain **nutrient content claims**, which are statements that highlight specific characteristics of a product that might be of interest to consumers, such as "fat free" or "low sodium." Standard definitions for these descriptors have been established by Canada's Food and Drug Regulations (FDR) (see **Table 2.2**). Because of the importance of many types of foods in disease prevention, food labels are also permitted to include some **diet-related health claims**. Health claims refer to a relationship between a nutrient, food, food component, or dietary supplement and the reduced risk of a disease or health-related condition. All health claims must be truthful and must not mislead or deceive consumers. There are two main types of diet-related health claims: **disease-reduction**

Nutrient content claims	Table 2.2
Claim	**Description**
Free	Used on products that contain such little amount of fat, saturated fat, cholesterol, sodium, sugars, or calories that health experts consider it insignificant. For example, "fat free" means <0.5 g per serving. Synonyms for *free* include *without, no,* and *zero*.
Low	Used for foods that can be eaten frequently without exceeding the Daily Value for fat, saturated fat, cholesterol, sodium, or calories. Specific definitions have been established for each of these nutrients. For example, *low-fat* means that the food contains ≤3 g of fat per serving, and *low-calorie* means that the food contains 120 kilocalories or less per 100 grams. Synonyms for *low* include *little, few,* and *low source of*.
Lean and extra lean	Used to describe the fat content of meat, poultry, seafood, and game meats. *Lean* means that the food contains <10% of fat. *Extra lean* is defined as containing <7.5% of fat.
High	Used to describe foods that contain 20% or more of the Daily Value for a particular nutrient. Synonyms for *high* include *rich in* and *excellent source of*.
Source	Contains a "significant" amount of the nutrient. For example, a source of calcium has 165 mg or more per serving, and a source of fibre has 2 or more grams of fibre.
Reduced	Used to describe food that contains a minimum of 25% less of that nutrient compared with a similar product. Synonyms include: ___-reduced or *lower in* ___ for products that have been altered, and *fewer* or *less* for all products.
Light	Used in different ways. First, it can be used on a nutritionally altered product that contains 25% fewer calories or fat than a reference food. Second, it can be used when the sodium content of a low-calorie, low-fat food has been reduced by 50% as in *lightly salted*. The term *light* can be used to describe properties such as texture and colour, as long as the label explains the intent—for example, *light and fluffy*.
More	Used when the food contains at least 25% more of the nutrient compared with a similar reference food. Synonyms for *more* are *fortified, enriched,* and *added*.

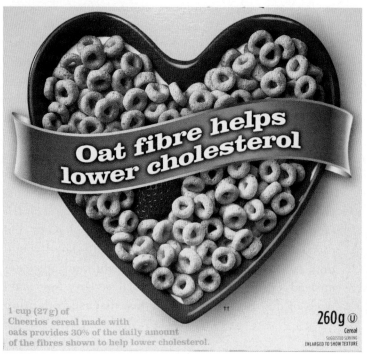

1 cup (27 g) of Cheerios cereal made with oats provides 30% of the daily amount of the fibres shown to help lower cholesterol.

†† 260 g Ⓤ Cereal
SUGGESTED SERVING
ENLARGED TO SHOW TEXTURE

Luisa Begani

a. Disease-reduction claims found on some labels make correlations between the nutrient content of a food and a decreased risk of disease.

b. Nutrient-content claims highlight the amounts of certain key nutrients that are found in the food product.

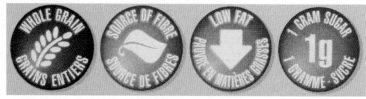

Luisa Begani

claims and **function claims** (Figure 2.13). Very few disease-reduction claims are approved by Health Canada (see **Table 2.3**), and a claim cannot place too much value on the ability of the product alone to improve health. For instance, it is acceptable for a label to claim, "A diet rich in vegetables and fruits reduces the risk of some types of cancer; product X is rich in vegetables and fruit." However, a label cannot explicitly state, "Product X, which is high in fruits and vegetables, lowers the risk of some types of cancers"; such a statement places too

much importance on consumption of the product itself, instead of on its health-promoting ingredients.

Unlike disease-reduction claims, function claims relate to the well-established beneficial effects of a specific food or food constituent on the *normal* function of the body or for good health. Examples include "Calcium helps promote strong bones and teeth," "Coarse wheat bran promotes laxation," and "Consumption of 250 mL (1 cup) of green tea has an antioxidant effect in blood." New health claims may be proposed at any time, so this list will expand. The most current information on label statements and claims can be found on the Canadian Food Inspection Agency website (www.inspection.gc.ca).

Natural Health Product Labels

Natural health products can range from multivitamin pills to herbal remedies, probiotics, and essential fatty acid and amino acid isolates. These products, which are sometimes also referred to as "complementary" or "alternative" medicines, are regulated by the National Health Products Directorate, a branch of Health Canada. Natural health products first require a licence before they can be sold in Canada. To obtain this licence, the manufacturers must provide detailed information about the product to Health

Permitted disease-reduction claims[14]   Table 2.3
"A healthy diet containing foods high in potassium and low in sodium may reduce the risk of high blood pressure. (Name of the food) is sodium-free."
"A healthy diet with adequate calcium and vitamin D may reduce the risk of osteoporosis. (Name of the food) is a good source of calcium."
"A healthy diet low in saturated and trans fats may reduce the risk of heart disease. (Name of the food) is free of saturated and trans fats."
"A healthy diet rich in a variety of vegetables and fruit may help reduce the risk of some types of cancer."
"Does not promote tooth decay."

THINKING IT THROUGH 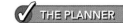 THE PLANNER

Using Food Labels to Make Healthy Choices

Scott is trying to improve his nutritional health. He has visited the Canada's Food Guide website and now knows how much food he should choose from each food group, but he sometimes has trouble making decisions when shopping for food.

For breakfast, he likes hot or cold cereal. Whether he eats oatmeal or granola, it is a serving from the grains group.

Refer to the labels shown here. Are they equivalent in terms of the amounts of saturated fat and added sugar? Which has more unsaturated fat?
▼

Old Fashioned Oats

Nutrition facts
Valeur nutritive
Per 1/2 cup (40 g), pour 1/2 tasse (40 g)

Amount / Teneur	% Daily Value / % valeur quotidienne
Calories / Calories 150	
Fat / Lipides 3 g	5 %
Saturated / saturés 0.5 g + Trans / trans 0 g	3 %
Cholesterol / Cholestérol 0 mg	
Sodium / Sodium 0 mg	0 %
Carbohydrate / Glucides 27 g	9 %
Fibre / Fibres 4 g	16 %
Sugars / Sucres 0 g	
Protein / Protéines 5 g	

INGREDIENTS: 100% rolled oats

Natural Granola

Nutrition facts
Valeur nutritive
Per 1/2 cup (51 g), pour 1/2 tasse (51 g)

Amount / Teneur	% Daily Value / % valeur quotidienne
Calories / Calories 230	
Fat / Lipides 3 g	13 %
Saturated / saturés 3.5 g + Trans / trans 1 g	22 %
Cholesterol / Cholestérol 0 mg	
Sodium / Sodium 20 mg	1 %
Carbohydrate / Glucides 34 g	11 %
Fibre / Fibres 3 g	12 %
Sugars / Sucres 16 g	
Protein / Protéines 5 g	

INGREDIENTS: Whole grain rolled oats, whole grain rolled wheat, brown sugar, raisins, dried coconut, almonds, partially hydrogenated cottonseed and soybean oils, nonfat dry milk, glycerin, honey

Your answer: _____
_____

Scott likes to have juice with his breakfast. He is deciding between plain orange juice and the less expensive juice drink, which claims to be an excellent source of vitamin C.

How much of the sugar in the orange juice is added?
▼

The only ingredients listed are water and concentrated orange juice. This ingredient list tells Scott that no sugar has been added. The 22 grams of sugars listed in the Nutrition Facts panel all come from the sugar found naturally in oranges.

Orange Juice

Nutrition Facts
Valeur nutritive
Per 250 mL / par 250 mL

Amount / Teneur	% Daily Value / % valeur quotidienne
Calories / Calories 110	
Fat / Lipides 0 g	0 %
Saturated / saturés 0 g + Trans / trans 0 g	0 %
Cholesterol / Cholestérol 0 mg	
Sodium / Sodium 0 mg	0 %
Potassium / Potassium 470 mg	13 %
Carbohydrate / Glucides 27 g	9 %
Sugars / Sucres 22 g	
Protein / Protéines 2 g	
Vitamin A / Vitamine A	0 %
Vitamin C / Vitamine C	120 %
Calcium / Calcium	2 %
Iron / Fer	0 %
Folate / Folate	25 %

Ingredients: Water, concentrated orange juice

Juice Drink

Nutrition Facts
Valeur nutritive
Per 1 cup (250 mL)/par 1 tasse (250 mL)

Amount / Teneur	% Daily Value / % valeur quotidienne
Calories / Calories 120	
Fat / Lipides 0 g	0 %
Saturated / saturés 0 g + Trans / trans 0 g	0 %
Cholesterol / Cholestérol 0 mg	0 %
Sodium / Sodium 160 mg	7 %
Carbohydrate / Glucides 29 g	10 %
Fibre / Fibres 0 g	0 %
Sugars / Sucres 28 g	
Protein / Protéines 0 g	
Vitamin A / Vitamine A	0 %
Vitamin C / Vitamine C	100 %
Calcium / Calcium	0 %
Iron / Fer	0 %

Ingredients: Water, glucose-fructose, pear and grape juice concentrates, citric acid, water-extracted orange and pineapple juice concentrates, ascorbic acid (vitamin C), natural flavour.

Which choice provides more vitamin C?
▼

Your answer: _____
_____

Other than water, what is the most abundant ingredient, by weight, in the juice drink? In the orange juice?
▼

Your answer: _____
_____

The added vitamin C increases the nutrient density of the juice drink, but does that make it a better choice than the orange juice?
▼

Your answer: _____
_____

What advice would you give Scott when choosing between more- and less-processed products?
▼

Your answer: _____
_____

(Check your answers in Appendix K.)

Natural health products • Figure 2.14

The labels of natural health products must contain a product license number, a list of medicinal and non-medicinal ingredients, a description of recommended doses, and, where applicable, any necessary cautionary statements. It may also include a health claim that has been authorized by Health Canada. What does *not* have to appear on an NHP label, however, is a nutrient facts panel.

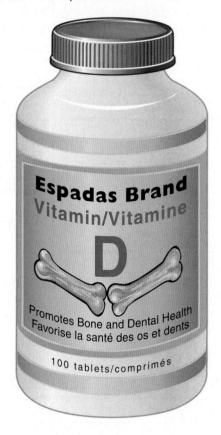

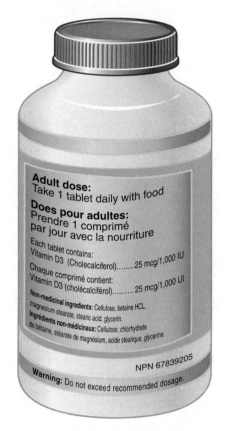

Espadas Brand
Vitamin/Vitamine

D

Promotes Bone and Dental Health
Favorise la santé des os et dents

100 tablets/comprimés

Adult dose:
Take 1 tablet daily with food

Does pour adultes:
Prendre 1 comprimé
par jour avec la nourriture

Each tablet contains:
Vitamin D3 (Cholecalciferol).........25 mcg/1,000 IU
Chaque comprimé contient:
Vitamin D3 (cholécalciférol)..........25 mcg/1,000 UI

Non-medicinal ingredients: Cellulose, betaine HCL, magnesium stearate, stearic acid, glycerin.
Ingrédients non-médicinaux: Cellulose, chlorhydrate de bétaine, stéarate de magnésium, acide stéarique, glycerine.

NPN 67839205

Warning: Do not exceed recommended dosage.

Canada, including the active medical ingredients, dose, potency, and non-medicinal ingredients. If approved, the product will then receive a Natural Product Number. The labels of these products must include the name, licence number, list of ingredients, recommended uses, and any cautionary statement (**Figure 2.14**).

CONCEPT CHECK

1. **Why** are serving sizes standardized on food labels?

2. **What** food label information will help you to find foods that are low in saturated fat and cholesterol?

3. **Where** should you look to see if a food contains nuts?

4. **How** can structure and function claims on dietary supplement labels be misleading?

Summary

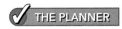

1 Background on Nutrition Recommendations 32

- Nutrition recommendations are designed to encourage consumption of a diet that promotes health and prevents disease. Some of the earliest nutrition recommendations in Canada were in the form of **food guides**, which translated **Recommended Nutrient Intakes (RNIs)** into food intake recommendations. The first set of Recommended Dietary Allowances, developed during World War II, focused on energy and the nutrients most likely to be deficient in a typical diet. Current recommendations focus on promoting health and preventing chronic disease and nutrient deficiencies.

- Dietary recommendations can be used as a standard for assessing the **nutritional status** of individuals and of populations. Records of dietary intake, together with information obtained from a physical examination, a medical history, and laboratory tests can be used to assess an individual's nutritional status. Collecting information about the food intake and the health of individuals in the population or surveying the foods available can help to identify potential and actual nutrient deficiencies and excesses within a population and help policymakers to develop improved nutrition recommendations.

Assessing nutritional status • Figure 2.2

		FOOD DIARY	
	Record all the food and beverages you eat. Include the food, how it was prepared, the amount you ate and the brand name. Don't forget to list all fats used in cooking and all spreads and sauces added.		
Time	**Food**	**Kind and how prepared**	**Amount**
7:00 A.M.	Eggs	scrambled	2
	Butter	in eggs	5 mL
	toast	whole wheat	2 slices
	Butter	on toast	10 mL
	Milk	non-fat	250 ml
	Orange juice	from frozen concentrate	250 ml
12:00 P.M.	Big Mac	Mc Donalds	1

2 Dietary Reference Intakes (DRIs) 34

- **Dietary Reference Intakes (DRIs)** are recommendations for the amounts of energy, nutrients, and other food components that should be consumed by healthy people to promote health, reduce the incidence of chronic disease, and prevent deficiencies. **Estimated Average Requirements**

(EARs) can be used to evaluate the adequacy of a population's nutrient intake. **Recommended Dietary Allowances (RDAs)** and **Adequate Intakes (AIs)** can be used by individuals as a goal for nutrient intake, and **Tolerable Upper Intake Levels (ULs)** indicate a safe upper intake limit.

- The DRIs make two types of energy-intake recommendations. **Estimated Energy Requirements (EERs)** provide an estimate of how many calories are needed to not gain or lose body weight. **Acceptable Macronutrient Distribution Ranges (AMDRs)** recommend the proportion of energy in a healthy diet that should be sourced from carbohydrate, fat, and protein.

The right amount of energy from the right sources • Figure 2.5

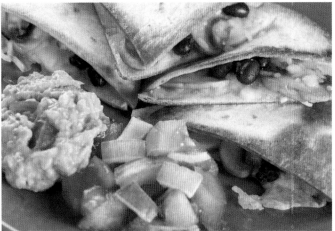

© Can Stock Photo Inc. / charlotteLake

3 Tools for Diet Planning 38

- *Eating Well with Canada's Food Guide* is Health Canada's current food guide. It recommends amounts from four food groups plus oils, based on individual energy needs and depending on an individual's life stage and gender. This food guide also now includes culturally relevant foods and examples of how to estimate portion size. It also stresses the concepts of using variety and moderation in choosing a healthy diet and promotes physical activity.

- The food guide also provides additional recommendations for how to choose wisely from each food group. These recommendations include eating one dark green and one orange vegetable a day, choosing more whole grain products, eating two servings of fish each week, and limiting the amount of fat, sugar, and salt in our food choices.

Eating Well with Canada's Food Guide: Messages and symbolism • Figure 2.7

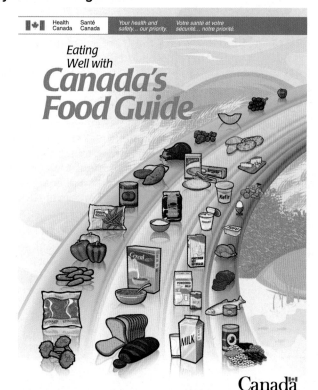

4 Food and Natural Health Product Labels 45

• Standardized food labels are designed to help consumers make healthy food choices by providing information about the nutrient composition of foods and about how a food fits into the overall diet. The **Nutrition Facts** panel presents information about the amount of various nutrients in a standard serving. For most nutrients, the amount is also given as a percentage of the **Daily Value**. A food label lists the contents of the product in order of prominence by weight. It will also feature the **common name** for the food, its **durable life date**, and a **net quantity declaration**, outlining the quantity of the product found in the package. Food labels often include terms whose definitions have been determined by Canada's Food and Drug Act, including **nutrient content claims**, such as *low fat* or *high fibre*. Food labels can also include two types of **diet-related health claims**, **disease-reduction claims** and **function claims**, which refer to a relationship between a nutrient, food, food component, or dietary supplement and the risk of a particular disease or health-related condition. All health claims are reviewed by the Canadian Food Inspection Agency and permitted only when they are supported by scientific evidence, but the level of scientific support for such claims varies.

• Supplements such as vitamins, minerals, and probiotics are considered natural health products by Health Canada and have a different set of restrictions and labelling requirements. Natural health products approved by Health Canada must include recommended uses, any cautionary statements, and a list of ingredients on their labels, but they do not need to include a Nutrition Facts panel.

Natural health products • Figure 2.14

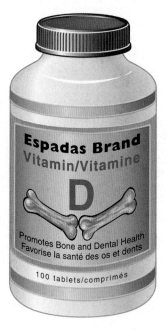
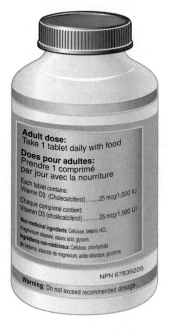

Key Terms

Critical and Creative Thinking Questions

1. The food guide recommends reducing the sugar, salt, and fat content of foods. Suggest some changes that the food industry can implement to support these nutrition recommendations.

2. If a food record indicates that Gina consumes less than the RDA for vitamin C and more than the RDA for vitamin A, what does this information mean in terms of her nutritional status? Does she have a vitamin C deficiency? Is she at risk of vitamin A toxicity? What other factors need to be considered before drawing any conclusions about her nutritional status?

3. If a survey indicates that the consumption of red meat, which is an excellent source of iron, has been declining over the past five years, what conclusion can be drawn about the iron intake of the population during that period? How might this decline affect public health? How might it affect public health policy?

4. Select three packaged foods that have food labels. What is the percentage of calories from fat in each product? How many grams of carbohydrate, fat, and fibre are in each serving? How does each product fit into your daily diet with regard to total carbohydrate recommended? Total fat? Dietary fibre? If you consumed a serving of each of these three foods, how much more saturated fat could you consume during the day without exceeding the recommendations? How much more total carbohydrate and fibre should you consume that day to meet recommendations for a 2,000-kilocalorie diet?

5. Vanessa is trying to increase her intake of calcium and vitamin D by taking a dietary supplement. How can she determine whether it contains enough of these nutrients to meet her needs but not so much that it will cause toxicity? If the product claims to build strong bones, does this mean that it will help reverse Vanessa's osteoporosis? Why or why not?

What is happening in this picture?

This man is snacking on chips while watching television.

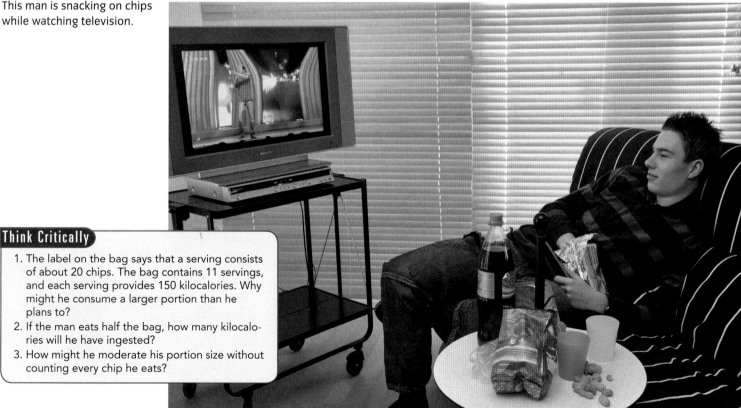

© imagebroker / Alamy

Think Critically

1. The label on the bag says that a serving consists of about 20 chips. The bag contains 11 servings, and each serving provides 150 kilocalories. Why might he consume a larger portion than he plans to?
2. If the man eats half the bag, how many kilocalories will he have ingested?
3. How might he moderate his portion size without counting every chip he eats?

Self-Test
(Check your answers in Appendix K.)

1. Which DRI standards can be used as goals for individual intake?
   a. AIs
   b. RDAs
   c. EARs
   d. A and B only

2. Based on the following graph, which shows one day's intake of selected nutrients, which of these statements about this person's nutrient intake is true?

Nutrient	Percent of recommendation 0%　　50%　　100%
Vitamin A	75%
Vitamin C	115%
Iron	54%
Calcium	75%
Saturated fat	134%

   a. She has an iron deficiency.
   b. She consumes the recommended amount of vitamin A.
   c. If she consumes this amount of iron every day, she is at risk for iron deficiency.
   d. She has osteoporosis.

3. Which DRI standard can help you determine whether a supplement contains a toxic level of a nutrient?
   a. RDA
   b. AI
   c. EAR
   d. UL

4. Which letter labels the DRI standard that represents the average needs of the population?

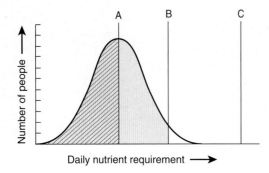

   a. A　　b. B　　c. C　　d. None of the above is correct.

5. Which of the following statements is false?
   a. An EER value gives the amount of energy needed to maintain body weight.
   b. Your EER stays the same when you gain weight.
   c. If you consume more calories than your EER, you will gain weight.
   d. Your EER depends on your age, gender, weight, height, and activity level.

6. Which of the following is *not* a food group in *Eating Well with Canada's Food Guide*?
   a. milk
   b. meat and alternatives
   c. vegetables and fruit
   d. fats and sweets

7. *Eating Well with Canada's Food Guide* recommends that _____ consume a daily supplement of vitamin D
   a. men and women over the age of 50
   b. women of childbearing age
   c. vegetarians
   d. people with osteoporosis

8. Which of the following is not a recommendation in the "Make each Food Guide Serving Count" section of *Eating Well with Canada's Food Guide*?
   a. Make at least half of each day's grain products whole grain.
   b. Consume at least two food guide servings of fish each week.
   c. Choose fresh vegetables and fruit over frozen.
   d. Select lower-fat milk alternatives.

9. Use the following label to determine which of the following statements about the amount of saturated fat in this product is true.

Nutrition Facts Valeur nutritive	
Per 1 cup (220 g)/par 1 tasse (225 g)	
Amount **Teneur**	**% Daily Value** **% valeur quotidienne**
Calories / Calories 250	
Fat / Lipides 12 g	18%
Saturated / saturés 3 g + Trans / trans 1.5 g	15%
Cholesterol / Cholestérol 30 mg	10 %
Sodium / Sodium 470 mg	20 %
Carbohydrate / Glucides 31 g	10%
Fibre / Fibres 0 g	0%
Sugars / Sucres 5 g	
Protein / Protéines 5 g	
Vitamin A / Vitamine A	4 %
Vitamin C / Vitamine C	2 %
Calcium / Calcium	20 %
Iron / Fer	4 %

a. This product contains 15% of the maximum daily recommended amount of saturated fat.

b. This product is high in saturated fat.

c. To meet nutritional needs, the other foods you consume during the day should provide 17 g of saturated fat.

d. This product is low in saturated fat.

10. In which order are the ingredients listed on a food label?

a. alphabetical

b. from largest to smallest, by volume

c. from largest to smallest, by weight

d. dry ingredients first, followed by liquid ingredients

11. Which of the following is used to assess nutritional status?

a. measurements of body dimensions

b. medical history and physical examination

c. laboratory tests

d. All of the above

12. Which of the following is a function claim?

a. Fibre maintains bowel regularity.

b. Soluble fibre helps reduce the risk of heart disease.

c. Calcium helps reduce the risk of osteoporosis.

d. Diets that are low in sodium can reduce the risk of high blood pressure.

13. What is meant by nutritional status?

a. how healthy a person's diet is relative to that of his or her peer group

b. the measure of a person's health in terms of his or her intake and utilization of nutrients

c. a person's blood values relative to normal levels

d. the quality of foods a family is able to afford

14. Which of the following is a permitted diet-related health claim?

a. Product X is sodium free.

b. It is recommended that men consume 38 g of fibre and women consume 25 g of fibre each day. Product X is an excellent source of fibre.

c. Consumption of product X is associated with a reduced risk of cardiovascular disease.

d. A healthy diet low in saturated and trans fats may reduce the risk of heart disease. Product X is low in saturated and trans fats.

15. Which of the following is not required on the label of a natural health product?

a. a list of ingredients

b. recommended uses

c. Nutrition Facts panel

d. a licence number

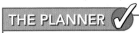

THE PLANNER

Review your Chapter Planner on the chapter opener and check off your completed work.

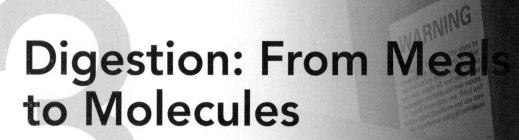

Digestion: From Meals to Molecules

The human body can be compared to a car: We fill the tank of our car with gasoline to get down the highway; we fill our body with food to get on with life. In both "machines," combustion combines with oxygen to release energy. In a car's engine, the explosion that releases energy is contained within a cylinder. In a human, the energy is released by reactions within a living cell.

Our bodies are machine-like in another way: They are virtually identical to one another. Like cars, we look different on the outside but are similar on the inside. Just as the internal combustion engine works in the same way, no matter where it's manufactured, the processes that drive human bodies are more similar than different because they are based on the same fundamental chemical reactions.

Like cars, the type of fuel that we put into our body and how well we take care of our body has a large effect on how long and how well our body will last. When a car breaks down, it costs money and time to repair. A breakdown in our body can lead to a chronic disease, which can cost time, money, and effort to repair. In both cases, the "machine" that is left rarely runs as effectively as it did before. That's why eating the right fuels and nutrients is essential to the proper functioning of our body.

Despite the similarities, human bodies and machines are also very different. For instance, an automobile cannot use gasoline to heal itself or to grow, but our body can heal and grow when provided with the proper nutrients. Cars are typically fuelled only by gasoline, but the human digestive system must process fuel from many sources for use by the "high-performance machine" that is the human body.

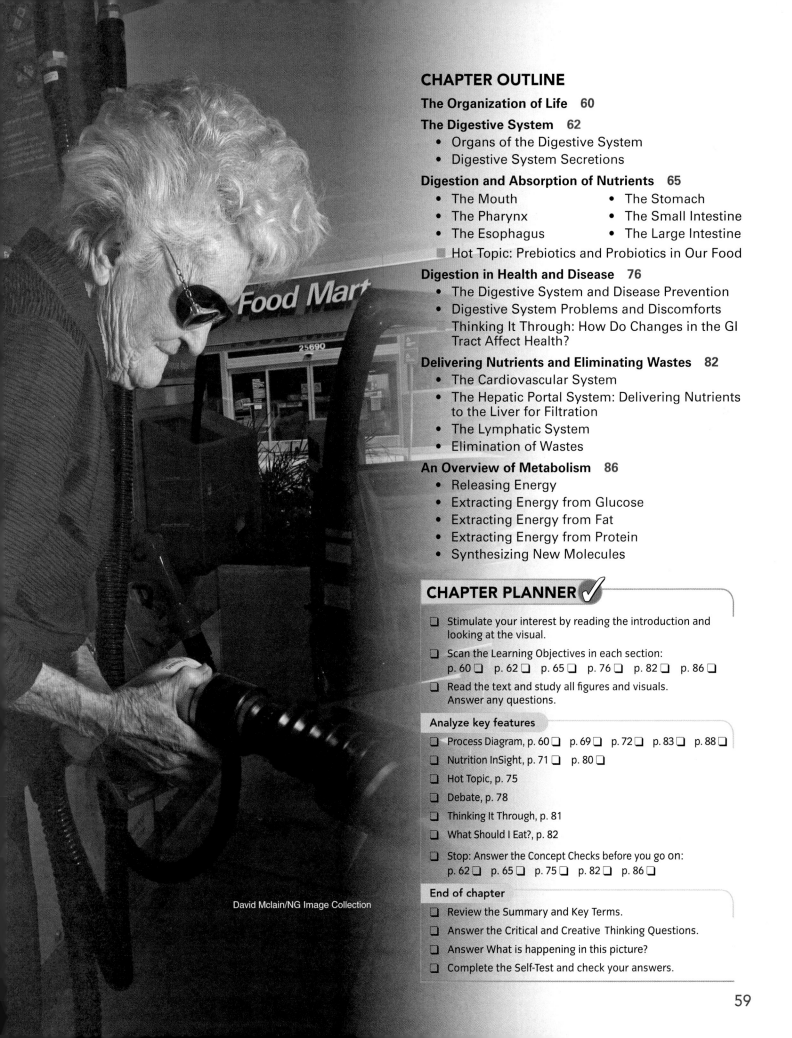

CHAPTER PLANNER ✔

- ❏ Stimulate your interest by reading the introduction and looking at the visual.
- ❏ Scan the Learning Objectives in each section:
  p. 60 ❏   p. 62 ❏   p. 65 ❏   p. 76 ❏   p. 82 ❏   p. 86 ❏
- ❏ Read the text and study all figures and visuals. Answer any questions.

Analyze key features

- ❏ Process Diagram, p. 60 ❏   p. 69 ❏   p. 72 ❏   p. 83 ❏   p. 88 ❏
- ❏ Nutrition InSight, p. 71 ❏   p. 80 ❏
- ❏ Hot Topic, p. 75
- ❏ Debate, p. 78
- ❏ Thinking It Through, p. 81
- ❏ What Should I Eat?, p. 82
- ❏ Stop: Answer the Concept Checks before you go on:
  p. 62 ❏   p. 65 ❏   p. 75 ❏   p. 82 ❏   p. 86 ❏

End of chapter

- ❏ Review the Summary and Key Terms.
- ❏ Answer the Critical and Creative Thinking Questions.
- ❏ Answer What is happening in this picture?
- ❏ Complete the Self-Test and check your answers.

David Mclain/NG Image Collection

The Organization of Life

LEARNING OBJECTIVES

1. **Describe** the organization of living things, from atoms to organisms.

2. **Name** the organ systems that work with the digestive system to deliver nutrients and eliminate wastes.

Matter is considered to be all substances in the world that have mass and occupy space, be it a meal, the plate you are about to eat it from, or even you, yourself. Matter is composed of miniscule, non-visible **atoms** (**Figure 3.1**). Atoms combine to form **molecules**, which can have different properties from the atoms they contain. In any living system, such as the human body or the plant and animal products you eat, the molecules are organized into **cells**, the smallest units of life. Cells that are similar in structure and function form **tissues**. The human body contains four types of tissue: muscle, nerve, epithelial, and connective. These tissues are

atoms The smallest units of an element that retain the properties of the element.

molecules Units of two or more atoms of the same or different elements bonded together.

cells The basic structural and functional units of living things.

PROCESS DIAGRAM

From atoms to organisms • Figure 3.1

The organization of life begins with atoms that form molecules, which are then organized into cells to form tissues, organs, organ systems, and whole organisms. The foods we eat contain nutrients, such as proteins, that are made up of atoms and may help in forming our final body structure.

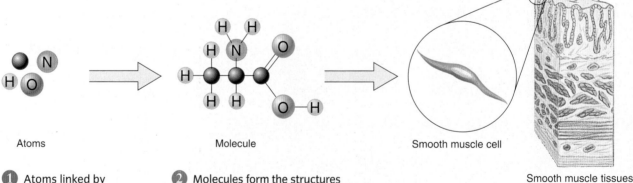

Atoms

Molecule

Smooth muscle cell

Smooth muscle tissues

1. Atoms linked by chemical bonds form molecules. Proteins are composed of carbon, hydrogen, oxygen, and nitrogen atoms, which are linked by bonds of different types and strengths to form a protein molecule.

2. Molecules form the structures that make up cells. Each cell is bounded by a membrane. In multicellular organisms, cells are usually specialized to perform specific functions. Proteins are found in different parts of the cell with varying functions depending on their nature. In muscle cells, muscle contractions are produced by two types of proteins: myosin and actin.

3. Groups of similar cells form tissues. Specific types of muscle cells can combine to make up smooth muscle tissue. Smooth muscle can be found in different sections of the gastrointestinal (GI) tract.

organs Discrete structures composed of more than one tissue that perform a specialized function.

organized in varying combinations to form **organs**. Most organs do not function alone but are part of an **organ system**, such as the digestive system, the cardiovascular system, or the endocrine system. An organ may be part of more than one organ system. For example, the pancreas is part of the endocrine system and also part of the digestive system.

The body's 11 organ systems interact to perform all the functions necessary for life (**Table 3.1**). For example, the digestive system, which is the primary organ system responsible for moving nutrients into the body, is assisted by the endocrine system, which secretes **hormones** that help regulate how much we eat

hormones Chemical messengers that are produced in one location in the body, released into the blood, and travel to other locations, where they elicit responses.

and how quickly food and nutrients travel through the digestive system. The digestive system is also aided by other organ systems: the nervous system, which sends nerve signals that help control the passage of food through the digestive tract; the cardiovascular system, which transports nutrients to individual cells in the body; and the urinary, respiratory, and integumentary systems, which eliminate wastes generated in the body. The foods we eat contain many nutrients, which in turn support the various organ systems in our body in various ways: by providing structure, as in the case of muscle protein or the iron found in blood; by supporting chemical reaction, as the B vitamins do during metabolism; or by providing the energy required for the body to do work, as is the role of carbohydrates, fats, and proteins.

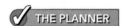

THE PLANNER

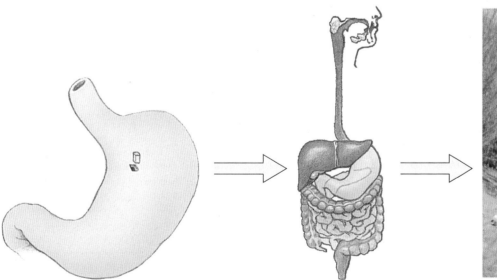

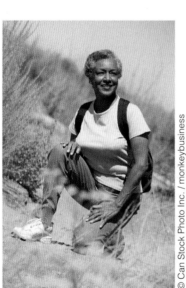

© Can Stock Photo Inc. / monkeybusiness

Organ | Organ system | Organism

4 Organs such as the heart, the kidneys, and the stomach are discrete structures that perform specific functions in the body and are composed of different tissue types. The stomach is primarily composed of smooth muscle tissue but also contains nervous, epithelial, and connective tissues, which work together to achieve the stomach's function.

5 A group of organs that work together to perform a particular function form an organ system. The stomach is one part of the digestive system, which functions in the digestion and absorption of nutrients.

6 The organ systems work together to ensure proper functioning of the entire organism. For example, the digestive system works with the circulatory system to provide cells with the required oxygen and nutrients needed for the human organism to move and function.

PROCESS DIAGRAM

The 11 major organ systems of the human body   Table 3.1

System	Main components	Main function
Circulatory	Heart, blood vessels	Transportation of blood, which carries oxygen, nutrients, and wastes etc.
Digestive	Digestive tract (mouth, pharynx, esophagus, stomach, intestines), accessory organs (salivary glands, pancreas, liver, gallbladder)	Digestion, absorption of meals
Endocrine	Pituitary, adrenal, thyroid, pancreas, and other ductless glands	Production and release of hormones (chemical messengers)
Integumentary	Skin, hair, glands, fingernails	Protection, glandular secretion, temperature regulation, regulation of body temperature
Lymphatic	Lymph nodes, lymph vessels, spleen	Drainage, immunity, transportation of fat-soluble nutrients
Muscular	Skeletal muscles	Movement, structure, and production of heat
Nervous	Sensory receptors, nerves, spinal cord, brain	Generation of response to stimuli from external and internal environments, transmission of impulses to activate muscles and glands, integration of activities of other systems
Reproductive	Ovaries, vagina, uterus, mammary glands (females)	Production of offspring
	Testes, penis (males)	Production of sex hormones
Respiratory	Lungs, air passageways, trachea, pharynx, larynx	Gas exchange with external environment
Skeletal	Bones, cartilage, joints	Structure, support, framework for the movement of muscles
Urinary	Kidney, bladder, urethra	Elimination of wastes, regulation of water, pH and electrolyte balance

---

CONCEPT CHECK **STOP**

1. **How** are atoms, molecules, and cells related to one another?

2. **How** do the endocrine and nervous systems interact with the digestive system?

The Digestive System
LEARNING OBJECTIVES

1. **Define** digestion and absorption.

2. **List** the organs that make up the digestive system.

3. **Describe** the tissues that make up the wall of the gastrointestinal tract.

4. **Explain** the roles of mucus, enzymes, nerves, and hormones in digestion.

The digestive system is the organ system that is primarily responsible for the **digestion** and **absorption** of nutrients. When you eat a taco, for example, the tortilla, meat, cheese, lettuce, and tomato are broken apart, releasing the nutrients and other food components they contain. Water,

digestion The process by which food is broken down into components small enough to be absorbed into the blood stream.

absorption The process of taking substances from the gastrointestinal tract into the interior of the body.

vitamins, and minerals are taken into the body without being broken into smaller units, but proteins, carbohydrates, and fats must be digested further before they can be absorbed. Proteins are broken down into amino acids, most of the carbohydrate is broken down into sugars like glucose, and most fats are digested to produce molecules with long carbon chains called fatty acids. The sugars, amino acids, and fatty acids can then be absorbed into the body. The fibre in whole grains, fruits, and vegetables that cannot be digested is not absorbed into the body. This fibre may, however, promote digestive health as it travels through us untouched.

It and other unabsorbed substances pass through the digestive tract and are eliminated in **feces**.

Organs of the Digestive System

The digestive system is composed of the **gastrointestinal tract** and accessory organs (**Figure 3.2a**). The gastrointestinal tract is a hollow tube, about 9 m (30 feet) long, running from the mouth to the

> **feces** Body waste, including unabsorbed food residue, bacteria, mucus, and dead cells, which is eliminated from the gastrointestinal tract by way of the anus.

Structure of the digestive system • Figure 3.2

Mouth: Chews food and mixes it with saliva

Salivary glands: Produce saliva, which contains a starch-digesting enzyme

Pharynx: Swallows chewed food mixed with saliva

Esophagus: Moves food to the stomach

Stomach: Churns and mixes food; secretes acid and a protein-digesting enzyme

Liver: Makes bile, which aids in digestion and absorption of fat

Pancreas: Releases bicarbonate to neutralize intestinal contents; produces enzymes that digest carbohydrate, protein, and fat

Gallbladder: Stores bile and releases it into the small intestine when needed

Small intestine: Absorbs nutrients into blood or lymph; most digestion occurs here

Large intestine: Absorbs water and some vitamins and minerals; home to intestinal bacteria; passes waste material

Colon
Rectum

Anus: Opens to allow waste to leave the body

a. The digestive system consists of the organs of the digestive tract—mouth, pharynx, esophagus, stomach, small intestine, and large intestine—plus four accessory organs—salivary glands, liver, gallbladder, and pancreas.

Contraction of the layers of smooth muscle—over which we do not have voluntary control—helps mix food, break it into small particles, and propel it through the digestive tract.

This external layer of connective tissue provides support and protection.

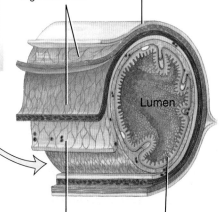

Lumen

Ask Yourself

Bile is made in the _____ and stored in the _____. It is released into the _____, where it is important for the digestion and absorption of _____.

Think Critically

Why is food in the lumen still outside the body?

b. This cross-section through the wall of the small intestine reveals the four tissue layers that make up the wall of the gastrointestinal tract.

This layer of connective tissue contains nerves and blood vessels. It provides support, nourishes the mucosa, and sends the nerve signals that control secretions and muscle contractions.

The mucosa, which lines the GI tract, is a type of epithelial tissue. Nutrients must pass through these mucosal cells before they can reach the blood or lymph.

anus. It is also called the gut, GI tract, alimentary canal, or digestive tract. The inside hole of the tube is the **lumen** (**Figure 3.2b**). Food in the lumen is not technically inside the body because it has not been absorbed. When you swallow something that cannot be digested, such as a whole sesame seed or an unpopped kernel of popcorn, it passes through your digestive tract and exits in the feces without ever entering your blood or cells. Only after substances have been absorbed into the cells that line the intestine can they be said to be inside the body.

The lumen is lined with a layer of **mucosal cells** called the **mucosa**, which contributes to both secretion and absorption. Because mucosal cells are in direct contact with churning food and harsh digestive secretions, they live only two to five days. The dead cells are sloughed off into the lumen, where some components are digested and absorbed, and the rest are eliminated in feces. New mucosal cells are formed continuously to replace those that die. To allow for this rapid replacement, the mucosa has high nutrient requirements and is one of the first parts of the body to be affected by nutrient deficiencies.

The time food takes to travel the length of the GI tract from mouth to anus is called the **transit time**. The shorter the transit time, the more rapidly material is passing through the digestive tract. In a healthy adult, transit time is 24 to 72 hours, depending on the composition of the individual's diet and his or her level of physical activity, emotional state, health status, and use of medications.

Digestive System Secretions

Digestion is aided by substances secreted into the digestive tract from cells in the mucosa and from some of the accessory organs. One of these substances is **mucus**, which moistens, lubricates, and protects the digestive tract.

Enzymes are also present in digestive system secretions. They accelerate the chemical reactions

mucus A viscous fluid secreted by glands in the digestive tract and other parts of the body. It lubricates, moistens, and protects cells from harsh environments.

enzymes Protein molecules that accelerate the rate of specific chemical reactions without being changed themselves.

Enzyme activity • Figure 3.3

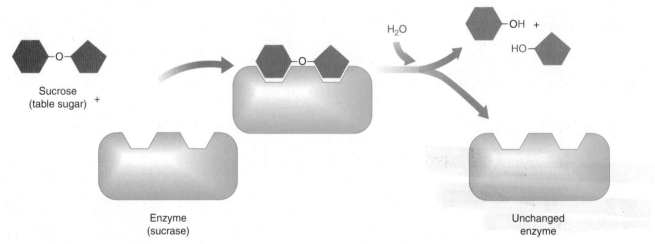

a. Hydrolysis uses water to break down larger molecules into their constituent components. Enzymes can facilitate this process, which is used to break down different food components. The enzyme shown here, *sucrase,* breaks apart the two-sugar molecule sucrose into its components, glucose and fructose. *Amylases* work on longer carbohydrate chains, but have no effect on fat. Conversely, enzymes called *lipases* digest fat and have no effect on carbohydrate.

b. A condensation reaction helps construct larger molecules from smaller ones, such as the joining of amino acids in the first stages of protein synthesis. The above condensation reaction leads to the removal of water. Both condensation and hydrolysis reactions can be facilitated by enzymes.

that break down food into units that can be absorbed. Enzymes help speed chemical reactions by establishing the optimal environment for these reactions to occur, such as by bringing different reactants together. In the gastrointestinal tract, enzymes play a large role in digestion by facilitating the process of **hydrolysis**, where an input of water helps split apart larger molecules into smaller molecules (**Figure 3.3a**). The opposite of a hydrolysis reaction is a **condensation** reaction (**Figure 3.3b**), where two molecules come together to form a larger molecule, typically resulting in the loss of water. Both condensation and hydrolysis reactions can occur with or without an enzyme, but most reactions do involve enzymes, as they vastly increase their speed.

> **hydrolysis** A reaction that uses water to break down larger molecules into their structural units.
>
> **condensation** A reaction in which two structural units combine to create a larger molecule, typically resulting in the loss of a water molecule.

The gastrointestinal tract is part of the endocrine system and part of the digestive system because it releases hormones. These hormones help prepare different parts of the gut for the arrival of food and thus regulate both digestion and the rate at which food moves through the digestive system. Some hormonal signals slow digestion, whereas others facilitate it. For example, when the nutrients from your lunch reach your small intestine, they trigger the release of hormones that signal the pancreas and gallbladder to secrete digestive substances into the small intestine.

CONCEPT CHECK   STOP

1. **What** happens during digestion and absorption?

2. **Which** organs make up the gastrointestinal tract?

3. **What** are mucosal cells?

4. **How** are enzymes important for digestion and absorption?

Digestion and Absorption of Nutrients

LEARNING OBJECTIVES

1. **Describe** what happens in each of the organs of the gastrointestinal tract.

2. **Discuss** factors that influence how quickly food moves through the GI tract.

3. **Explain** how the structure of the small intestine aids in its function.

4. **Distinguish** passive diffusion from active transport.

Imagine warm slices of freshly baked bread smeared with melting butter. Is your mouth watering? You don't even need to put food in your mouth for activity to begin in the digestive tract. Sensory input alone—the sight of the bread being lifted out of the oven, the smell of the bread, the clatter of the butter knife—may promote appetite. Your mouth may water and your stomach may begin to secrete digestive substances. These responses occur when the nervous system signals the digestive system to ready itself for a meal. For food to be used by the body, however, you need to do more than smell your meal. The food must be consumed and digested, and the nutrients must be absorbed and transported to the body's cells. This process involves the combined functions of all the organs of the digestive system and the help of some other organ systems.

The Mouth

Digestion involves chemical and mechanical processes, both of which begin in the mouth. The presence of food in the mouth stimulates the flow of **saliva** from various salivary glands. Saliva is primarily composed of water, which moistens the food and carries dissolved food molecules to thousands of taste buds, most of which are located on the tongue. Human taste buds are responsive to five tastes: sweet, salty, sour, bitter, and savoury (umami). Foods with more than one of these tastes will stimulate more than one taste bud. Signals from the taste buds, along with the aroma of food, allow us to enjoy the taste of the food we eat. Saliva also contains two enzymes: **salivary amylase**, which breaks starch molecules into shorter

> **saliva** A watery fluid that is produced and secreted into the mouth by the salivary glands. It contains lubricants, enzymes, and other substances.

carbohydrate chains, and lingual lipase, which initiates the digestion of fat. Using chemicals such as enzymes to help break down food is known as **chemical digestion**. Saliva also helps protect against tooth decay because it washes away food particles and contains antibacterial substances, such as the enzyme lysozyme, which inhibits the growth of bacteria that cause tooth decay.

Chewing food begins the process of **mechanical digestion**. Adult humans typically have 32 teeth, which are specialized for biting, tearing, grinding, and crushing foods. Chewing breaks food into pieces that are small enough to be swallowed and increases the surface area in contact with digestive juices. The strong muscular force of the tongue helps mix food with saliva and aids chewing by constantly repositioning food between the teeth. Chewing also breaks up fibre, which traps nutrients. If the fibre is not broken up, some of the nutrients in the food cannot be absorbed. For example, if the fibrous skin of corn is not broken open by the teeth, the nutrients inside the corn remain inaccessible, and it travels, undigested, through the intestines for elimination in the feces.

The Pharynx

The **pharynx**, more commonly known as the throat, is the part of the gastrointestinal tract responsible for swallowing. It is also part of the respiratory tract and is responsible for bringing air into the lungs. As we prepare to swallow, the mass of chewed food mixed with saliva, called a **bolus**, is directed to the back of the mouth by the tongue. During swallowing, the air passages are blocked by a valve-like flap of tissue called the epiglottis so that food goes to the next segment of the gastrointestinal tract, the esophagus, and not to the lungs (**Figure 3.4**). Eating too quickly or talking while eating can interfere with the closing of the epiglottis. As a result, food can "go down the wrong tube," passing into an upper air passageway instead of entering the digestive tract. This food can usually be dislodged with a cough.

> **epiglottis** A piece of elastic connective tissue that covers the opening to the lungs during swallowing.

The Esophagus

The esophagus does not actively participate in digestion; it instead provides a passageway and mechanical assistance for moving food between the pharynx and the stomach. In the esophagus, the bolus is moved along by rhythmic contractions of the smooth muscles, an action called peristalsis (**Figure 3.5a**). The contractions of peristalsis are strong enough so that even if you ate while standing on your head, food would reach your stomach. This contractile movement, which is controlled automatically by the nervous system, also occurs at different points throughout the gastrointestinal tract, pushing digesting food from the pharynx through the large intestine. Another major type of movement found in the digestive tract is segmentation (**Figure 3.5b**), which occurs in the small intestine and will be further discussed later in this chapter.

> **peristalsis** Coordinated muscular contractions that move material through the GI tract.

To leave the esophagus and enter the stomach, food must pass through a **sphincter**, a layer of muscle that encircles the tube of the digestive tract and acts as a valve. When the sphincter contracts, the valve is closed; when it relaxes, the valve is open (**Figure 3.6**). The **lower esophageal sphincter**, located between the esophagus and the stomach, prevents food from moving from the stomach back into the esophagus. Stomach contents can move in this direction during what is commonly known as heartburn (as discussed later in this chapter): Some of the acidic stomach contents leak up through a weakened sphincter into the esophagus, causing a burning sensation.

Swallowing • Figure 3.4

When a bolus is swallowed, it normally pushes the epiglottis down over the opening to the passageway that leads to the lungs.

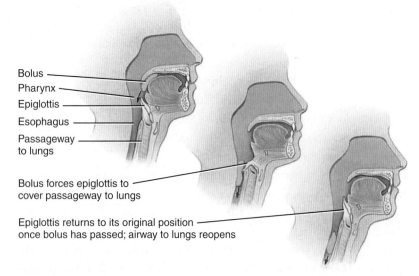

Bolus
Pharynx
Epiglottis
Esophagus
Passageway to lungs

Bolus forces epiglottis to cover passageway to lungs

Epiglottis returns to its original position once bolus has passed; airway to lungs reopens

Moving food through the GI tract • Figure 3.5

The food we swallow doesn't just fall down the esophagus and into the stomach. It is pushed along by muscular contractions and enters the stomach in response to the opening and closing of the sphincter located where the esophagus meets the stomach.

a. Peristalsis in the small intestine allows the chyme to be pushed forward toward the large intestine.

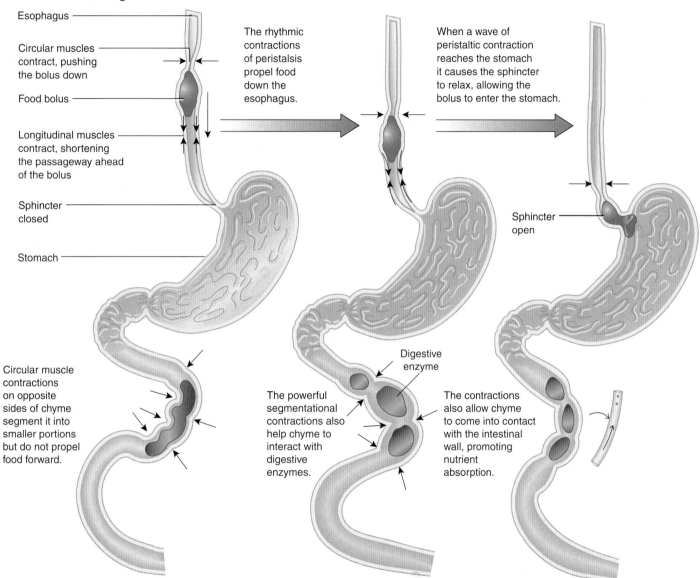

Esophagus

Circular muscles contract, pushing the bolus down

Food bolus

Longitudinal muscles contract, shortening the passageway ahead of the bolus

Sphincter closed

Stomach

Circular muscle contractions on opposite sides of chyme segment it into smaller portions but do not propel food forward.

The rhythmic contractions of peristalsis propel food down the esophagus.

When a wave of peristaltic contraction reaches the stomach it causes the sphincter to relax, allowing the bolus to enter the stomach.

Sphincter open

Digestive enzyme

The powerful segmentational contractions also help chyme to interact with digestive enzymes.

The contractions also allow chyme to come into contact with the intestinal wall, promoting nutrient absorption.

b. Segmentation helps section chime, mix chime with digestive enzymes, and leads to interactions with the intestinal wall that promote absorption.

The Stomach

The stomach is an expanded portion of the gastrointestinal tract that serves as a temporary storage site for food. Here the bolus is mashed and mixed with highly acidic stomach secretions to form a semiliquid food mass called **chyme**. The mixing of food in the stomach is aided by an extra layer of smooth muscle in the stomach wall (Figure 3.6a). Some digestion takes place in the stomach, but, with the exception of some water, alcohol, and a few drugs, such as acetylsalicylic acid (Aspirin) and acetaminophen (Tylenol), very little absorption occurs here.

Gastric juice Chemical digestion in the stomach is caused by **gastric juice** produced by gastric glands

Stomach structure and function • Figure 3.6

a. Most of the gastrointestinal tract is surrounded by two layers of smooth muscle, one running longitudinally and one running horizontally, but the stomach contains a third smooth muscle layer running diagonally. The presence of all three layers allows for the powerful contractions that churn and mix the stomach contents. The pyloric sphincter at the bottom of the stomach controls the flow of chyme into the small intestine.

b. The lining of the stomach is covered with valleys called gastric pits. Inside these pits are the gastric glands, made up of different types of cells that produce the mucus, hydrochloric acid (parietal cells), and the inactive form of pepsin (chief cells) contained in gastric juice.

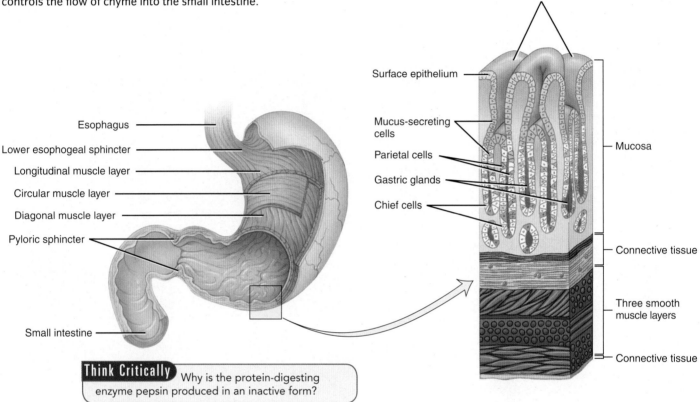

Think Critically Why is the protein-digesting enzyme pepsin produced in an inactive form?

in pits that dot the stomach lining (Figure 3.6b). Gastric juice is a mixture of water, mucus, hydrochloric acid, and pepsinogen, an inactive form of the protein-digesting enzyme **pepsin**. Hydrochloric acid begins protein digestion by unfolding proteins and activating pepsin from its inactive form. This enzyme is secreted in the inactive pepsinogen form so that it will not damage the gastric glands that produce it. The hydrochloric acid in gastric juice also kills most of the bacteria present in food and stops the activity of the carbohydrate-digesting enzyme salivary amylase. To ensure that the contents of gastric juice don't digest the protein found in the cells of the stomach wall, a thick layer of mucus protects the protein that makes up the stomach wall from the hydrochloric acid and pepsin in gastric juice.

Regulation of stomach activity How much your stomach churns, how much gastric juice is released, and

how fast material empties out of the stomach are regulated by signals from both nerves and hormones. These signals originate from three sites—the brain, the stomach, and the small intestine (**Figure 3.7**).

When the brain is stimulated by the site, smell, or thought of food, it prepares the stomach to receive food by increasing gastric secretions. The presence of a bolus of food in the stomach further regulates stomach action by increasing stomach churning and gastric secretions. When food then enters the small intestine, hormones released from the small intestine increase the secretions of enzymes and substances into the small intestine. These enzymes will help digest the food further and create the perfect environment for this digestion. Chyme also signals to the stomach to delay its emptying so the small intestine has enough time to digest that chyme before more enters the small intestine. As chyme begins to enter the small intestine from the stomach, the small intestine provides various forms of

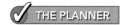

The regulation of stomach motility and secretion • Figure 3.7

Stomach activity is affected by food that has not yet reached the stomach, by food that is in the stomach, and by food that has left the stomach.

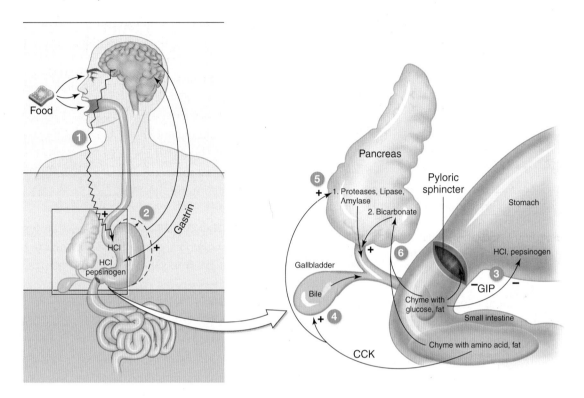

1 Before food enters the stomach, the thought, smell, sight, or taste of food causes the brain to send nerve signals (indicated by the zigzag lines) that stimulate gastric secretions and increase the rate of stomach churning or motility, thereby preparing the stomach to receive food.

2 Food entering the stomach causes the stomach to stretch, which signals the brain to stimulate the secretion of gastrin, a hormone that triggers an increase in the release of gastric juice.

3 When fat and glucose-rich chyme enter the small intestine, they trigger the release of the hormone GIP (glucose-dependent insulinotroptic peptide), which leads to the contraction of the pyloric sphincter, delaying gastric emptying and slowing the secretion of gastric juice. This process ensures that the amount of chyme entering the small intestine does not exceed the intestine's ability to process it.

4 If the chyme that enters the small intestine contains amino acids and fats, cholecystokinin (CCK) is released. CCK stimulates the contraction of the gallbladder, which then releases bile into the small intestine to help digest fat.

5 CCK also stimulates the pancreas to secrete proteases, lipases, and amylase into the small intestine to aid in the digestion of protein, fats, and carbohydrates, respectively.

6 Acidic chyme entering the small intestine also leads to the secretion of the hormone secretin. Secretin stimulates the pancreas to secrete bicarbonate into the small intestine to neutralize the acidity of chyme.

feedback to the stomach to regulate how quickly it empties (see Figure 3.7). Chyme normally empties from the stomach within two to six hours, but this rate varies depending on the size and composition of the meal that has been consumed. A large meal takes longer to leave the stomach than does a small meal. Liquids empty quickly; solids, however, leave the stomach more slowly than liquids, lingering until they are well mixed with gastric juice and liquefied.

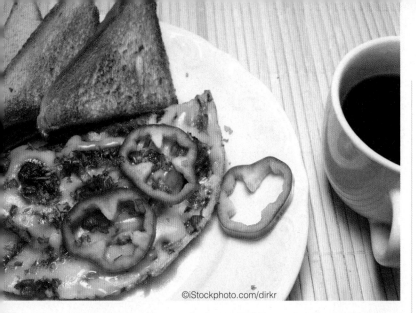

©iStockphoto.com/dirkr

Hunger and meal composition • Figure 3.8

What you choose for breakfast can affect how soon you become hungry for lunch. A small, carbohydrate-rich meal of toast and coffee will leave your stomach far more quickly than a larger meal containing more protein, fibre, and fat, such as a vegetable-and-cheese omelette with whole-wheat toast and butter.

The nutritional composition of a meal also affects how long it stays in the stomach. A meal that consists primarily of carbohydrate from starch and sugar leaves quickly, but a meal that is high in fibre or protein takes longer to leave the stomach. A high-fat meal stays in the stomach the longest. The longer a meal stays in the stomach, the fuller you will typically feel. Therefore, meals with a greater nutrient mixture may help to control your desire to eat. If you are trying to regulate your energy intake, select voluminous meals with a good mixture of nutrients, especially foods that are higher in fibre. Fibre promotes fullness, is a very low source of energy, and promotes digestive health (**Figure 3.8**).

The Small Intestine

The small intestine, a narrow tube about 6 m (20 feet) long, is the main site for the chemical digestion of food, completing the process that the mouth and stomach start. The small intestine is composed of three different segments: the duodenum (25–30 cm), the jejunum (2–3 m), and the ileum (2–4 m). Even though the duodenum is one of the smallest parts of the gastrointestinal tract, most digestion occurs here. The absorption of water, vitamins, minerals, and the products of carbohydrate, fat, and protein digestion occur primarily along the large surface area of the remainder of the small intestine, but also occur in the duodenum.

The small intestine has unique structural features that contribute to its digestive function and increase the amount of surface area, such as its long length and various

folds (**Figure 3.9**). Together, these features provide a surface area that is about the size of a tennis court (250 square metres), maximizing the available area for various chemical reactions and absorption to occur.

Peristalsis in the small intestine allows the chyme to be pushed forward toward the large intestine. The small intestine also produces other muscular contractions called **segmentation**. Segmentation is not meant to propel chyme forward, but rather to divide up this chyme, mix it with digestive enzymes, and help that chyme encounter the walls of the small intestine, where digested molecules can be absorbed (see Figure 3.5).

> **segmentation**
> Coordinated, periodic muscular contractions that aid in digestion and absorption, but do not significantly propel chyme forward.

Secretions that aid digestion In the small intestine, secretions from the pancreas, the gallbladder, and the small intestine itself aid digestion (see Figure 3.7). The pancreas secretes **pancreatic juice**, which contains digestive enzymes and **bicarbonate**, the latter of which helps regulate pH. When chyme enters the small intestine, it is acidic but the small intestine requires a fairly neutral environment for enzymes to function. Intestinal cells therefore release the hormone secretin, which stimulates the pancreas to secrete bicarbonate back into the small intestine. Bicarbonate, a base, neutralizes the acid in the chyme, making the environment in the small intestine as neutral or slightly basic as required for maximum enzymatic activity.

When amino acids and fats enter the small intestine, the hormone cholecystokinin (CCK) is released. CCK delays stomach emptying and regulates the secretion of digestion-promoting molecules into the small intestine. CCK stimulates the pancreas to secrete **pancreatic amylase,** an enzyme that continues the job of breaking down starches into sugars, which was started in the mouth by salivary amylase. Pancreatic **proteases** (protein-digesting enzymes), such as trypsin and chymotrypsin, break protein into shorter and shorter chains of amino acids, and fat-digesting enzymes called **lipases** break down fats into fatty acids, glycerol, and mono-glycerides. The pancreatic pro-teases, like the pepsin produced by the stomach, are released in an inactive form so that they will not digest the glands that produce them. CCK also stimulates the release of **bile**, which aids in the

> **bile** A digestive fluid made in the liver and stored in the gallbladder that is released into the small intestine, where it aids in fat digestion and absorption.

a. The wall of the small intestine is arranged in large circular folds, which increase the surface area in contact with nutrients. ▼

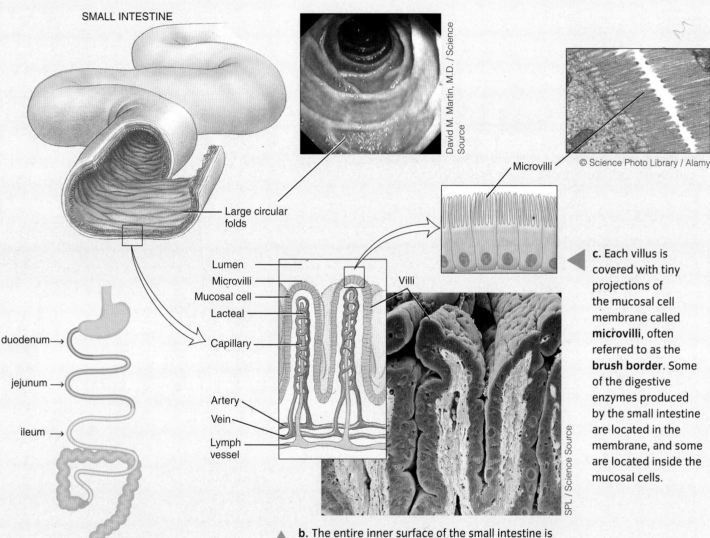

SMALL INTESTINE

David M. Martin, M.D. / Science Source

Microvilli

© Science Photo Library / Alamy

Large circular folds

Lumen
Microvilli
Mucosal cell
Lacteal
Capillary

Villi

duodenum →

jejunum →

ileum →

Artery
Vein
Lymph vessel

SPL / Science Source

c. Each villus is covered with tiny projections of the mucosal cell membrane called **microvilli**, often referred to as the **brush border**. Some of the digestive enzymes produced by the small intestine are located in the membrane, and some are located inside the mucosal cells.

b. The entire inner surface of the small intestine is covered with finger-like projections called **villi** (the singular is *villus*). Each villus contains a **capillary** (a small blood vessel) and a **lacteal** (a small lymph vessel). Nutrients must cross only the single-cell layer of the mucosa to reach the blood or lymph for delivery to the tissues of the body.

d. The small intestine is divided into three segments: the duodenum, the jejunum, and the ileum. Most digestion in the GI tract occurs in the duodenum, while absorption occurs along the entire length of the small intestine.

Ask Yourself

What are the structural features of the small intestine that increase its surface area?

digestion and absorption of fats. Bile is first produced in the liver, but stored in the gallbladder for quick release when required. Bile that is secreted into the small intestine mixes with fat and divides it into small globules, allowing lipases to access and digest the fat molecules more efficiently. The bile and digested fats then form small droplets that facilitate the absorption of fat into the mucosal cells. As they move through and then leave the mucosal cells, the products of fat digestion are incorporated into transport particles. These are then absorbed into the lymph before passing into the blood (**Figure 3.10**).

Intestinal digestive enzymes, found in the cell membranes or inside the cells lining the small intestine, aid the digestion of double sugars (two sugar units) into single sugar units and the digestion of short amino acid chains into single amino acids. The sugars from carbohydrate digestion and the amino acids from protein digestion pass into the blood and are delivered to the liver (see Figure 3.10).

Absorption After our ingested meal has been broken down into nutrient subunits, the gastrointestinal tract must absorb these nutrients into a circulatory system so they can be stored, excreted, or transported to where they are needed in the body. The small intestine is the main site for the absorption of nutrients. To be absorbed, nutrients must pass from the lumen of the GI tract, through the mucosal cells lining the tract, and then into

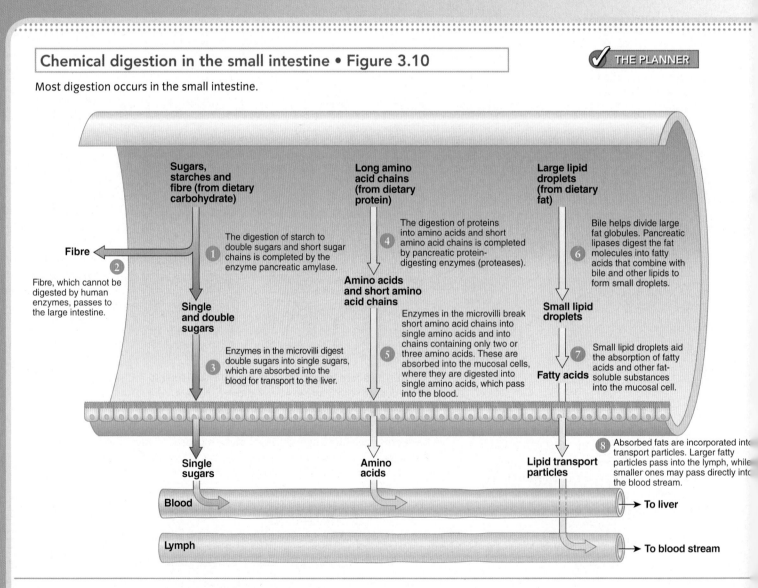

Chemical digestion in the small intestine • Figure 3.10

THE PLANNER

Most digestion occurs in the small intestine.

Sugars, starches and fibre (from dietary carbohydrate)

Fibre

Fibre, which cannot be digested by human enzymes, passes to the large intestine.

1 The digestion of starch to double sugars and short sugar chains is completed by the enzyme pancreatic amylase.

2

Single and double sugars

3 Enzymes in the microvilli digest double sugars into single sugars, which are absorbed into the blood for transport to the liver.

Long amino acid chains (from dietary protein)

4 The digestion of proteins into amino acids and short amino acid chains is completed by pancreatic protein-digesting enzymes (proteases).

Amino acids and short amino acid chains

5 Enzymes in the microvilli break short amino acid chains into single amino acids and into chains containing only two or three amino acids. These are absorbed into the mucosal cells, where they are digested into single amino acids, which pass into the blood.

Large lipid droplets (from dietary fat)

6 Bile helps divide large fat globules. Pancreatic lipases digest the fat molecules into fatty acids that combine with bile and other lipids to form small droplets.

Small lipid droplets

7 Small lipid droplets aid the absorption of fatty acids and other fat-soluble substances into the mucosal cell.

Fatty acids

8 Absorbed fats are incorporated into transport particles. Larger fatty particles pass into the lymph, while smaller ones may pass directly into the blood stream.

Single sugars

Amino acids

Lipid transport particles

Blood → To liver

Lymph → To blood stream

simple diffusion The unassisted diffusion of a substance across the cell membrane.

osmosis The unassisted diffusion of water across the cell membrane.

facilitated diffusion The assisted diffusion of a substance across the cell membrane with the help of a protein carrier.

active transport The transport of substances across a cell membrane with the aid of a protein carrier and the expenditure of energy.

either the blood or the lymph. Several different mechanisms are involved (**Figure 3.11**). Some rely on **diffusion**, which is the net movement of substances from an area of higher concentration to an area of lower concentration. The mechanisms that move substances into and out of cells without an input of energy include simple diffusion, in which material moves freely across the cell membrane; osmosis, which is the diffusion of water; and facilitated diffusion, in which a carrier molecule is needed for the substance to cross the membrane. Conversely, active transport requires both energy and a carrier molecule. This process can transport material from an area

of lower concentration to an area of higher concentration. Much of our resting energy expenditure each day is used for the many processes that require active transport to occur.

The Large Intestine

Materials not absorbed in the small intestine pass through a sphincter between the small intestine and the large intestine. This sphincter prevents material from the large intestine from re-entering the small intestine.

The large intestine is about 1.5 m (5 feet) long and is divided into the ceacum; the colon, which makes up the majority of the large intestine; the rectum; and the anus (**Figure 3.12**). The ceacum connects the small intestine to the colon and is the attachment point for the appendix. The function of the appendix, however, is not fully known. Some scientists argue that it is a remnant of a structure our ancestors used to digest leaves and foliage, while others argue that it helps to promote the bacterial health of the large intestine. The colon is the largest portion

Absorption mechanisms • Figure 3.11

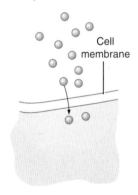
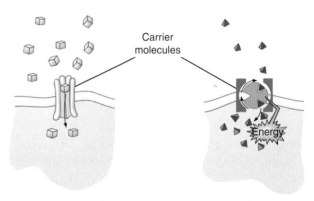

a. In **simple diffusion**, substances pass freely across a cell membrane from an area of higher concentration to an area of lower concentration, and no energy is required. Here the purple balls represent molecules that move by means of simple diffusion. Vitamin E and fatty acids are absorbed into mucosal cells by simple diffusion.

b. **Osmosis** is the passage of water molecules (indicated by the purple arrow) from an area with a lower concentration of dissolved substances (indicated by blue dots) to an area with a higher concentration of dissolved substances. Water can move both into and out of the lumen of the GI tract by osmosis.

c. **Facilitated diffusion** is a type of passive diffusion that requires a carrier molecule. Here the yellow cubes represent molecules that move from an area of higher concentration to an area of lower concentration, with the help of a carrier molecule. The sugar fructose found in fruit is absorbed by facilitated diffusion.

d. **Active transport** requires energy and a carrier molecule. The red pyramids represent molecules that are transported from an area of lower concentration to an area of higher concentration. Active transport allows glucose and amino acids to be absorbed even when they are present in higher concentrations in the mucosal cell than in the lumen.

Ask Yourself

1. Which absorption mechanism(s) can move nutrients only from an area with a higher concentration of that nutrient to an area with a lower concentration?
2. Which absorption mechanism(s) require(s) a carrier molecule?
3. Which absorption mechanism(s) require(s) energy?

The large intestine is the final section of the GI tract • Figure 3.12

Some material that is not absorbed in the small intestine can be broken down by colonic bacteria in the large intestine and then absorbed. The remaining undigested or unabsorbed material is packaged into feces for excretion into the external environment via the anus.

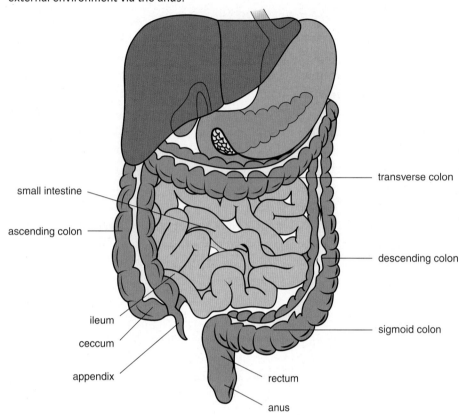

small intestine

ascending colon

ileum

ceccum

appendix

transverse colon

descending colon

sigmoid colon

rectum

anus

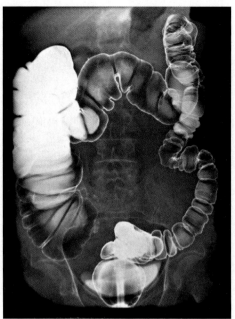

© PHOTOTAKE Inc. / Alamy

of the large intestine and is composed of four segments: the ascending colon, the transverse colon, the descending colon, and the sigmoid colon. Here, meal remnants that cannot be processed in the small intestine may be digested and absorbed or, more likely, are finally packaged into a form that can be excreted from the body. Although most nutrient absorption occurs in the small intestine, water and some vitamins and minerals are also absorbed in the colon. The last portions of the large intestine are the rectum, a temporary holding point for feces and the anus, where the digestive tract opens to the exterior of the body.

Peristalsis occurs more slowly in the large intestine than in the small intestine. Water, nutrients, and fecal matter may spend 24 hours in the large intestine, in contrast to the three to five hours it takes these materials to move through the small intestine. This slow movement favours the growth of bacteria called the **intestinal**

microbiota, which are permanent, beneficial residents of this part of the gastrointestinal tract (see *Hot Topic: Prebiotics and Probiotics in Our Food*). These bacteria break down unabsorbed portions of food, such as fibre, producing nutrients that can be used by the microbiota or, in some cases, are absorbed into the body. For example, the microbiota synthesize small amounts of certain B vitamins and vitamin K, some of which can be absorbed. As the microbiota break down material in the colon, they produce gas, which causes flatulence. If your small intestine lacks the appropriate enzymes, such as those that break down some of the carbohydrates in beans or milk, colonic microbiota might take over the task, making you more likely to feel the bloating and flatulent effects of the gas they produce. In a healthy adult, between 200 and 2,000 mL of gas is produced in the intestine each day, depending on the intestinal environment and the types of food consumed.

HOT TOPIC

✓ THE PLANNER

Prebiotics and probiotics in our food

The human gut is home to 300 to 500 species of bacteria. The right mix of bacteria is important for immune function, proper growth and development of colon cells, and optimal intestinal motility and transit time.[1] A healthy bacterial environment, or microbiota, can inhibit the growth of harmful bacteria and has been shown to both prevent the diarrhea associated with antibiotic use and reduce the duration of diarrhea resulting from intestinal infections and other causes.[2] Evidence also suggests that a healthy microbiota may relieve constipation, reduce allergy symptoms, modify the risk of colon cancer, and affect body weight.[3,4,5] Consuming these beneficial bacteria, called **probiotics**, is one way of promoting a healthy microbiota. Another way is to consume **prebiotics**, substances that serve as a food supply for beneficial bacteria.

Health Canada recognizes the potential benefits of consuming probiotics. The Food Directorate therefore allows certain function claims pertaining to probiotics. For example, manufacturers can state that their products contain probiotics and that probiotics promote regularity, improve nutrient absorption, and aid digestion.[6]

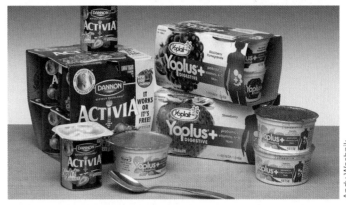

Andy Washnik

a. Ads claim that eating yogurt will help regulate the digestive system. Consumers see these products as a tasty way to provide nutrients and help regulate digestion.

● Beneficial bacteria   ● Harmful bacteria

Colon mucosa

Without probiotics   With probiotics

b. Scientists recognize that yogurt contains beneficial bacteria, including *Lactobacillus* and *Bifidobacterium*. When these living micro-organisms are consumed in adequate amounts, they live temporarily in the colon, where they inhibit the growth of harmful bacteria and confer other health benefits on the host. However, the bacteria must be consumed frequently because they are flushed out in the feces.

Think Critically Why might consuming a prebiotic increase the numbers of healthy bacteria in the gut?

Material that is not absorbed in the colon is divided into feces with the help of the unique segmental structure of the large intestine and muscle contractions that force the food to be sectioned. The remaining matter then passes into the rectum, where it is stored temporarily and then evacuated through the anus as feces. The feces are a mixture of undigested, unabsorbed matter, dead cells, secretions from the GI tract, water, and bacteria. The amount of bacteria varies but can comprise more than half the weight of the feces. The amount of water in the feces is affected by fibre and fluid intake. Because fibre retains water, when adequate fibre and fluids are consumed, feces have a higher water content and are more easily passed, promoting digestive health.

A summary of the function of the large intestine and other digestive organs can be found in **Table 3.2**.

CONCEPT CHECK STOP

1. **How** does food move through the GI tract?

2. **What** are the functions of the stomach?

3. **How** do the villi and microvilli aid absorption?

4. **Why** is active transport needed for the complete absorption of some nutrients?

Digestive tract summary   Table 3.2

Organ	Main function	Main secretions
Mouth	Mechanical digestion (teeth, tongue) Chemical digestion (carbohydrate, fats)	Saliva: water, electrolytes, mucus, enzymes (amylase, lipase, lysozyme)
Pharynx	Conduit for food and inspired air	
Esophagus	Conduit for food	
Stomach	Chemical digestion (proteins)	Hydrochloric acid, pepsinogen, mucus, intrinsic factor (vitamin B12 absorption), hormones (gastrin, GIP)
Small Intestine	Chemical digestion (carbohydrates, fats, proteins)	Hormones (secretin, CCK), brush border enzymes
Large Intestine	Removal of water and packaging of wastes into feces, bacterial digestion of some nutrients, absorption of some vitamins	
Accessory Organs		
Liver	Production of bile (fat digestion)	Bile
Gallbladder	Storage of bile	Bile
Pancreas	Production of digestive enzymes	Amylase, lipase, proteases, bicarbonate

Digestion in Health and Disease

LEARNING OBJECTIVES

1. **Explain** how the gastrointestinal tract protects us from infection.

2. **Describe** the causes of food allergies.

3. **Discuss** the causes and consequences of ulcers, heartburn, and GERD.

4. **Explain** how dental problems and gallstones might affect food intake.

The health of the GI tract is essential to our overall health. The gut acts as a defence against invasion by disease-causing organisms and other contaminants and allows us to obtain nutrients efficiently. Food allergies, which can be life-threatening, have their origins in the GI tract, but most common gastrointestinal problems are minor and do not affect long-term health.

The Digestive System and Disease Prevention

Food almost always contains bacteria and other contaminants, but it rarely makes us sick. This is because the mucosa of the GI tract contains tissue that is part of the immune system. This tissue prevents disease-causing bacteria and toxins from taking over the GI tract and invading the body.

Invading micro-organisms such as viruses and bacteria have a structure on their surfaces called an **antigen**, which tells the body that it is a foreign invader. When this antigen enters the lumen or is absorbed into the mucosa, the immune system can destroy it using one of several weapons, such as various types of white blood cells, which circulate

antigen A substance found on disease-causing agents that identifies them as foreign from the body's cells. When introduced into the body, it stimulates an immune response.

in the blood and reside in the mucosa of the gastrointestinal tract. There, they can quickly destroy most infectious agents that enter the body through the mucosa.

When an antigen is present, **phagocytes** are the first type of white blood cell to come to the body's defence by eliminating or "eating" the micro-organism. If the invader is not eliminated by the phagocytes, more specific white blood cells called **lymphocytes** join the battle. Some lymphocytes (cytotoxic T-cells) destroy foreign micro-organisms by binding to them. This type of lymphocyte helps eliminate foreign tissue and cells that have been infected by viruses and bacteria. Other lymphocytes (B cells) produce and secrete protein molecules called **antibodies**. Each antibody is specific for the antigen it will then bind to. The antigen–antibody complex prevents the micro-organism from entering body cells where it can cause damage; it also signals phagocytes to come and eliminate the micro-organism. Once antibodies for a specific antigen have been made, the immune system remembers and is ready to fight its associated infectious agent when it attempts to re-enter the body. This characteristic explains why an adult who had chicken pox as a child rarely has it again as an adult despite being exposed to it. The body recognizes the chicken pox virus and can produce a large number of antibodies for it quickly, eliminating it before the signs and symptoms of disease are experienced.

> **antibodies** Proteins, released by a type of lymphocyte, that interact with antigens and promote the removal of foreign invaders from the body.

If harmful organisms infect the GI tract, the body may help the immune system by using diarrhea or vomiting to flush them out.

Food allergies

Food allergies are very serious concern to the 7% of Canadians who suffer from them.[7] They are an issue both because they can limit consumable foods and cause discomfort and because some allergies are so severe that even consuming a small amount of the ingredient can lead to death. To protect consumers, Canadian food manufacturers are required to clearly state on the label whether a product contains any major ingredient that is likely to cause allergic reactions, such as peanuts, tree nuts, milk, eggs, fish, shellfish, soy, and wheat.

Our immune system protects us from many invaders without us even knowing. Unfortunately, the response of the immune system to a foreign substance is also to blame for allergic reactions. An allergic reaction occurs when the immune system produces antibodies to a substance, called an allergen, which is present in our diet or environment. **Food allergies** occur when the body sees proteins present in food as foreign substances and initiates an immune response. The immune response causes symptoms that range from hives to life-threatening reactions, such as breathing difficulties or a drop in blood pressure.

> **allergen** A substance that causes an allergic reaction.

The first time a food is consumed, it does not trigger an allergic reaction, but in a susceptible person, this first exposure begins the process. As the food is digested, tiny fragments of undigested protein trigger the production of antibodies. When the food protein is eaten again, it binds to the antibodies, signalling the release of chemicals that cause redness, swelling, and other allergy symptoms. When the protein enters the mouth, the allergic person may experience an itching or tingling sensation on the tongue or lips. As the protein travels down to the stomach and intestines, the allergic response may lead to vomiting and cramps. After the protein fragments are absorbed and travel through the blood, they may cause a drop in blood pressure, hives, and breathing difficulties. The best way to avoid allergy symptoms is to avoid foods that cause an allergic reaction.

Food allergies differ from food intolerances (e.g., lactose-intolerance), which are adverse reactions to substances in food, and typically do not involve the immune system.

Celiac disease

Celiac disease is a condition in which the protein gluten, found in wheat, barley, and rye, triggers an immune system response that damages or destroys the villi of the small intestine. For most of us, the gluten in our foods is digested and absorbed like other proteins. However, for people with celiac disease, consuming even a tiny amount of gluten can cause abdominal pain, diarrhea, and fatigue. Eventually, this damage can lead to malnutrition, weight loss, anemia, osteoporosis, intestinal cancer, and other chronic illnesses.[8] Celiac disease is similar to gluten-intolerance, but the symptoms of celiac disease are more severe. Celiac disease is an inherited condition that affects an estimated 1 in 133 people in Canada.[9] Although gluten-intolerance is currently a trendy condition (see *Debate: Should You Be Gluten Free?*), it and celiac disease can be diagnosed only by a blood test or an intestinal biopsy. For people with celiac disease, consuming a diet that eliminates gluten provides relief from symptoms. A gluten-free diet means eliminating products made from wheat, barley, or rye, including most breads, crackers, pastas, cereals, cakes, and cookies. It also requires eliminating foods ranging from packaged gravies to soy sauce that are processed with these grains.

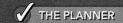
The Issue: You see the term "gluten free" on breakfast cereals, cake mixes, pastas, soups, and many other products. Gluten-free diets are essential for people with celiac disease, but a gluten-free diet has also been promoted for weight loss and to treat a host of other ailments. Is gluten free a healthy alternative for everyone?

The increase in the number of gluten-free foods over the past few years is partly due to greater awareness and better diagnosis of celiac disease; however, a switch to gluten-free products has also been promoted as a healthier way of eating for everyone. Advocates claim that a gluten-free diet will promote weight loss and help those who have joint pain, rheumatoid arthritis, osteoporosis, anemia, and diabetes. They contend that individuals with these symptoms have undiagnosed celiac disease. Although a small number of people may benefit from a gluten-free diet because they have celiac disease but no obvious symptoms, eating a gluten-free diet is unlikely to cure these conditions in people who do not have celiac disease, despite the suggestion of celebrity endorsements.

What about going gluten free for weight loss? Gluten-free foods are not any lower in calories than other foods, but eliminating everything that contains gluten from your diet—most types of cereal, bread, pasta, cakes, and cookies—will help cut calories. Gluten-free foods are also not nutritionally superior to other foods, but if you are trying to lose weight, carefully choosing everything you put in your mouth will force you to plan your diet carefully and may help with weight loss.

Is a gluten-free diet harmful? Eliminating gluten involves carefully checking each ingredient in the foods you eat to eliminate products made not only from wheat, which is both the major grain in the Canadian diet and one of our major exports, but also from barley and rye, and the myriad of foods that have wheat added as a thickener (see the figure). The major problem with a gluten-free diet is that it eliminates most flours, breads, pasta, and breakfast cereals, which are important sources of B vitamins and iron. Eliminating these foods creates a risk for nutrient deficiencies. A gluten-free diet is not harmful as long as it provides enough of all the nutrients typically consumed in gluten-containing foods. People diagnosed with celiac disease can work with a dietitian to ensure they have a well-balanced, varied diet that meets all their nutrient needs, whereas a dietitian is generally not consulted by people who eat a gluten-free diet for other reasons.

So, although current research does not support the benefits of eliminating gluten if you do not have celiac disease, anything that makes you consider your diet carefully can be beneficial. Individuals with gluten sensitivity benefit from the gluten-free craze, which has increased the availability and quality of gluten-free foods, improved the labelling of gluten-free products, and heightened awareness of celiac disease. Proponents believe a gluten-free diet will improve everyone's health. Skeptics consider gluten-free diets to be another trend like the low-carb fad of a few years back.

Think Critically

Neither potatoes nor onions contain gluten. If you had celiac disease, based on the ingredients shown here, which would be a safer choice: the French fries or the onion rings?

French Fries

INGREDIENTS: POTATOES, VEGETABLE OIL (PALM, SUNFLOWER, SOYBEAN, AND/OR CANOLA), SALT, DEXTROSE, DISODIUM DIHYDROGEN PYROPHOSPHATE, ANNATTO (VEGETABLE COLOUR).

Onion Rings

INGREDIENTS: ONIONS, BLEACHED WHEAT FLOUR, SOYBEAN OIL AND/OR CANOLA OIL, YELLOW CORN FLOUR, SUGAR, SALT, SOY FLOUR, WHEY, DEXTROSE, LEAVENING (MONOCALCIUM PHOSPHATE, SODIUM BICARBONATE), YEAST, POLYSORBATE 80, CALCIUM PROPIONATE (PRESERVATIVE).

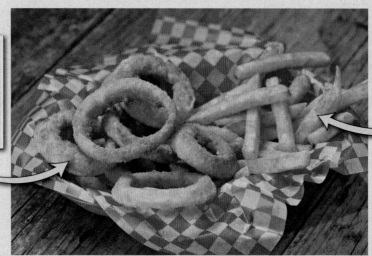

©iStockphoto.com/DebbiSmirnoff

Digestive System Problems and Discomforts

Almost everyone experiences digestive system problems from time to time. These problems often cause discomfort and frequently limit the types of foods that can be consumed (**Figure 3.13a**). Digestive system problems can also interfere with nutrient digestion and absorption. Problems may occur anywhere in the digestive tract, from the mouth to the anus, and can affect the accessory organs that provide the secretions that are essential for proper GI function.

Heartburn and GERD

Heartburn occurs when the acidic contents of the stomach leak back past the lower esophageal sphincter into the esophagus (**Figure 3.13b**).

> **heartburn** A burning sensation in the middle chest caused when acidic stomach contents leak back into the esophagus.
>
> **gastroesophageal reflux disease (GERD)** A chronic condition in which acidic stomach contents leak into the esophagus, causing pain and damaging the esophagus.
>
> **peptic ulcers** Open sores in the lining of the stomach, esophagus, or upper small intestine.

Heartburn has nothing to do with the heart, but this term relates to the proximity of the esophagus to the heart, where some believe the discomfort originates. The medical term for the leakage of stomach contents into the esophagus is *gastroesophageal reflux*, also commonly known as acid reflux. Occasional heartburn is common, but if it occurs more than twice a week, it may indicate a condition called **gastroesophageal reflux disease (GERD)**. If left untreated, GERD can eventually lead to more serious health problems, such as bleeding, ulcers, and cancer.

The discomforts of heartburn and GERD can be avoided by limiting the amounts and types of foods consumed. Eating small meals and consuming beverages between meals rather than with meals prevents heartburn by reducing the volume of material in the stomach. Symptoms can be minimized by avoiding fatty and fried foods, chocolate, peppermint, and caffeinated beverages, which increase stomach acidity or slow stomach emptying. Other behaviours that are helpful for preventing heartburn include remaining upright after eating, wearing loose clothing, avoiding smoking and alcohol, and losing weight. For many people, medications that neutralize acid or reduce acid secretion are needed to manage symptoms.

Peptic ulcers

Peptic ulcers occur when the mucus barrier protecting the stomach, esophagus, or upper small intestine is penetrated and the acid and pepsin in digestive secretions damage the gastrointestinal lining (**Figure 3.13c**). Mild ulcers cause abdominal pain; more severe ulcers can cause life-threatening bleeding.

Peptic ulcers can result from GERD or from misuse of medications such as acetylsalicylic acid (Aspirin) or non-steroidal anti-inflammatory drugs (Motrin, Advil) but are more often caused by infection with the bacterium *Helicobacter pylori* (*H. pylori*). These bacteria burrow into the mucus and destroy the protective mucosal layer.[10] More than half of the world's population is infected with *H. pylori*, but not everyone who is infected develops ulcers.[11] *H. pylori* can be treated using antibiotics.

Gallstones

Clumps of solid material that accumulate in either the gallbladder or the bile duct are referred to as **gallstones** (**Figure 3.13d**). They can cause pain when the gallbladder contracts in response to fat in the intestine. Gallstones can interfere with bile secretion and reduce fat absorption. They are usually treated by removing the gallbladder. After the gallbladder has been removed, bile, which is produced in the liver, drips directly into the intestine as it is produced rather than being stored and squeezed out in large amounts when fat enters the intestine. This process compromises fat absorption.

Diarrhea, constipation, and hemorrhoids

Diarrhea, constipation, and hemorrhoids are common discomforts that are related to problems in the intestines. **Diarrhea** refers to frequent, watery stools. It occurs when material moves through the colon too quickly for sufficient water to be absorbed or when water is drawn into the lumen from cells lining the intestinal tract.

Diarrhea can be caused by bacterial or viral infections, irritants that inflame the lining of the GI tract, the passage of undigested food into the large intestine, medications, and chronic intestinal diseases. Diarrhea causes loss of fluids and minerals. Severe diarrhea lasting more than a day or two can be life-threatening.

Constipation refers to hard, dry stools that are difficult to pass; it occurs when the water content of the stool is too low. Constipation can be caused by a diet that contains insufficient fluid or fibre, lack of exercise, a weakening of the muscles of the large intestine, and a variety of medications (**Figure 3.13e**). It can be prevented by drinking plenty of fluids, consuming a high-fibre diet, and getting enough exercise (see *What Should I Eat?* and *Thinking It Through*).

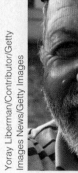

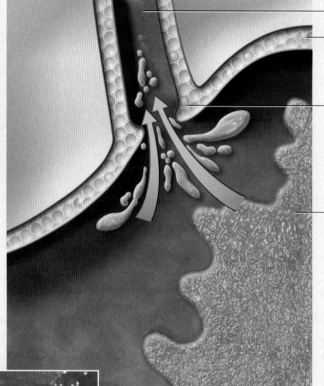

a. Tooth loss and dental pain can make chewing difficult. Poorly chewed food may not be completely digested, thereby limiting the intake of certain foods and reducing nutrient absorption. Tooth decay and gum disease are more likely when saliva production is reduced or when dental hygiene is neglected. Reduced saliva production is a side effect of many medications and can cause changes in taste and difficulty in swallowing.

Esophagus

Stomach wall

Sphincter

Acidic stomach contents

b. Heartburn and GERD occur when stomach acid leaks back through the lower esophageal sphincter and irritates the lining of the esophagus. Stomach contents also pass through this sphincter during vomiting. Vomiting may be caused by an illness, a food allergy, medication, an eating disorder, or pregnancy.

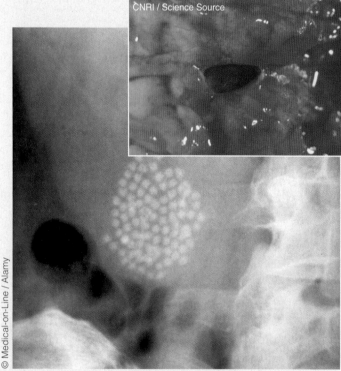

CNRI / Science Source

© Medical-on-Line / Alamy

c. Peptic ulcers occur when the mucosa is destroyed, exposing underlying tissues to gastric juices. Damage that reaches the nerve layer causes pain, and bleeding can occur if the small blood vessels of the mucosa are damaged. If the stomach or esophagus wall is perforated because of an ulcer, a serious abdominal infection can occur.

e. Constipation, in which the feces are hard and dry, is often due to a diet that is too low in fibre and fluids. It increases pressure in the colon and can lead to outpouches in the colon wall, shown here, called diverticula (discussed further in Chapter 4).

Colon wall

Dr. Larpent / CNRI / Science Source

Diverticula

d. Gallstones, visible in this image of the abdomen, are deposits of cholesterol, bile pigments, and calcium in the gallbladder or the bile duct. They can block bile from entering the small intestine, causing pain when the gallbladder contracts and reducing fat digestion and absorption.

Frequent episodes of diarrhea and constipation can irritate the blood vessels that surround the anal canal, leading to a condition commonly referred to as **hemorrhoids**.

This condition can lead to pain or bleeding in the anus, especially when trying to excrete feces.

THINKING IT THROUGH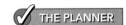

How Do Changes in the GI Tract Affect Health?

Kara is a registered dietitian. Patients often approach her to ask about their gastrointestinal problems. For each patient described here, think about how their digestion and absorption of nutrients are affected and the consequences for their nutritional health.

A 50-year-old man is taking medication that reduces the amount of saliva he produces.

What effect might this side effect of medication have on his nutrition and health?

▼

Your answer: _____

_____

An 80-year-old woman who wears poorly fitting dentures likes raw carrots but can't chew them thoroughly.

How might her poorly fitting dentures affect the digestion and absorption of nutrients contained in the carrots?

▼

Your answer: _____

_____

A 47-year-old woman undergoes treatment for colon cancer, which requires that most of her large intestine be surgically removed.

How does this surgery affect the amount of fluid she needs to consume?

▼

Your answer: _____

_____

A 56-year-old man has gallstones, which cause pain when his gallbladder contracts.

What foods should he avoid and why?

▼

Your answer: _____

_____

A 40-year-old woman weighing 160 kg (350 lb.) has undergone a surgical procedure called gastric bypass. The diagram shows how her stomach and small intestine were altered.

Why can't she eat as much food as before or absorb all the nutrients from the food she eats?

▼

Your answer: _____

_____

(Check your answers in Appendix I.)

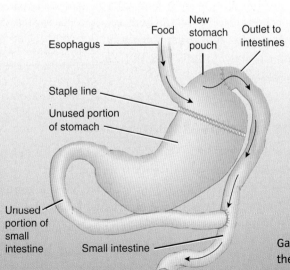

Gastric bypass surgery involves stapling off the top portion of the stomach and attaching it directly to the small intestine.

WHAT SHOULD I EAT?
For Digestive Health

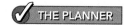

Reduce the chances of heartburn
- Eat enough to satisfy your hunger but not so much that you are stuffed.
- Wait 10 minutes between your first and second courses to see how full you feel.
- Stay upright after you eat—don't flop on the couch in front of the television.
- Avoid overconsumption of caffeine, chocolate, peppermint, and fatty foods, all of which may provoke the problem.

Avoid constipation by consuming enough fibre and fluid
- Choose whole-grain cereals such as oatmeal or raisin bran.
- Double your servings of vegetables at dinner.
- Eat two pieces of fruit with your lunch.
- Choose whole-grain bread.
- Drink one or two beverages with or before each meal.

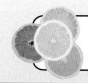

Use iProfile to find the fibre content of your favourite fruits and vegetables.

CONCEPT CHECK	STOP

1. **Why** is the immune function of the GI tract so important?

2. **How** can food allergy symptoms be prevented?

3. **What** foods should be avoided by people with heartburn? By people with gallstones?

4. **When** can ulcers be treated with antibiotics?

Delivering Nutrients and Eliminating Wastes

LEARNING OBJECTIVES

1. **Trace** the path of blood circulation.

2. **Discuss** how blood flow is affected by eating and activity.

3. **Explain** the functions of the lymphatic system.

4. **List** four ways that waste products are eliminated from the body.

After food has been digested and the nutrients absorbed, the nutrients must be delivered to the cells. This delivery is handled by the **cardiovascular system**, which consists of the heart and blood vessels. **Capillaries** in the villi of the small intestine absorb amino acids from protein, single sugars from carbohydrate, and small products of fat digestion, which are then transported via the blood to the liver (see Figure 3.9b). The products of digestion that are too large, such as cholesterol and large fatty acids, are absorbed into **lacteals**, which are part of the **lymphatic system**, and then eventually drain into the blood.

lacteals Lymph vessels in the villi of the small intestine that pick up particles containing the larger products of fat digestion.

capillaries Small, thin-walled blood vessels through which blood and the body's cells exchange gases and nutrients.

The Cardiovascular System

The cardiovascular system circulates blood throughout the body. Blood carries nutrients from the foods we consume and oxygen from the air we breathe to the body cells where the nutrients and oxygen are required. Blood also removes carbon dioxide and other waste products from these body cells. Other substances, such as hormones, are moved by the blood from one part of the body to another.

Blood circulation • Figure 3.14

Blood pumped to the lungs picks up oxygen and delivers nutrients. Blood pumped to the rest of the body delivers oxygen and nutrients.

① Oxygen-poor blood that reaches the heart from the rest of the body is pumped through the arteries to the capillaries of the lungs.

② In the capillaries of the lungs, oxygen from inhaled air is picked up by the blood, and carbon dioxide is released into the lungs and exhaled.

③ Oxygen-rich blood returns to the heart from the lungs via veins.

④ Oxygen-rich blood is pumped out of the heart into the arteries that lead to the rest of the body.

⑤ In the capillaries of the body, nutrients and oxygen move from the blood to the body's tissues, and carbon dioxide and other waste products move from the tissues to the blood, to be carried away.

⑥ Oxygen-poor blood returns to the heart via veins.

⑦ The hepatic portal circulation delivers small, water-soluble nutrients to the liver. These substances are first absorbed into the capillaries of the villi and eventually drain into the hepatic portal vein, which moves absorbed nutrients into the liver.

⑧ Absorbed nutrients that are in transit to the rest of the body are filtered by the liver and then drain into a vein close to the heart.

⑨ Larger nutrients that cannot pass into the blood are absorbed into the lymphatic system via lacteals. These nutrients bypass liver filtration en route to direct deposition into the blood stream.

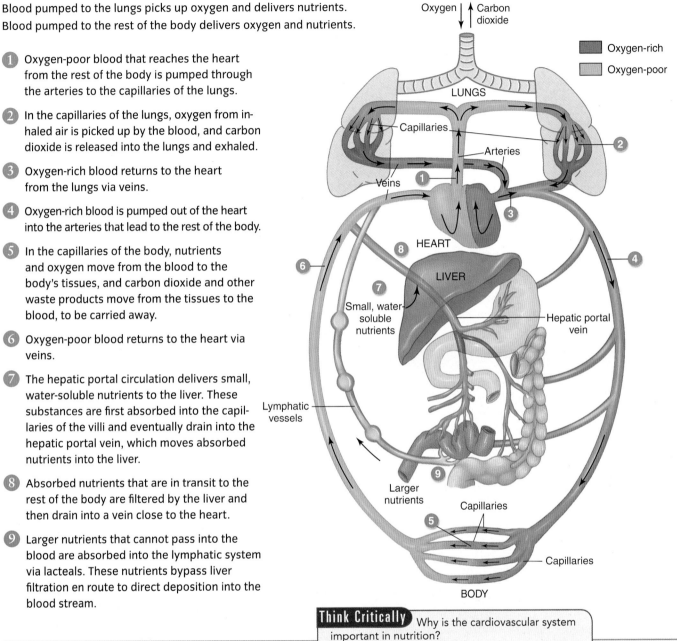

Think Critically Why is the cardiovascular system important in nutrition?

The heart is the workhorse of the cardiovascular system. It is a muscular pump with two circulatory loops—one that carries blood to and from the lungs and one that carries blood to and from the rest of the body (**Figure 3.14**).

The blood vessels that transport blood and dissolved substances toward the heart are called **veins**, and those that transport blood and dissolved substances away from the heart are called **arteries**. As arteries carry blood away from the heart, they branch many times to form smaller and smaller blood vessels. The smallest arteries are called **arterioles**. Arterioles branch to form capillaries. Blood from capillaries then flows into the smallest veins, the **venules**, which converge to form larger and larger veins for returning blood to the heart.

The exchange of nutrients and gases occurs across the thin walls of the capillaries. In most body tissues, oxygen and nutrients carried by the blood pass from the capillaries into the cells, and carbon dioxide and other waste products pass from the cells into the capillaries. In the capillaries of the lungs, blood releases carbon dioxide to be exhaled and picks up oxygen to be delivered to the cells. In the capillaries of the GI tract, blood delivers oxygen and picks up water-soluble nutrients absorbed from the diet then delivers them to the liver for filtration before sending the remaining nutrients to the rest of the body.

The amount of blood, and hence the amounts of nutrients and oxygen, delivered to a specific organ or tissue depends on the need. When you are resting, about 25% of your blood goes to your digestive system, about 20% to your skeletal muscles, and the rest to the heart, kidneys, brain, skin, and other organs.[12] This distribution changes when you eat or exercise. When you have eaten a large meal, a greater proportion of your blood goes to your digestive system to provide the oxygen and nutrients needed by the GI muscles and glands for digestion of the meal and absorption of nutrients. When you are exercising strenuously, about 70% of your blood is directed to your skeletal muscles to deliver nutrients and oxygen and remove carbon dioxide and other waste products (**Figure 3.15**).

Blood flow at rest and during exercise • Figure 3.15

a. At rest between meals, the amount of blood directed to the abdomen, which includes the organs, muscles, and glands of the digestive system, is similar to the amount that goes to the skeletal muscles.[12]

b. During exercise, the demands of the muscles take priority, and only a small proportion of the blood is directed to the abdomen.[12] This distribution of blood flow explains why you may get cramps if you exercise right after eating a big meal: Your body cannot direct enough blood to both the intestines and the muscles at the same time. The muscles win out, and food remains in your intestines, where it can lead to cramps.

© Can Stock Photo Inc. / Paha_L

© Can Stock Photo Inc. / colorcarnival

Abdomen

Skeletal muscles

Other organs

Distribution of blood flow at rest

Distribution of blood flow during exercise

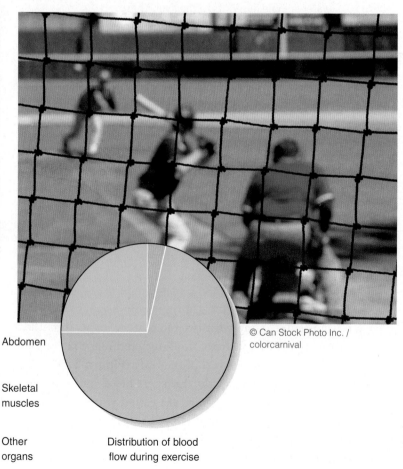

The Hepatic Portal System: Delivering Nutrients to the Liver for Filtration

Water-soluble molecules in the small intestine, including amino acids, sugars, water-soluble vitamins, and the water-soluble products of fat digestion, cross the mucosal cells of the villi and enter the capillaries (see Figure 3.10). Once in the capillaries, these absorbed nutrients first travel to the liver via the **hepatic portal vein** (see Figure 3.14).

The liver acts as a gatekeeper between the body and substances absorbed from the intestine. It decides what to do with the nutrients that have been absorbed. Some nutrients are stored in the liver, some are changed into different forms, and others are allowed to pass through unchanged. Depending on the body's needs, the liver determines whether individual nutrients are stored or delivered immediately to the cells. The liver is also important in the synthesis and breakdown of amino acids, proteins, and lipids. It modifies the products of protein breakdown to form molecules that can be safely transported to the kidney for excretion. The liver also helps detoxify substances absorbed from the intestines that could potentially harm the body, such as alcohol, through the action of various enzymes.

Organ systems involved in elimination of wastes • Figure 3.16

Both the nutrients taken in by the digestive system and the oxygen taken in by the respiratory system are distributed to all the cells in the body by the circulatory system. Unabsorbed materials are eliminated in the feces. Metabolic wastes found in the blood are transferred to the outside environment by the skin and the urinary and respiratory systems.

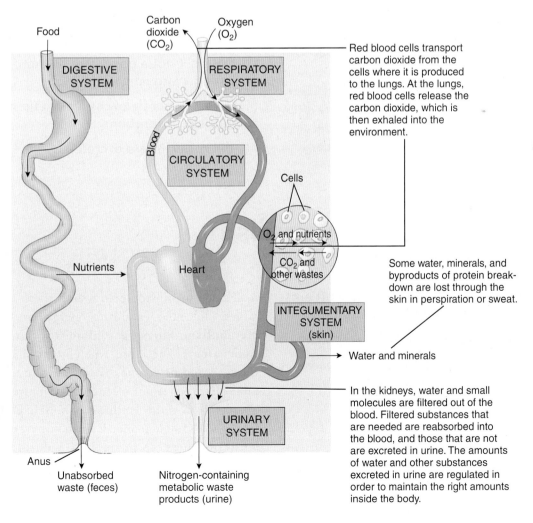

EXTERNAL ENVIRONMENT

Food

Carbon dioxide (CO_2)

Oxygen (O_2)

DIGESTIVE SYSTEM

RESPIRATORY SYSTEM

Blood

CIRCULATORY SYSTEM

Cells

Red blood cells transport carbon dioxide from the cells where it is produced to the lungs. At the lungs, red blood cells release the carbon dioxide, which is then exhaled into the environment.

O_2 and nutrients

CO_2 and other wastes

Nutrients

Heart

Some water, minerals, and byproducts of protein breakdown are lost through the skin in perspiration or sweat.

INTEGUMENTARY SYSTEM (skin)

Water and minerals

In the kidneys, water and small molecules are filtered out of the blood. Filtered substances that are needed are reabsorbed into the blood, and those that are not are excreted in urine. The amounts of water and other substances excreted in urine are regulated in order to maintain the right amounts inside the body.

URINARY SYSTEM

Anus

Unabsorbed waste (feces)

Nitrogen-containing metabolic waste products (urine)

The Lymphatic System

The lymphatic system is a circulatory system in the body that is less intricate than the cardiovascular system. It consists of a network of tubules (lymph vessels) and lymph organs that contain infection-fighting cells. In addition to its immune function, the lymphatic system contributes to the absorption of fat and drains fluid that could potentially build up at the tissues, thereby preventing swelling.

The lymphatic system is an important part of the immune system. Fluid collected in the lymph vessels is filtered past a collection of infection-fighting cells before being returned to the blood. If some of these cells detect an antigen, an immune response is triggered. White blood cells and antibodies produced by this response enter the blood and help destroy the foreign substance.

Since they do not dissolve in water, fat-soluble substances such as cholesterol, fatty acids, and fat-soluble vitamins cannot be absorbed directly into the blood. Once they have been packaged into a transporter, the lymph system assumes the responsibility of absorbing and transporting these substances, which are now too large to enter the blood stream (see Figure 3.14). They pass from the intestinal mucosa into the lacteals located in the villi (see Figure 3.9b). The lacteals drain into larger lymph vessels. Lymph vessels from the intestine and most other organs drain into the thoracic duct, which empties into the blood near the neck. Therefore, unlike the products of protein and carbohydrate digestion, which are absorbed into the blood stream, substances absorbed into the lymphatic system are not first filtered by the liver before entering the general blood circulation.

Elimination of Wastes

Material that is not absorbed from the gut into the body is eliminated from the gastrointestinal tract in the feces. Wastes that are generated in the body, such as carbon dioxide, minerals, and nitrogen-containing wastes, must also be eliminated and are done so at one of three sites: the lungs, the skin, or the kidneys. Carbon dioxide and some water are lost via the lungs, whereas water, minerals, and nitrogen-containing wastes are lost through the skin, but the kidney is the primary site for the excretion of metabolic wastes. As blood passes through the kidneys, it filters out some water, minerals, and the nitrogen-containing by-products of protein breakdown to be excreted in urine. **Figure 3.16** illustrates the circulatory system's role in both the delivery of nutrients and oxygen and the elimination of wastes.

CONCEPT CHECK 🛑 STOP

1. **Where** does blood go after it leaves the lungs?

2. **Why** is it not a good idea to exercise after eating a large meal?

3. **What** is the role of the lymphatic system in nutrient absorption?

4. **What** wastes are excreted by the kidney? The lungs?

An Overview of Metabolism

LEARNING OBJECTIVES

1. **Discuss** the two general ways in which nutrients can be used after they have been absorbed.

2. **Describe** what happens in cellular respiration.

3. **List** the types of molecules that can be made from glucose, from fatty acids, and from amino acids.

Once nutrients are inside the body's cells, they are used either for energy or to synthesize all the structural and regulatory molecules needed for growth and maintenance. Together, the chemical reactions that break down molecules to provide energy and those that synthesize larger molecules requiring energy are referred to as **metabolism**. Energy is contained within the bonds between atoms. Therefore, when larger molecules are synthesized and new bonds are formed, in a process called **anabolism**, an input of energy is required. An example of anabolism is the synthesis of muscle protein from the amino acids found in blood. Anabolism requires, and thus burns up, energy in the process, reducing the likelihood for energy storage as fat. Conversely, when molecules are broken down, such as when we break down nutrients absorbed from our meals at our cells, energy is released.

This breakdown of molecules is called **catabolism.** Unfortunately, if too many energy-yielding nutrients are ingested, our body will only use the energy it requires, and may store excesses as fat tissue. Many of the reactions of metabolism occur in series known as **metabolic pathways.** Molecules that enter these pathways are modified at each step with the help of enzymes. Reactions that synthesize molecules occur in different cellular compartments from those that break down molecules for energy. For example, ribosomes are cellular structures that specialize in the synthesis of proteins, and **mitochondria** are cell organs that are responsible for breaking down molecules to release energy.

Releasing Energy

After glucose, fatty acids, and amino acids (derived from carbohydrates, fats, and proteins, respectively), arrive at the tissues, they can then help to fuel the energy needs of the cell. Even though these nutrients have lots of energy

> **ATP (adenosine triphosphate)**
> A high-energy molecule that the body uses to power activities that require energy.

trapped within their bonds, our cells cannot easily extract this energy for use as is. The main energy form that our body *can* readily use is called **adenosine triphosphate (ATP)** (**Figure 3.17**). The energy trapped within the bonds of these energy-yielding nutrients must first be transferred to the high-energy bonds of ATP before it can be used.

In the most common pathway that produces ATP, glucose is broken down with the help of oxygen. As the bonds between glucose are broken down through a complex series of reactions, the energy trapped between its bonds is released and eventually captured as ATP (**Figure 3.18**). This process produces two waste products: water and carbon dioxide, which then enter the blood stream to be excreted. This overall process is called **cellular respiration** and occurs primarily in the mitochondria of the cell. It is summarized in the following formula:

$$C_6H_{12}O_6 \ + \ 6O_2 \ = \ 6H_2O \ + \ 6CO_2 \ + \ ATP$$

Glucose + Oxygen = Water + Carbon + Energy
Dioxide

Cells with higher energy demands have more mitochondria. When your muscle cells are challenged through physical activity, they adapt to become more efficient by

ATP is the main energy currency of the cell. It has two high energy bonds between phosphate molecules. When one of the phosphate groups is broken off of ATP, energy is released and this released energy can be used immediately to fuel the energy demands of the cell. The remaining products are ADP and a phosphate group. If energy is released elsewhere in the cell, it can be used to create another high-energy bond between the remaining ADP and a phosphate group, creating another molecule of ATP.

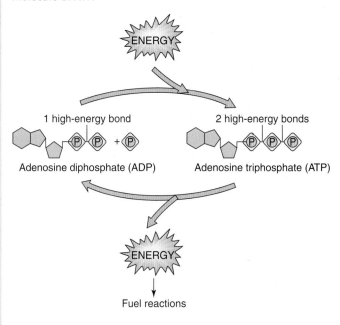

increasing the number of mitochondria they have. This increase in mitochondria enhances the muscle cells' ability to break down nutrients for ATP, thus increasing the natural energy expenditure of the body!

Extracting Energy from Glucose

Since our cells cannot directly use the energy found in glucose to fuel processes, great efforts are made to ensure that the energy found in glucose is converted into a form our cells can use, typically ATP. Two very important molecules, NAD+ and FAD, participate in this process by accepting electrons at different points to become NADH + H^+ and $FADH_2$, respectively. They then shuttle these electrons to the final step, the electron transport chain, where they can be used to generate ATP.

Step 1: Glycolysis Glycolysis is the breakdown of glucose and is the only metabolic pathway in this series that occurs in the cytoplasm of the cell. Because the breakdown of glucose does not require oxygen, it is termed an **anaerobic**

Extracting energy from glucose, fats, and amino acids • Figure 3.18

To form ATP, glucose needs to be catabolized through a complex series of reactions that leads to the production of more than 30 molecules of this energy currency. Fats and amino acids can also be used to produce ATP, by entering the same metabolic pathway glucose undergoes at varying points. The point at which these nutrients enter the pathway depends on the specific fat component or amino acid.

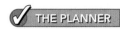
THE PLANNER

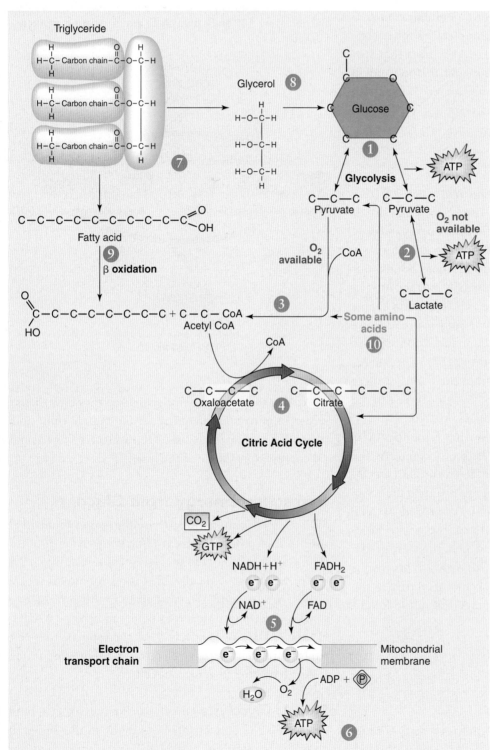

Extracting Energy from Glucose

1. Glucose is first broken down into two molecules of pyruvate; a small amount of ATP is produced.

2. If oxygen is not available, pyruvate is then converted into lactate; a small amount of ATP is produced. When oxygen becomes available again, lactate is converted back into pyruvate.

3. If oxygen is available, pyruvate is converted into acetyl coA, following an input of coenzyme A.

4. Acetyl coA then enters the citric acid cycle, where a main outcome is the capture of electrons by $FADH_2$ and $NADH + H^+$.

5. These electron transporters then carry electrons to the mitochondrial membrane, where a series of oxidation and reduction reactions occur.

6. The energy released during the electron transport chain is captured within more than 30 molecules of ATP.

Extracting Energy from Fat

7. A triglyceride molecule is first broken down into glycerol and three fatty acids.

8. The glycerol molecule can be converted into glucose, which then proceeds through steps 1-6.

9. The fatty acid molecule is broken down, bit by bit, into two carbon molecules by the process of beta-oxidation. These two-carbon molecules can then be used to form acetyl coA, which proceeds through steps 4-6.

Extracting Energy from Amino Acids

10. Before amino acids can enter cellular respiration, they need to have their nitrogen group removed. The remaining skeleton can be used to form either pyruvate, acetyl coA, or a citric acid cycle intermediate, and proceeds through the appropriate remaining steps of cellular respiration.

process. During glycolysis, a six-carbon glucose molecule is broken down into two molecules of the three-carbon pyruvate. This process leads to the production of ATP, but it is minimal. Also, because an initial input of energy is required for the process to occur, the total amount of energy produced is insufficient to fuel all the various reactions in our cells. Pyruvate therefore undergoes further catabolism to produce more ATP.

Step 2: The Breakdown of Pyruvate

What happens next to pyruvate depends on the amount of oxygen available in the cells.

(a) The aerobic breakdown of pyruvate: During periods of low energy demand or during rhythmic, repetitive activities such as running, your body can effectively time the maximal oxygen delivery to match your cellular needs. This oxygen can then be used to convert pyruvate to a molecule called acetyl CoA. This process requires coenzyme A, which is derived from vitamin B5, pantothenic acid. This process is not reversible.

(b) The anaerobic breakdown of pyruvate: Although the above process is preferred by your cells, in the first couple of minutes after exercising begins or when activity is very intense such as intense weightlifting, your body cannot perfectly match its oxygen needs with oxygen delivery. Your cells therefore need to employ another strategy to break down pyruvate to form ATP: anaerobic metabolism. In this reaction, pyruvate is converted into a molecule called **lactate** without the use of oxygen. Although this process results in a net production of ATP, the level of ATP is too low to sustain longer activities. This condition is also unsustainable because the buildup of lactate promotes an acidic environment in the tissues. The burning sensation sometimes experienced during intense activities is due to this acidic environment. Luckily, the conversion of pyruvate to lactate is reversible, so if oxygen becomes available again, lactate can be converted back into pyruvate, then to acetyl CoA and proceed to the next step in the series: the citric acid cycle.

Step 3: The Citric Acid Cycle

Acetyl CoA next enters a very involved set of reactions called the citric acid cycle (also known as Kreb's cycle or the Tricarboxylic acid, or TCA, cycle). In the first step, acetyl CoA combines with a four-carbon sugar called **oxaloacetate** to form the six-carbon sugar **citrate** (from where the cycle gets its name). Citrate then proceeds through a complex set of reactions during which bonds between molecules and atoms are both formed and broken, leading to a net release of energy and electrons. This energy is captured as GTP, a molecule similar in structure and function to ATP, and the electrons are captured to form NADH + H$^+$ or FADH$_2$, which will be used to synthesize ATP in the next and final step.

Step 4: The Electron Transport Chain

During the final step, the electron carriers, NADH + H$^+$ and FADH$_2$, proceed to the inner mitochondrial membrane where they donate their electrons at different stages to drive the **electron transport chain (ETC)**. In the ETC, a set of oxidation reactions (i.e., the loss of electrons) and reduction reactions (i.e., the gain of electrons) shuttle electrons across several donor and acceptor molecules. As this process occurs, energy is released, which is finally captured by more than 30 molecules of ATP. This step completes the process of converting glucose (food energy) into ATP (chemical energy our cells can use). The cells now have the energy they require to drive their various active reactions.

Extracting Energy from Fat

Fats can also be converted into ATP, but they first need to be broken down into their two parts: glycerol and fatty acids (see Figure 3.18). Glycerol can then be converted into glucose and proceed through the following steps. Fatty acids contain the bulk of the energy from fat. To enter the process of cellular respiration, these multi-carbon structures first need to be broken down into two-carbon structures. This step is accomplished through the process of **beta-oxidation**, which requires oxygen and Coenzyme A to produce the two-carbon molecule acetyl CoA. Acetyl CoA can then enter step 3: the citric acid cycle. Canadian diets are typically high in 18-carbon fatty acids, which can accordingly be converted into nine two-carbon molecules of acetyl CoA.

An important side note to this process is that carbohydrates are needed so that our cells can extract energy from fat. Although cells can produce acetyl CoA from fatty acids, before acetyl CoA can proceed through the citric acid cycle, it must first combine with oxaloacetate, a carbohydrate. This process explains why it is said that "fat burns in a carbohydrate flame." If a diet is deficient in carbohydrates, as a result of either starvation or an extremely low-carbohydrate diet, the incomplete metabolism of fatty acids produces molecules called **ketone bodies**. Ketone bodies can be used for fuel in the heart and the brain, but their acidic nature may lower the pH of the blood.

Extracting Energy from Protein

As you will learn in Chapter 6, our body prefers to use absorbed amino acids not for energy but to construct body proteins such as hormones, enzymes, and muscle protein. Energy can be extracted from amino acids, but it is a wasteful process and is not the preferred energy-producing pathway of the cell. Nevertheless, even at rest, a small proportion of the ATP we generate comes from protein. Unlike glucose and fatty acids, amino acids contain nitrogen, which first needs to be removed through the process of **deamination** before it can proceed through the above pathways.

There are 20 different amino acids, which can enter the breakdown pathway at different points, depending on their unique structure. They can be used to form either pyruvate, acetyl CoA, citric acid cycle intermediates, or ketone bodies.

Synthesizing New Molecules

Glucose, fatty acids, and amino acids that are not broken down for energy are used, with the input of energy from ATP, to synthesize structural, regulatory, or storage molecules. Glucose molecules are used to synthesize the glucose-storage molecule glycogen, which is a small energy reserve located in muscle and liver tissue. Excess carbohydrates may also be used to synthesize fatty acids and stored as fat, but this synthesis is a minor process. Excess fatty acids are used to make cell membranes and regulatory molecules, but are mostly used to create body fat. This function does not mean that dietary fat consumption is entirely responsible for increasing unwanted fat stores in the body. If fats are consumed within your total energy needs, they will not be converted to body fats. If your total energy consumption from *all three* sources is greater than your needs, then your body will preferentially use glucose for required energy and will convert the now immediately unnecessary fatty acids into body fat, intended for future energy needs. Amino acids are used to synthesize the various proteins that the body needs and, when necessary, to make glucose. Excess amino acids can also be converted into fatty acids and stored as body fat if total caloric intake exceeds body needs.

CONCEPT CHECK STOP

1. **How** are nutrients used to produce ATP?

2. **Why** can cellular respiration be thought of as cell breathing?

3. **What** types of molecules can be made from amino acids?

Summary

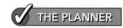 THE PLANNER

1 The Organization of Life 60

- Our bodies and the foods we eat are all made from the same building blocks—**atoms**. Atoms are linked together by chemical bonds to form **molecules**. Molecules can form **cells**, the basic unit of life. Cells with similar structures and functions are organized into **tissues**, and tissues are organized into the **organs** and **organ systems** that make up an organism. The 11 body organ systems work together; the passage of food through the digestive system and the secretion of digestive substances and various **hormones** are regulated by the nervous and endocrine systems.

From atoms to organisms • Figure 3.1

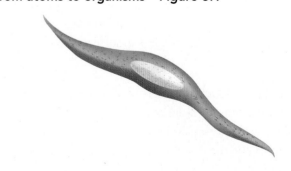

2 The Digestive System 62

- The digestive system has two major functions: **digestion** and **absorption**. Digestion breaks down food and nutrients into units that are small enough to be absorbed. Absorption transports nutrients into the body. Food substances that are not absorbed are packaged into **feces** for elimination.

- The main component of the digestive system is the **gastrointestinal tract**, which consists of a hollow tube that begins at the mouth and continues through the pharynx, esophagus, stomach, small intestine, and large intestine, ending at the anus. The walls of this tube contain a layer called the **mucosa**. **Mucosal cells** secrete molecules into the **lumen**, the centre of the tube, to aid digestion. Accessory organs outside the gastrointestinal tract, such as the pancreas, liver, gallbladder, and various glands, also participate in digestion and absorption by producing and/or secreting molecules that aid in digestion and absorption once secreted into the GI tract. They can all affect the total **transit time** through the digestive tract.

- The digestion of food and absorption of nutrients are aided by the secretion of **mucus** and **enzymes**. Enzymes can catalyze **condensation** and **hydrolysis** reactions. In hydrolysis, an input of water helps break a larger molecule into a smaller one. During condensation, two smaller molecules come together to form a larger molecule and water is released.

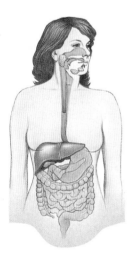

Structure of the digestive system • Figure 3.2

3 Digestion and Absorption of Nutrients 65

- The processes involved in digestion begin in response to the smell or sight of food and continue as food enters the digestive tract at the mouth. Here, food is broken down into smaller pieces by the teeth during the process of **mechanical digestion** and mixed with **saliva** to promote **chemical digestion**. Carbohydrate digestion is begun in the mouth by **salivary amylase**.

- From the mouth, the combination of chewed food mixed with saliva, called the **bolus**, passes through the **pharynx** and into the esophagus. The **epiglottis** ensures that swallowed food passes into the esophagus and not into the windpipe, where it can cause choking.

- The rhythmic contractions of **peristalsis** propel the bolus down the esophagus to the stomach. The **sphincters** found throughout the digestive tract have circular muscle that allows them to open and close and regulate movement from one segment of the tract to another. For instance, the **lower esophageal sphincter** closes so the acidic contents of the stomach don't enter into the esophagus.

- The stomach is a temporary storage site for food. The muscles of the stomach mix the food into a semiliquid mass called **chyme**, and **gastric juice**, which contains hydrochloric acid and **pepsin**, begins the digestion of protein. The rate at which the stomach empties varies with the amount and composition of food consumed and is regulated by nervous and hormonal signals.

- The small intestine is the primary site for nutrient digestion and absorption. The structural features of the small intestine, such as the **villi** and **microvilli**, ensure a large absorptive surface area. **Segmentation** is a type of movement that helps mix luminal contents together to promote digestion. In the small intestine, **bicarbonate** from the pancreas neutralizes stomach acid, and **pancreatic juices** containing **pancreatic amylase, proteases, and lipases** digest carbohydrate, fat, and protein. **Brush border** enzymes secreted from the intestinal walls further promote digestion. The digestion and absorption of fat in the small intestine are aided by **bile** from the gallbladder. Larger fat molecules are first packaged, and then absorbed into **lacteals** for transport.

- The absorption of food across the intestinal mucosa occurs by means of several different transport mechanisms. **Simple diffusion** and **facilitated diffusion** are types of **diffusion** that do not require energy and move substances from an area of high concentration to an area of low concentration. **Osmosis** involves the movement of water to balance out the concentration differences of solutes. **Active transport** requires an input of energy to move substances from an area of low concentration to an area of high concentration.

- Components of chyme that are not absorbed in the small intestine pass on to the large intestine, where some water and nutrients are absorbed. The large intestine is populated by **intestinal microbiota** that digest some of the unabsorbed materials. **Probiotics** found in food are bacteria that promote healthy intestinal microbiota. **Prebiotics** further support this environment by acting as food for bacteria. These bacteria in the large intestine can digest fibre, producing small amounts of nutrients and gas. Anything that cannot be digested further in the large intestine is eliminated in the feces.

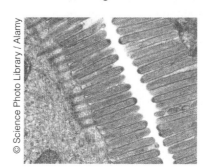

The structure of the small intestine • Figure 3.9

4 Digestion in Health and Disease 76

- Immune system cells and tissues located in the gastrointestinal tract help prevent disease-causing organisms and chemicals from entering the body. An **antigen** entering the digestive tract is attacked first by **phagocytes**. If it is not eliminated by the phagocytes, **lymphocytes** respond specifically to the antigen by producing **antibodies**. The immune system protects us from disease but can also cause **food allergies**. These allergies occur when a substance in food is recognized as an **allergen** and incorrectly triggers an immune response. **Celiac disease** is also caused by an overactive immune system, in response to the protein gluten. It can lead to severe damage of the small intestine wall.

- Diseases or discomforts at any point in the digestive system can interfere with food intake, digestion, or nutrient absorption. Common problems include tooth decay, reduced saliva production, **heartburn**, **GERD**, **peptic ulcers**, **gallstones**, vomiting, **diarrhea**, **hemorrhoids**, and **constipation**.

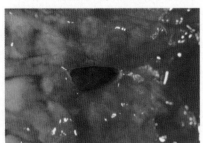

Digestive disorders
• Figure 3.13

CNRI / Science Source

5 Delivering Nutrients and Eliminating Wastes 82

- Absorbed nutrients are delivered to the cells by the **cardiovascular system**. The heart pumps blood to the lungs to pick up oxygen and release carbon dioxide. From the lungs, blood returns to the heart and is then pumped to the rest of the body to deliver oxygen and nutrients and remove carbon dioxide and other wastes before returning to the heart. Exchange of nutrients and gases occurs at the **capillaries**. The fat-soluble products of digestion enter **lacteals** in the intestinal villi. Lacteals join larger lymph vessels. The nutrients absorbed via the **lymphatic system** enter the blood without first passing through the liver.

- The cardiovascular system is a complex transport system that shuttles blood and the nutrients and wastes around the body. **Arteries** and **arterioles** transport blood away from the heart, while **veins** and **venules** transport blood toward the heart.

- The products of carbohydrate and protein digestion and the water-soluble products of fat digestion enter capillaries in the intestinal villi and are transported to the liver via the **hepatic portal vein**. The liver removes the absorbed

substances for storage, converts them into other forms, or allows them to pass unaltered. The liver also protects the body from toxic substances that may have been absorbed.

- The **lymphatic system** aids digestion through its involvement with fat absorption. It also helps the immune system defend against infections, and is involved in maintaining fluid balance.

- Unabsorbed materials are eliminated in the feces. The waste products of metabolism are excreted by the lungs, skin, and kidneys.

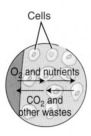

Cells

O_2 and nutrients

CO_2 and other wastes

Organ systems involved in elimination of wastes • Figure 3.16

6 An Overview of Metabolism 86

- **Metabolism** is the sum of all the chemical reactions that take place in your body. It is broken down into two subtypes: **anabolism,** which builds larger molecules, and **catabolism,** which breaks down those larger molecules. The **metabolic pathways** involved in producing usable energy in our body occur in the **mitochondria**.

- In the cells, glucose, fatty acids, and amino acids absorbed from the diet can be broken down by means of **cellular respiration** to provide energy in the form of **adenosine triphosphate (ATP)**.

- During the main pathway of cellular respiration, glucose is converted to two molecules of pyruvate, which is then converted to acetyl CoA when oxygen is present. During **anaerobic** conditions when oxygen is not present, pyruvate is converted into **lactate**. Acetyl CoA enters the citric acid cycle where it combines with **oxaloacetate** to form **citrate**. As bonds are being broken during the citric acid cycle, the electron carriers NADH+, H+, and FADH$_2$ pick up electrons and transport them to the **electron transport chain (ETC)**, where they are donated and accepted by various molecules, and energy is captured between the bonds of ATP.

- Fatty acids can undergo **beta-oxidation**, where two-carbon structures are split off one at a time from the longer fatty acid chain. These structures combine with coenzyme A to form acetyl CoA, which can enter the breakdown pathway. If the body lacks carbohydrates, the newly formed acetyl CoA cannot proceed through the citric acid cycle and is instead used to synthesize **ketone bodies**, which the heart and lungs can use as fuel.

- Amino acids must first be removed through a process of **deamination** to lose their nitrogen structures so they can be converted to ATP. The remaining carbon skeleton can then be used in the breakdown pathway at several different points, depending on its unique structure.

- In the presence of ATP, glucose, fatty acids, and amino acids can be used either to synthesize structural or regulatory molecules or to synthesize energy-storage molecules.

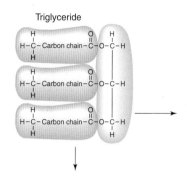

Extracting energy from glucose, fats, and amino acids • Figure 3.18

Key Terms

- absorption 62
- active transport 73
- allergen 77
- anabolism 86
- anaerobic 87
- antibodies 77
- antigen 76
- arteries 83
- arterioles 83
- atoms 60
- ATP (adenosine triphosphate) 87
- beta-oxidation 89
- bicarbonate 70
- bile 70
- bolus 66
- brush border 71
- capillaries 82
- capillary 71
- cardiovascular system 82
- catabolism 87
- celiac disease 77
- cells 60
- cellular respiration 87

- chemical digestion 66
- chyme 67
- citrate 89
- condensation 65
- constipation 79
- deamination 90
- diarrhea 79
- diffusion 73
- digestion 62
- electron transport chain (ETC) 89
- enzymes 64
- epiglottis 66
- facilitated diffusion 73
- feces 63
- food allergies 77
- gallstones 79
- gastric juice 67
- gastroesophageal reflux disease (GERD) 79
- gastrointestinal tract 63
- heartburn 79
- hemorrhoids 81
- hepatic portal vein 85

- hormones 61
- hydrolysis 65
- intestinal microbiota 74
- ketone bodies 90
- lactate 89
- lacteal 71
- lacteals 82
- lipases 70
- lower esophageal sphincter 66
- lumen 64
- lymphatic system 82
- lymphocytes 77
- mechanical digestion 66
- metabolic pathways 87
- metabolism 86
- microvilli 71
- mitochondria 87
- molecules 60
- mucosa 64
- mucosal cells 64
- mucus 64
- organ system 61
- organs 61

- osmosis 73
- oxaloacetate 89
- pancreatic amylase 70
- pancreatic juice 70
- pepsin 68
- peptic ulcers 79
- peristalsis 66
- phagocytes 77
- pharynx 66
- prebiotics 75
- probiotics 75
- proteases 70
- saliva 65
- salivary amylase 65
- segmentation 70
- simple diffusion 73
- sphincter 66
- tissues 60
- transit time 64
- veins 83
- venules 83
- villi 71

Critical and Creative Thinking Questions

1. For lunch, a student has a smoothie made with blended fruit and juice. His friend has a burger, fries, and a milkshake. Which person's stomach will empty faster? Why?

2. After reading about the benefits of a high-fibre diet, a 23-year-old man decides to double his fibre intake by taking a fibre supplement that provides 15 g of fibre. How might this dramatic increase affect the feces? How might it affect the amount of intestinal gas produced?

3. Starting in the esophagus, trace the path of food through the digestive system. At each organ, indicate anatomical adaptations of the general GI tract tube structure that enable the

functions of that organ. For example, how does the structure of the small intestine aid absorption?

4. Water is absorbed from the small intestine and colon by osmosis. What might happen to the body's water balance if a large number of small, unabsorbed molecules ended up in the colon?

5. What path does an amino acid follow from absorption to delivery to a cell? Compare this path with the path followed by a large fatty acid.

6. During your vacation, you feasted and went beyond your energy needs consuming excess carbohydrates, proteins, and fats. What is the fate of each of these molecules in the body?

What is happening in this picture?

This man's digestive tract is not working. Nutrients are being infused into his blood through a process called total parenteral nutrition (TPN).

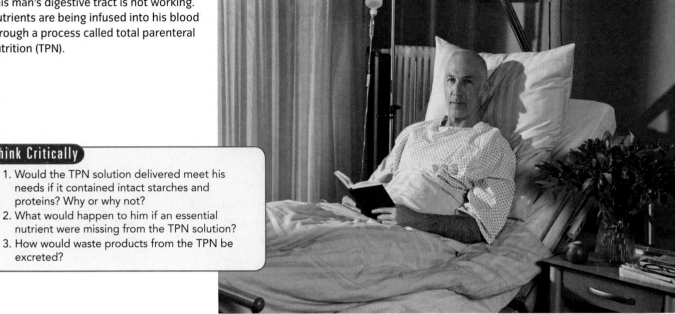

©iStockphoto.com/fStop_Images

Think Critically

1. Would the TPN solution delivered meet his needs if it contained intact starches and proteins? Why or why not?
2. What would happen to him if an essential nutrient were missing from the TPN solution?
3. How would waste products from the TPN be excreted?

Self-Test

(Check your answers in Appendix J.)

1. Which of the following is the smallest unit of life?

   a. atom   c. cell   e. organism

   b. molecule   d. tissue

2. Which of the following statements about saliva is false?

   a. It lubricates the mouth.

   b. It helps protect the teeth from decay.

   c. It moistens food so that it can be tasted and swallowed.

   d. It contains the enzyme salivary amylase.

   e. It contains the protein-digesting enzyme pepsin.

Use the diagram to answer questions 3 and 4.

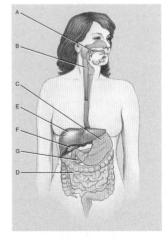

3. Which letter in this illustration points to the organ where carbohydrate digestion begins?

   a. A   b. B   c. C   d. D   e. E

4. Which letter in this illustration points to the organ where bile is stored?

   a. A   b. C   c. E   d. F   e. G

5. The tissue layer labelled C _____.

   a. secretes mucus

   b. contains nerves and blood vessels

   c. mixes and propels food through the GI tract

   d. provides external support to the gut

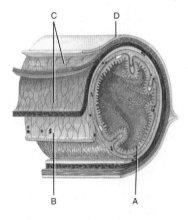

6. The _____ prevents food from entering the passageway to the lungs during swallowing.

a. gallbladder

b. pancreas

c. epiglottis

d. tongue

7. The secretion of digestive juices does not begin until food enters the mouth.

a. True

b. False

8. The rhythmic contractions that propel food through the GI tract are called _____.

a. peristalsis

b. enzymatic digestion

c. swallowing

d. gastroesophageal reflux

e. chewing

9. Which of the following is most likely to inhibit stomach secretions and stomach motility?

a. the release of gastrin

b. the smell of freshly baked cookies

c. the entry of food into the small intestine

d. the entry of food into the stomach

10. The diffusion of water across a membrane is called _____.

a. simple diffusion

b. osmosis

c. facilitated diffusion

d. active transport

11. Which of the following is not true of the microvilli?

a. They help increase the surface area available for absorption.

b. They contain digestive enzymes.

c. Each contains a capillary and a lacteal.

d. They are referred to as the brush border.

12. This diagram could represent all the following except _____.

a. heartburn

b. diarrhea

c. GERD

d. vomiting

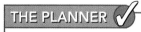

13. Which of the numbers on this illustration label blood that is rich in oxygen?

a. 1 and 2

b. 2 and 5

c. 3 and 4

d. 5 and 6

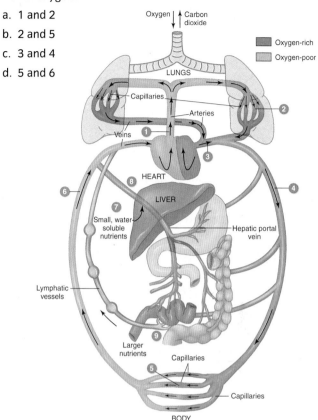

14. Most digestion and absorption occur in the _____.

a. small intestine

b. stomach

c. mouth

d. large intestine

15. All absorbed nutrients go directly to the liver.

a. True

b. False

THE PLANNER ✓

Review your Chapter Planner on the chapter opener and check off your completed work.

Carbohydrates: Sugars, Starches, and Fibres

A fragrant loaf of bread fresh from the oven, a plate of *al dente* pasta, a steaming bowl of sticky rice, piping hot noodles. What quality do these tantalizing foods share? All are important dietary basics produced from high-carbohydrate grains.

Wheat and other grains are so fundamental to the world's food supply that every culture relies on them as a readily available, inexpensive source of calories. In Canada, grains not only provide us with an essential part of our diet but they are also a fundamental component of our agricultural output. Specifically, wheat exports from Canada account for 20% of the world wheat market, and the harvesting of this grain and others is essential to the livelihood of many local farmers.

Grains such as barley, oats, corn, and wheat are important carbohydrate sources that can be transformed into noodles, tortillas, couscous, and breakfast cereals or baked into breads, cakes, crackers, and chips. We smother them with sauces; we wrap and hold them around fillings, both savoury and sweet. Carbohydrates also come from fruits, milk, and starchy vegetables, such as potatoes, peas, and beans. Altogether, carbohydrate-rich foods provide more than half the calories in the Canadian diet.

Many of us in Western societies have a love–hate relationship with carbohydrates. We're told to "carbo-load" before serious, sustained exercise, such as a marathon, yet we're admonished by health and fitness authorities to moderate our intake of carbohydrate-rich foods. Many people have come to fear carbohydrates as a cause of unwanted weight gain and other health problems. Can such a fundamental dietary staple contribute to today's chronic diseases? Or is it the *type* of carbohydrates in our diet that we should be concerned about? Can't humans and carbohydrates just learn to get along?

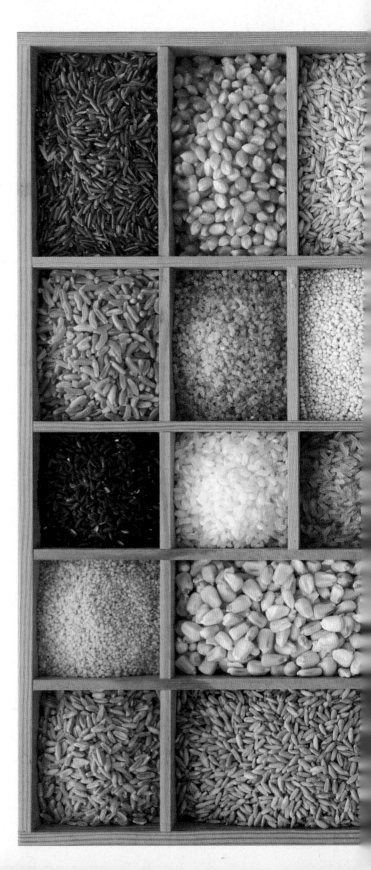

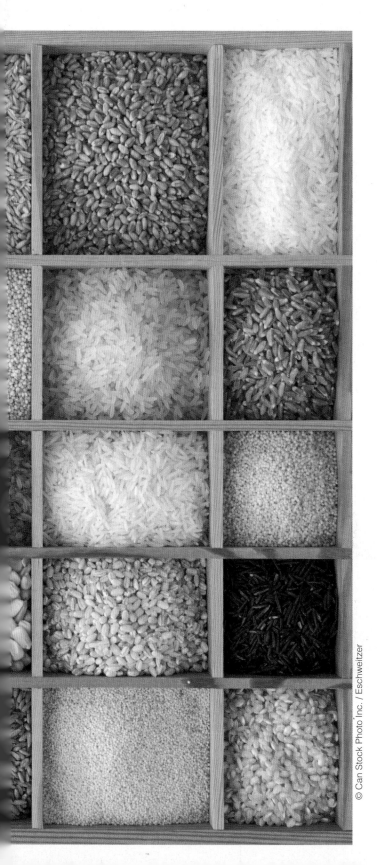

© Can Stock Photo Inc. / Eschweitzer

CHAPTER PLANNER ✓

- ❏ Stimulate your interest by reading the introduction and looking at the visual.
- ❏ Scan the Learning Objectives in each section:
  p. 98 ❏   p. 100 ❏   p. 103 ❏   p. 107 ❏   p. 110 ❏   p. 119 ❏
- ❏ Read the text and study all figures and visuals. Answer any questions.

Analyze key features
- ❏ Nutrition InSight, p. 100 ❏   p. 105 ❏
- ❏ Process Diagram, p. 104
- ❏ Hot Topic, p. 106
- ❏ Thinking It Through, p. 120
- ❏ What Should I Eat?, p. 121
- ❏ Stop: Answer the Concept Checks before you go on:
  p. 103 ❏   p. 107 ❏   p. 110 ❏   p. 118 ❏   p. 123 ❏

End of chapter
- ❏ Review the Summary and Key Terms.
- ❏ Answer the Critical and Creative Thinking Questions.
- ❏ Answer What is happening in this picture?
- ❏ Complete the Self-Test and check your answers.

Carbohydrates in Our Food

LEARNING OBJECTIVES

1. **Distinguish** refined carbohydrates from unrefined carbohydrates.

2. **Define** enrichment.

3. **Explain** how added refined sugars and naturally occurring sugars differ from each other.

Our hunter-gatherer ancestors ate very differently from the way we eat. Their diet consisted almost entirely of **unrefined foods**—foods eaten either just as they were found in nature or with only minimal processing, such as cooking. Today, we still consume some unrefined sources of carbohydrate, but many of the foods we consume are made with **refined** grains, contain added refined sugar, and often have fewer or different nutrients from those found in the original source (**Figure 4.1**).

> **refined** Refers to foods that have undergone processing to remove the coarse parts of the original food.

The world's increased consumption of refined carbohydrates over the past few decades has been implicated as one of the many causes of the current obesity epidemic and the rising incidence of chronic diseases. Recommendations for a healthy diet suggest that we select more unrefined sources of carbohydrates, including whole grains, vegetables, and fruits, and that we limit foods high in refined carbohydrates, such as candies, cookies, and sweetened beverages. So it's not so much a matter of limiting carbohydrates, but of being wise about the carbohydrates we choose to eat.

What Is a Whole Grain?

When you eat a bowl of oatmeal or a slice of whole-wheat toast, you are typically consuming a **whole-grain product**. Whole-grain products include the entire kernel of the grain: the **germ**, the **bran**, and the **endosperm** (**Figure 4.2a**). Refined grain products, such as white bread and even some brown breads, include just the endosperm. The bran and germ are discarded during refining and, along with them, fibre, phytochemicals, and some vitamins and minerals are lost. To make up some of these losses, refined grains sold in Canada are enriched. **Enrichment**, which is a type of **fortification**, adds back some, *but not all*, of the nutrients lost in processing (**Figure 4.2b**). For example, thiamin and iron are lost when grains are milled, but, through enrichment, they are later added

> **enrichment** The addition of specific amounts of thiamin, riboflavin, niacin, and iron to refined grains. Since 1998, folic acid has also been added to enriched grains.
>
> **fortification** The addition of nutrients to foods.

Unrefined and refined foods • Figure 4.1

Corn is an unrefined source of carbohydrate, but it can be refined by washing, cooking, extruding, and drying to eventually end up as cornflakes in your cereal bowl. The sugar you sprinkle on cornflakes is also a refined carbohydrate; it has been refined from sugar cane or sugar beets.

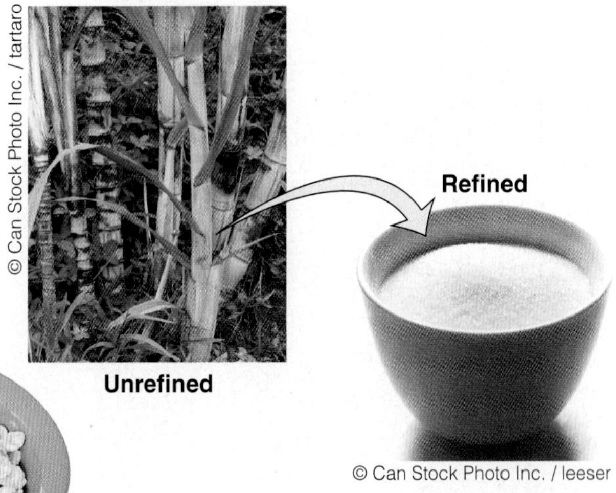

© Can Stock Photo Inc. / StephanieFrey

Unrefined

Refined

© Can Stock Photo Inc. / stepanov

© Can Stock Photo Inc. / tartaro

Unrefined

Refined

© Can Stock Photo Inc. / leeser

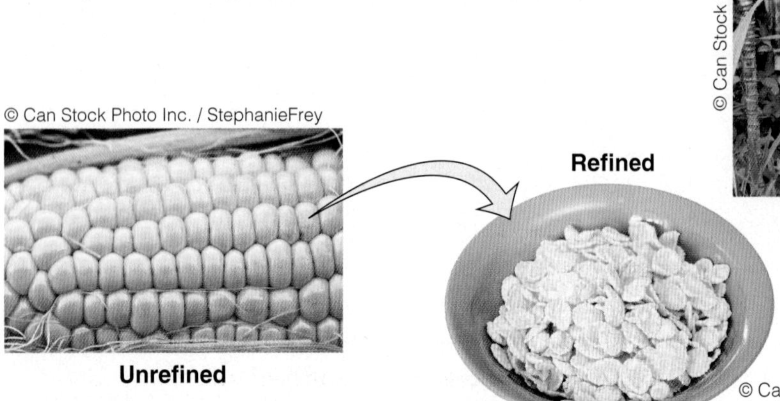

Whole grains • Figure 4.2

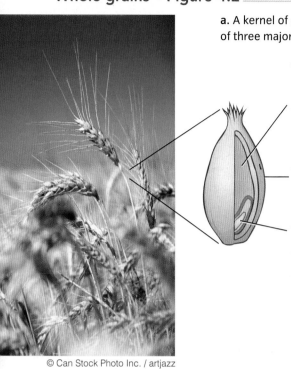
© Can Stock Photo Inc. / artjazz

a. A kernel of grain is made up of three major parts.

The **endosperm** is the largest part of the kernel. It is made up of primarily starch, but it also contains most of the kernel's protein, along with some vitamins and minerals.

The outermost **bran** layers contain most of the fibre and are a good source of many vitamins and minerals.

The **germ**, located at the base of the kernel, is the embryo where spouting occurs. It is a source of oil and is rich in vitamin E.

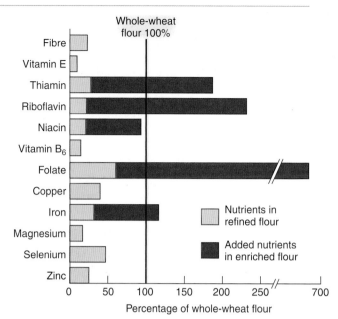

b. The amounts of many nutrients in refined flour (yellow bars) are much lower than the amounts originally present in the whole grain (100% line). In enriched flour, thiamin, riboflavin, niacin, iron, and folate have been added back in amounts that equal or exceed the original levels (red bars).

back at even higher levels. Fibre, vitamin E, and vitamin B$_6$ are also removed by milling, but they are rarely added back. Therefore, compared with foods made from whole grains, foods made with refined grains contain more of some nutrients and less of others.

What Is Added Refined Sugar?

Refined sugars are commonplace in the typical Canadian diet. Refined sugars are chemically similar to natural sugar sources, and they can be similarly used to provide energy. However, the common sources of refined sugar in Canada, such as cookies, candy, and pop, typically lack the same healthy micronutrients and phytochemicals contained in natural sources. When separated from their plant sources, refined sugars no longer comprise the same fibre, vitamins, minerals, and phytochemicals found in the original plant. They are accordingly less likely to promote health in the same way that unrefined sugar sources can and contribute **empty calories** to the diet. Foods that naturally contain sugars, such as fruits and milk, provide vitamins, minerals, and phytochemicals along with the calories from the sugar, making them higher in nutrient density (**Figure 4.3**).

empty calories
Energy with few additional nutrients.

Nutrient density • Figure 4.3

A 355-mL (12-oz) can of pop contains about 140 Calories from sugar but almost no other nutrients. Three medium kiwis also provide about 140 Calories and plenty of other nutrients, including vitamin C, folate, and calcium, making the kiwis more nutrient dense than the pop.

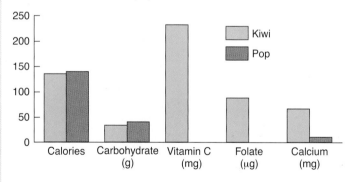

CONCEPT CHECK **STOP**

1. **What** is the difference between a whole-grain product and a product made with a refined grain?

2. **Why** are foods high in added refined sugars said to contribute empty calories?

Types of Carbohydrates

LEARNING OBJECTIVES

1. **Name** the basic unit of carbohydrate.

2. **Classify** carbohydrates as simple or complex.

3. **Describe** the types of complex carbohydrates.

4. **Distinguish** soluble fibre from insoluble fibre.

C hemically, carbohydrates are a group of compounds made up of one or more **sugar units** that contain carbon (*carbo*) as well as hydrogen and oxygen in the same two-to-one proportion found in water (*hydrate*, H_2O). A carbohydrate made up of only one sugar unit is called a **monosaccharide**,

sugar unit The smallest unit of a carbohydrate molecule.

monosaccharide A carbohydrate made up of a single sugar unit.

a carbohydrate made up of two sugar units is called a **disaccharide**, and a carbohydrate made up of more than two sugar units is called a **polysaccharide**.

disaccharide A carbohydrate made up of two sugar units.

polysaccharide A carbohydrate made up of two or more sugar units linked together.

Nutrition InSight   Carbohydrates • Figure 4.4

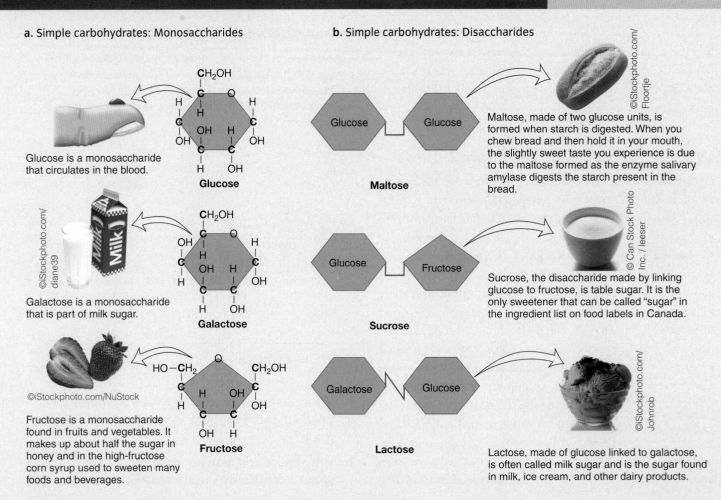

a. Simple carbohydrates: Monosaccharides

Glucose is a monosaccharide that circulates in the blood.

Glucose

Galactose is a monosaccharide that is part of milk sugar.

©iStockphoto.com/ diane39

Galactose

©iStockphoto.com/NuStock

Fructose is a monosaccharide found in fruits and vegetables. It makes up about half the sugar in honey and in the high-fructose corn syrup used to sweeten many foods and beverages.

Fructose

b. Simple carbohydrates: Disaccharides

Glucose + Glucose

Maltose

©iStockphoto.com/ Floortje

Maltose, made of two glucose units, is formed when starch is digested. When you chew bread and then hold it in your mouth, the slightly sweet taste you experience is due to the maltose formed as the enzyme salivary amylase digests the starch present in the bread.

Glucose + Fructose

Sucrose

© Can Stock Photo Inc. / leeser

Sucrose, the disaccharide made by linking glucose to fructose, is table sugar. It is the only sweetener that can be called "sugar" in the ingredient list on food labels in Canada.

Galactose + Glucose

Lactose

©iStockphoto.com/ Johnrob

Lactose, made of glucose linked to galactose, is often called milk sugar and is the sugar found in milk, ice cream, and other dairy products.

Simple Carbohydrates

Monosaccharides and disaccharides are classified as **simple carbohydrates**. The three most common monosaccharides in our diet are glucose, **fructose**, and **galactose**. Each contains six carbon, 12 hydrogen, and six oxygen atoms ($C_6H_{12}O_6$), but these three sugars differ in the arrangement of these atoms (**Figure 4.4a**). Glucose, often called *blood sugar*, is the most important carbohydrate fuel for the human body. Under normal conditions, the brain and red blood cells rely solely on glucose to fuel their activity.

glucose A six-carbon monosaccharide that is the primary form of carbohydrate used to provide energy in the body.

The most common disaccharides in our diet are **maltose**, **sucrose**, and **lactose** (**Figure 4.4b**).

Complex Carbohydrates

Complex carbohydrates are polysaccharides; they are generally not sweet-tasting the way simple carbohydrates are. They include glycogen in animals and starches and fibres in plants (**Figure 4.4c**). Glycogen is the storage form of glucose in humans and other animals. It is found in the liver and muscles, but we don't consume it in our diet because the glycogen in animal muscles is broken down soon after the animal is slaughtered.

Starch is made up of glucose molecules linked together

glycogen The storage form of carbohydrate in animals, made up of many glucose molecules linked together in a highly branched structure.

starch A carbohydrate found in plants, made up of many glucose molecules linked in straight or branched chains.

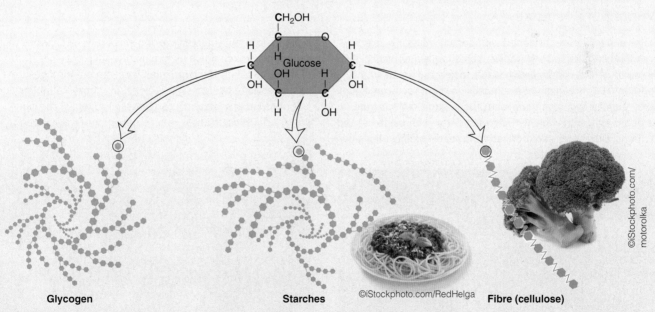

c. Complex carbohydrates

Glucose

©iStockphoto.com/RedHelga

©iStockphoto.com/motorolka

Glycogen

The polysaccharide glycogen is made of highly branched chains of glucose. This branched structure allows glycogen, which is found in muscle and liver, to be broken down quickly when the body needs glucose.

Starches

Different types of starch consist of either straight chains or branched chains of glucose. We consume a mixture of starches in grain products, legumes, and other starchy vegetables.

Fibre (cellulose)

Most fibre is made of either straight or branched chains of monosaccharides, but the bonds that link the sugar units cannot be broken by human digestive enzymes. For example, **cellulose**, shown here, is a fibre made up of straight chains of glucose molecules. It is found in wheat bran and broccoli.

Think Critically How do the bonds that link the glucose units in a molecule of starch differ from those in a molecule of cellulose fibre?

Photosynthesis • Figure 4.5

Glucose is produced in plants through the process of **photosynthesis**, which uses energy from the sun to convert carbon dioxide and water to glucose. Plants most often convert glucose to starch. When a human eats plants, digestion converts the starch back to glucose.

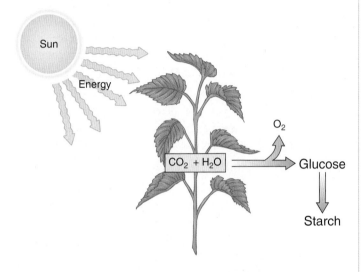

in either straight or branched chains (see Figure 4.4c). It is the storage form of carbohydrate found in the endosperm of plants and provides energy for plant growth and reproduction. When we eat plants, we consume the energy stored in the starch (**Figure 4.5**).

Fibre is a type of complex carbohydrate that cannot be broken down by human digestive enzymes. Thus, fibre cannot be absorbed in the human small intestine and passes relatively unchanged into the large intestine. Fibre includes several chemical substances, some of which are soluble in water. **Soluble fibre**, found around and inside plant cells, dissolves in water to form viscous solutions. Although human enzymes can't digest soluble fibre, it is estimated that it still provides approximately 2 kcal per gram of energy. Bacteria in the large intestine can ferment soluble fibre to produce short-chain fatty acids,

> **soluble fibre** Fibre that dissolves in water or absorbs water and can be broken down by intestinal microbiota. It includes pectins, gums, and some hemicelluloses.

which, once absorbed, add to energy intake. Foods containing soluble fibre include oats, apples, beans, and seaweed (**Figure 4.6**). Soluble fibre is considered to be heart healthy because it binds cholesterol-containing compounds in the small intestine promoting their excretion, and limiting their absorption; this leads to lower blood cholesterol levels. It also regulates blood sugar levels by delaying gastric emptying, which may help to reduce the risk of type-2 diabetes.

Soluble fibre • Figure 4.6

a. Jams and jellies are thickened with pectin, which is a soluble fibre found in fruits and vegetables. Some foods are thickened with gums, which combine with water to keep solutions from separating. Gums you might see in an ingredient list include gum arabic, gum karaya, guar gum, locust bean gum, xanthan gum, and gum tragacanth, which are extracted from shrubs, trees, and seedpods. Other gums are derived from seaweed, including agar, carrageenan, and alginates.

© Can Stock Photo Inc. / brozova

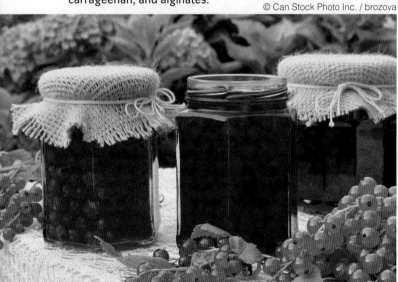

b. Beans contain soluble fibre and small polysaccharides that cannot be broken down by human digestive enzymes. Both of these pass into the large intestine, where their digestion by bacteria creates gas. Over-the-counter enzyme tablets and solutions (such as Beano®) can be taken to digest the small polysaccharides and thus reduce the amount of gas produced.

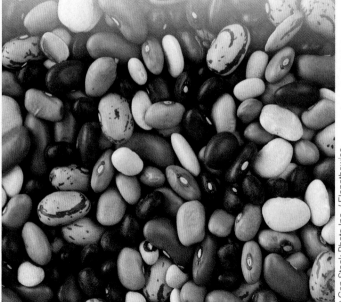

© Can Stock Photo Inc. / Elenathewise

Fibre that does not dissolve in water is called **insoluble fibre**. Insoluble fibre comes primarily from structural parts of plants, such as cell walls. Food sources of insoluble fibre include wheat and rye bran, broccoli, and celery. Insoluble fibre helps promote intestinal health by speeding passage through the intestines, while binding toxic waste products. It accordingly promotes regular bowel movements and prevents constipation. Insoluble fibre is believed to pass relatively unchanged through the digestive tract, thus contributing a negligible amount of calories to the diet.

Foods that contain fibre typically don't comprise only soluble fibre or only insoluble fibre, but both fibres.

> **insoluble fibre**
> Fibre that, for the most part, does not dissolve in water and cannot be broken down by bacteria in the large intestine. Insoluble fibre includes cellulose, some hemicelluloses, and lignin, which can all be found in the cell walls of plants.

CONCEPT CHECK

1. **Which** monosaccharide circulates in the blood?
2. **What** is glycogen?
3. **Which** type of fibre is plentiful in beans?

Carbohydrate Digestion and Absorption

LEARNING OBJECTIVES

1. **Describe** the steps of carbohydrate digestion.
2. **Explain** how low levels of lactase can cause abdominal discomfort.
3. **Discuss** the health benefits of indigestible carbohydrates.
4. **Draw** a graph that illustrates the glycemic response of both pop and beans.

D isaccharides such as sucrose (table sugar) and complex carbohydrates such as starch must be digested to monosaccharides before they can be absorbed into the body. Carbohydrates that cannot be completely digested cannot be absorbed but still have an impact on the gastrointestinal tract and overall health. Once absorbed, carbohydrates travel in the blood to the liver.

Carbohydrate Digestion

Carbohydrate digestion begins in the mouth, with the action of salivary amylase, the enzyme that breaks down the amylose form of starch. Most carbohydrate digestion occurs downstream in the small intestine, where digestive enzymes help break down disaccharides and more complex carbohydrates into monosaccharides, which can then be absorbed (**Figure 4.7**). Pancreatic amylase in the small intestine helps to further digest amylose, whereas disaccharides are each digested by a specific enzyme: Maltase digests maltose, sucrase digests sucrose, and lactase digests lactose. If the body does not produce the specific enzyme needed to break down a disaccharide or a more complex carbohydrate, these carbohydrates pass unchanged into the colon, where intestinal bacteria may break them down further. Unfortunately, this process can lead to the production of uncomfortable bloating and gas, which is evidenced during lactose intolerance. Material that cannot be absorbed is then excreted in the feces.

Lactose intolerance The disaccharide lactose is broken down by the enzyme lactase in the small intestine. We are all born with adequate levels of lactase, but for many people, these levels decline so much with age that lactose cannot be completely digested, a condition called **lactose intolerance**. When these individuals consume dairy products, the lactose passes into the large intestine, where it draws in water and is metabolized by bacteria, producing gas and potentially causing abdominal distension, bloating, cramping, and diarrhea. Lactose intolerance affects approximately 7 million Canadians and its incidence is more common in non-Caucasian ethnicities.[1]

> **lactose intolerance** The inability to digest lactose due to a reduction in the levels of the enzyme lactase.

Because milk is the primary source of calcium in the Canadian diet, lactose-intolerant individuals may have difficulty meeting their calcium needs. Those who can tolerate small amounts of lactose can meet their calcium

Carbohydrate digestion • Figure 4.7

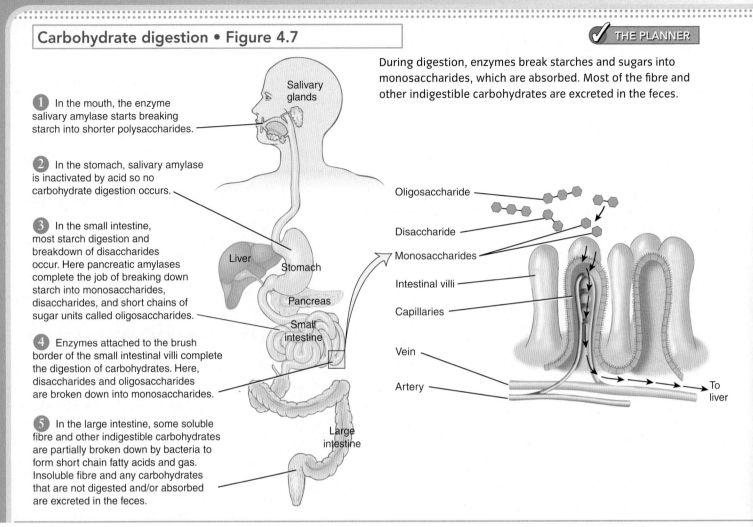

During digestion, enzymes break starches and sugars into monosaccharides, which are absorbed. Most of the fibre and other indigestible carbohydrates are excreted in the feces.

1 In the mouth, the enzyme salivary amylase starts breaking starch into shorter polysaccharides.

2 In the stomach, salivary amylase is inactivated by acid so no carbohydrate digestion occurs.

3 In the small intestine, most starch digestion and breakdown of disaccharides occur. Here pancreatic amylases complete the job of breaking down starch into monosaccharides, disaccharides, and short chains of sugar units called oligosaccharides.

4 Enzymes attached to the brush border of the small intestinal villi complete the digestion of carbohydrates. Here, disaccharides and oligosaccharides are broken down into monosaccharides.

5 In the large intestine, some soluble fibre and other indigestible carbohydrates are partially broken down by bacteria to form short chain fatty acids and gas. Insoluble fibre and any carbohydrates that are not digested and/or absorbed are excreted in the feces.

Salivary glands
Liver
Stomach
Pancreas
Small intestine
Large intestine

Oligosaccharide
Disaccharide
Monosaccharides
Intestinal villi
Capillaries
Vein
Artery
To liver

needs by consuming smaller portions of milk throughout the day. Cheese and yogurt may also be tolerated because some of the lactose originally present in the milk is either digested by bacteria or lost in processing. Those who cannot tolerate any lactose can get their calcium from tofu and fish consumed with bones. Another option is to take lactase tablets with or before consuming milk products to digest the lactose before it passes into the large intestine.

Calcium-fortified foods and supplements and lactase-treated (i.e., lactose-free) milk are also available. People who consume lactose-free beverages such as soy milk that have been fortified with calcium may not be consuming the same amounts of calcium in their diet as advertised on the Nutrition Facts panel because fortified calcium can sink to the bottom of a container. The availability of calcium from soy milk, specifically unrefrigerated soy milk, can be improved by shaking the container before consumption.[2]

Indigestible carbohydrates Fibre and some **oligo-saccharides** are not digested because they cannot be broken down by human enzymes. **Resistant starch** is also not digested, either because the natural structure of the grain protects the starch molecules or because cooking and processing alter their digestibility. Legumes, unripe bananas, cold cooked potatoes, rice, and pasta are high in resistant starch.

oligosaccharides
Short carbohydrate chains containing 3 to 10 sugar units.

resistant starch
Starch that escapes digestion in the small intestine.

As indigestible carbohydrates pass through the gastrointestinal tract, they slow the rate at which nutrients are absorbed (**Figure 4.8a**). Fibre can also bind to certain minerals, preventing their absorption. For example, wheat bran fibre binds to zinc, calcium, magnesium, and iron. Indigestible carbohydrates also speed transit through the intestine by increasing the amount of fluid and the volume of material in the intestine, which stimulates peristalsis, causing the muscles of the large intestine to work more and to function better (**Figure 4.8b**).

a. The bulk and volume of a fibre-rich meal dilutes the gastrointestinal contents. This dilution slows the digestion of food and absorption of nutrients (green dots), causing a delay and a blunting of the rise in blood glucose that occurs after a meal. When a low-fibre meal is consumed, the nutrients are more concentrated; thus, digestion and absorption occur more rapidly, causing a quicker, sharper rise in blood glucose. Also, a fibre-rich meal stretches the stomach more, which is one of the main feedback messages to the brain, signalling fullness from a meal, potentially decreasing caloric consumption. ▼

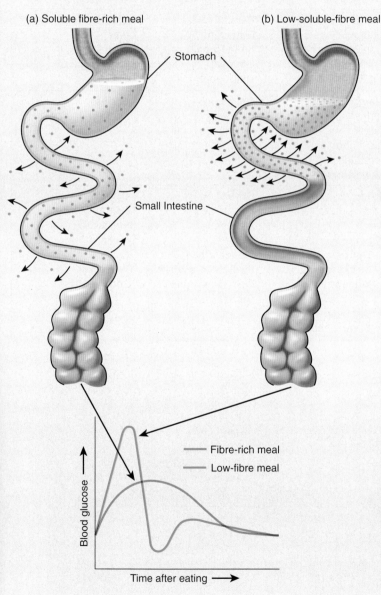

(a) Soluble fibre-rich meal   (b) Low-soluble-fibre meal

Stomach

Small Intestine

Fibre-rich meal
Low-fibre meal

Blood glucose

Time after eating ⟶

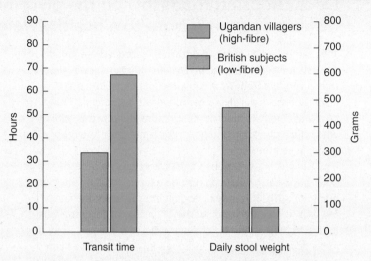

▲ **b.** Stool weights are greater and transit times shorter for Ugandan villagers, who consume a diet high in fibre, than for British subjects, who consume a more refined, low-fibre diet. (Source: Adapted from Burkitt, D.P., Walker, A.R.P., and Painter, N.S. Dietary fiber and disease. *JAMA* 229:1068–1074, 1974.)

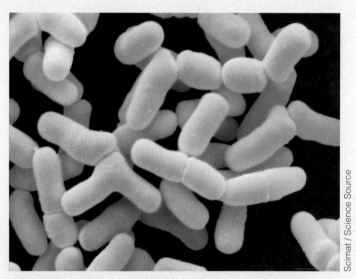

Scimat / Science Source

▲ **c.** Indigestible carbohydrates are a food source for the bacteria in the colon. When bacteria break down these carbohydrates, fatty acids are formed. The acidic conditions inhibit the growth of undesirable bacteria and favour the growth of healthy bacteria, such as the *Bifidobacteria* shown here.[3] In addition to inhibiting the growth of disease-causing bacteria, these fatty acids may help protect against colon cancer and may prevent and treat inflammation in the bowel, which causes diarrhea.[4,5]

Some carbohydrates that are not digested by human enzymes are digested by intestinal bacteria when they reach the large intestine, producing fatty acids and gas. The fatty acids can be used as a fuel source for cells in the colon and other body tissues, where they may play a role in regulating cellular processes (**Figure 4.8c**).

Carbohydrate Digestion and Absorption 105

HOT TOPIC

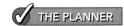

Does choosing foods low on the glycemic index reduce risk of disease and contribute to a healthy weight?

Potatoes are a source of unrefined carbohydrate, but scientists know that potatoes have an effect on blood glucose that is very different from the effect of beans. Beans are also a source of unrefined carbohydrate but, compared with potatoes, they are much higher in fibre and protein, both of which slow digestion and absorption and therefore reduce the glycemic response.

The glycemic response of beans versus potatoes is shown here graphically, but it can also be expressed using the **glycemic index (GI)**. This index was first introduced in the early 1980s by a research team at the University of Toronto, led by Dr. David Jenkins and his colleague Dr. Tom Wolever. They originally developed the concept to identify which foods helped people with diabetes manage their condition. The glycemic index is a relative ranking of how a food affects blood glucose relative to the effect of an equivalent amount of carbohydrate from a reference food, such as white bread or pure glucose.[6] For example, on a glycemic index scale on which white bread is 100, potatoes are 90, and kidney beans are about 25. A shortcoming of the glycemic index is that it is measured using a portion of food that contains a set amount of carbohydrate (usually 50 g), not a typical food portion. To overcome this shortcoming, **glycemic load** can be used to rank the effect of a food on blood sugar. This method considers the glycemic response of a typical portion of food.

A shortcoming of both the glycemic index and glycemic load is that they are determined for individual foods rather than for meals, which contain mixtures of foods. What do you think the glycemic response graph would look like for a stew containing potatoes, beef, carrots, and onions?

LOW GI (55 OR LESS) Choose most often ✓✓✓	MEDIUM GI (56-69) Choose more often ✓✓	HIGH GI (70 OR MORE) Choose less often ✓
Breads: 100% stone ground whole wheat Heavy mixed grain Pumpernickel	**Breads:** Whole wheat Rye Pita	**Breads:** White bread Kaiser roll Bagel, white
Cereal: All Bran™ Bran Buds with Psyllium™ Oat Bran™	**Cereal:** Grapenuts™ Puffed wheat Oatmeal Quick oats	**Cereal:** Bran flakes Corn flakes Rice Krispies™
Grains: Barley Bulgar Pasta/noodles Parboiled or converted rice	**Grains:** Basmati rice Brown rice Couscous	**Grains:** Short-grain rice
Other: Sweet potato Yam Legumes Lentils Chickpeas Kidney beans Split peas Soy beans Baked beans	**Other:** Potato, new/white Sweet corn Popcorn Stoned Wheat Thins™ Ryvita™ (rye crisps) Black bean soup Green pea soup	**Other:** Potato, baking (Russet) French fries Pretzels Rice cakes Soda crackers

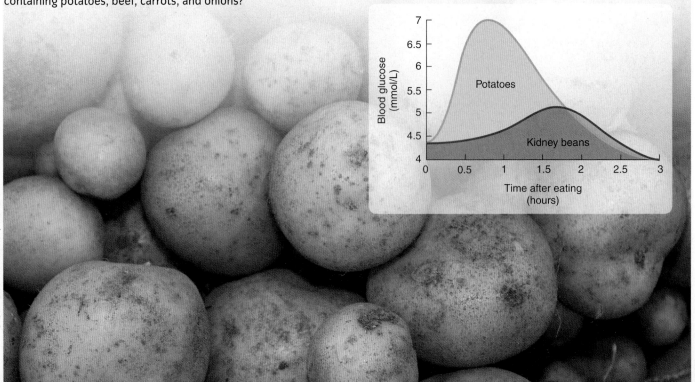

Carbohydrate Absorption

After a meal, the monosaccharides from carbohydrate digestion enter the portal circulation and travel to the liver. The liver uses fructose and galactose for energy. Glucose can be used for energy, stored as liver glycogen, or delivered via the general blood circulation to other body tissues, causing blood glucose levels to rise. **Glycemic response** is a measure of how quickly and how high blood glucose levels rise after carbohydrate is consumed. Glycemic response is affected by the time it takes for a food to leave the stomach and by how quickly it is digested and the glucose absorbed.

glycemic response The rate, magnitude, and duration of the rise in blood glucose that occurs after food is consumed.

Refined sugars and starches generally cause a greater glycemic response than unrefined carbohydrates because sugars and starches consumed alone leave the stomach quickly and are rapidly digested and absorbed. For example, when you drink a can of sugary pop, your blood glucose increases within minutes. Because fibre takes longer to leave the stomach and slows absorption in the small intestine, fibre-containing foods cause a lower glycemic response (see *Hot Topic*). When carbohydrate, fat, and protein are consumed together, stomach emptying is slowed, delaying both digestion and absorption of carbohydrate; as a result, blood glucose rises more slowly than when carbohydrate is consumed alone. For instance, after a meal of chicken, brown rice, and green beans, which contains carbohydrate, fat, protein, and fibre, blood glucose doesn't begin to rise for 30 to 60 minutes.

CONCEPT CHECK

1. **What** steps are involved in starch digestion?

2. **What** foods are good sources of calcium for someone with lactose intolerance?

3. **Why** is fibre essential to your health if it isn't an essential nutrient?

4. **How** does fibre affect glycemic response?

Carbohydrate Functions

LEARNING OBJECTIVES

1. **Name** the main function of carbohydrate in the body.

2. **Explain** how insulin and glucagon help regulate blood glucose levels.

3. **Compare** anaerobic and aerobic metabolism.

4. **Discuss** what happens to protein and fat metabolism when dietary carbohydrate is insufficient.

The main function of carbohydrates is to provide energy, but carbohydrates also play other roles in the body. The sugar galactose, for example, is needed by nerve tissue; and, in breastfeeding women, galactose combines with glucose to produce the milk sugar lactose. The monosaccharides ribose and deoxyribose play non-energy roles as components of RNA and DNA, respectively, the two molecules that contain the cell's genetic information. Ribose is also a component of the B vitamin riboflavin. Oligosaccharides are associated with cell membranes, where they help signal information about cells, and large polysaccharides found in connective tissue provide cushioning and lubrication.

Getting Enough Glucose to Cells

Glucose is an important fuel for body cells. Many body cells can use energy sources other than glucose, but under normal conditions, the brain and red blood cells specifically require glucose for fuel. To provide a steady supply of glucose, the concentration of glucose in the blood is regulated by the liver and by hormones secreted by the pancreas. The rise in blood glucose levels after eating stimulates the pancreas to secrete the hormone **insulin**, which allows glucose to be taken into body cells, causing blood glucose levels to drop. Once inside cells, glucose can be used immediately for energy or converted into

insulin A hormone made in the pancreas that allows glucose to enter cells, where it can stimulate the synthesis of fat and liver and muscle glycogen.

energy-storage molecules for future use. In both muscle cells and liver cells, insulin promotes the conversion of glucose into glycogen for storage. In the liver and in fat-storing cells, insulin promotes the conversion of glucose to fat for storage (**Figure 4.9**).

> **glucagon** A hormone made in the pancreas that raises blood glucose levels by stimulating the breakdown of liver glycogen and the synthesis of glucose.

A few hours after eating, blood glucose levels—and consequently the amount of glucose available to the cells—begin to decrease. This decrease triggers the pancreas to secrete the hormone **glucagon** (see Figure 4.9). Glucagon raises blood glucose by signalling the liver cells to break down glycogen into glucose, which is released into the blood. At the same time, glucagon signals the liver to synthesize new glucose molecules from lactate, glycerol, and some amino acids, a process called gluconeogenesis. These glucose molecules are also released into the blood, bringing blood glucose levels back to normal.

Glucose as a Source of Energy

Cells use glucose to provide energy via cellular respiration (see Chapter 3). Cellular respiration uses oxygen to convert glucose to carbon dioxide and water and to provide energy in the form of adenosine triphosphate (ATP).

Blood glucose regulation • Figure 4.9

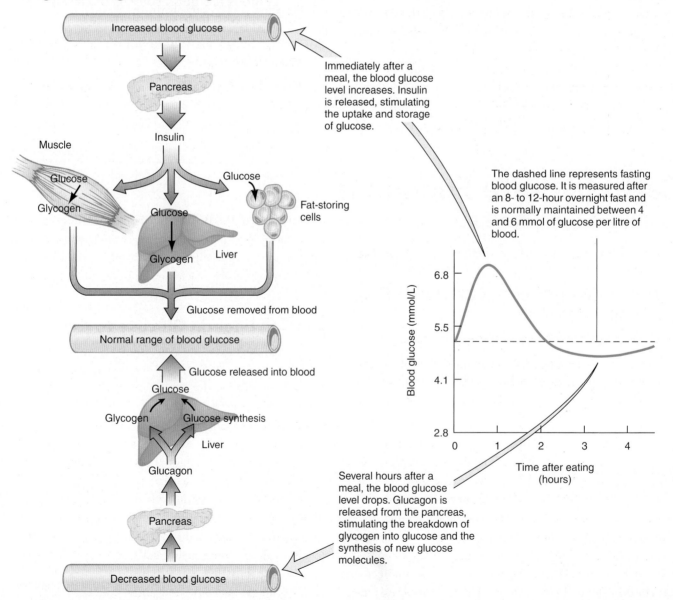

glycolysis An anaerobic metabolic pathway that splits glucose into two three-carbon pyruvate molecules; the energy released from one glucose molecule is used to make two molecules of ATP.

anaerobic metabolism Metabolism in the absence of oxygen.

aerobic metabolism Metabolism in the presence of oxygen. It can completely break down glucose to yield carbon dioxide, water, and energy in the form of ATP.

The first step in cellular respiration is **glycolysis**. Because oxygen isn't needed for this reaction, glycolysis is sometimes called anaerobic glycolysis, or **anaerobic metabolism**. Glycolysis can rapidly produce two molecules of ATP from each glucose molecule. When oxygen is limited, no further metabolism of glucose and production of ATP occurs. Instead, anaerobic metabolism occurs, leading to the production of lactic acid, which is responsible for the "burn" experienced during intense activities such as weightlifting. When oxygen is available, the complete breakdown of glucose can proceed. This **aerobic metabolism** produces more than 30 molecules of ATP for each glucose molecule.

Carbohydrate and protein breakdown Glucose is the primary source of energy for the brain and red blood cells. If adequate amounts are not available, glucose can

be synthesized from three-carbon molecules. Fatty acids cannot be used to make glucose because the reactions that break them down produce two-carbon, rather than three-carbon, molecules. Amino acids from protein breakdown can supply the three-carbon molecules through the process of gluconeogenesis. However, because protein is not stored in the body, this use of amino acids takes away functioning body proteins. Body proteins that are broken down to make glucose are no longer available to do their job, whether that job is to speed up a chemical reaction or contract a muscle. Sufficient dietary carbohydrate ensures that protein is not utilized in this way; carbohydrate is therefore said to *spare* protein.

Carbohydrate and fat breakdown Most of the energy stored in the body is stored as fat. To fully access the energy from fatty acids, the diet must also contain carbohydrates. If carbohydrate is not available, molecules called either **ketones** or **ketone bodies** are formed (**Figure 4.10**). Small amounts of ketones can be used for energy by the heart, muscle, and kidney. Even the brain, which prefers glucose, can obtain a portion of its energy from ketones.

ketones or **ketone bodies** Acidic molecules formed when the body has insufficient carbohydrate to completely metabolize the acetyl CoA produced from fatty acid breakdown.

Ketone formation • Figure 4.10

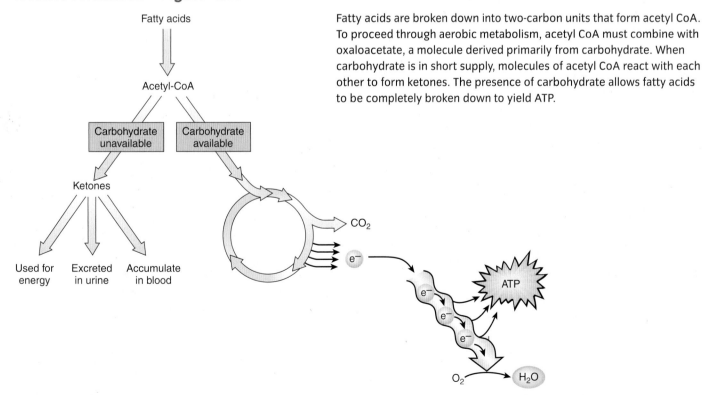

Fatty acids are broken down into two-carbon units that form acetyl CoA. To proceed through aerobic metabolism, acetyl CoA must combine with oxaloacetate, a molecule derived primarily from carbohydrate. When carbohydrate is in short supply, molecules of acetyl CoA react with each other to form ketones. The presence of carbohydrate allows fatty acids to be completely broken down to yield ATP.

Ketones not used for energy can be excreted in the urine. However, if ketones build up in the blood to high

ketosis High levels of ketones in the blood.

levels, a condition known as **ketosis**; they can increase the blood's acidity so much that normal body processes are disrupted. Mild ketosis can occur during starvation or when consuming a low-carbohydrate weight-loss diet, causing symptoms such as reduced appetite, headaches, dry mouth, and odd-smelling breath. Severe ketosis can occur with untreated diabetes and can cause coma and even death.

1. **Why** is it important to keep blood glucose levels in the normal range?

2. **How** do insulin and glucagon affect blood glucose levels?

3. **What** process breaks down glucose in the presence of oxygen to yield ATP?

4. **Why** is carbohydrate said to spare protein?

Carbohydrates in Health and Disease

LEARNING OBJECTIVES

1. **Discuss** the causes and health consequences of diabetes.

2. **Describe** how carbohydrates contribute to the development of dental caries.

3. **Discuss** the role of carbohydrates in weight control.

4. **Explain** how fibre may help protect health.

Are carbohydrates good for you or bad for you? On the one hand, carbohydrates have been blamed for everything from diabetes to obesity. On the other hand, Canadian guidelines for a healthy diet recommend that people base their diet on carbohydrate-rich foods to reduce disease risk. This incongruity relates to the health effects of different types of dietary carbohydrates: Diets high in whole grains, fruits, and vegetables are associated with a lower incidence of a variety of chronic diseases, whereas diets high in refined carbohydrates, such as refined grains and foods high in added sugars, may contribute to chronic disease risk.

Diabetes

Diabetes mellitus, commonly referred to simply as diabetes, is a disease characterized by

diabetes mellitus A disease characterized by elevated blood glucose due to either insufficient production of insulin or decreased sensitivity of cells to insulin.

high blood glucose levels (**Figure 4.11**). Although some glucose in the blood is necessary, chronically elevated levels can be toxic. Approximately 2 million Canadians are currently living with diagnosed diabetes, and this number is

expected to rise significantly in the near future.[7] Diabetes not only affects lifestyle but is also associated with other health issues. In fact, compared with people who do not have diabetes, Canadians living with diabetes are hospitalized four times more often with heart failure, six times more often with kidney disease, and nineteen times more often for a lower limb amputation.[7] If the cases of diabetes rise, an according increase may occur in all of these comorbidities, placing an increased burden on the Canadian health care system. The incidence of diabetes is not uniform among all Canadians, but is greater in people of Aboriginal, Hispanic, Asian, South Asian, or African descent (**Figure 4.12**).[7]

Types of diabetes Type-1 diabetes is an unpreventable autoimmune disease in which the insulin-secreting pancreatic cells are destroyed by the body's immune system. This form of diabetes accounts for only 5 to 10% of diagnosed cases and is usually diagnosed before age 30. Because no insulin is produced,

type-1 diabetes The form of diabetes caused by autoimmune destruction of insulin-producing cells in the pancreas, usually leading to absolute insulin deficiency.

autoimmune disease A disease that results from immune reactions that destroy normal body cells.

Blood glucose levels in diabetes • Figure 4.11

Normal blood glucose is less than 6 mmol/L blood after an eight-hour fast; a fasting blood level of 6.1–6.9 mmol/L is defined as prediabetes; a fasting level of 7 mmol/L or greater is defined as diabetes. Two hours after consuming 75 g of glucose, normal blood levels are less than 7.8 mmol/L; prediabetes levels are between 7.8 and 11 mmol/L; and diabetes levels are 11.1 mmol/L or greater.

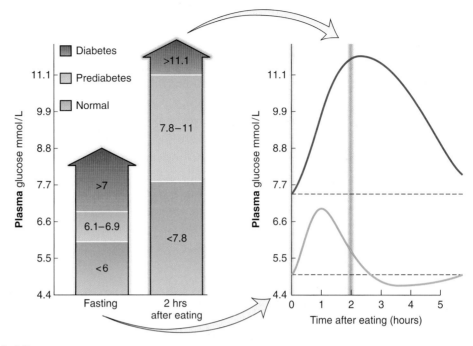

Incidence of diabetes • Figure 4.12

The incidence of diabetes in Canada is rising and not all provinces and territories are affected equally. Newfoundland and Labrador, Nova Scotia, Manitoba, Ontario, and New Brunswick have the highest rates of diabetes, while Alberta, British Columbia, and Quebec have the lowest rates. Across most provinces, rates in men are higher than in women, but rates are higher in women in Yukon and the Northwest Territories.[8]

Age-standardized prevalence percentages[a] of diagnosed diabetes among people aged 1 year and older, by sex, province, and territory, Canada,[b] 2006-07

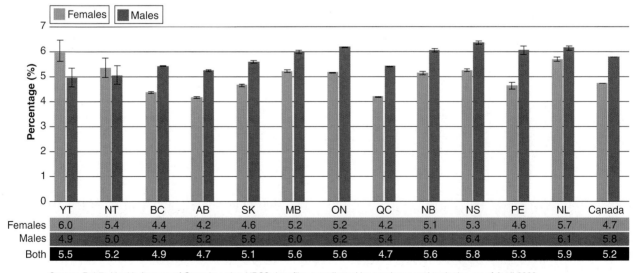

	YT	NT	BC	AB	SK	MB	ON	QC	NB	NS	PE	NL	Canada
Females	6.0	5.4	4.4	4.2	4.6	5.2	5.2	4.2	5.1	5.3	4.6	5.7	4.7
Males	4.9	5.0	5.4	5.2	5.6	6.0	6.2	5.4	6.0	6.4	6.1	6.1	5.8
Both	5.5	5.2	4.9	4.7	5.1	5.6	5.6	4.7	5.6	5.8	5.3	5.9	5.2

Source: Public Health Agency of Canada, using NDSS data files contributed by provinces and territories, as of April 2009
[a]Age-standardized to the 1991 Canadian population. [b]Data for Nunavut were unavailable.
[‡]The 95% Confidence Interval shows an estimated range of values which is likely to include the true prevalence rate 19 times out of 20.

Ask Yourself

Why do you believe the incidence of diabetes tends to be higher in men than women?

people with type-1 diabetes must inject insulin to keep their blood glucose levels in the normal range.

The more common form of diabetes is **type-2 diabetes**, which accounts for 90 to 95% of all cases. It occurs either

> **type-2 diabetes**
> The form of diabetes characterized by insulin resistance and relative (rather than absolute) insulin deficiency.

when the body does not produce enough insulin or when body cells lose their sensitivity to it, a condition called **insulin resistance**. Therefore, the amount of insulin released is insufficient to allow enough glucose to enter the cells, and blood glucose levels remain high and, thus, toxic to the heart, blood vessels, kidneys, and nerves (**Figure 4.13**). Type-2 diabetes is believed to be due to both genetic and lifestyle factors. It is a progressive disease that usually begins with **prediabetes**, a condition in which glucose levels are above normal but not high enough to be diagnosed as diabetes (see Figure 4.11). In many cases, adjustments in diet and lifestyle can keep prediabetes from progressing to type-2 diabetes.

Gestational diabetes is an elevation of blood sugar that is first recognized during pregnancy. The high levels of glucose in the mother's blood are passed to the fetus, frequently resulting in a baby who is large for gestational age and at increased risk of complications. Gestational diabetes usually resolves after the pregnancy, but women with gestational diabetes are at increased risk of developing type-2 diabetes later in life. It is therefore important that pregnant women regulate their blood glucose by not excessively over-consuming nutrients during pregnancy.

Diabetes complications • Figure 4.13

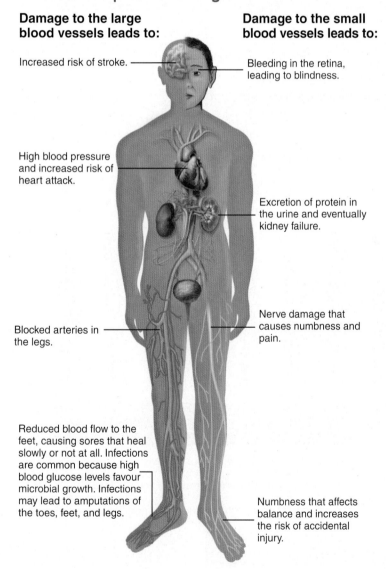

Damage to the large blood vessels leads to:

Increased risk of stroke.

High blood pressure and increased risk of heart attack.

Blocked arteries in the legs.

Reduced blood flow to the feet, causing sores that heal slowly or not at all. Infections are common because high blood glucose levels favour microbial growth. Infections may lead to amputations of the toes, feet, and legs.

Damage to the small blood vessels leads to:

Bleeding in the retina, leading to blindness.

Excretion of protein in the urine and eventually kidney failure.

Nerve damage that causes numbness and pain.

Numbness that affects balance and increases the risk of accidental injury.

Symptoms and complications of diabetes

The symptoms and complications of all types of diabetes result from the inability to use glucose normally and from high glucose levels in the blood. Cells that require insulin to take up glucose are starved for glucose, and cells that can use glucose without insulin are exposed to damaging high levels.

The early symptoms of diabetes include frequent urination, excessive thirst, blurred vision, and weight loss. Frequent urination and excessive thirst occur because, as blood glucose levels rise, the kidneys excrete the extra glucose and, as a result, must also excrete extra water, increasing the volume of urine. The additional loss of water from the body makes the individual thirsty. Blurred vision occurs when excess glucose enters the lens of the eye, drawing in water and causing the lens to swell. Weight loss may also occur because cells are unable to use glucose for energy and so the body must break down fat to obtain the energy it needs.

The long-term complications of diabetes include damage to the heart, blood vessels, kidneys, eyes, and nerves (see Figure 4.13), which are believed to be caused by chronic exposure to high glucose levels from the blood.

Managing blood glucose Although diabetes is a very damaging disease, proper lifestyle intervention can successfully help manage diabetes, minimize the negative long-term effects, and even reduce some of the financial costs associated with its treatment. The goal in treating diabetes is to maintain blood glucose levels within the normal range. The Canadian Diabetes Association accordingly recommends a program of diet, exercise, and, in many cases, medication, along with frequent monitoring of blood glucose levels.[9] Carbohydrate intake must be coordinated with exercise and medication schedules so that glucose and insulin are available in the right proportions.

Dietary management involves limiting the amount of carbohydrate consumed to prevent a rapid or prolonged rise in blood glucose.[10] A diet providing unrefined carbohydrates such as whole grains and vegetables is recommended because these carbohydrate sources cause a slower rise in blood glucose than refined carbohydrates. Diets for individuals with diabetes should also be limited in saturated fat, *trans* fat, and cholesterol to reduce the risk for cardiovascular disease. Weight management is an important component of diabetes care because excess body fat increases the resistance of body cells to insulin. Exercise is important not only because it helps to achieve and maintain a healthy body weight but also because it increases the sensitivity of body cells to insulin.[10,11]

Canadians living with diabetes face both the likelihood of more health complications and the increased medical costs associated with treating these ailments. Medications and supplies to treat diabetes can cost an individual anywhere from $1,000 to $15,000 a year.[7] Recent research suggests that lifestyle intervention is not only less costly but also more effective than the use of medications (**Figure 4.14**).

Type-1 diabetes presents different management challenges, as insulin is not being effectively secreted, if at all, from the pancreas. Historically, patients with type-1 diabetes faced a shorter life expectancy and increased risk of complications without insulin in their system. This bleak forecast changed in the 1920s, when Frederick Banting; his lab assistant, Charles Best; and a colleague, J Macleod, all working out of the University of Toronto, were able to isolate insulin. Once this insulin was given to patients, the severe symptoms of type-1 diabetes were dramatically alleviated almost immediately upon administration! Now, patients with type-1 diabetes can live long and healthy lives if they continually inject this hormone under prescribed intervals. The isolation of insulin was recently voted the top Canadian invention of all times by viewers of the Canadian Broadcasting Corporation (CBC).[13] In addition to taking their insulin injections as prescribed, patients with type-1 diabetes should also follow similar lifestyle behaviours as are recommended for patients with type-2 diabetes.

Managing type-2 diabetes • Figure 4.14

A multi-clinic and multi-state intervention program involving more than 3,000 people called the Diabetes Prevention Program, took place in the United States over 2–3 years.[12] Patients with prediabetes were assigned to one of three groups: an intensive lifestyle intervention group, where patients accumulated 150 minutes of weekly physical activity, reduced their dietary fat and caloric intake, and lost at least 7% of their body weight; a group that received only the diabetes-reducing drug, metformin; and a control group that received a placebo (fake version) of the metformin drug. Compared to the control group, the lifestyle intervention group and the metformin group had a 58% and 31% reduction in diabetes incidence respectively. The lifestyle intervention group also had the lowest rates of hospitalization and gastrointestinal symptoms. A 10-year follow up of the study showed that over time, diabetes incidence increased in all groups, but the lifestyle intervention and metformin groups still respectively had a 34% and 18% lower risk of diabetes incidence compared to the control group. These results show that the risk of type-2 diabetes is reduced most significantly through lifestyle modification.

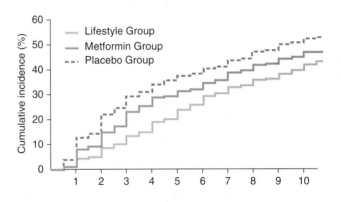

Carbohydrate intake and the risk of diabetes

Evidence is accumulating that carbohydrate consumption may play a role in the development of type-2 diabetes in susceptible individuals.[14,15] Populations where the diet is high in whole grains show a lower risk of developing type-2 diabetes than populations where the diet is high in refined starches and added sugars.[16,17] The reason for this relationship is not fully understood. However, some suggest that because insulin needs are increased when the diet is high in refined carbohydrates, the insulin-producing cells in the pancreas may wear out over time.[12]

Hypoglycemia

Another condition that involves blood glucose is **hypoglycemia**. Symptoms of hypoglycemia include low blood sugar (less than

> **hypoglycemia**
> Abnormally low blood glucose levels.

4 mmol glucose/litre blood), irritability, sweating, shakiness, anxiety, rapid heartbeat, headache, hunger, weakness, and sometimes seizures and coma. Hypoglycemia occurs most frequently in people with diabetes as a result of overmedication. It can also be caused by abnormalities in insulin production or by abnormalities in the way the body responds to insulin or to other hormones.

Fasting hypoglycemia, which occurs when an individual has not eaten, is often related to an underlying condition, such as excess alcohol consumption, hormonal deficiencies, or tumours. Treatment involves identifying and treating the underlying disease. **Reactive hypoglycemia** occurs in response to the consumption of high-carbohydrate foods. The rise in blood glucose from the high-carbohydrate meal stimulates insulin release. However, when too much insulin is secreted, the result can be a rapid fall in blood glucose to abnormally low levels. To prevent the rapid changes in blood glucose that occur with reactive hypoglycemia, the diet should consist of small, frequent meals that are low in carbohydrate and high in protein and fibre.

Dental Caries

Dental caries, or cavities, are the best documented health problem associated with carbohydrate intake. Eighty-five percent of people age 18 years and older have had caries. They occur when bacteria on the teeth metabolize carbohydrates, producing tooth-damaging acids (**Figure 4.15**). Simple carbohydrates, especially sucrose, are easiest for the bacteria to metabolize into acids, but starchy foods also promote tooth decay. In fact, *any* carbohydrate-rich food can promote the action of tooth-decaying bacteria, even milk, vegetables, and bread. The longer teeth are exposed to carbohydrates—for example, through frequent snacking, consuming foods that stick to the teeth, sucking hard candy, and slowly sipping pop—the greater the risk of caries. Limiting intake of sweet or sticky foods and proper dental hygiene can help prevent dental caries. Fluoride has also been shown to lower the action of these plaque-causing bacteria. The Canadian Dental Association accordingly recommends brushing twice daily with a fluoride-containing toothpaste.[18] Sugar substitutes, specifically sugar alcohols such as xylitol, may also be used to minimize bacterial action, as they are not fermented by bacteria.

Weight Management

As low-carbohydrate diets have gained in popularity, carbohydrates have received a bad reputation for being

Tooth decay • Figure 4.15 _____

The regions on these teeth that are stained brown indicate the presence of dental plaque. The main component of dental plaque is bacterial colonies. If the plaque is not brushed, flossed, or scraped off, the bacteria metabolize the carbohydrates in food, producing acid. This acid can dissolve tooth enamel and the underlying tooth structure, forming dental caries.

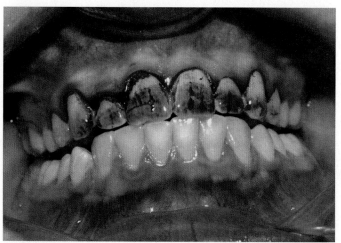

SPL / Science Source

fattening. In reality, carbohydrates are no more fattening than other nutrients. Weight gain is primarily caused by excess intake of total calories, no matter whether the excess is from carbohydrate, fat, or protein. Carbohydrates provide only 4 kilocalories per gram, less than half the 9 kilocalories per gram provided by fat (**Figure 4.16**).

Carbohydrates and weight loss The type of carbohydrates you consume can affect how hungry you feel and may determine whether you lose or gain weight. A diet high in unrefined carbohydrates is high in fibre, which is filling, allowing you to feel satisfied with less food. This type of diet may help promote weight loss by decreasing appetite. However, diets high in fibre may be problematic for children, who have a small stomach capacity, because they may become satiated before meeting their nutrient requirements.

Foods high in refined carbohydrates cause a rapid rise in blood glucose and therefore stimulate release of insulin. The more insulin you produce, the more fat you store, so a diet high in refined carbohydrates may shift metabolism toward fat storage. In contrast, a low-carbohydrate diet causes less insulin release and hence does not promote fat storage. Low-carbohydrate diets tend to lead to weight loss because they reduce insulin levels and raise blood ketone levels, both of which suppress appetite. In addition, these diets limit food choices to such an extent that the

a. It is often the fat we add to high-carbohydrate foods that increases their calorie count. A medium-sized baked potato provides about 160 kilocalories. Adding 30 mL (2 tablespoons) of sour cream brings the total to more than 200 kilocalories, and adding 30 mL (2 tablespoons) of butter more than doubles the total number of calories.

b. A diet high in sugar-sweetened beverages may increase caloric intake because beverages do not induce satiety to the same extent as solid forms of carbohydrate.[19] A diet high in unrefined, whole-grain carbohydrates may help reduce total food intake because the fibre in these foods increases the sense of fullness by adding bulk and slowing digestion.

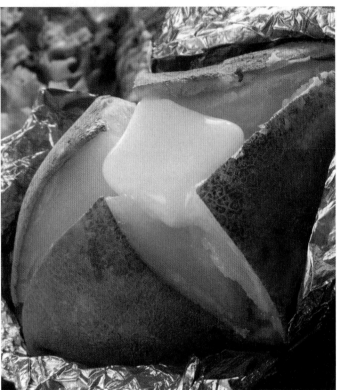

©iStockphoto.com/EasyBuy4u

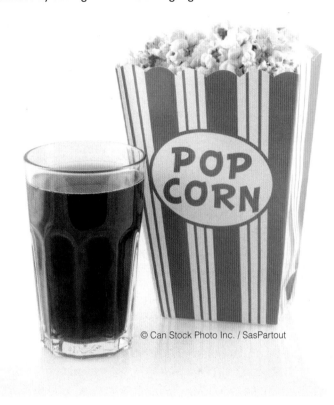

© Can Stock Photo Inc. / SasPartout

monotony may result in a spontaneous reduction in calorie intake.[20] The weight loss achieved with these diets, as with any other weight-loss diet, is therefore caused by consuming less energy than the body expends, not necessarily because carbohydrates are limited. A major issue with very restrictive low-carbohydrate diets is that they may be difficult to maintain long term, and cravings for carbohydrates may promote future binging. Here, the dietary planning principle of moderation—not too much and not too little—is especially applicable.

Non-nutritive sweeteners One way to reduce the amount of refined sugar in the diet is to replace sugar with a **non-nutritive sweetener** (also called **artificial sweetener**), which provides no calories. The Canadian Food and Drugs Act and Regulations has approved aspartame, sucralose, acesulfame K, neotame, cyclamate, and various sugar alcohols, such as sorbitol and xylitol,

as non-nutritive sweeteners and has defined **acceptable daily intakes (ADIs)**—levels that should not be exceeded when using these products.[21] Saccharin, the oldest of the non-nutritive sweeteners, is available in the United States, but in Canada is available only at the pharmacy. It was once considered a carcinogen, but substantial evidence now suggests that saccharin does not promote cancer in humans. Accordingly, a proposal to reinstate saccharin as an acceptable sweetener is currently under review.

Aspartame and sucralose are the products typically available to sweeten coffee (**Figure 4.17**). Aspartame is made of two amino acids: aspartic acid and phenylalanine. Because aspartame breaks down when heated, it is typically used in cold products or added after cooking. Much attention has been given to aspartame and its potential association with cancer, but this claim has never been fully proven. Health Canada will continue to review all data concerning the safety of aspartame as it becomes available.

Non-nutritive sweeteners
• Figure 4.17 _____

Consumers often recognize their favourite non-nutritive sweetener by the colour of the packet.

Sucralose, the sweetener in Splenda, is 600 times sweeter than sucrose. The ADI is 5 mg/kg of body weight/day, and one packet contains about 12 mg of sucralose. A 70-kg (154-lb.) person could consume 29 packets without exceeding the ADI.

In the United States, Sweet'n Low is primarily composed of saccharine, which is 300 times sweeter than sucrose. In Canada, since saccharin is still not approved for use, Sweet'n Low's main ingredient is cyclamate, which is 30-50 times sweeter than sugar. Its ADI is approximately 5 mg/kg of body weight/day. It is not recommended for pregnant women.

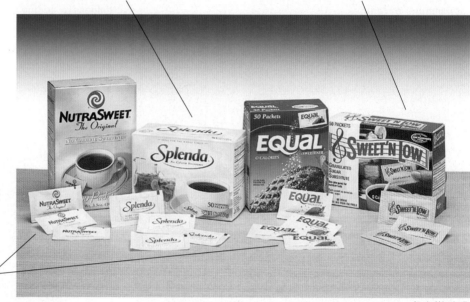

Aspartame, the sweetener in NutraSweet and Equal, is 200 times sweeter than sucrose. The ADI is 50 mg/kg of body weight/day, and one packet contains 37 mg of aspartame. To exceed the ADI, a 70-kg (154-lb.) person would have to consume 95 packets or 16 355-mL (12-oz) aspartame-sweetened beverages.

Andy Washnik

It maintains that the large body of evidence on aspartame is in line with its inclusion of aspartame as an acceptable and safe sweetener for purchase.[21] Sucralose is sucrose that has been modified so that it cannot be digested or absorbed. It is marketed under the brand name Splenda. Because it is heat stable, it can be used in cooking, and no negative health effects have been shown, even in larger doses. Acesulfame K, used in the sweetener Sunette, is also heat stable. It is 200 times sweeter than sucrose and is often used in combination with other sweeteners, such as aspartame. Neotame, like aspartame, is made from two amino acids, but because the bond between them is harder to break than the bond in aspartame, neotame is heat stable and can be used in baking. It was approved for sale in Canada in 2007. Cyclamate is marketed under the brand names Sweet'n Low and Sugar Twin and is 30 times sweeter than sucrose. The newest sweetener on the market in the United States is rebiana, which is a natural sweetener made from the leaf of the stevia plant.[22] It is about 300 times sweeter than sugar and is marketed as Truvia and PureVia. This sweetener is still under review in Canada, and is currently not on the list of approved food additives. It is nonetheless approved for use in certain natural health products, which undergo an approval system different from that for food additives.[23]

Sugar alcohols are a family of sweeteners that occur naturally in fruits and vegetables and can be manufactured from common sources of sugars. Health Canada has concluded that their addition to foods is safe. These sugar alcohols, which include mannitol, sorbitol, xylitol, and maltitol, are commonly found in chewing gum. Because bacteria do not ferment sugar alcohols, the use of sugar alcohols may help prevent dental caries. Sugar alcohols tend to pull fluid into the digestive tract, and if consumed in large amounts, they can cause intestinal discomfort including diarrhea and gas.

When these sweeteners are used instead of sugar, calorie intake is reduced. Over time, using them may help with weight loss. However, because foods that are high in added sugar tend to be nutrient poor, replacing them with artificially sweetened alternatives does not necessarily increase the nutrient density or overall quality of the diet. Also the increased use of non-nutrient sweeteners in Canada raises an important question: if non-nutritive sweeteners are readily available in many products, why haven't we seen an associated decrease in either caloric intake or the incidence of obesity in Canada and the United States? Replacing natural sugar sources with artificial sweeteners is not itself enough to promote significant weight loss over the long term and should be used in addition to overall caloric reduction if the goal is weight loss or weight maintenance. Although the usefulness of non-nutritive sweeteners for weight loss depends on whether the calories they replace are added back from other food sources, these sweeteners can help reduce the incidence of dental caries and manage blood sugar levels.

Heart Disease

The impact of carbohydrates on heart disease risk depends on the type of carbohydrate. There is evidence that a diet high in sugar can raise blood lipid levels and thereby increase the risk of heart disease,[24] whereas diets high in fibre have been found to reduce the risk of heart disease.[25]

Foods containing soluble fibre, such as legumes, oats, flaxseed, and brown rice, may reduce blood cholesterol levels. High blood cholesterol promotes the accumulation of fatty deposits in the arteries, which can promote both heart attacks and strokes. In the digestive tract, soluble fibre binds dietary cholesterol and bile acids, which are made from cholesterol, preventing them from being absorbed (**Figure 4.18**). Soluble fibre may also help lower blood cholesterol because the by-products of the bacterial breakdown of the fibre may inhibit cholesterol synthesis in the liver or increase its removal from the blood.[26]

Insoluble fibres, such as wheat bran and cellulose, do not lower blood cholesterol, but a diet high in any type of fibre may help lower blood pressure, normalize blood glucose levels, prevent obesity, and affect a number of other parameters that help reduce the risk of heart disease.[27]

The Heart and Stroke Foundation of Canada recommends that Canadians avoid low-carbohydrate diets for the purposes of weight loss, as these diets may be higher in

Cholesterol and soluble fibre • Figure 4.18

a. When the diet is low in soluble fibre, dietary cholesterol and bile, which contain cholesterol and bile acids made from cholesterol, are absorbed into the blood and transported to the liver, where they are reused.

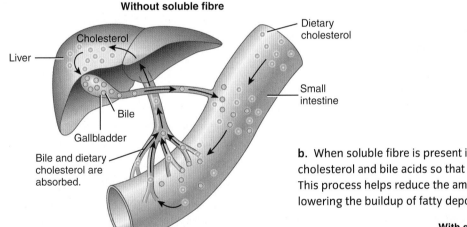

b. When soluble fibre is present in the digestive tract, the fibre binds cholesterol and bile acids so that they are excreted rather than absorbed. This process helps reduce the amount of cholesterol in the body, thus lowering the buildup of fatty deposits in the arteries.

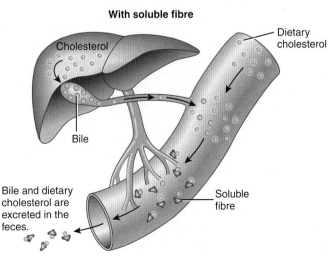

Diverticula • Figure 4.19

Diverticula (the singular is *diverticulum*) are outpouches in the wall of the colon that form at weak points due to pressure exerted when the colon contracts. Fecal matter can accumulate in these pouches, causing irritation, pain, and inflammation—a condition known as **diverticulitis**. Diverticulitis may lead to infection. Treatment usually includes antibiotics to eliminate the infection and a low-fibre diet to prevent irritation of inflamed tissues. Once the inflammation is resolved, a high-fibre diet is recommended to ease stool elimination and reduce future attacks of diverticulitis.

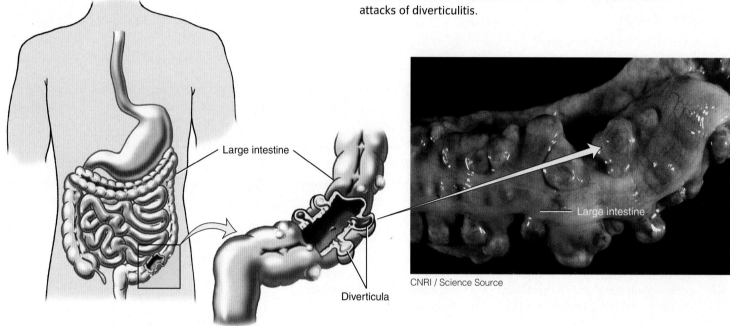

Large intestine

Diverticula

Large intestine

CNRI / Science Source

saturated and *trans* fats. Instead, they recommend a high-fibre, low-fat diet including five to ten servings of fruits and vegetables per day. Physical activity is further recommended as a mechanism to lose weight and promote overall heart health.[28]

Bowel Health

Fibre and other indigestible carbohydrates add bulk and absorb water in the gastrointestinal tract, making the feces larger and softer and reducing the pressure needed for defecation. The result is a reduced risk of developing **diverticulosis** (**Figure 4.19**) and a reduced incidence of constipation and **hemorrhoids**, the swelling of veins in the rectal or anal area.

> **diverticulosis**
> A condition in which outpouches (or sacs) form in the wall of the large intestine.

When choosing a high-fibre diet to promote health, an important side note is to ensure fluid intake is also adequate. Although fibre speeds movement of the intestinal contents, when the diet is low in fluid, fibre can contribute to constipation. The more fibre in the diet, the more water is needed to keep the stool soft. When too little fluid is consumed, the stool becomes hard and difficult to eliminate.

In severe cases of excessive fibre intake and low fluid intake, intestinal blockage can occur.

A diet high in fibre, particularly from whole grains, may reduce the risk of colon cancer, although not all studies support this finding.[29-32] Fibre reduces contact between the cells lining the colon and potentially cancer-causing substances in the feces. Fibre in the colon also affects the intestinal microbiota and their by-products. These by-products may directly affect colon cells or may change the environment of the colon in a way that can affect the development of colon cancer. Some of the protective effect may also be due to antioxidant vitamins and phytochemicals present in fibre-rich whole grains.

CONCEPT CHECK

1. **What** health problems are common in people with uncontrolled diabetes?

2. **Why** does frequent carbohydrate snacking promote dental caries?

3. **When** does a low-carbohydrate diet promote weight loss?

4. **How** does fibre benefit colon health?

Meeting Carbohydrate Needs

LEARNING OBJECTIVES

1. **Discuss** how Canadians' carbohydrate intake compares with recommendations.

2. **Calculate** the percentage of calories from carbohydrate in a food or in a diet.

3. **Use** food labels to identify foods high in fibre and low in added sugar.

Recommendations for carbohydrate intake focus on two main points: getting enough carbohydrate to meet the need for glucose and choosing the types that promote health and prevent disease.

Carbohydrate Recommendations

The RDA for carbohydrate is 130 g/day, based on the average minimum amount of glucose used by the brain.[33] In a diet that meets energy needs, this amount provides adequate glucose and prevents ketosis. Additional carbohydrate provides an important source of energy in the diet and nutrient-dense carbohydrate sources can add vitamins, minerals, fibre, and phytochemicals. Therefore, the Acceptable Macronutrient Distribution Range (AMDR) for carbohydrate is 45 to 65% of total calorie intake. A diet within this range meets energy needs without excessive amounts of protein or fat (**Figure 4.20**).

The typical Canadian diet meets the recommendation for the amount of carbohydrate, but most of this carbohydrate comes from refined sources, making the diet lower in fibre and higher in added sugar than recommended (see *Thinking It Through*). The Adequate Intake (AI) for fibre is 38 g/day for men and 25 g/day for women; the typical intake is only about 12.5 g/day.

There is no RDA or Daily Value for added sugar, and such sugar is not found explicitly in Canada's Food Guide. A small amount of added sugars can be part of an otherwise healthy diet as long as they do not increase caloric intake beyond recommended levels, which is often the case. In fact, added sugars currently account for 12% of total energy consumption in Canada.[34]

Because no specific toxicity is associated with high intake of any type of carbohydrate, no upper limit (UL) has been established for total carbohydrate intake, for fibre intake, or for added sugar intake.

Choosing Carbohydrates Wisely

To promote a healthy, balanced diet, *Eating Well with Canada's Food Guide* recommends increasing consumption of whole grains, vegetables, and fruits and limiting bakery products, candy, soft drinks, and other foods high in added sugars.

How much carbohydrate do you eat? • Figure 4.20

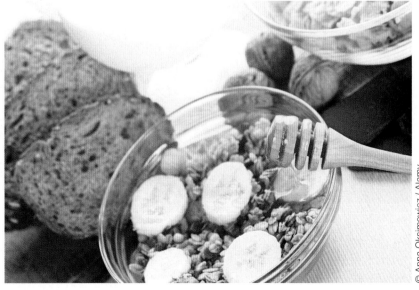

To calculate the percentage of calories from carbohydrate in a diet, first determine the number of grams of carbohydrate and multiply this value by 4 kilocalories per gram. For example, this vegetarian diet provides about 300 grams of carbohydrate:

300 g × 4 kilocalories/g = 1,200 kilocalories from carbohydrate

Next divide the number of kilocalories from carbohydrate by the total number of kilocalories in the diet and multiply by 100 to convert it to a percentage. In this example, the diet contains 2,000 total kilocalories, and so it provides:

(1,200 kilocalories from carbohydrate/2,000 kilocalories total) × 100 = 60% of kilocalories from carbohydrate. This value is between the AMDR of 45–65% daily energy from carbohydrates.

© Anna Oksimowicz / Alamy

THINKING IT THROUGH

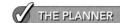

Becoming Less Refined

Lucia thinks a good diet is important. She is concerned that she eats too much added refined sugar and not enough fibre. To determine whether this is a problem, she records what she eats for a day and uses iProfile to determine her energy and nutrient intake. Lucia finds that her daily diet provides 2,340 kcal, 67 grams of protein, 80 grams of fat, 350 grams of carbohydrate, and 12 grams of fibre.

How does her intake compare with the recommended amounts of carbohydrate and fibre?
▼

Your answer: _____

_____

By calculating the percentage of calories from carbohydrate (350 grams carbohydrate × 4 kcal/gram ÷ 2,340 kcal × 100 = 60%), Lucia finds that she is within the recommended range of 45 to 65%. Her fibre intake is low, however. She eats 12 grams of fibre, which is 13 grams less than the 25 grams recommended for women her age.

Lucia is 23 years old and exercises 30 to 60 minutes per day. Each day, she eats about six servings of grain products, three servings of vegetables, and one serving of fruit.

How does her intake of grains, fruits, and vegetables compare with *Eating Well with Canada's Food Guide*?
▼

Your answer: _____

_____

To increase her fibre intake Lucia looks at the grains, fruits, and vegetables in her diet. She decides to switch to whole-grain bread and cereal but is not sure which fruits and vegetables are the best sources of fibre. She therefore looks up the fibre content of some of her favourites.

Choose a combination of fruits and vegetables from this list that will add at least 13 grams of fibre to Lucia's diet.
▼

Food	Fibre (grams)	Food	Fibre (grams)
Black beans, 125 mL (½ cup)	7.5	Canned pears, 125 mL (½ cup)	3
Green beans, 125 mL (½ cup)	2	Kiwi, 2 small	5
Iceberg lettuce, 250 mL (1 cup)	0.8	Broccoli, 125 mL (½ cup)	2.4
Apple, 1 medium	3.7	Banana, 1 medium	2.8
Asparagus, 125 mL (½ cup)	1.4	Raw spinach, 250 mL (1 cup)	0.8
Orange, 1 medium	3	Watermelon, 250 mL (1 cup)	0.8

Your answer: _____

_____

Lucia sees that much of the added sugar in her diet comes from pop and candy. She decides she can reduce her intake of added sugar and boost her fibre intake by drinking water and eating dried fruit and granola bars as snacks.

What are the carbohydrate pros and cons of these two choices?
▼

Your answer: _____

_____

(Check your answers in Appendix I.)

Nutrition Facts
Valeur nutritive
Per 1/4 cup (40 g)/par 1/4 tasse (40 g)

Amount Teneur	% Daily Value % valeur quotidienne
Calories / Calories 110	
Fat / Lipides 0 g	0 %
Saturated / saturés 0 g + Trans / trans 0 g	0 %
Cholesterol / Cholestérol 0 mg	0 %
Sodium / Sodium <5 mg	0 %
Carbohydrate / Glucides 26 g	9 %
Fibre / Fibres 2 g	8 %
Sugars / Sucres 15 g	
Protein / Protéines 1g	
Vitamin A / Vitamine A	15 %
Vitamin C / Vitamine C	2 %
Calcium / Calcium	2 %
Iron / Fer	0 %

Ingredients: Dried apricots, natural flavours, sulphur dioxide added as a preservative.

Nutrition Facts
Valeur nutritive
Per 1 bar (42 g) / par 1 barre (42 g)

Amount Teneur	% Daily Value % valeur quotidienne
Calories / Calories 180	
Fat / Lipides 6 g	9 %
Saturated / saturés 0.5 g + Trans / trans 0 g	3 %
Cholesterol / Cholestérol 0 mg	0 %
Sodium / Sodium 167 mg	7 %
Carbohydrate / Glucides 29 g	10 %
Fibre / Fibres 2 g	8 %
Sugars / Sucres 11 g	
Protein / Protéines 4 g	
Vitamin A / Vitamine A	0 %
Vitamin C / Vitamine C	0 %
Calcium / Calcium	4 %
Iron / Fer	4 %
Riboflavin / Riboflavine	2 %
Niacin / Niacine	4 %

Ingredients: Whole grain rolled oats, sugar, canola oil, crisp rice with soy protein (rice flour, soy protein concentrate, sugar malt, salt), honey, brown sugar syrup, soy lecithin, baking soda, natural flavour, peanut flour, almond flour, pecan flour.

Healthy Canada's Food Guide carbohydrate choices • Figure 4.21

Carbohydrates are the main nutrient found in grain products and vegetables and fruits, but sources of carbohydrates can be found in every food group. Unrefined, nutrient dense sources should be favoured, while heavily processed sources and those that are high in added sugars, salt, and fat should be limited.

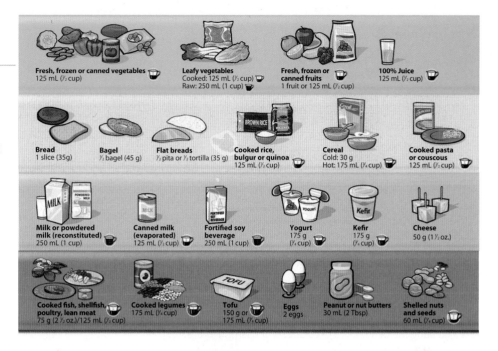

Fresh, frozen or canned vegetables 125 mL (½ cup)

Leafy vegetables Cooked: 125 mL (½ cup) Raw: 250 mL (1 cup)

Fresh, frozen or canned fruits 1 fruit or 125 mL (½ cup)

100% Juice 125 mL (½ cup)

Bread 1 slice (35g)

Bagel ½ bagel (45 g)

Flat breads ½ pita or ½ tortilla (35 g)

Cooked rice, bulgur or quinoa 125 mL (½ cup)

Cereal Cold: 30 g Hot: 175 mL (¾ cup)

Cooked pasta or couscous 125 mL (½ cup)

Milk or powdered milk (reconstituted) 250 mL (1 cup)

Canned milk (evaporated) 125 mL (½ cup)

Fortified soy beverage 250 mL (1 cup)

Yogurt 175 g (¾ cup)

Kefir 175 g (¾ cup)

Cheese 50 g (1 ½ oz.)

Cooked fish, shellfish, poultry, lean meat 75 g (2 ½ oz.)/125 mL (½ cup)

Cooked legumes 175 mL (¾ cup)

Tofu 150 g or 175 mL (¾ cup)

Eggs 2 eggs

Peanut or nut butters 30 mL (2 Tbsp)

Shelled nuts and seeds 60 mL (¼ cup)

Using *Eating Well with Canada's Food Guide*

For most Canadians, the vegetables and fruits and grain products food groups provide us with the majority of our carbohydrate intake. For a 2,000-kilocalorie diet, the food guide recommends that adult females consume six to seven servings and adult males consume eight servings of grain products a day (at least half of which should be whole grains). These females should also be consuming seven to eight servings of vegetables and fruits a day, while men should be consuming eight to ten servings. As **Figure 4.21** suggests, refined carbohydrates can be replaced with unrefined ones to make the diet healthier. For example, an apple provides about 80 kilocalories and 3.7 grams of fibre, making it a better choice than a cup of apple juice, which has the same amount of energy but almost no fibre (0.2 gram).

WHAT SHOULD I EAT?
Carbohydrates

✓ THE PLANNER

Choose more unrefined carbohydrates
- Pass on the white bread and instead have your sandwich on whole wheat, oat bran, rye, or pumpernickel.
- Add extra vegetables to your stir fry and serve it over brown rice.
- Satisfy your sweet tooth with a fresh fruit salad.

Increase your fibre
- Don't forget beans—kidney beans, chickpeas, black beans, and others have more fibre and resistant starch than any other vegetables.

- Add berries, bananas, and oats to cereal and desserts.
- Eat air-popped popcorn instead of potato chips.

Limit added sugars
- Switch to a 355-mL (12-oz) can instead of a 591-mL (20-oz) bottle when you grab some pop or, better yet, have a glass of low-fat milk.
- Use one-quarter less sugar in your recipe next time you bake.
- Snack on a piece of fruit instead of a chocolate bar.
- Switch to an unsweetened breakfast cereal.

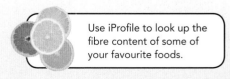

Use iProfile to look up the fibre content of some of your favourite foods.

Whole Wheat Bread

Nutrition Facts
Valeur nutritive
Per 1 slice (27 g) / par 1 tranche (27 g)

Amount Teneur	% Daily Value % valeur quotidienne
Calories / Calories 70	
Fat / Lipides 1 g	2 %
Saturated / saturés 0 g + Trans / trans 0 g	0 %
Cholesterol / Cholestérol 0 mg	0 %
Sodium / Sodium 10 mg	0 %
Carbohydrate / Glucides 12 g	4 %
Fibre / Fibres 2 g	8 %
Sugars / Sucres 2 g	
Protein / Protéines 2 g	
Iron / Fer	8 %

The Nutrition Facts panel of a food label lists the number of grams of total carbohydrate, fibre, and sugars. The total carbohydrate and fibre values are also given as a percentage of the Daily Value.

*Percent Daily Values (DV) are based on a 2,000-calorie diet. Your daily values may be higher or lower depending on your calorie needs:

	Calories:	2,000	2,500
Total Fat	Less than	65g	80g
Sat Fat	Less than	20g	25g
Cholesterol	Less than	300mg	300mg
Sodium	Less than	2,400mg	2,400mg
Total Carbohydrate		300g	375g
Dietary Fibre		25g	30g

NOT A SODIUM FREE FOOD

The Daily Value for total carbohydrate is 60% of the diet's energy content, or 300 g for a 2,000-Calorie diet. The Daily Value for fibre in a 2,000-Calorie diet is 25 g for men and 38 g for women.

INGREDIENTS: WHOLE WHEAT FLOUR, WATER, SWEETENERS (GLUCOSE/FRUCTOSE, MOLASSES), WHEAT GLUTEN, SOYBEAN CONTAINS 2% OR LESS OF THE FOLLOWING: YEAST DOUGH CONDITIONERS (MONO DIGLYCERIDES, ETHOXYLATED MONO & GLYCERIDES, CALCIUM STEAROYL-2-LACTYLATE), YEAST NUTRIENTS (CALCIUM SULFATE, MONO- CALCIUM PHOSPHA CALCIUM PROPIONATE (A PRESERVATIVE).

To identify products made mostly from *whole* grains, look for the word "whole" before the name of the grain. If this is the first ingredient listed, the product is made from mostly whole grain. "Wheat flour" simply means it was made with wheat, not whole wheat. Note that foods labelled with the words "multigrain," "stone-ground," "100% wheat," "cracked wheat," "seven-grain," or "bran" are not necessarily 100% whole-grain products and may also contain refined grains.

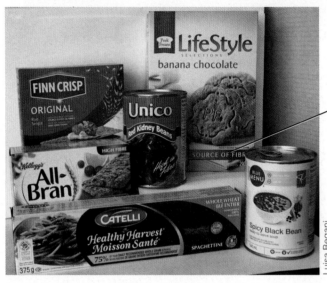

Food labelled "source of fibre," "high source of fibre," and "very high source of fibre" must respectively contain at least 2, 4, and 6 grams of fibre per serving.

The ingredient list helps identify added sugars. Many products have more than one added sweetener. The closer the name of each sweetener appears to the beginning of the list, the more of it has been added.

INGREDIENTS: CULTURED PASTEURIZED GRADE A REDUCED FAT MILK, SUGAR, NONFAT MILK, GLUCOSE/FRUCTOSE, STRAWBERRY PUREE, MODIFIED CORN STARCH, KOSHER GELATIN, TRI-CALCIUM PHOSPHATE, NATURAL FLAVOUR COLOURED WITH CARMINE, VITAMIN A ACETATE, VITAMIN D₃

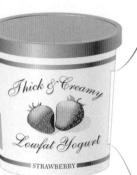

On the ingredient list, all these mean added sugar: Brown sugar, corn sweetener, corn syrup, dextrose, fructose, fruit juice, glucose, glucose/fructose, honey, invert sugar, lactose, maltose, malt syrup, molasses, raw sugar, sucrose, and sugar syrup concentrates.

Products labelled "reduced sugar" contain 25% less sugar than the regular, or reference, product.

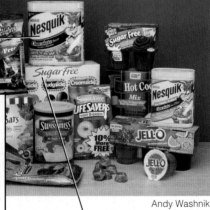

Andy Washnik

Foods labelled "sugar free" contain less than 0.5 g of sugar per serving.

Nutrition Facts
Valeur nutritive
Per 125 mL (87 g) / par 125 mL (87g)

Amount Teneur	% Daily Value % valeur quotidienne
Calories / Calories 190	
Fat / Lipides 3.5 g	5 %
Saturated / saturés 2 g + Trans / trans 0 g	10 %
Cholesterol / Cholestérol 15 mg	4 %
Sodium / Sodium 100 mg	4 %
Carbohydrate / Glucides 32 g	11 %
Fibre / Fibres 0 g	0 %
Sugars / Sucres 28 g	
Protein / Protéines 7 g	
Vitamin A / Vitamine A	15 %
Vitamin C / Vitamine C	0 %
Calcium / Calcium	30 %
Iron / Fer	0 %

The number of grams of sugars listed under Nutrition Facts tells you the total amount of mono-saccharides plus disaccharides in a food, but this number does not distinguish between added sugar and the sugar occurring naturally in the food.

Interpreting food labels Food labels can help in choosing the right mix of carbohydrates (**Figure 4.22**). The Nutrition Facts panel helps find foods that are good sources of fibre. The ingredient list helps identify whole-grain products and sources of added sugar. Health claims and nutrient content claims such as "high in fibre" or "no sugar added" identify foods that help meet the recommendations for fibre and added sugar intake (see *What Should I Eat? Carbohydrates*).

CONCEPT CHECK

1. **How** does the Canadian diet compare with recommendations for fibre and added sugar?

2. **What** types of carbohydrate are recommended by *Eating Well with Canada's Food Guide*?

3. **Where** on a food label can you find information about added sugars?

Summary

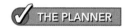

1 Carbohydrates in Our Food   98

- **Unrefined foods** such as whole grains, fruits, and vegetables are good sources of fibre and micronutrients. When these foods are **refined**, nutrients and fibre are lost.

- Whole grains contain the **bran**, **germ**, and **endosperm**; refined grains include only the endosperm. **Enrichment**, one type of **fortification**, adds back some but not all of the nutrients lost in refining. Unrefined **whole grain products** are therefore typically more nutrient dense than refined ones.

- Refined sugars contain **empty calories** with few nutrients; for this reason, foods high in added refined sugar are low in nutrient density.

Whole grains • Figure 4.2

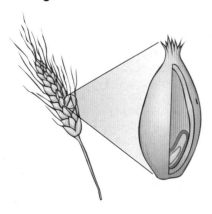

2 Types of Carbohydrates   100

- Carbohydrates contain carbon and also contain hydrogen and oxygen in the same proportion as in water. Carbohydrates include **monosaccharides**, **disaccharides**, and **polysaccharides**, which, respectively, comprise one, two, and more than two **sugar units**.

- **Simple carbohydrates** are those with only one or two sugar units per molecule. Monosaccharides are composed of a single sugar unit and include **glucose**, **fructose**, and **galactose**. Disaccharides have two sugar units in a chain. **Maltose**, **sucrose**, and **lactose** are examples of disaccharides.

- **Complex carbohydrates** are those composed of longer chains of sugar units. **Glycogen** is the type of complex carbohydrate used to store glucose in the body. **Starch** is made in plants through the process of **photosynthesis** and is our main dietary source of complex carbohydrates. **Fibre** is a complex carbohydrate that cannot be digested in the stomach or small intestine. **Soluble fibre** dissolves in water to form a viscous solution and is digested by bacteria in the colon; **insoluble fibre** is not digested by bacteria and adds bulk to fecal matter.

Carbohydrates • Figure 4.4

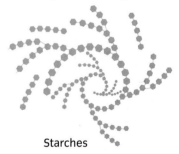

Starches

3 Carbohydrate Digestion and Absorption   103

- Disaccharides and starches must be digested to monosaccharides before they can be absorbed. In individuals with **lactose intolerance**, low levels of the enzyme lactase allow lactose to pass into the colon undigested, causing cramps, gas, and diarrhea. Indigestible complex carbohydrates, including fibre, some **oligosaccharides**, and **resistant starch**, can increase intestinal gas, but they benefit health by increasing bulk in the stool, promoting growth of healthy microbiota, and slowing nutrient absorption.

- After a meal, blood glucose levels rise. The rate and duration of this rise are referred to as the **glycemic response**. Glycemic response is affected by the amount and type of carbohydrate consumed and by other nutrients ingested with the carbohydrate. The **glycemic index** ranks foods on their likelihood to trigger a glycemic response. Its major shortcoming is that it is measured using a portion of food with a set amount of carbohydrate. The **glycemic load** considers the glycemic response of a more typical food portion and is therefore often used instead of the glycemic index.

Carbohydrate digestion • Figure 4.7

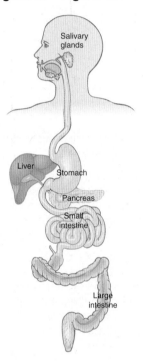

Ketone formation • Figure 4.10

glucose. Therefore, adequate carbohydrate intake is said to spare protein. Limited carbohydrate intake also results in the formation of **ketones** (or **ketone bodies**) by the liver. These can be used as an energy source by other tissues. Ketones that accumulate in the blood can lead to **ketosis**. Symptoms of this condition range from headache and lack of appetite to coma and even death if levels of ketones are extremely high.

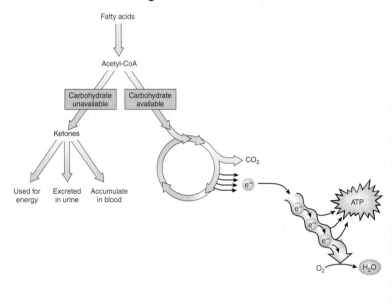

- **Diabetes mellitus**, commonly called diabetes, is characterized by high blood glucose levels. It occurs either because insufficient insulin is produced due to a genetic **autoimmune disease (type-1 diabetes)** or because of **insulin resistance** in the body (**type-2 diabetes**). People who have type-2 diabetes begin with an elevated blood glucose state called **prediabetes**. If lifestyle medication and treatment cannot promote healthy blood glucose levels and the body becomes **insulin resistant**, type-2 diabetes can fully manifest. Over time, high blood glucose levels damage tissues and contribute to the development of heart disease, kidney failure, blindness, and infections that may lead to amputations. Pregnant women are also at risk for **gestational diabetes**, which increases pregnancy-related risks and the risk of developing type-2 diabetes after the child is born.

- **Hypoglycemia**, or low blood glucose, causes symptoms such as sweating, headaches, and rapid heartbeat. **Fasting hypoglycemia** occurs when blood glucose levels drop in response to a lack of dietary carbohydrate. **Reactive hypoglycemia** can occur after a meal that is very high in carbohydrates. In this situation, the high glycemic response triggers a large release of insulin, which promotes a large uptake of glucose into the cells and drops blood glucose levels dramatically.

- Carbohydrate, primarily as glucose, provides energy to the body. Blood glucose levels are maintained by the hormones **insulin** and **glucagon**. When blood glucose levels rise, insulin from the pancreas allows cells to take up glucose from the blood and promotes the synthesis of glycogen and fat. When blood glucose levels fall, glucagon increases them by causing glycogen breakdown and glucose synthesis.

- Glucose is metabolized through cellular respiration. It begins with **glycolysis**, which breaks each six-carbon glucose molecule into two three-carbon pyruvate molecules, producing ATP even when oxygen is unavailable. The complete breakdown of glucose through **aerobic metabolism** requires oxygen and produces carbon dioxide, water, and more ATP than glycolysis. Glucose can also be broken down through **anaerobic metabolism**, which doesn't require oxygen, but much less energy is derived this way.

- When carbohydrate intake is limited, amino acids from the breakdown of body proteins can be used to synthesize

- Diets high in carbohydrate, particularly refined sugars, increase the risk of dental caries. The carbohydrate provides a food supply for bacteria that form plaque on the teeth.

- Gram for gram, carbohydrates provide less energy than fat. High-fibre diets may prevent weight gain by making you feel full longer so that you eat less. Low-carbohydrate diets promote weight loss by causing a spontaneous reduction in food intake. **Non-nutritive sweeteners** aid weight loss if the sugar calories they replace are not added back from other food sources. While non-nutritive sweeteners can be included in a healthy diet, it is recommended that people stay below the **acceptable daily intakes (ADIs)** for these products.

- Diets high in unrefined carbohydrates from whole grains, vegetables, fruits, and legumes may reduce the risk of heart disease. Soluble fibre helps prevent heart disease by lowering blood cholesterol.

- Fibre is involved in promoting bowel health. If a diet lacks fibre, it can lead to damage of the walls of the large intestine, resulting in outpouchings, or **diverticula**. A person who has **diverticulosis** will typically have many diverticula

throughout their colon. These diverticula can become inflamed and irritated, a condition known as **diverticulitis**. A high-fibre diet can reduce the risk of developing diverticulosis and reduce the incidence of both constipation and **hemorrhoids**, the swelling of veins in the rectal or anal area.

6 Meeting Carbohydrate Needs 119

- Guidelines for a healthy diet recommend 45 to 65% of energy from carbohydrates. Most of this dietary carbohydrate should come from whole grains, legumes, fruits, and vegetables. Foods high in added sugar should be consumed in moderation.

- The recommendations of *Eating Well with Canada's Food Guide* and the information on food labels can be used to select healthy amounts and sources of carbohydrate.

Choosing carbohydrates from the label • Figure 4.22

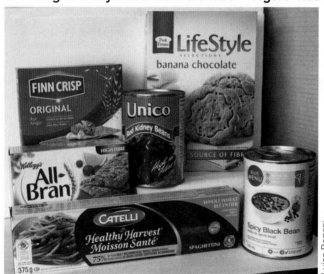

Luisa Begani

Cholesterol and soluble fibre • Figure 4.18

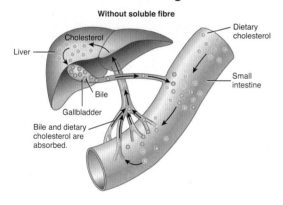

Key Terms

Critical and Creative Thinking Questions

1. Adam is 14 and plays basketball. Recently, he has been thirsty all the time, and he needs to get up several times a night to urinate. He has lost 4.5 kg (10 lb.) and is so tired that he has been missing basketball practice. What type of diabetes is most likely affecting Adam? How does it need to be managed? Why is it important to keep blood sugar levels within the normal range in both type-1 and type-2 diabetes?

2. Are carbohydrates good for you? Explain why or why not.

3. Imagine that you have gained 9 kg (20 lb.) over the past five years, and you decide to use a low-carbohydrate diet to return to a healthy weight. You are happy with your initial weight loss but begin to have headaches and bad breath. What is causing these symptoms and why?

4. Your breakfast cereal provides 20% of the Daily Value for fibre and lists whole oats as the first ingredient and brown sugar as the second ingredient. What does this information tell you about whether it is a whole-grain product? What does this information tell you about the amount of added sugar it contains? Would you recommend this product to a friend? Why or why not?

5. Record everything you eat for three days. Next to each high-carbohydrate food, record whether the food is unrefined, minimally processed, or highly processed. Suggest some changes to increase your intake of less refined carbohydrates. List some foods in your diet that are high in added sugars. Suggest some changes to reduce your intake of these sugars. How can you increase your fibre intake?

What is happening in this picture?

These students are choosing fruit drinks because they believe these beverages are healthier choices than pop.

Think Critically

1. How does the amount of added sugar in fruit drinks, sports drinks, and iced tea compare to the amount in soft drinks?
2. Do these beverages provide significant amounts of any essential nutrients?
3. Suggest beverage alternatives that would be lower in added sugar.

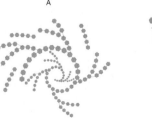

altrendo images/Altrendo/Getty Images, Inc.

Self-Test

(Check your answers in Appendix J.)

1. Which of the following is a source of unrefined carbohydrate?
   a. white bread
   b. white rice
   c. corn on the cob
   d. donut

2. Which of the following is most likely to occur soon after you eat a large carbohydrate-rich meal?
   a. You break down body fat stores.
   b. Your pancreas releases insulin.
   c. Your pancreas releases glucagon.
   d. Your liver breaks down glycogen.

3. Which of the molecules in the figure below is a disaccharide?

   a. A   b. B   c. C   d. D

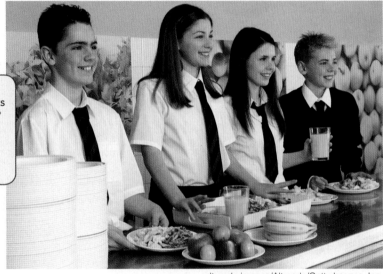

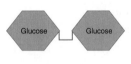

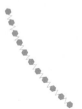

4. If curve B on the graph shows the glycemic response after eating kidney beans, which of the following foods is most likely to cause a glycemic response similar to that shown by curve A?

   a. saltine crackers   b. pat of butter

   c. egg   d. bowl of bran cereal

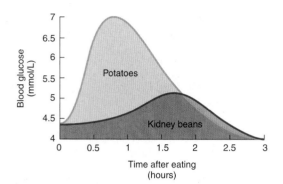

5. A diet that provides about half of its calories from carbohydrate _____.

   a. contains too much carbohydrate to be healthy

   b. is bad for your heart

   c. increases the risk of diabetes

   d. contains the recommended percentage of carbohydrate

6. In the figure below, which part of a whole grain contains most of the grain's fibre and many vitamins?

   a. A   b. B   c. C

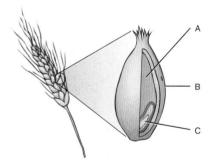

7. Foods high in added sugar provide _____.

   a. many vitamins in each calorie

   b. empty calories

   c. soluble fibre

   d. insoluble fibre

8. Which statement about simple carbohydrates is false?

   a. Fructose is found in fruit.

   b. Lactose is milk sugar.

   c. Glucose is blood sugar.

   d. Maltose is table sugar.

9. The digestive enzymes that break disaccharides into monosaccharides are located in the _____.

   a. stomach   b. saliva

   c. brush border   d. colon

10. When blood glucose levels drop, which of the following does not occur?

   a. Glucagon is released.

   b. Glycogen is broken down.

   c. Fatty acids are used to make glucose.

   d. Amino acids from protein are used to make glucose.

11. Which of the following statements about soluble fibre is false?

   a. It holds water in the gastrointestinal tract.

   b. It is not digested by bacteria in the colon.

   c. It dissolves in water and forms a viscous solution.

   d. It slows the absorption of nutrients.

12. People who are lactose intolerant do not produce enough of the enzyme _____.

   a. lactase   b. lactose

   c. galactose   d. amylase

13. The graph below shows an individual's glycemic response after consuming a sugar-sweetened beverage. Which of the following individuals does this graph represent?

   a. a person who has a normal glycemic response

   b. a person who has hypoglycemia

   c. a person who has prediabetes

   d. a person who has diabetes

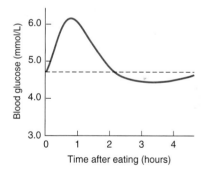

14. Which of the following is an anaerobic process?

   a. glycolysis

   b. the conversion of pyruvate to acetyl CoA

   c. the citric acid cycle

   d. the electron transport chain

15. A high-fibre diet may help protect against which of the following?

   a. heart disease

   b. diverticulosis

   c. large swings in blood glucose

   d. all of the above

THE PLANNER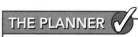

Review your Chapter Planner on the chapter opener and check off your completed work.

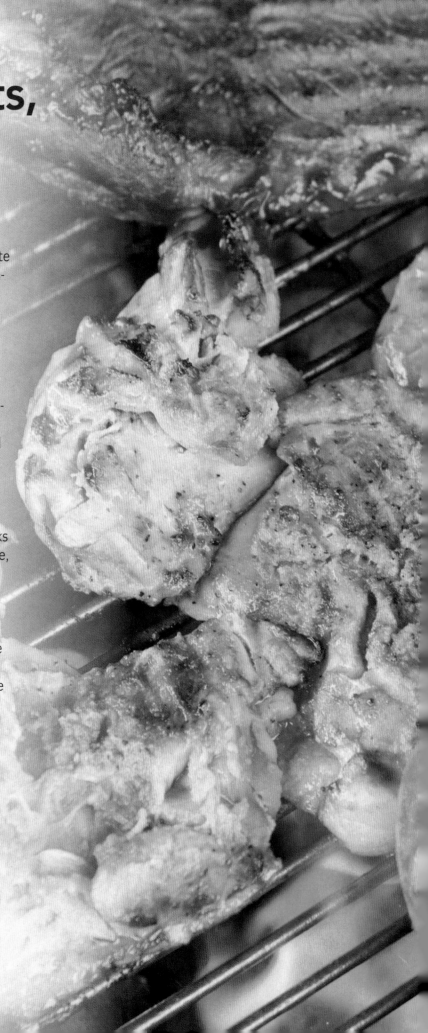

Lipids: Oils, Fats, Phospholipids, and Sterols

"**S**ausages taste good. Pork chops taste good," wrote filmmaker Quentin Tarantino in the original screenplay of *Pulp Fiction*. Fat makes foods taste good, smell good, and feel good to our palate. Tarantino understands the appeal of fat. As for its function, we have to rely on study, not entertainment.

The word *fat* has come to be associated with unhealthiness, unfitness, and obesity. Fitness gurus and enthusiastic celebrities declare that "fat is bad," whether you are considering which fast-food meal to choose or trying to remove it from your waist. Their 30-second commercial or half-hour program for a new diet regimen or exercise contraption—or both—gives little consideration to the vital role that fats play in healthy nutrition. There is, in reality, nothing intrinsically "bad" about dietary fats. The body uses fats as building blocks for other molecules, for vitamin absorbtion and storage, as a source of energy, and for energy storage. Fats are as important to a well-balanced diet as carbohydrates, proteins, and vitamins; without fats, the body cannot function.

Unfortunately, the amount of dietary fat we require and the amount we desire are often two very different things. In the case of the body's requirements for these substances, moderation is key. Whatever our bodies don't use remains in reserves of stored fat. Depending on our lifestyle choices, these abundant unused reserves may become not only unnecessary but harmful to our health.

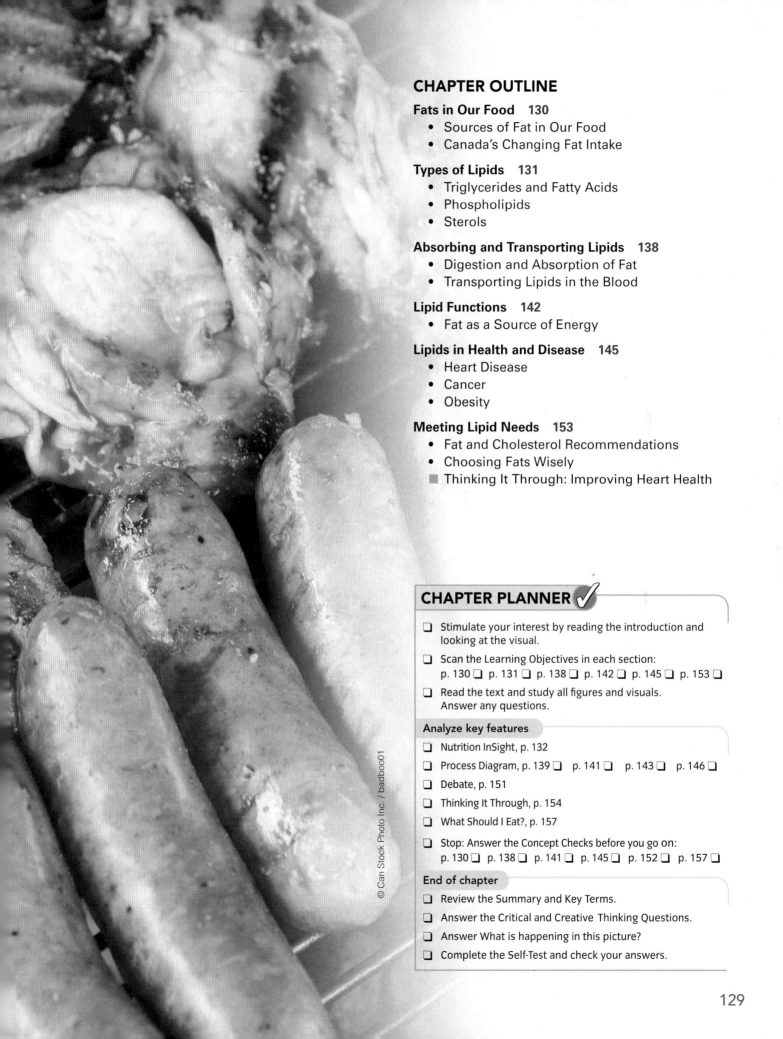

CHAPTER OUTLINE

© Can Stock Photo Inc. / badboo01

CHAPTER PLANNER ✓

- ❑ Stimulate your interest by reading the introduction and looking at the visual.
- ❑ Scan the Learning Objectives in each section:
  p. 130 ❑   p. 131 ❑   p. 138 ❑   p. 142 ❑   p. 145 ❑   p. 153 ❑
- ❑ Read the text and study all figures and visuals. Answer any questions.

Analyze key features
- ❑ Nutrition InSight, p. 132
- ❑ Process Diagram, p. 139 ❑   p. 141 ❑   p. 143 ❑   p. 146 ❑
- ❑ Debate, p. 151
- ❑ Thinking It Through, p. 154
- ❑ What Should I Eat?, p. 157
- ❑ Stop: Answer the Concept Checks before you go on:
  p. 130 ❑   p. 138 ❑   p. 141 ❑   p. 145 ❑   p. 152 ❑   p. 157 ❑

End of chapter
- ❑ Review the Summary and Key Terms.
- ❑ Answer the Critical and Creative Thinking Questions.
- ❑ Answer What is happening in this picture?
- ❑ Complete the Self-Test and check your answers.

Fats in Our Food

LEARNING OBJECTIVES

1. **Describe** the qualities that fat adds to foods.

2. **Identify** sources of hidden fat in the diet.

3. **Discuss** how fat intake in Canada has changed since the 1970s.

The fats in our foods contribute to their texture, flavour, and aroma. It is the fat that gives ice cream its smooth texture and rich taste. Olive oil imparts a unique flavour to salads and many traditional Italian and Greek dishes. Sesame oil gives egg rolls and other Chinese foods their distinctive aroma. But while the fats in our foods contribute to their appeal, they also add to their caloric content and can affect our health both positively and negatively.

Sources of Fat in Our Food

Sometimes the fat in our food is obvious. For example, you can see the strips of fat in a slice of bacon sizzling in a frying pan or the layer of fat around the outside of your steak. Other visible sources of fat in our diets are the fats we add to foods at the table—the pat of butter melting on your steaming baked potato and the dressing you pour over your salad.

Some other sources of fat are less obvious. Cheese, ice cream, and whole milk are high in fat, and foods such as crackers, doughnuts, cookies, and muffins, which we think of as sources of carbohydrates, may also be quite high in fat (**Figure 5.1**). We also add invisible fat when we fry foods: French fries start as potatoes, which are low in fat, but when they are immersed in hot oil for frying, they become higher sources of fat.

Canada's Changing Fat Intake

Eating patterns in Canada have changed significantly over time, moving away from issues of inadequacies, which occurred in the pre-war period, towards issues of excesses, occurring now. The consumption of fats has also changed, from the total amounts we eat, to the types of fat we eat, to the sources of fat in our diet. Exactly how much fat Canadians consume is difficult to determine, but Statistics Canada estimates that the average fat intake has risen

Visible and hidden fats • Figure 5.1

The amount of fat in a food is not always obvious. The two strips of bacon in this breakfast provide a total of 8 g of fat, and the muffin provides 16 g.

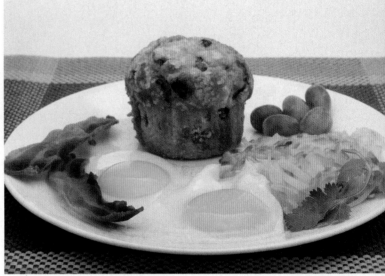

© iStockphoto.com/Donald Erickson

from 85 grams per day in 1981 to 91 grams per day in 2009. This latest estimate is down from an all-time high of 101 grams per day in 2001.[1] We are eating more fat overall, but because our caloric intake has also increased over the past three decades, the proportion of fat in our diet has remained relatively constant (**Figure 5.2c**).[1] In general, Canadians are doing better in terms of the types of fat we eat: We are eating less *trans* fats, saturated fats, and cholesterol, and we are increasing our consumptions of heart-healthy unsaturated fats. While red meats continue to be a main source of fat in the diet, a good portion of our fat intake comes from items such as pizza, sandwiches, burgers, cakes, cookies, and doughnuts (**Figure 5.2b**).[2]

CONCEPT CHECK

1. **How** does the fat in ice cream contribute to its appeal?

2. **What** are some invisible sources of fat in the diet?

3. **How** have the sources of fat in the Canadian diet changed since the 1980s?

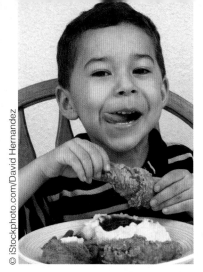

Canadian food intake then and now • Figure 5.2

b. Today, we drink low-fat milk and eat leaner meats, but we eat more fat from creams, cheese, sauces, and take-out food.[2]

c. In 1981, it is estimated that Canadians consumed an average of 2,214 kilocalories and 85 grams of fat per day. This rose to 2,358 kilocalories and 91 grams of fat in 2009. While our total fat consumption has increased, since our caloric intake has also increased, the proportion of calories from fat in our diet has stayed relatively constant.[1]

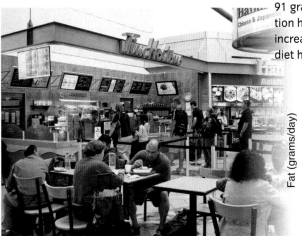

© B. O'Kane / Alamy

a. In the 1970s, a typical dinner included high-fat meat, bread with butter, and mashed potatoes with lots of gravy, and it was usually served with a glass of whole milk.

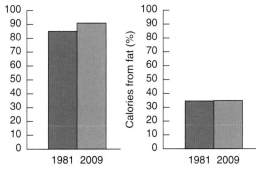

Types of Lipids
LEARNING OBJECTIVES

1. **Describe** the functions of triglycerides, phospholipids, and cholesterol.

2. **Compare** the structures of saturated, monounsaturated, polyunsaturated, omega-6, omega-3, and *trans* fatty acids.

3. **Name** foods that are sources of saturated, monounsaturated, polyunsaturated, omega-6, omega-3, and *trans* fatty acids.

4. **Explain** why some fatty acids are considered essential.

Lipids are hydrophobic substances, meaning they do not dissolve in water. We tend to use the term *fat* to refer to lipids, but we are usually referring to types of lipids called **triglycerides**. Triglycerides make up most of the lipids in our food and in our bodies. The structure of triglycerides includes three lipid molecules called **fatty acids** attached to a backbone of glycerol, another hydrophobic molecule.

lipids A group of organic molecules, most of which do not dissolve in water. They include fatty acids, triglycerides, phospholipids, and sterols.

Two other types of lipids that are important in nutrition but are present in the body in smaller amounts are **phospholipids** and **sterols**.

Triglycerides and Fatty Acids

A triglyceride consists of the three-carbon molecule glycerol with three fatty acids attached to it (**Figure 5.3a**). A fatty acid is a chain of carbon atoms with an acid group at one end of the chain (**Figure 5.3b**). Fatty acids vary in the length of their carbon chains and the types and locations of carbon–carbon bonds within the chain. Triglycerides may contain different combinations of fatty acids. The fatty acids in a triglyceride determine the triglyceride's function in the body and the properties it gives to food.

triglycerides The major form of lipids in food and the body; consist of three fatty acids attached to a glycerol molecule.

fatty acids Molecules made up of a chain of carbons linked to hydrogen, with an acid group at one end of the chain.

phospholipids Types of lipids whose structure includes a phosphorus atom.

sterols Types of lipids with a structure composed of multiple chemical rings.

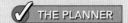

a. A triglyceride contains glycerol and three fatty acids. The carbon chains of the fatty acids vary in length from short-chain fatty acids (4 to 7 carbons) to medium-chain (8 to 12 carbons) and long-chain fatty acids (more than 12 carbons). The types of fatty acids in triglycerides determine their texture, taste, physical characteristics, and actions in the body.

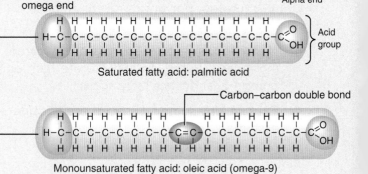

Glycerol — Fatty acids

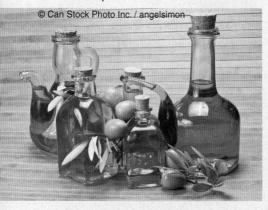

© Can Stock Photo Inc. / angelsimon

Oils are fats that are liquid at room temperature. The properties of the fatty acids in vegetable oil allow it to remain a liquid.

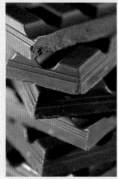

© iStockphoto.com/peepo

The amounts and types of fatty acids in the triglycerides of chocolate allow it to remain brittle at room temperature, snap when bitten into, and then melt quickly and smoothly in your mouth.

b. Most fatty acids in plants and animals contain between 14 and 22 carbons. Each carbon atom in the carbon chain is attached to up to four other atoms. At the omega (also called methyl) end of the carbon chain, three hydrogen atoms are attached to the carbon (CH_3). At the other end of the chain, the alpha end, an acid group (COOH) is attached to the carbon. Each of the carbon atoms in between is attached to two carbon atoms and up to two hydrogen atoms. If only one hydrogen atom is attached to adjacent carbon atoms, a double bond forms between them, and the fat is unsaturated; that is, it is less saturated with hydrogen atoms.

A **saturated fat** when each carbon atom is attached to as many hydrogen atoms as possible so that no double bonds form. The fat on the outside of a steak is solid at room temperature because it is high in saturated fatty acids.

A **monounsaturated fatty acid** contains one carbon–carbon double bond. Canola, olive, and peanut oils, as well as nuts and avocados, are high in monounsaturated fatty acids.

A **polyunsaturated fatty acid** contains more than one carbon–carbon double bond. When the first double bond occurs between the sixth and seventh carbon atoms (from the omega end), the fatty acid is called an **omega-6 (ω-6) fatty acid**. Corn oil, safflower oil, soybean oil, and nuts are sources of omega-6 polyunsaturated fatty acids.

If the first double bond in a polyunsaturated fatty acid occurs between the third and fourth carbon atoms (from the omega end), the fatty acid is an **omega-3 (ω-3) fatty acid**. Fish oils, flaxseed, soybean and canola oils, nuts, and leafy green vegetables are sources of omega-3 polyunsaturated fatty acids.

Methyl or omega end — Alpha end

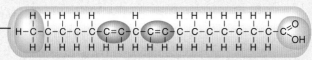

Acid group

Saturated fatty acid: palmitic acid

Carbon–carbon double bond

Monounsaturated fatty acid: oleic acid (omega-9)

Polyunsaturated fatty acid: linoleic acid (omega-6)

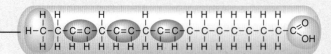

Polyunsaturated fatty acid: alpha-linolenic acid (omega-3)

Fatty acids are classified as **saturated fatty acids** or **unsaturated fatty acids**, depending on whether they contain carbon–carbon double bonds (see Figure 5.3b).

> **saturated fatty acid** A fatty acid in which the carbon atoms are bonded to as many hydrogen atoms as possible; it therefore contains no carbon–carbon double bonds.
>
> **unsaturated fatty acid** A fatty acid that contains one or more carbon–carbon double bonds; may be either monounsaturated or polyunsaturated.

Saturated fats have no double bonds and are thus "saturated" with hydrogen atoms. Unsaturated fatty acids have one or more double bonds, leaving less room for hydrogen atoms, making them "less saturated" or "unsaturated" with these atoms. The number, location, and type of double bonds affect both the characteristics that fatty acids give to food and the health effects they have in the body. Triglycerides that are high in saturated fatty acids, such as those found in butter and lard, tend to be solid at room temperature, whereas triglycerides that are higher in unsaturated fatty acids, such as those found in corn, canola, and sunflower oils, are liquid at room temperature.

Saturated fats Saturated fatty acids are more plentiful in animal foods, such as meat and dairy products, than in plant foods. Plant oils are generally low in saturated fatty acids (**Figure 5.4**). The long-chain saturated fats found in animal sources have long been implicated in the development of cardiovascular disease due to their association with increased levels of LDL ("bad") cholesterol in the blood. Diets that replace saturated fat intake with unsaturated fat intake, especially polyunsaturated fat, are believed to offer a modestly reduced risk of heart disease.[3]

Medium-chain saturated fats Most of the fatty acids we consume come from longer chain fatty acids, such as stearic acid, which is 18 carbons long. Medium chain fatty acids (6–10 carbons in length) behave differently and may have more beneficial effects compared to their longer counterparts. Since these fats are shorter and relatively water-soluble, they are quickly digested and absorbed into the blood stream (Note: not the lymph). They then bypass peripheral fat tissue, making them less likely to be stored as fat. Since they are also used for fuel more quickly than longer chain fatty acids, choosing these tropical oils over animal fats may promote a healthier body weight. Saturated plant oils are also useful in food processing because they are less susceptible to spoilage than are more unsaturated oils. Spoilage of fats and oils, referred to as *rancidity*, occurs when the unsaturated bonds in fatty acids are

Fatty acid composition of foods • Figure 5.4

The fats and oils in our diets contain combinations of saturated, monounsaturated, and polyunsaturated fatty acids. Vegetable oils are good sources of mono- and polyunsaturated fatty acids. The fats found in salmon, ground flax seeds, walnuts, and canola oil are good sources of the heart healthy omega-3 fatty acids. Animal fats, coconut oil, and other tropical oils are high in saturated fatty acids, and processed foods often contain *trans* fatty acids.

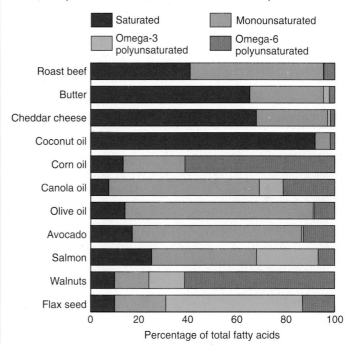

damaged by oxygen. When fats go rancid, they give food an "off" flavour. Sources of medium chain fatty acids include coconut oil, palm kernel oil, and palm oil. They are often called **tropical oils** because they are found in plants that are common in tropical climates.

Unsaturated fats

Monounsaturated fatty acids Monounsaturated fatty acids (MUFAs) have a single double bond and are found in a variety of foods such as meat, olive oil, avocados, and nuts. These fatty acids have historically been thought to be cardioprotective, due to the association between high MUFA intake and lowered LDL cholesterol. However, new research questions this long-held belief, and more research is required before we have a clear understanding of the effects of MUFAs on the body and on health.[3,4]

Essential fatty acids: omega-3 and omega-6 polyunsaturated fatty acids The body is capable of synthesizing most of the fatty acids it needs from glucose or other sources of carbon, hydrogen, and oxygen. However, humans are not able to synthesize fatty acids that have double bonds in the omega-6 and omega-3 positions (see Figure 5.3b). Therefore, the two polyunsaturated fatty acids (PUFAs), **linoleic acid (LA)** (omega-6) and **alpha-linolenic acid (ALA)** (omega-3),

> **essential fatty acids (EFAs)** Fatty acids that must be consumed in the diet because they cannot be made by the body or cannot be made in sufficient quantities to meet needs.

are considered essential fatty acids (EFAs). Practically all of the PUFAs in the human diet are these EFAs. They must be consumed in the diet if they are to carry out their essential functions and make other omega-6 and omega-3 fatty acids needed by the body (**Figure 5.5**). If the diet is low in LA and/or ALA, any fatty acids that the body would normally synthesize from them also become dietary essentials. Essential fatty acids, specifically omega-3 fatty acids, have health benefits beyond the normal physiological roles of fats in the body.

Essential fatty acids are important for the formation of the phospholipids that give cell membranes their structure and functional properties. As such, they are important for growth, skin integrity, fertility, and maintaining red blood cell structure. They are particularly important in cell membranes in the retina of the eye and in the central nervous system. Arachidonic acid (omega-3) and DHA (omega-6) are necessary for normal brain development in infants and young children. Essential fatty acids also serve as regulators of fatty acid and glucose metabolism through their role in gene expression.

Longer-chain omega-6 and omega-3 polyunsaturated fatty acids made from linoleic and alpha-linolenic acid, respectively, are used to make hormone-like molecules called **eicosanoids**. Eicosanoids help regulate blood clotting, blood pressure, immune function, and other body processes. The effect of an eicosanoid on these functions depends on the fatty acid from which it is made. For example, when the omega-6 fatty acid arachidonic acid is the starting material, its eicosanoid

> **eicosanoids** Regulatory molecules that can be synthesized from omega-3 and omega-6 fatty acids.

increases blood clotting; when the eicosanoid is made from the omega-3 fatty acid EPA, it decreases blood clotting.

Increasing consumption of foods that are rich in omega-3 fatty acids increases the proportion of omega-3 eicosanoids, which, in turn, reduces the risk of heart disease by decreasing inflammation, lowering blood pressure, and reducing blood clotting. *Eating Well with Canada's Food*

Essential fatty acids • Figure 5.5

Linoleic acid is an omega-6 fatty acid that is found in vegetable oils, such as corn and safflower oils. **Arachidonic acid** is an omega-6 fatty acid that is found in both animal and vegetable fats. It is essential only when the diet does not provide enough linoleic acid for the body to synthesize adequate amounts of it. Alpha-linolenic acid (ALA) is an omega-3 fatty acid that is found in ground flaxseed, canola oil, and nuts. **Eicosapentaenoic acid**

(EPA) and **docosahexaenoic acid (DHA)** are omega-3 fatty acids that are synthesized from alpha-linolenic acid; in our diet they are found in fatty fish. Many products found at the grocery store are now fortified with essential fatty acids such as omega-3 eggs and DHA milk. These technologies were both originally developed at the University of Guelph in Ontario.

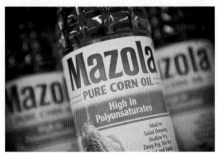
© PSL Images / Alamy

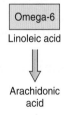
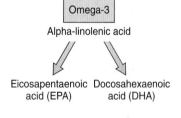

Omega-6
Linoleic acid
↓
Arachidonic acid

Omega-3
Alpha-linolenic acid
↙ ↘
Eicosapentaenoic acid (EPA) Docosahexaenoic acid (DHA)

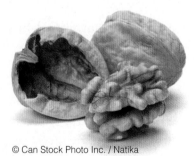
© Can Stock Photo Inc. / Natika

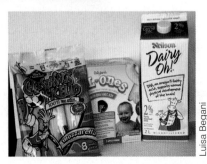
Luisa Begani

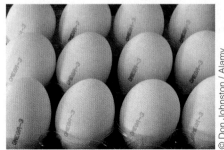
© Don Johnston / Alamy

Guide accordingly recommends eating two or more servings per week of fish, which is a good source of EPA and DHA.[5] Omega-3 can also be found in walnuts, canola oil, ground flaxseed, and in many fortified products available at the grocery store (see Figure 5.5).

If adequate amounts of LA and ALA are not consumed, an essential fatty acid deficiency will result. Symptoms include scaly, dry skin, liver abnormalities, poor healing of wounds, impaired vision and hearing, and growth failure in infants. Because the requirement for essential fatty acids is well below Canadians' typical intake, essential fatty acid deficiencies are rare in this country. However, deficiencies have occurred in infants and young children consuming low-fat diets and in individuals who are unable to absorb lipids.

Trans fatty acids Food manufacturers can increase the shelf life of oils by using a process called **hydrogenation**, which makes unsaturated oils more saturated. Hydrogenation improves the storage properties of the oils and makes them more solid at room temperature. Products such as some hard margarines and shortening have undergone hydrogenation. A disadvantage of this process is that in addition to converting some double bonds into saturated bonds, some double bonds are transformed from the *cis* to the *trans* configuration (**Figure 5.6**). Most *trans* fats we consume are those made through the process of hydrogenation.

> **hydrogenation**
> A process whereby hydrogen atoms are added to the carbon–carbon double bonds of unsaturated fatty acids, making them more saturated.

Cis and *trans* fatty acids • Figure 5.6

a. The orientation of hydrogen atoms around the double bond distinguishes *cis* fatty acids from **trans fatty acids**. Most unsaturated fatty acids found in nature have double bonds in the *cis* configuration.

In *trans* fatty acids the hydrogens are on opposite sides of the double bond, making the carbon chain straighter, similar to the shape of a saturated fatty acid.

In *cis* fatty acids, the hydrogens are on the same side of the double bond and cause a bend in the carbon chain.

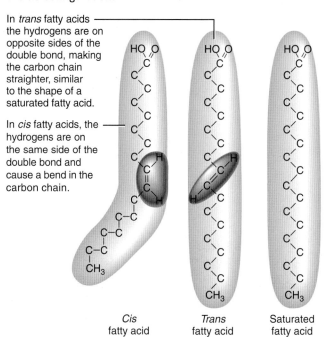

Cis fatty acid   *Trans* fatty acid   Saturated fatty acid

b. Small amounts of *trans* fatty acids occur naturally, and larger amounts are generated by hydrogenation. In 2007, Health Canada called on food manufacturers to voluntarily reduce the amount of *trans* fat in their products to less than 5% of total fat, which the majority of manufacturers have now complied with.[6]

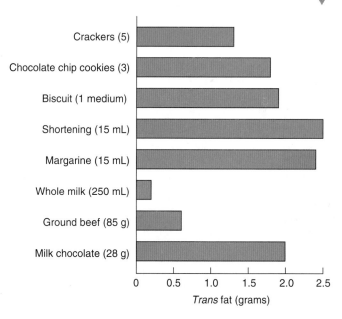

Trans fat (grams)

- Crackers (5)
- Chocolate chip cookies (3)
- Biscuit (1 medium)
- Shortening (15 mL)
- Margarine (15 mL)
- Whole milk (250 mL)
- Ground beef (85 g)
- Milk chocolate (28 g)

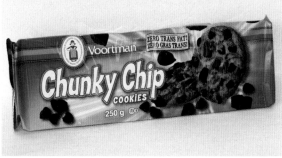

Luisa Begani

c. Four years before Health Canada's call for a reduction in the amounts of *trans* fats in processed foods, the Canadian company Voortman voluntarily elected to eliminate *trans* fats from all its products. Voortman was the first company in Canada and one of the first in North America to do so. Many manufacturers have now followed suit, and the amount of *trans* fats in processed foods has decreased significantly, as has the consumption of *trans* fats in Canada.[6]

Ask Yourself

Which of the foods shown here contain only natural sources of *trans* fatty acids?

Phospholipids • Figure 5.7

a. Like a triglyceride, a phospholipid has a backbone of glycerol, but it contains two fatty acids rather than three. Instead of the third fatty acid, a phospholipid has a chemical group containing phosphorus, called a **phosphate group**. The fatty acids at one end of a phospholipid molecule are hydrophobic: insoluble in water, but soluble in fat; whereas the phosphate-containing region at the other end is hydrophilic: soluble in water, but insoluble in fat.

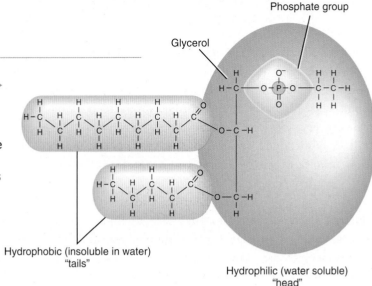

Phosphate group

Glycerol

Hydrophobic (insoluble in water) "tails"

Hydrophilic (water soluble) "head"

b. Since dietary lipids are hydrophobic ("water-hating"), they cannot dissolve readily in water, making them difficult to transport in water-based environments such as the blood. Phospholipids help suspend lipids in watery environments by acting as emulsifiers. The salad dressing shown here does not contain an emulsifier, so it separates into a layer of oil and vinegar and must be shaken before it is poured on your salad. Ranch salad dressings are emulsified so that they do not separate when left standing.

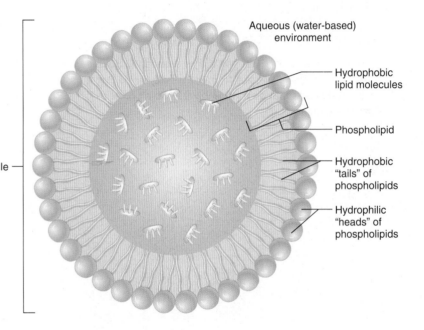

Aqueous (water-based) environment

Hydrophobic lipid molecules

Phospholipid

Hydrophobic "tails" of phospholipids

Hydrophilic "heads" of phospholipids

Micelle

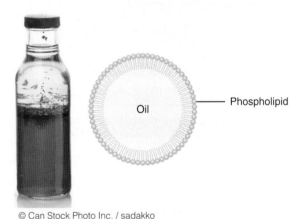

Oil

Phospholipid

© Can Stock Photo Inc. / sadakko

c. Phospholipids are an important component of cell membranes. They form a double-layered sheet called the **lipid bilayer** by orienting the hydrophilic, phosphate-containing "heads" toward the aqueous (water) environments inside and outside the cell and the hydrophobic fatty acid "tails" toward each other to form the lipid centre of the membrane. The lipid bilayer is a critical component of the cell, as it limits what substances can easily move into and out of it.

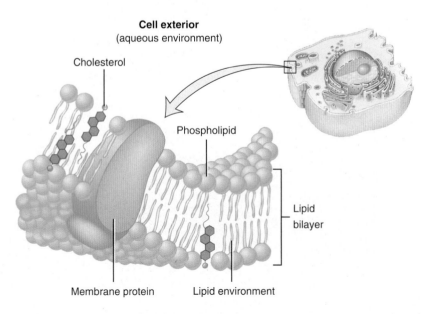

Cell exterior
(aqueous environment)

Cholesterol

Phospholipid

Lipid bilayer

Membrane protein

Lipid environment

Cytoplasm
(aqueous environment)

Although *trans* fatty acids are technically unsaturated fatty acids, they afford a risk of heart disease greater than any other type of dietary fat. This effect is due to their association with higher levels of LDL ("bad") cholesterol and lower levels of HDL ("good") cholesterol in the blood. Sources of *trans* fat made through the process of hydrogenation should be minimized or even eliminated from the diet.

Phospholipids

Phospholipids are critically essential to the structure and function of our body. Although they are present in very small amounts in our food, our body is able to make its own phospholipids to meet the body's needs. Phospholipids found in the body play various essential roles due to their abilities to allow water and fat to mix. They can do this because of their hydrophilic end, which dissolves in water, and the hydrophobic end, which dissolves in fat (**Figure 5.7a**).

In foods, substances that allow fat and water to mix are referred to as **emulsifiers**. For example, the phospholipids in egg yolks allow the oil and water in cake batter to mix; phospholipids in salad dressings prevent the oil and vinegar in the dressing from separating. One of the best-known phospholipids is **lecithin**. Eggs and soybeans are natural sources of lecithin. The food industry uses lecithin as an emulsifier in margarine, salad dressings, chocolate, frozen desserts, and baked goods to prevent oil from separating from the other ingredients. In the body, lecithin is a major constituent of cell membranes (**Figure 5.7c**). It is also used to synthesize the neurotransmitter acetylcholine, which activates muscles and plays an important role in memory.

Sterols

Sterols are a type of lipid with distinct ring structures in their chain. They are found in plant foods and both the lean and fatty parts of animal foods, as well as in every cell in the human body. The best-known sterol is **cholesterol** (**Figure 5.8**). Cholesterol is needed in the body, but because the liver manufactures it, it is not required from the diet. More than 90% of the cholesterol in the body is found in cell membranes

> **cholesterol** A sterol, produced by the liver and consumed in the diet, which is needed to build cell membranes and make hormones and other essential molecules.

Cholesterol • Figure 5.8

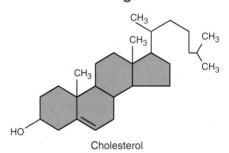

a. The cholesterol structure shown here illustrates the four interconnected rings of carbon atoms that form the backbone structure that is common to all sterols.

Cholesterol

b. Egg yolks and organ meats such as liver and kidney are high in cholesterol. Lean red meats and skinless chicken are low in total fat but still contain some cholesterol. Cholesterol is not found in plant cell membranes, so even high-fat plant foods, such as nuts, peanut butter, and vegetable oils, do not contain cholesterol.

Where's the cholesterol?

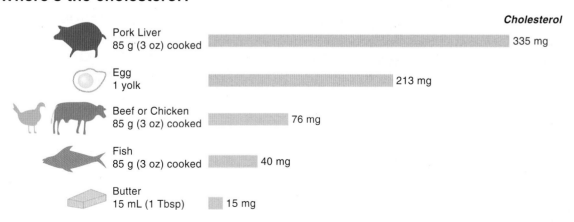

	Cholesterol
Pork Liver 85 g (3 oz) cooked	335 mg
Egg 1 yolk	213 mg
Beef or Chicken 85 g (3 oz) cooked	76 mg
Fish 85 g (3 oz) cooked	40 mg
Butter 15 mL (1 Tbsp)	15 mg

(see Figure 5.7c). It is also part of myelin, the insulating coating on many nerve cells. Cholesterol is needed to synthesize other sterols, including vitamin D; bile acids, which are emulsifiers in bile; cortisol, which is a hormone that regulates our physiological response to stress; and testosterone and estrogen, which are hormones necessary for reproduction.

High levels of blood cholesterol are one of the leading risk factors for heart disease. That being said, since the body can make its own cholesterol, high dietary cholesterol is not the leading risk factor for high blood cholesterol. A diet high in saturated fats, and *trans* fats especially, is associated with high levels of unhealthy cholesterol in the blood, increasing a person's risk for heart disease.

In the diet, cholesterol is found only in foods from animal sources. Plant foods do not typically contain cholesterol unless it has been added in the course of cooking or processing. Plants do contain other sterols, however, and these **plant sterols** have a role similar to that of cholesterol in animals: They help form plant cell membranes. Plant sterols are found in small quantities in most plant foods; when consumed in the diet, they may help reduce cholesterol levels in the body, potentially promoting heart health.

CONCEPT CHECK

1. **What** is the structural difference between saturated and unsaturated fatty acids?

2. **Where** are most phospholipids found in the body?

3. **Why** is cholesterol not a dietary essential?

4. **Which** is higher in cholesterol: a 15-mL spoonful of peanut butter or an egg?

Absorbing and Transporting Lipids

LEARNING OBJECTIVES

1. **Discuss** the steps involved in the digestion and absorption of lipids.

2. **Describe** how lipids are transported in the blood and delivered to cells.

3. **Compare** the functions of LDLs and HDLs.

The fact that oil and water do not mix poses a problem for the digestion of lipids in the watery environment of the small intestine and their transport in the blood, which is mostly water. Therefore, the body has special mechanisms that allow it to digest and transport lipids.

Digestion and Absorption of Fat

In healthy adults, most fat digestion and absorption occur in the small intestine (**Figure 5.9**). Here, bile acts as an emulsifier, breaking down large lipid droplets into small globules by orientating its hydrophilic ends to the water-based environment and its hydrophobic ends toward the lipids. The triglycerides in the globules can then be digested by enzymes from the pancreas. The resulting mixture of fatty acids, partially digested triglycerides, cholesterol, and bile forms smaller droplets called **micelles**, which facilitate absorption (see Figure 5.9). The bile in the micelles is also absorbed and returned to the liver to be reused.

> **micelles** Particles that are formed in the small intestine when the products of fat digestion are surrounded by bile. They are an aggregation of lipid molecules as a droplet that facilitates the absorption of lipids.

Once inside the mucosal cells of the intestine, the fatty acids, cholesterol, and other fat-soluble substances must be processed further before they can be transported in the blood.

The fat-soluble vitamins (A, D, E, and K) are absorbed through the same process as other lipids. These vitamins are not digested but must be incorporated into micelles to be absorbed. The amounts absorbed can be reduced if dietary fat is very low or if disease, medications, or other dietary components interfere with fat absorption.

Lipid digestion and absorption • Figure 5.9

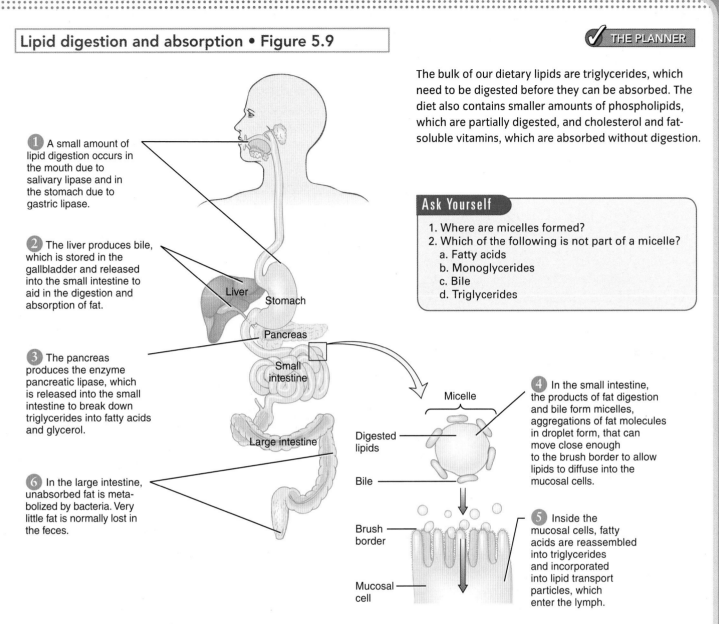

The bulk of our dietary lipids are triglycerides, which need to be digested before they can be absorbed. The diet also contains smaller amounts of phospholipids, which are partially digested, and cholesterol and fat-soluble vitamins, which are absorbed without digestion.

Ask Yourself

1. Where are micelles formed?
2. Which of the following is not part of a micelle?
   a. Fatty acids
   b. Monoglycerides
   c. Bile
   d. Triglycerides

1 A small amount of lipid digestion occurs in the mouth due to salivary lipase and in the stomach due to gastric lipase.

2 The liver produces bile, which is stored in the gallbladder and released into the small intestine to aid in the digestion and absorption of fat.

3 The pancreas produces the enzyme pancreatic lipase, which is released into the small intestine to break down triglycerides into fatty acids and glycerol.

6 In the large intestine, unabsorbed fat is metabolized by bacteria. Very little fat is normally lost in the feces.

Liver
Stomach
Pancreas
Small intestine
Large intestine

Micelle
Digested lipids
Bile
Brush border
Mucosal cell

4 In the small intestine, the products of fat digestion and bile form micelles, aggregations of fat molecules in droplet form, that can move close enough to the brush border to allow lipids to diffuse into the mucosal cells.

5 Inside the mucosal cells, fatty acids are reassembled into triglycerides and incorporated into lipid transport particles, which enter the lymph.

Transporting Lipids in the Blood

Lipids that are consumed in the diet are absorbed into the intestinal mucosal cells. From here, small fatty acids, which are soluble in water, are absorbed into the blood and travel to the liver for further processing. Long-chain fatty acids, cholesterol, and fat-soluble vitamins, which are not soluble in water, are not absorbed directly into the blood and must be packaged for transport. They are covered with a water-soluble envelope of protein, phospholipids, and cholesterol to form particles called lipo-proteins (**Figure 5.10**). Different types of lipoproteins transport dietary lipids from the small intestine to body cells, from the liver to body cells, and from body cells back to the liver for disposal. Some of these lipoproteins (low-density lipoproteins, or LDL) are associated with heart disease, while others (high-density lipoproteins, or HDL) actually improve heart health.

Transport from the small intestine After long-chain fatty acids (from the digestion of triglycerides) have been absorbed into the mucosal cells, they are reassembled into triglycerides. These triglycerides, along with cholesterol and fat-soluble vitamins, are packaged with

lipoproteins Particles that transport lipids in the blood.

Lipoprotein structure • Figure 5.10

Lipoproteins consist of a core of triglycerides and cholesterol surrounded by a shell of protein, phospholipids, and cholesterol. Phospholipids orient with their fat-soluble "tails" toward the interior of the lipoprotein and their water-soluble "heads" toward the watery environment outside the lipoprotein.

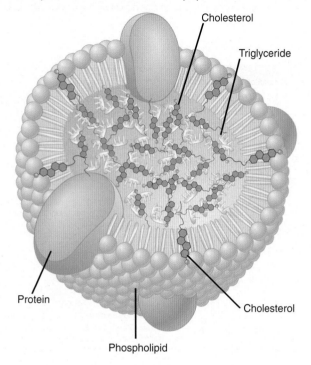

Cholesterol

Triglyceride

Protein

Cholesterol

Phospholipid

to differentiate between cholesterols that are heart healthy and those that are not. These terms are actually a bit of misnomer, however, because they actually refer to transport molecules called lipoproteins, composed of a protein and phospholipid shell that transports triglycerides and cholesterol through the bloodstream. The density of the lipoprotein depends on how much protein (high in density) it has compared with the remaining triglycerides, cholesterol, and phospholipids (low in density). A high-density lipoprotein therefore has more protein and less fatty substances compared with a low-density lipoprotein. The relative amounts of these substances in the lipoproteins determine their function and, in the case of high-density lipoproteins and low-density lipoproteins (the so-called good cholesterol and bad cholesterol), their likelihood to reduce or increase the risk of heart disease.

The liver can synthesize lipids, which are then transported from the liver in **very-low-density lipoproteins (VLDLs)**. Like chylomicrons, VLDLs are lipoproteins primarily consisting of triglycerides that circulate in the blood, delivering these fatty substances to body cells. When the triglycerides have been removed from the VLDLs, a denser, smaller particle remains. About two-thirds of these particles are returned to the liver, and the rest are transformed in the blood into **low-density lipoproteins (LDLs)**. LDLs are the primary cholesterol delivery system for cells. They contain a higher proportion of cholesterol than do chylomicrons or VLDLs (see Figure 5.11). High levels of LDLs in the blood have been associated with an increased risk for heart disease, leading to the term *bad cholesterol*.

> **low-density lipoproteins (LDLs)**
> Lipoproteins that transport cholesterol to cells. They are not consumed from the diet; they are made by the body.

Eliminating cholesterol Because most body cells have no system for breaking down cholesterol, it must be returned to the liver to be eliminated from the body. This reverse cholesterol transport is accomplished by **high-density lipoproteins (HDLs)**. HDL cholesterol is often called *good cholesterol* because high levels of HDL in the blood are associated with a reduction in the risk of heart disease because they lower the cholesterol content of blood.

> **high-density lipoproteins (HDLs)**
> Lipoproteins that pick up cholesterol from cells and transport it to the liver so that it can be eliminated from the body. They are not consumed from the diet; they are made by the body.

> **chylomicrons**
> Lipoproteins that transport lipids from the mucosal cells of the small intestine and deliver triglycerides to other body cells.

phospholipids, cholesterol, and protein to form lipoproteins called **chylomicrons**. Chylomicrons are too large to enter the capillaries in the small intestine, so they pass from the intestinal mucosa into the lymph, which then delivers them to the blood (**Figure 5.11**). They circulate in the blood, delivering triglycerides to body cells. The enzyme **lipoprotein lipase**, found in adipose tissue, the heart, and muscles, then promotes the uptake of triglycerides from chylomicrons and other lipoproteins, into body cells. Lipoprotein lipase must first break down the triglycerides into fatty acids and glycerol, which can diffuse across the cell membrane to enter cells. Once inside the cells, fatty acids can either be used to provide energy or reassembled into triglycerides for storage.

Transport from the liver All cholesterol in the blood was once believed to be negative for heart health. Now we use the terms *good cholesterol* and *bad cholesterol*

Lipid transport and delivery • Figure 5.11

THE PLANNER

Chylomicrons and very-low-density lipoproteins (VLDLs) transport triglycerides and deliver them to body cells. Low-density lipoproteins transport and deliver cholesterol, while high density lipoproteins help return cholesterol to the liver for reuse or elimination.

1 Chylomicrons formed in the mucosal cells pass first into the lymph, which drains into the blood. They circulate in the blood, delivering triglycerides to body cells.

Dietary fat

Chylomicron

Lymph vessel

INTESTINE

Bile

3 What remains of the chylomicrons consists mostly of cholesterol and protein. These particles travel to the liver to be disassembled.

Cholesterol

Lipoprotein lipase

2 The enzyme lipoprotein lipase, which is present on the surface of cells lining the blood vessels, breaks down the triglycerides in chylomicrons into fatty acids and glycerol. These can then enter the surrounding cells to be used or stored.

LIVER

Fatty acids

Body cells

Blood vessels

VLDL

LDL receptor

Fatty acids

Lipoprotein lipase

7 HDLs pick up cholesterol from other lipoproteins and body cells and return it to the liver. Some of this cholesterol is broken down and some is transferred to organs with high requirements for cholesterol, such as those that synthesize steroid hormones.

HDL

LDL

LDL receptor

4 VLDLs are made in the liver and transport lipids away from the liver. They function similarly to chylomicrons because both particles deliver triglycerides to body cells with the help of the enzyme lipoprotein lipase.

5 What remains of the VLDL particles after the triglycerides are removed is either returned to the liver or transformed in the blood into LDL particles.

Cholesterol

Body cells

6 To deliver cholesterol, LDL particles bind to a protein on the cell membrane called an **LDL receptor**. This binding allows the whole LDL particle to be removed from circulation and enter the cell, where the cholesterol and other components can be used.

☐ Triglyceride
☐ Cholesterol
☐ Phospholipid
☐ Protein

Chylomicron
Chylomicrons are the largest lipoproteins and contain the greatest proportion of triglycerides.

VLDL
VLDLs are smaller than chylomicrons but still contain a high proportion of triglycerides.

LDL
LDLs contain a higher proportion of cholesterol than do other lipoproteins.

HDL
HDLs are high in cholesterol and are the densest lipoproteins due to their high protein content.

CONCEPT CHECK   STOP

1. **How** does bile help in the digestion and absorption of lipids?

2. **Why** are lipoproteins needed to transport lipids?

3. **What** is the primary function of LDL cholesterol?

Lipid Functions

LEARNING OBJECTIVES

1. **List** the functions of lipids in the body.

2. **Explain** why we need the right balance of omega-3 and omega-6 fatty acids.

3. **Summarize** how fatty acids are used to provide energy.

4. **Describe** how fat is stored and how it is retrieved from storage.

Fat is necessary to maintain health. In our diet, fat is needed to absorb fat-soluble vitamins and is a source of essential fatty acids and energy. In our bodies, lipids form structural and regulatory molecules and are broken down to provide adenosine triphosphate (ATP). As discussed earlier, cholesterol plays both regulatory and structural roles: It is used to make steroid hormones, and it is an important component of cell membranes and the myelin coating that is necessary for brain and nerve function.

Most lipids in the body are triglycerides stored in **adipose tissue**, which is the fat that lies under the skin and around internal organs (**Figure 5.12**). The triglycerides in our adipose tissue provide a lightweight energy-storage molecule, help cushion our internal organs such as the heart and kidneys, and insulate us from changes in temperature. Unfortunately, the amount of adipose tissue in the average Canadian has increased significantly over time. This excess adipose tissue, or "body fat," is associated with the three leading causes of death in Canada: cancer, cardiovascular disease, and stroke. Triglycerides are also found in oils that lubricate body surfaces, keeping the skin soft and supple.

Fat as a Source of Energy

Fat is an important source of energy in the body (**Figure 5.13**). Because each gram of fat provides 9 kilocalories, compared with only 4 kilocalories per gram from carbohydrate or protein, a large amount of energy can be stored

Adipose tissue • Figure 5.12

a. Adipose tissue is an important source of stored energy. It also insulates the body from changes in temperature and provides a cushion to protect against shock. The amount and location of adipose tissue affect our physical appearance, specifically our body size and shape. This tissue is preferentially deposited in some body areas, such as your abdominal region, rather than other areas, such as your thighs and shoulders. Where adipose tissue is stored varies across both male and female populations and is based almost entirely on individual genetics. Thus, a specific diet or exercise regime cannot honestly promise results for fat loss from one specific location over another.

b. Adipose tissue cells contain large droplets of triglyceride that push the other cell components to the perimeter of the cell. As weight is gained, the triglyceride droplets enlarge and, once they reach their maximum size, they divide, forming new **adipocytes**, or fat cells. When weight is lost and total body fat is lowered, fat cells can only shrink, not disappear. Once fat cells have been added to the body, they remain, making it more difficult to achieve the pre-fat gain state and appearance.

Ed Reschke

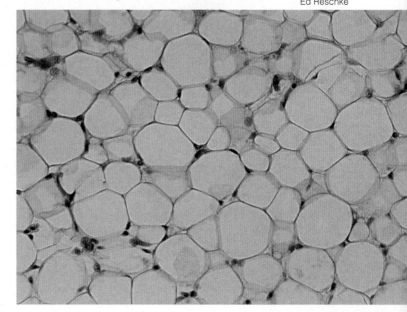

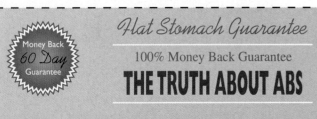

Metabolism of fat • Figure 5.13

Digestion of dietary triglycerides yields fatty acids and a small amount of glycerol. Fatty acids provide most of the energy stored in a triglyceride molecule. Inside the mitochondria, the fatty acid chains are broken down to form acetyl CoA, which can be further metabolized to generate carbon dioxide, water, and ATP. The glycerol molecules, which contain three carbon atoms, can also be used to produce ATP or small amounts of glucose or pyruvate, which can then proceed through aerobic metabolism.

1. A triglyceride molecule is broken down into glycerol and three fatty acids.

2. Glycerol can be used to synthesize glucose or pyruvate, which will then proceed through the following stages of aerobic metabolism to produce ATP.

3. Beta-oxidation splits off two carbons at a time from the long fatty acid molecule, yielding a two-carbon molecule, which will combine with coenzyme A to produce acetyl coA. The remaining fatty acid chain will further undergo beta-oxidation to yield additional molecules of acetyl coA.

4. If oxygen and enough carbohydrate are available, acetyl CoA enters the citric acid cycle, releasing two molecules of carbon dioxide and high-energy electrons, which are captured by NADH + H+ and FADH₂.

5. In the final step of aerobic metabolism, the electron carriers enter the electron transport chain, which results in the production of ATP and water.

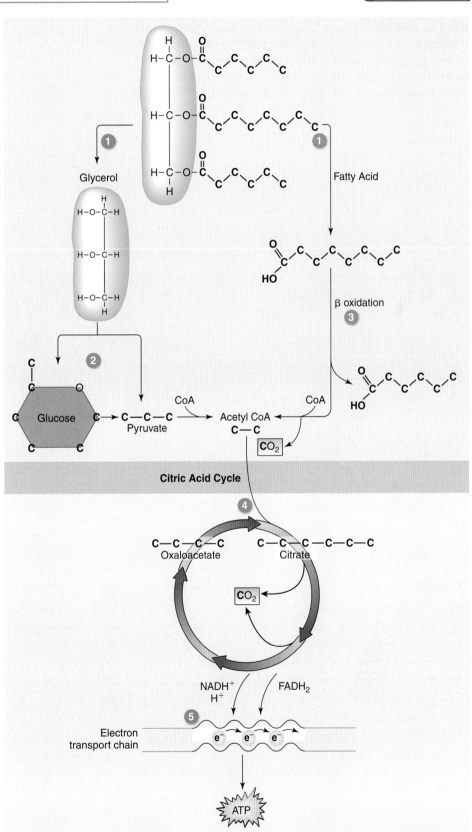

Storing and retrieving energy from fat stores • Figure 5.14

When we consume too many calories, excess energy is stored in the form of triglycerides. When the energy needs of our body are insufficient to fuel body processes and physical activity, triglycerides in adipose tissue are broken down, releasing fatty acids, which can be used to provide energy.

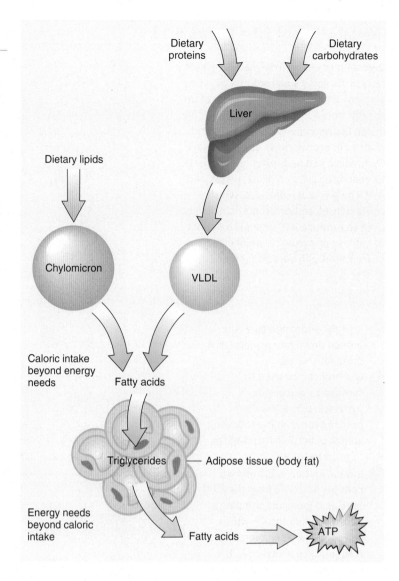

in the body as fat without a great increase in body size or weight. Even a lean man stores more than 50,000 kilocalories of energy in the form of triglycerides, which equates to about 6 kg (14 lb.) of fat.

Triglycerides that are consumed in the diet can be either used immediately to fuel the body or stored in adipose tissue. Throughout the day, triglycerides are continuously stored and then retrieved from storage to be broken down, depending on the body's current energy needs. For example, after a meal, some triglycerides will be stored; then, between meals, some of the stored triglycerides will be broken down to provide energy. When the energy consumed in the diet equals the body's energy requirements, the net amount of body fat does not change.

Storing triglycerides Regardless of whether excess calories come from fat, carbohydrates, or protein, when they

are consumed in the diet, fat deposition is promoted. When these excess calories come from fat, chylomicrons directly transport that majority of them from the intestines to adipose tissue for storage. This process is demonstrated by the fact that the fatty acid composition of your adipose tissue varies, depending on the types of fatty acids in the food you eat. Excess calories that are consumed as carbohydrate or protein must first go to the liver, where they can be used to synthesize fatty acids, which are then assembled into triglycerides and transported in VLDLs to adipose tissue (**Figure 5.14**).

The ability of the body to store excess triglycerides is theoretically limitless! Cells in your adipose tissue can increase in weight by about 50 times, and new fat cells can be made when existing cells reach their maximum size.

Retrieving energy from fat stores When you eat fewer calories than you need, your body takes energy from its fat stores. In this situation, an enzyme inside the fat cells receives a signal to break down stored triglycerides. The fatty acids and glycerol that result are released directly into the blood and circulate throughout the body. They are taken up by cells and used to produce ATP (see Figure 5.14).

If the diet, and thus the blood, lacks carbohydrate, the acetyl CoA produced by fatty acid breakdown cannot enter aerobic metabolism. These fatty acids will instead be used to make *ketones* (see Chapter 4). Muscle and adipose tissue can use ketones as an energy source. During prolonged starvation or fasting, the brain can adapt itself to use ketones to meet about half of its energy needs. For the other half, it continues to require glucose. Fatty acids cannot be used to make glucose, and only a small amount of glucose can be made from the glycerol released from triglyceride breakdown.

CONCEPT CHECK

1. **What** is the function of adipose tissue?
2. **How** are fatty acids used to produce ATP?
3. **What** happens to dietary fat after it has been absorbed?

Lipids in Health and Disease

LEARNING OBJECTIVES

1. **Define** essential fatty acid deficiency.
2. **Describe** the events that lead to the development of atherosclerosis.
3. **Evaluate** your risk of heart disease.
4. **Discuss** the role of dietary fat in promoting weight gain.

The amount and types of fat you eat can affect your health. A diet that is too low in fat can reduce the absorption of fat-soluble vitamins, slow growth, and impair the functioning of the skin, eyes, liver, and other body organs. Eating the wrong types of fat, specifically *trans* and animal fats, can contribute to chronic diseases such as heart disease and cancer. Consuming too much fat can increase calorie intake and contribute to extra body fat storage and therefore weight gain. Excess body fat, in turn, is associated with an increased risk of diabetes, cardiovascular disease, and high blood pressure.

Heart Disease

In 2009, the Public Health Agency of Canada estimated that at least 1.6 million Canadians suffer from diagnosed heart disease or the effects of a stroke.[9] Both of these conditions are classified as **cardiovascular disease** (CVD), as are high blood pressure, peripheral artery disease, and any disease that affects the heart (*cardio*) and/or blood vessels (*vascular*). For many years, cardiovascular disease was the number-one cause of death in Canada, but cancer rates are now more similar to those of CVD, as mortality rates from CVD have deceased. This decrease is likely due to advances in the detection and treatment of cardiovascular disease in Canada.

Atherosclerosis is a type of cardiovascular disease in which cholesterol and other deposits enter the artery walls, reducing their elasticity and eventually limiting the flow of blood. For example, if the flow of blood is completely stopped by a blood clot, the lack of oxygen and nutrient delivery to downstream cells can lead to a heart attack or a stroke, depending on whether the blood clot occurs in the heart or brain, respectively. The development of atherosclerosis has been linked to diets that are high in *trans* fat, saturated fat, and cholesterol.[10] Dietary cholesterol increases blood cholesterol in only about a third of individuals who are sensitive to cholesterol.[11] The main dietary fats associated with cardiovascular disease, however, are saturated fats and, more significantly, *trans* fats because they cause unhealthy

> **atherosclerosis**
> A type of cardiovascular disease that involves the buildup of fatty material in the artery walls.

Development of atherosclerosis • Figure 5.15

The inflammation that occurs in response to an injury to the artery wall precipitates the development of atherosclerotic plaque. The presence of plaque can eventually lead to a heart attack or stroke.

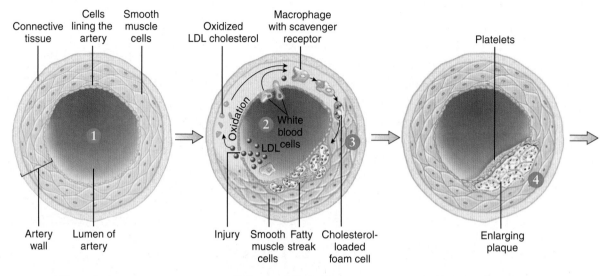

Normal artery

1. The wall of a normal, healthy artery consists of a layer of epithelial cells surrounded by smooth muscle.

2. Plaque formation begins when the lining of the artery is damaged. An injury makes the lining more permeable to LDL particles, which migrate into the artery wall, where they are retained. Here, they are modified to form oxidized LDL cholesterol, which promotes inflammation.

Fatty streak formation

3. Oxidized LDL cholesterol causes white blood cells to stick to and migrate into the artery wall, where they mature into large cells called macrophages that consume LDL. As macrophages fill with oxidized LDL cholesterol, they become **foam cells**. These cholesterol-filled cells accumulate in the artery wall and then burst, forming a fatty streak.[7,8]

Plaque accumulation

4. Macrophages and foam cells in the artery wall secrete chemicals that continue the inflammatory process and promote growth of the plaque, narrowing the artery and worsening the condition. Smooth muscle cells migrate into the fatty streak and secrete fibrous proteins. Platelets, which are cell fragments involved in blood clotting, clump together around the plaque. As plaque builds up, it causes the artery to narrow further and lose its elasticity.

---

lipid levels in the body. Because of the dangerous effects of *trans* fats, Health Canada was the first government agency in the world to implement the mandatory labelling of *trans* fats on prepackaged foods.

How atherosclerosis develops Inflammation, the process whereby the body responds

atherosclerotic plaque Cholesterol-rich material that is deposited in the arteries of individuals with atherosclerosis. It consists of cholesterol, smooth muscle cells, fibrous tissue, and eventually calcium.

to injury, drives the formation of **atherosclerotic plaque**. For example, cutting yourself triggers an inflammatory response. White blood cells, which are part of the immune system, rush to the injured area, blood clots form, and soon new tissue grows to heal the wound. Similar inflammatory responses occur when an artery is injured, but instead of resulting in healing, they

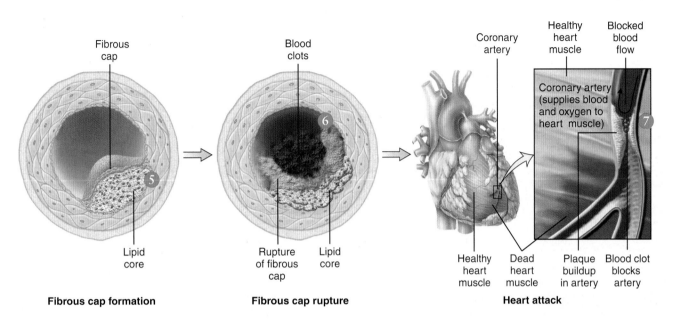

Fibrous cap formation

Fibrous cap rupture

Heart attack

⑤ As the process progresses, a cap of smooth muscle cells and fibrous proteins forms over the plaque, walling it off from the lumen of the artery. If the inflammation continues, substances secreted by immune system cells can cause the cap to degrade.[7,8]

⑥ If the cap ruptures or erodes, exposing the inner core, blood clots can rapidly form around it. The blood clots can completely block the artery at that spot or break loose and block an artery elsewhere.

⑦ If blood flow in a coronary artery is blocked, the result is a heart attack. Heart muscle cells that are cut off from their blood supply die, causing pain and reducing the heart's ability to pump blood. If the blood flow to the brain is interrupted, a stroke results. Brain cells are cut off from their blood supply and die.

lead to the development of atherosclerotic plaque (**Figure 5.15**). Therefore, the atherosclerotic process begins with an injury, and the response to this injury causes changes in the lining of the artery wall.

The exact cause of the injuries that initiate the development of atherosclerosis is not known but may be related to elevated blood levels of LDL cholesterol, glucose, or the amino acid homocysteine, or to high blood pressure,

smoking, diabetes, genetic alterations, or infection.[8] The specific cause may differ depending on the individual.

Risk factors for heart disease High LDL cholesterol, smoking high blood pressure, physical inactivity, obesity, and diabetes are considered primary risk factors for heart disease. Other factors that affect risk include age, gender, genetics, stress, and alcohol consumption (**Table 5.1**).

What's your risk of heart disease? Table 5.1

Risk factor	How it affects your risk
Blood lipid level	Blood levels of total cholesterol, LDL cholesterol, HDL cholesterol, and triglycerides are all used to assess risk.

	Low risk/optimal	Near optimal	Borderline high risk	High risk
Cholesterol (mmol/L)	< 5.2		5.2–6.2	> 6.2
LDL cholesterol (mmol/L)	< 2.6	2.6–3.3	3.4–4.1	> 4.1
HDL cholesterol (mmol/L)	≥ 1.6			< 1 (for men)
				< 1.3 (for men)
Triglycerides (mmol/L)	< 1.7		1.7–2.2	≥ 2.3

Risk factor	How it affects your risk
High blood pressure	High blood pressure can damage blood vessel walls, initiating atherosclerosis. It forces the heart to work harder, causing it to enlarge and weaken over time.
Obesity	Obesity increases blood pressure, blood cholesterol levels, and the risk of developing diabetes. It also increases the amount of work the heart must do to pump blood throughout the body. Obese people also have higher risks because their diet and lifestyle patterns favour an increased risk of heart disease.
Diabetes	High blood glucose damages blood vessel walls, initiating atherosclerosis.
Lifestyle	Smoking increases risk. Regular exercise decreases risk by reducing blood pressure, increasing healthy HDL cholesterol levels, reducing the risk of diabetes, and promoting a healthy weight. Diet, including the types of lipids and the amounts of fibre, antioxidants, B vitamins, salt, sugar, and alcohol included in the diet, can affect the risk of heart disease.
Age	Risk is increased in men age 45 and older and in women age 55 and older.
Gender	Men and women are both at risk for heart disease, but men are generally affected a decade earlier than are women. This difference is due in part to the protective effect of the hormone estrogen in women. As women age, the effects of menopause—including a decline in estrogen level and a gain in weight—increase heart disease risk. The difference between genders may also be more behavioural in nature, as smoking, stress, and high-fat diets are more prevalent in the male population.
Family history	Individuals with a male family member who exhibited heart disease before age 55 or a female family member who exhibited heart disease before age 65 are considered to be at increased risk. In Canada, South Asians have a higher risk than white or Chinese Canadians.[12] Although we know that cardiovascular disease affects ethnicities differently, evidence on the rates in all of Canada's ethnic groups is currently unavailable.

Diet and heart disease risk Heart disease risk is affected by individual nutrients, such as *trans* and total fats; some whole foods, such as nuts and fish; and dietary patterns, such as diets that are high in plant foods. For example, diets that are high in fibre, **antioxidants**, and B vitamins can reduce the risk of developing heart disease. On the other hand, too much sodium or *trans* fat can increase heart disease risk. Intake of fish, nuts, and whole grains may decrease risk, while diets that are high in red meat may increase risk. More important than any

antioxidants Substances that are able to neutralize reactive oxygen molecules and thereby prevent cell damage.

individual dietary factor, though, are overall dietary and lifestyle patterns. The importance of these patterns is exemplified by the fact that historically, the incidence of heart disease has been lower in Asian and Mediterranean countries than in Canada (**Figure 5.16**). The heart-protective effect of these traditional diets has prompted nutrition experts to promote a Mediterranean dietary pattern to reduce the risk of heart disease in Canada.

Frequently, diet affects heart disease risk because it alters blood cholesterol levels. High intakes of saturated fat and cholesterol from high-fat meats and many processed foods can cause an increase in blood levels of total cholesterol and of LDL cholesterol. High intakes of *trans* fat from products

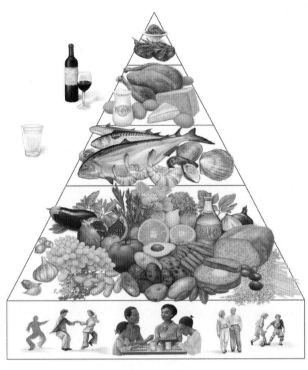

Mediterranean Diet Pyramid
A contemporary approach to delicious, healthy eating

Illustration by George Middleton. © 2009 Oldways Preservation & Exchange Trust. www.oldwayspt.org

a. In the Mediterranean region, the main source of dietary fat is olive oil, and the typical diet is high in nuts, vegetables, and fruits. Fish is consumed routinely and red meat, rarely. Despite a fat intake that is similar to that of the Canadian diet, the incidence of heart disease is much lower. This diet pyramid is based on the dietary patterns of Crete, Greece, and southern Italy around 1960, when the rates of chronic disease in this region were among the lowest in the world.

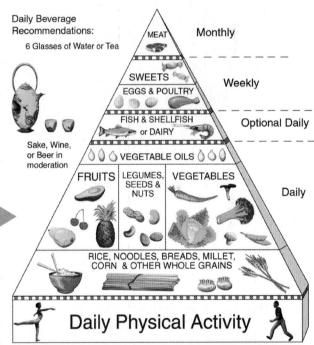

The Traditional Healthy Asian Diet Pyramid

Daily Beverage Recommendations:
6 Glasses of Water or Tea

Sake, Wine, or Beer in moderation

MEAT — Monthly

SWEETS
EGGS & POULTRY — Weekly

FISH & SHELLFISH or DAIRY — Optional Daily

VEGETABLE OILS

FRUITS | LEGUMES, SEEDS & NUTS | VEGETABLES — Daily

RICE, NOODLES, BREADS, MILLET, CORN & OTHER WHOLE GRAINS

Daily Physical Activity

© 2001 Oldways Preservation & Exchange Trust. www.oldwayspt.org

b. In Asian countries, plant foods that are rich in fibre and antioxidants form the base of the diet, and animal products are more peripheral. Traditional Asian diets include more fish and seafood than red meat. Combined with small amounts of vegetable oil, this pattern produces a balance of omega-3 to omega-6 fatty acids that helps prevent heart disease.[13] Routine consumption of green tea, which is high in antioxidants, may also contribute to the low rate of chronic disease in the region.[17] This diet pyramid was inspired by the traditional cuisines of southern and eastern Asia.

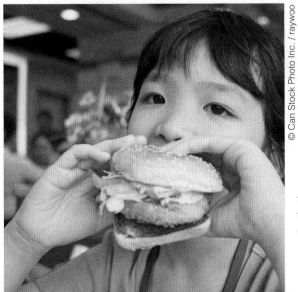

© Can Stock Photo Inc. / raywoo

c. Traditional Asian and Mediterranean diets often protect against heart disease, but as younger generations abandon these long-established dietary patterns for more modern options, the incidence of high blood pressure, elevated blood lipids, diabetes, and obesity is likely to rise.

such as shortening that contain hydrogenated vegetable oils increase blood levels of LDL cholesterol and the risk of heart attack. Replacing these unhealthy fats with monounsaturated and polyunsaturated fats from nuts and vegetable oils lowers total and LDL cholesterol.[10] Consuming less dietary cholesterol, however, may be less important in decreasing heart disease risk (see *Debate: Good Egg, Bad Egg*). Consuming plant sterols reduces cholesterol absorption in the small intestine, lowering total and LDL cholesterol levels.[10] Small quantities of plant sterols are present in many fruits, vegetables, nuts, seeds, cereals, legumes, and vegetable oils. Larger amounts have been added to products such as margarines, salad dressings, and orange juice.

Diet can also affect heart disease risk through mechanisms unrelated to blood cholesterol level. Much of the heart-protective effect of omega-3 fatty acids, such as those found in fish, is due to the eicosanoids made from them, which prevent the growth of atherosclerotic plaque, reduce blood clotting and blood pressure, and decrease inflammation (**Figure 5.17**).[13] Diets that are high in soluble

Eating to reduce the risk of heart disease • Figure 5.17

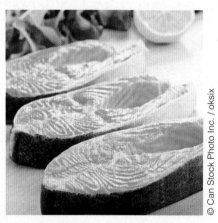

© Can Stock Photo Inc. / oksix

a. Omega-3 fatty acids found in fish, ground flaxseed, and vegetable oils reduce the risk of heart disease and decrease mortality from heart attacks. In addition to lowering triglyceride levels, they protect against heart disease by decreasing the stickiness of platelets, lowering blood pressure, improving the function of the cells lining blood vessels, reducing inflammation, and modulating heartbeats.[13]

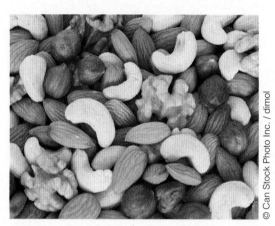

© Can Stock Photo Inc. / dimol

b. Nuts are high in omega-3 fatty acids, fibre, vegetable protein, antioxidants, and plant sterols. Diets containing nuts may lower heart disease risk by decreasing total and LDL cholesterol, increasing HDL, and improving the functioning of cells lining the artery wall.[18,19]

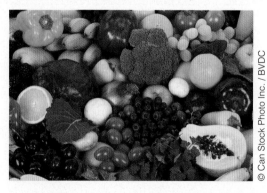

© Can Stock Photo Inc. / BVDC

c. Diets that are high in fruits, vegetables, and whole grains reduce the risk of heart disease.[20] If unprocessed, they typically contribute negligible amounts of cholesterol, saturated fats, and *trans* fats to the diet. Fruits and vegetables also add fibre, antioxidants, and phytochemicals. Whole grains provide fibre, omega-3 fatty acids, B vitamins, and antioxidants, as well as other phytochemicals that may protect against heart disease.

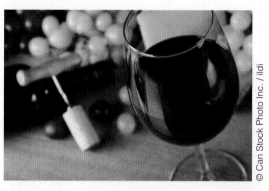

© Can Stock Photo Inc. / ildi

d. Moderate alcohol consumption—that is, one drink a day for women and two a day for men (one drink is equivalent to 140 mL (5.2 oz) wine, 355 mL (12.5 oz) beer, or 42 mL (1.5 oz) distilled spirits)—reduces blood clotting and increases HDL cholesterol but also raises blood triglyceride levels. Higher alcohol intake increases the risk of heart disease and can lead to other health and societal problems.

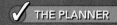
The Issue: Does consuming eggs increase your risk of heart disease?

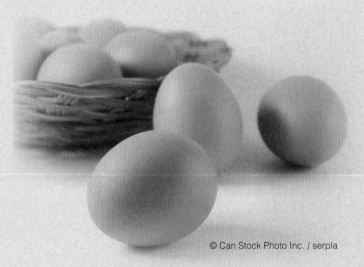

© Can Stock Photo Inc. / serpla

High blood cholesterol is one of the leading risk factors for heart disease. Many people therefore believe that consuming diets high in cholesterol will lead to higher levels of cholesterol in the blood and an increased susceptibility to disease. Since eggs are high in cholesterol, they have been a topic of debate among nutritionists and the media for some time. Many people who are concerned with their heart disease risk choose to limit or avoid this food and other high-cholesterol sources altogether. On the other hand, eggs are an excellent source of high-quality protein, are nutrient dense, satiating, and relatively low in calories, leading others to believe that eggs can be an important dietary staple. So, should you limit your consumption of eggs, or can they form part of a healthy diet?

Those who believe eggs should be limited cite the fact that one egg has more than 200 mg of cholesterol, while 28 g (1 oz) of lean meat has only about 30 mg of cholesterol. In the United States, the dietary guidelines recommend consuming less than 300 mg of cholesterol per day; consuming two eggs would therefore put you over your daily cholesterol limit. In Canada, no such upper limit exists because a direct association between cholesterol intake and heart disease risk has not been established. The cholesterol in our body comes both from what we eat and from cholesterol synthesized by our liver. Even if you don't eat any cholesterol, your liver will make all you need. For many people, when they eat cholesterol, their liver production slows, so blood levels of cholesterol don't rise; others are missing this regulation. For them, an increase in dietary cholesterol results in an increase in blood cholesterol. However, the increase is typically due to increases in both "good" HDL cholesterol and "bad"

LDL cholesterol, so the risk of atherosclerosis and heart disease does not change.[21] Furthermore, the LDL particles that form when dietary cholesterol increases are large. These larger LDL particles are thought to be less of a cardiovascular risk than smaller ones.[21]

Currently, the vast majority of epidemiological studies do not find a relationship between dietary cholesterol or egg consumption and cardiovascular disease.[21,22] For example, an evaluation of more than 20,000 male physicians participating in the Physicians' Health Study found that eating up to six eggs per week did not affect their risk or incidence of cardiovascular disease.[23] However, eating seven or more eggs per week caused an increased risk of death from cardiovascular disease, and eating any eggs was found to increase the risk of cardiovascular disease in people with type-2 diabetes.[23,24]

Nutrition professionals recognize that it is the overall dietary pattern, not the avoidance of particular foods, that is most important for health and wellness. Eggs are part of the Asian and Mediterranean dietary patterns, which are both associated with good cardiovascular health. One large egg contains 6 g of high-quality protein, and, unlike many other sources of cholesterol, eggs are low in cholesterol-raising saturated fat (see table). Eggs are also a good source of zinc, B vitamins, vitamin A, and iron. The yolk is rich in lutein and zeaxanthin, two phytochemicals that help protect against age-related eye disorders. Eggs may also help you maintain your weight. One study found that people who ate an egg-based breakfast ate fewer overall calories during the day than people who ate a bagel-based breakfast.[25]

Canadian guidelines align with the fact that lowering dietary cholesterol is less important for heart health than lowering *trans* and saturated fats and adopting a more plant-based diet. Many nutritional experts in the United States believe their recommendations should change to eliminate an upper limit for dietary cholesterol, putting their recommendation in line with those of Canada, Europe, Australia, New Zealand, Korea, and India.

Cholesterol and saturated fat content of foods		
Food	Cholesterol (mg)	Saturated fat (g)
Egg, one	212	1.6
Shrimp, 85 g (3 oz), raw	129	0.3
Salmon, 85 g (3 oz), cooked	57	0.6
Hamburger patty, 85 g (3 oz), broiled	71	7.5
Chicken breast, 85 g (3 oz), roasted, no skin	72	0.9
Bacon, 85 g (3 oz), pan fried	94	11.7
Pork sausage, 85 g (3 oz), cooked	71	7.8
Butter, 30 mL (2 Tbsp)	61	14.6
Milk, whole, 250 mL (8 fluid oz)	24	4.6
Cheese, cheddar, 28 g (1 oz)	30	6.0
Ice cream, vanilla, 125 mL (½ cup)	32	4.9

Think Critically Other than eggs, what food or foods in this table are high in cholesterol but low in saturated fat? How might these foods affect the risk of cardiovascular disease?

fibre may reduce heart disease risk by lowering cholesterol or by helping to lower triglyceride levels, blood pressure, and body weight.[11]

Diets that are high in plant foods are good sources of fibre, vitamins, minerals, and phytochemicals, some of which protect against heart disease because they perform antioxidant functions. Antioxidants decrease the oxidation of LDL cholesterol and, therefore, the development of plaque in artery walls.[14] Adequate intakes of vitamin B_6, vitamin B_{12}, and folic acid may also help protect against heart disease because they help maintain low blood levels of the amino acid homocysteine (discussed further in Chapter 7). Elevated homocysteine levels are associated with a higher incidence of heart disease.[15]

Focusing on healthy dietary patterns, as opposed to focusing on the consumption of single nutrients, seems to be more indicative of cardiovascular disease risk. Nutrition scientists therefore often recommend Mediterranean- or Asian-style diets, which are associated with a healthier heart (see Figure 5.16a and b). Another dietary pattern that is gaining in popularity is the Portfolio Diet. This dietary pattern first originated at St Michael's Hospital and the University of Toronto in Ontario. It has been found to be more effective than a low-fat diet at lowering blood cholesterol. The portfolio diet is a "dietary portfolio of cholesterol-lowering foods" that recommends a diet high in plant sterols, almonds, and soy protein and high in sources of soluble fibre, such as oats, barley, psyllium, okra, and eggplant. In one 24-week study, during the same 24-week period, this diet was able to lower blood cholesterol by 13%, whereas a low-fat diet lowered LDL by only 3%. The portfolio diet showed the added benefit of lowering triglycerides and blood pressure, while not lowering healthy HDL levels.[16] Accordingly, many physicians now recommend this diet for individuals with unhealthy blood cholesterol levels or increased heart disease risk.

Cancer

Cancer is a leading cause of death in Canada. Deaths from cardiovascular disease and cancer account for approximately 60% of all deaths.[26] There is evidence that the risk of cancer can be reduced by making changes to diet and activity patterns.[27] Populations consuming diets that are high in fruits and vegetables tend to have a lower risk of cancer than populations with lower intakes. Fruits and vegetables are rich in antioxidants such as vitamin C, vitamin E, and beta carotene. In contrast, the incidence of cancer is higher in populations that consume diets that are high in fat, particularly animal fats.

The good news is that the same type of diet that protects you from cardiovascular disease may also reduce the risk of certain forms of cancer. For example, the incidence of breast cancer in Mediterranean women, whose diet is high in unsaturated fat, is low despite a total fat intake similar to that in Canada and the United States.[28] *Trans* fatty acids, on the other hand, not only raise LDL cholesterol levels but have also been studied for their potential to increase the risk of prostate cancer, colon cancer, and breast cancer. Evidence linking *trans* fats to cancer is, however, inconsistent and insufficient; more study is needed to determine whether a potential association exists.[29] On the other hand, diets that are high in omega-3 fats from fish are associated with a lower incidence of colon cancer.[30]

Obesity

Excess dietary fat consumption contributes to weight gain and obesity. One reason is that fat contains 9 kilocalories per gram, more than twice the calorie content of carbohydrate or protein. Therefore, a high-fat meal contains more calories in the same volume than does a lower-fat meal. Because people have a tendency to eat a certain weight or volume of food, consuming meals that are high in fat causes more calories to be consumed.[31,32] Dietary fat may also contribute to weight gain because it is stored very efficiently as body fat.

Despite dietary fat's contribution to body fat storage, the fat content of the Canadian diet is not the sole reason for the high rate of obesity in Canada.[33] Weight gain typically occurs when energy intake exceeds energy expenditure, regardless of whether the extra energy comes from fat, carbohydrate, or protein. The increasing prevalence of overweight and obesity in Canada and worldwide is likely primarily due to a general increase in calorie intake combined with a decrease in energy expenditure.[34]

CONCEPT CHECK

1. **Why** does a deficiency of essential fatty acids cause health problems?

2. **How** does oxidized LDL cholesterol affect the formation of atherosclerotic plaque?

3. **What** are three dietary factors that increase the risk of heart disease?

4. **Why** might eating a high-fat diet increase the number of calories you consume?

Meeting Lipid Needs

LEARNING OBJECTIVES

1. **Discuss** the recommendations for fat and cholesterol intake.

2. **Classify** fats as either healthy or unhealthy.

3. **Name** a food that is high in cholesterol, saturated fat, or *trans* fat.

4. **Use** food labels to choose healthy fats.

The amount of fat the body requires from the diet is small, but a diet that provides only the minimum amount would be very high in carbohydrate, not very palatable, and not necessarily any healthier than diets with more fat. Therefore, the recommendations for fat intake focus on getting enough to meet the need for essential fatty acids and choosing the amounts and types of fat that will promote health and prevent disease.

Fat and Cholesterol Recommendations

The dietary reference intakes (DRIs) recommend a total fat intake of 20 to 35% of calories for adults. Of this amount, a small portion needs to come from the essential fatty acids. The adequate intake (AI) for linoleic acid is 12 g per day for women and 17 g per day for men. You can meet your requirement by consuming 125 g (½ cup) of walnuts or 30 mL (2 Tbsp) of safflower oil. For alpha-linolenic acid, the AI is 1.1 g per day for adult women and 1.6 g per day for adult men. Your requirement can be met by eating 62 g (¼ cup) of walnuts or 15 mL (1 Tbsp) of ground flaxseeds. Consuming these amounts provides the recommended ratio of linoleic to alpha-linolenic acid of between 5:1 and 10:1.[35]

The DRIs recommend that cholesterol, saturated fat, and *trans* fat intake be kept to a minimum because the risk of heart disease increases with higher intakes (see *Thinking It Through*). The Daily Values used on food labels give more specific recommendations.

Because children need more fat than adults do, to allow for growth and development, their acceptable ranges of fat intake are higher: 30 to 40% of calories for ages 1 to 3 and 25 to 35% of calories for ages 3 to 18. Like adults, adolescents and children over age 2 should consume a diet that is low in saturated fat, cholesterol, and *trans* fat.[36]

Choosing Fats Wisely

The majority of Canadians have fat intakes within the recommended 20 to 35% of calories from fat, but about 25% of Canadian adults consume fats above their acceptable macronutrient distribution range (AMDR).[37] Our *trans* fat intake is still well above recommended levels, but has improved significantly over the past two decades. In the 1990s, our *trans* fat intake was one of the highest in the world, more than four times above recommended levels![6] As a result of increased awareness of the risks of *trans* fats, mandatory labelling, and a challenge to food producers to reduce the *trans* fats in their products, this number has dropped to less than two times the recommended maximum level, which still represents a major cause for concern.[6] The main sources of *trans* fats in the Canadian diet are cakes, cookies, crackers, doughnuts, and potato chips.[38]

You can improve the proportion of healthy fats in your diet by shifting the sources of dietary fat. For example, limiting solid fats such as those in red meat and cheese will reduce your intake of saturated fat and cholesterol. Avoiding hydrogenated fats from foods such as hard margarines and baked goods will limit your intake of *trans* fats. Eating more nuts and avocados and cooking with canola and olive oils will boost your intake of monounsaturated fat, and eating more fish will boost your omega-3 intake.

Making wise food guide choices Your choices from each food group can have a significant impact on the amounts and types of fats in your diet (**Figure 5.18**). Generally, grains, fruits, and vegetables are low in total fat and saturated fat and they contain no cholesterol. However, choices from these groups need to be made with care to avoid fats that are added in processing or preparation. In Canada's Food Guide, the section "Make Each Food Serving Count" recommends choosing lower-fat options in all food groups. For example, smart choices from the meat and meat alternatives and the milk and

THINKING IT THROUGH

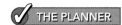
✓ THE PLANNER

Improving Heart Health

Tony is a financial advisor who spends much of his day sitting at his computer. When he is home with his family, he enjoys watching his children play soccer and basketball but rarely finds time to exercise himself. Tony's doctor recently told him that his blood cholesterol levels are elevated. His blood lipids and other information about his medical history are given below:

Sex	Male
Age	35
Family history	Mother had heart attack at age 60
Height/weight	173 cm (68 in.)/73 kg (160 lb.)
Blood pressure	145/80 (optimal is < 120/80)
Smoker	Yes
Activity level	Sedentary
Blood values	
Total cholesterol	5.4 mmol/L
LDL cholesterol	4.2 mmol/L
HDL cholesterol	0.9 mmol/L
Triglycerides	1.6 mmol/L

Which of the factors listed above increase Tony's risk of developing cardiovascular disease?
▼

Your answer: _____

_____

Tony meets with a dietitian. A diet recall reveals that his breakfast typically consists of a bagel with cream cheese and coffee with cream and sugar. For lunch, he goes out with his colleagues for fast food. Dinner at home with his family consists of beef or chicken, a green or orange vegetable, and rice or potatoes.

An analysis of his diet indicates that his total fat intake is within the recommended range of 20 to 35% of calories, but he consumes more saturated fat than is recommended, and his intake of omega-3 and monounsaturated fatty acids is low.

To reduce Tony's intake of saturated fat, the dietitian suggests that he switch to cereal with low-fat milk for breakfast and make better fast-food choices at lunchtime. For lunch, he frequents a burger fast-food restaurant, a taco shop, or a pizza restaurant.

What could he choose at his favourite fast-food restaurants to reduce his intake of saturated fat?
▼

Your answer: _____

_____

At home, to decrease consumption of saturated fats and increase consumption of unsaturated ones, the family switches to canola oil instead of butter for cooking and serves fish or seafood twice a week. Because these changes have reduced the calories in Tony's diet and he did not need to lose weight, he starts taking fruit and other healthy snacks to work.

Which of the snack choices pictured below is more heart healthy? Give two reasons.
▼

Your answer: _____

_____

(Check your answers in Appendix I.)

Cheese sandwich crackers

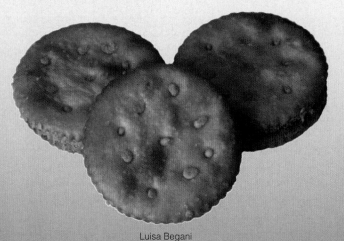

Luisa Begani

Dried fruit and nut mix

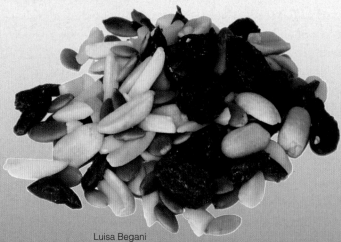

Luisa Begani

Healthy food guide choices • Figure 5.18

Eating Well with Canada's Food Guide now offers specific recommendations about fats, which are depicted outside the four food groups graphic. These recommendations mark a major change in the guide, as critics had argued that previous versions were flawed for their lack of recommendations regarding fat consumption. The Food Guide now advises using small amounts of unsaturated fats and limiting *trans* fats and sources of saturated fats.

Oils and Fats

* Include a small amount – 30 to 45 mL (2 to 3 Tbsp) – of unsaturated fat each day. This includes oil used for cooking, salad dressings, margarine and mayonnaise.
* Use vegetable oils such as canola, olive and soybean.
* Choose soft margarines that are low in saturated and trans fats.
* Limit butter, hard margarine, lard and shortening.

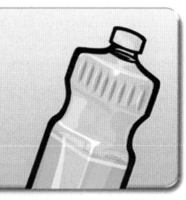

Limit trans fat

When a Nutrition Facts table is not available, ask for nutrition information to choose foods lower in trans and saturated fats.

Selecting lean meats • Figure 5.19

Fresh meats are not required to carry Nutrition Facts labels, but they often provide information about the fat content of the meat. The terms *lean* and *extra lean* are used to describe the fat content of packaged meats, such as hot dogs and lunch meat, and fresh meats, such as pork chops and steaks. The term *lean* refers to meat containing less than 10% fat by weight, and *extra lean* refers to meat containing less than 5% fat by weight. A general rule of thumb is to also look for meat that is more red than it is white. More white marbling means more fat.

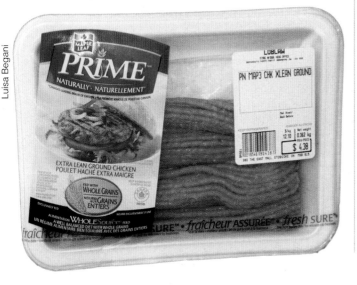

Luisa Begani

milk alternatives groups can reduce your intake of unhealthy fats (**Figure 5.19**).

The most concentrated sources of fat in the diet are the oils, butter, margarine, fatty sauces, and salad dressings used in cooking or added at the table. The fat and calories consumed from these sources can be easily underestimated. Limiting your consumption of these fat sources can reduce your total fat and calorie intake, and choosing liquid oils rather than solid fat can increase the proportion of unsaturated fats in your diet.

Referring to food labels Food labels are an accessible source of information about the fat content of packaged foods. The Nutrition Facts panel shows the amounts of total fat, saturated fat, and *trans* fat, and the ingredient list indicates the source of the fat—for example, whether a food contains corn oil, soybean oil, coconut oil, or partially hydrogenated vegetable oil. The unsaturated fat content of the product can be determined by subtracting the amount of saturated and *trans* fat from the amount of total fat. Nutrient content claims on food labels such as "low fat," "fat free," and "low cholesterol" can also be used to identify foods that help you meet the recommendations for fat intake. Be careful, however, that the lower-fat version of the product you are consuming doesn't compensate for the removed fat by adding other flavourings that increase the total caloric content or decrease the nutritional quality. Health claims can also help you choose foods that will meet your nutritional goals. For example, foods that are low in saturated fat and

Lipids on food labels • Figure 5.20

a. Understanding how to use food labels can help you make more informed choices about the foods you include in your diet. By noting the grams of fat and the total number of calories, you can determine the percentage of calories from fat in a product as follows:

1. Multiply the grams of fat by 9 kilocalories/gram. For example, this product provides 11 grams of fat:

$$11 \text{ grams} \times 9 \text{ kilocalories/gram} = 99 \text{ kilocalories from fat}$$

2. Divide kilocalories from fat by total kilocalories and multiply by 100 to obtain the percentage.

For example, this food contains 100 kilocalories/serving and 99 kilocalories from fat:

$$99 \text{ kilocalories} \div 100 \text{ kilocalories} \times 100 = 99\% \text{ kilocalories from fat}$$

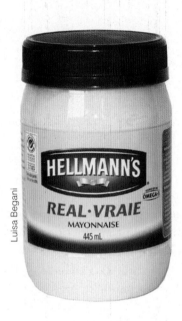

Nutrition Facts
Valeur nutritive
Per 1 Tbsp (15 mL)/par 1 cuillière à soupe (15 mL)

Amount Teneur	% Daily Value % valeur quotidienne
Calories / Calories 100	
Fat / Lipides 10 g	5 %
Saturated / saturés 1 g	
+ Trans / trans 0 g	10 %
Polyunsaturated Fat 3 g	
Monounsaturated Fat 6 g	
Cholesterol / Cholestérol 5 mg	2 %
Sodium / Sodium 95 mg	4 %
Carbohydrate / Glucides 0 g	0 %
Fibre / Fibres 0 g	0 %
Sugars / Sucres 0 g	
Protein / Protéines 0.1 g	
Vitamin A / Vitamine A	0 %
Vitamin C / Vitamine C	0 %
Calcium / Calcium	0 %
Iron / Fer	0 %

INGREDIENTS: CANOLA OIL, WATER, LIQUID WHOLE EGG, VINEGAR, SALT, LIQUID YOLK, SUGAR, SPICES, CONCENTRATED LEMON JUICE AND CALCIUM DISODIUM EDTA

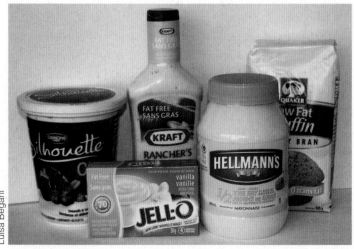

b. Food labelling regulations have developed standard definitions for descriptors such as "low fat" and "low cholesterol," and such terms can be used only in ways that will not confuse the consumer. For example, because saturated fat in the diet raises blood cholesterol, to be labelled "low cholesterol," a food must contain ≤20 mg cholesterol per serving and ≤2g saturated fat per serving. So crackers containing coconut oil, which are low in cholesterol but are high in saturated fat, cannot be labelled "low cholesterol."

WHAT SHOULD I EAT?
Fats and Cholesterol

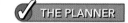

Limit your intake of cholesterol, *trans* fat, and saturated fat
- Use low-fat dairy products.
- Trim the fat from your meat before you cook it and serve chicken and fish but don't eat the skin.
- Reduce your usual amount of butter by half and use soft margarine rather than stick margarine.
- Use beans instead of meat in your chili, soups, and casseroles.
- Use a spray bottle to grease frying pans with unsaturated oil.

Increase the proportion of polyunsaturated and monounsaturated fats
- Use olive, peanut, or canola oil for cooking and salad dressing.
- Use corn, sunflower, or safflower oil for baking.

- Snack on nuts and seeds.
- Add olives and avocados to your salads.

Up your omega-3 intake
- Bake flaxseeds into breads and sprinkle them on your cereal or yogurt.
- Add another serving of fatty fish, such as mackerel, lake trout, herring, sardines, tuna, or salmon, to your weekly menu.
- Serve a leafy green vegetable with dinner.
- Add walnuts to your salad or cereal.
- Choose products fortified with omega-3 fatty acids such as omega-3 eggs or DHA milk.

 Use iProfile to find the varieties of nuts and fish that are highest in omega-3 fatty acids.

cholesterol may state that they help reduce the risk of heart disease (**Figure 5.20**).

Will using low-fat and reduced-fat products improve your diet? Some low-fat foods make an important contribution to a healthy diet. Low-fat dairy products are recommended because they provide all the essential nutrients contained in the full-fat versions but have fewer calories and less saturated fat and cholesterol. Using these products increases the nutrient density of the diet as a whole. However, not all reduced-fat foods are nutrient dense. Some are just lower-fat versions of nutrient-poor choices such as baked goods and chips. If these reduced-fat desserts and snack foods replace whole grains, fruits, and vegetables, the resulting diet could be low in fat but also low in fibre, vitamins, minerals, and phytochemicals (see *What Should I Eat?*).

Using low-fat foods does not necessarily transform a poor diet into a healthy one or improve overall diet quality, but if used appropriately, fat-modified foods can be part of a healthy diet.[39] For example, if you use a low-fat salad dressing to replace a full-fat version, you enhance the appeal of a nutrient-rich salad without as much added fat

and calories from the dressing. Low-fat products can also be used in conjunction with weight-loss diets because they are often lower in calories. But check the label: Although low-fat foods are generally lower in calories, they are by no means calorie free and cannot be consumed liberally without adding calories to the diet and possibly contributing to weight gain.

CONCEPT CHECK

1. **How** much fat is recommended in a healthy diet?

2. **Why** is fatty fish a healthier choice than fatty beef?

3. **Which** food groups contribute the most foods that are high in saturated fat and cholesterol?

4. **How** can labels help you identify foods that are low in cholesterol and saturated fat?

Summary

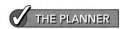

1 Fats in Our Food 130

- Fat adds calories, texture, and flavour to foods. Some of the fats we eat are visible, but others are hidden.

- Over the past 40 years, Canadians have changed the sources of fat in their diets, but the percentage of calories from fat has changed little, and the incidence of obesity and other chronic diseases has continued to rise.

Canadian food intake in the 1970s and today • Figure 5.2

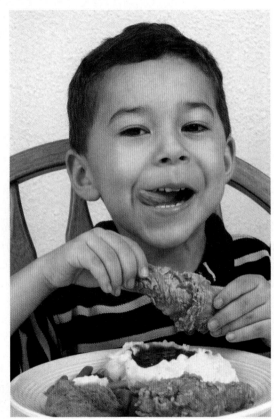

© iStockphoto.com/David Hernandez

2 Types of Lipids 131

- **Lipids** are a diverse group of organic compounds, most of which do not dissolve in water. **Triglycerides**, commonly referred to as fat, are the type of lipid that is most abundant in our food. A triglyceride contains three **fatty acids** attached to a molecule of glycerol. **Sterols** and **phospholipids** are minor sources of fat in the diet.

Triglycerides and fatty acids • Figure 5.3

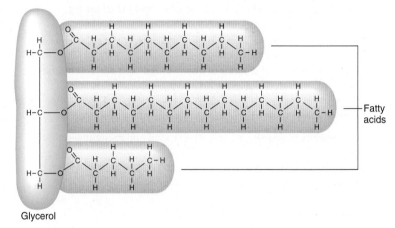

Glycerol

Fatty acids

- The structure of fatty acids affects their chemical properties and functions in the body. Each carbon atom in the carbon chain of a **saturated fatty acid** is attached to as many hydrogen atoms as possible, so no carbon–carbon double bonds form. Saturated fatty acids are found primarily in animal products. Exceptions include saturated plant oils, often called **tropical oils**. A **monounsaturated fatty acid** contains one carbon–carbon double bond. A **polyunsaturated fatty acid** contains more than one carbon–carbon double bond. The location of the first double bond determines whether it is an **omega-3 (ω-3) fatty acid**, such as **alpha-linolenic acid**, **eicosapentaenoic acid (EPA)**, or **docosahexaenoic acid (DHA)**, or an **omega-6 (ω-6) fatty acid**, such as **linolenic acid** or **arachidonic acid**. Omega-3 and Omega-6 fatty acids are **essential fatty acids** used to synthesize **eicosanoids**, which help regulate blood clotting, blood pressure, immune function, and other body processes. The orientation of hydrogen atoms around a carbon–carbon double bond distinguishes *cis* fatty acids from *trans* **fatty acids**. **Hydrogenation** transforms some carbon–carbon double bonds to the *trans* configuration.

- A phospholipid contains a **phosphate group** and two fatty acids attached to a backbone of glycerol. One end of the molecule is water soluble, and one end is lipid soluble. Phospholipids therefore make good **emulsifiers**, such as the emulsifier **lecithin**, which is found in many food products. In the human body, they are an important structural component of lipoproteins and cell membranes where they form a **lipid bilayer.**

- Sterols, of which **cholesterol** is the best known, are made up of multiple chemical rings. Cholesterol is made by the body and consumed in animal foods in the diet. In the body, it is a component of cell membranes and is used to synthesize vitamin D, bile acids, and some hormones. **Plant sterols** are found in most plant foods and may reduce cholesterol levels in the blood.

3 Absorbing and Transporting Lipids 138

- In the small intestine, muscular churning mixes chyme with bile from the gallbladder to break fat into small globules. This process allows pancreatic lipase to access these fats for digestion. The products of triglyceride digestion, cholesterol, phospholipids, and other fat-soluble substance combine with bile to form **micelles**, which facilitate the absorption of these materials.

- Lipids absorbed from the intestine are packaged with protein to form **chylomicrons**, a type of **lipoprotein**. The triglycerides in chylomicrons are broken down by **lipoprotein lipase** on the surface of cells lining the blood vessels. The fatty acids released are taken up by surrounding cells, and what remains is taken up by to the liver.

- **Very-low-density lipoproteins (VLDLs)** are synthesized by the liver. With the help of lipoprotein lipase, they deliver triglycerides to body cells. **Low-density lipoproteins (LDLs)** deliver cholesterol to tissues by binding to **LDL receptors** on the cell surface. **High-density lipoproteins (HDLs)** help remove cholesterol from cells and transport it to the liver for disposal.

Lipid digestion and absorption • Figure 5.9

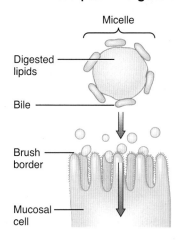

4 Lipid Functions 142

- Dietary fat is needed for the absorption of fat-soluble vitamins and to provide essential fatty acids. In the body, triglycerides in the **adipocytes** of **adipose tissue** provide a concentrated source of energy and insulate the body against shock and temperature changes.

- Throughout the day, triglycerides are continuously stored in adipose tissue and then broken down to release fatty acids,

depending on the immediate energy needs of the body. To generate ATP from fatty acids, the carbon chain is broken into two carbon units that form acetyl CoA, which can then be metabolized by aerobic pathways.

Storing and retrieving energy from fat stores • Figure 5.14

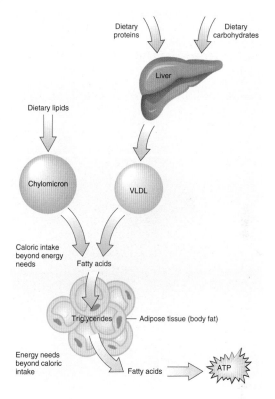

5 Lipids in Health and Disease 145

- **Atherosclerosis** is a type of **cardiovascular disease** characterized by the formation of **atherosclerotic plaque** in the artery wall. It begins with an injury to the artery wall that triggers **inflammation**, leading to plaque formation. A key event in the process is the oxidation of LDL cholesterol in the artery wall. Oxidized LDL cholesterol promotes inflammation and attracts white blood cells, which fill with cholesterol, forming **foam cells** that deposit in the artery wall. High blood levels of total and LDL cholesterol are risk factors for heart disease. High blood HDL cholesterol protects against heart disease. The risk of atherosclerosis is also increased by diabetes, high blood pressure, and obesity.

- Diets high in saturated fat, *trans* fat, and cholesterol may increase the risk of heart disease. Diets that reduce the risk of heart disease are high in omega-6 and omega-3 polyunsaturated fatty acids; monounsaturated fatty acids; certain B vitamins; and plant foods containing **antioxidants,** fibre, and phytochemicals. For reducing heart disease risk, the total dietary and lifestyle pattern is more important than any individual dietary factor.

• Diets high in fat correlate with an increased incidence of certain types of cancer. In general, the same types of lipids and other dietary components that protect you from heart disease will also protect you from certain forms of cancer.

• Fat contains 9 kilocalories per gram. A high-fat diet may therefore increase energy intake and promote weight gain, but such a diet is not the primary cause of obesity. Consuming more energy than expended leads to weight gain, regardless of whether the energy is from fat, carbohydrate, or protein.

Development of atherosclerosis • Figure 5.15

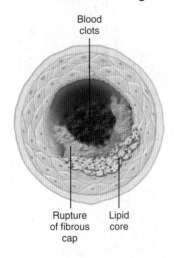

Blood clots

Rupture of fibrous cap

Lipid core

6 Meeting Lipid Needs   153

• The DRIs recommend that adults consume a diet that provides 20 to 35% of energy from fat and is low in cholesterol, saturated fat, and *trans* fat.

• Most Canadians consume the correct amount of energy from fat, but their diet does not always contain the healthiest types of fats. To reduce saturated fat and cholesterol intake, limit solid fats and choose liquid oils, fish, and nuts and seeds often. Use food labels to avoid processed foods that are high in saturated and *trans* fat. A diet that is based on whole grains, fruits, vegetables, and lean meats and low-fat dairy products will meet the recommendations for fat intake.

Selecting lean meats • Figure 5.19

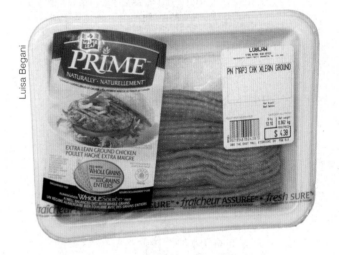

Luisa Begani

Key Terms

- adipocytes 142
- adipose tissue 142
- alpha-linolenic acid (ALA) 134
- antioxidants 148
- arachidonic acid 134
- atherosclerosis 145
- atherosclerotic plaque 146
- cardiovascular disease 145
- cholesterol 137
- chylomicrons 140
- docosahexaenoic acid (DHA) 134

- eicosanoids 134
- eicosapentaenoic acid (EPA) 134
- emulsifiers 137
- essential fatty acids (EFAs) 134
- fatty acids 131
- foam cells 146
- high-density lipoproteins (HDLs) 140
- hydrogenation 135
- inflammation 146
- lecithin 137

- linoleic acid (LA) 134
- lipid bilayer 136
- lipids 131
- lipoprotein lipase 140
- lipoproteins 139
- LDL receptor 141
- low-density lipoproteins (LDLs) 140
- micelles 138
- monounsaturated fatty acid 132
- omega-3 (ω-3) fatty acid 132
- omega-6 (ω-6) fatty acid 132

- phosphate group 136
- phospholipids 131
- plant sterols 138
- polyunsaturated fatty acid 132
- saturated fatty acids 133
- sterols 131
- *trans* fatty acids 135
- triglycerides 131
- tropical oils 133
- unsaturated fatty acids 133
- very-low-density lipoproteins (VLDLs) 140

Critical and Creative Thinking Questions

1. The percentage of calories from fat in the typical Canadian diet hasn't changed much since the 1980s. Nevertheless, this same period has seen an increase in the incidence of obesity in Canada. Discuss how it is possible that Canadians haven't changed the percentage of the fat in their diet, but are still gaining weight.

2. Record everything you eat for three days or refer to a previous food record. List the dairy products in your diet and indicate whether they are full fat or reduced fat. List the grain products you typically consume. How many of them are baked goods with added fats? How many of them are eaten with an added high-fat spread or sauce? Suggest changes you could make to reduce the fats added to your carbohydrates. List the vegetables in your diet. Underline those that are cooked or prepared in a way that increases their fat intake. For example, are they fried or topped with butter or margarine? List the high-protein foods in your diet. Use iProfile to determine the types and amounts of lipids they provide. Substitute some high-protein foods that would increase your intake of mono-unsaturated and omega-3 fatty acids.

3. Ka Ming is 54 years old and has lived in Canada since 1964. A physical exam reveals that his total blood cholesterol is 6.4 mmol/L and his HDL cholesterol is 0.7 mmol/L. He is at a healthy weight and does not smoke. He gets little exercise and consumes a diet that is a mixture of American foods and traditional Chinese foods. A medical history reveals that none of Ka Ming's relatives in China have had cardiovascular disease. Why might the lack of cardiovascular disease in his family history not be a true indication of Ka Ming's risk?

4. Compare and contrast the structure and functions of chylomicrons and VLDLs.

5. What are the similarities and differences in how the body responds to a cut on the finger and to an injury to the inside of an artery wall?

6. Why might taking fish oil supplements reduce the rate at which your blood clots?

7. How can a person who is a vegan and therefore consumes no dietary cholesterol still have elevated blood cholesterol?

What is happening in this picture?

This individual has familial hypercholesterolemia, a rare genetic disease in which there are no LDL receptors on cells. It causes cholesterol levels so high that the cholesterol deposits in body tissues, seen here as raised lumps.

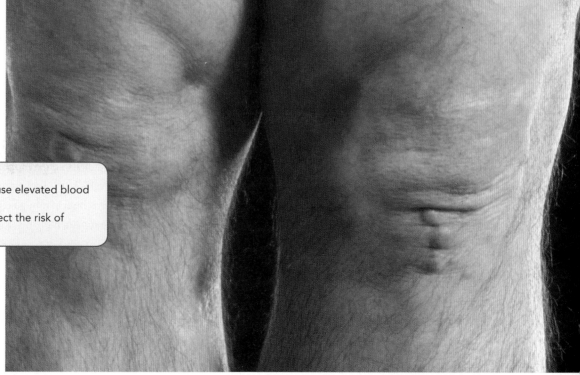

Bart's Medical Library/Phototake

Think Critically

1. Why would this condition cause elevated blood cholesterol?
2. How would this condition affect the risk of developing heart disease?

Self-Test

(Check your answers in Appendix J.)

1. What type of fatty acid is labelled C in the illustration?

   a. saturated

   b. monounsaturated

   c. omega-3 polyunsaturated

   d. omega-6 polyunsaturated

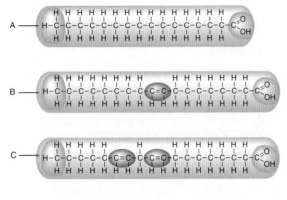
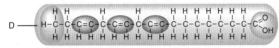

2. In the illustration, which figures represent essential fatty acids?

   a. A and D

   d. C and D

   b. A and B

   e. All of the above

   c. B and C

3. Which one of the following is unlikely to occur after you eat a fatty meal?

   a. Fatty acids stored in adipose tissue are released into the blood and taken up by body cells as an energy source.

   b. The gallbladder releases bile into the small intestine.

   c. Micelles are formed in the small intestine.

   d. Pancreatic lipase releases fatty acids from triglycerides.

   e. The concentration of chylomicrons in the blood increases.

4. Omega-3 fatty acids have a beneficial effect on blood lipid levels but also reduce the risk of cardiovascular diseases because they _____.

   a. inhibit the absorption of cholesterol from the diet

   b. increase the formation of oxidized LDL cholesterol

   c. cause mutations in cellular DNA

   d. break down *trans* fatty acids

   e. are converted into eicosanoids

5. Which of the following statements about cholesterol is false?

   a. It is used to synthesize vitamin D.

   b. It is needed to make bile.

   c. It is an essential component of animal cell membranes.

   d. It is found in peanut butter, leafy green vegetables, and avocados.

   e. It is needed to make the hormones estrogen and testosterone.

6. Which two fatty acids are considered essential?

   a. saturated and unsaturated

   b. linoleic and α-linolenic

   c. stearic and palmitic

   d. EPA and DHA

   e. short and medium chain

Use the diagram below to answer questions 6 and 7.

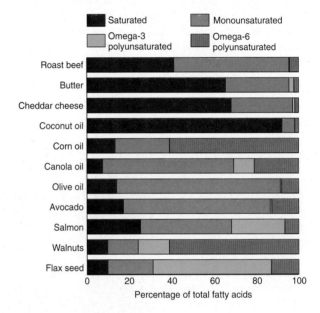

7. Which of the following statements about dietary sources of fat is true?

   a. Coconut oil is high in polyunsaturated fat.

   b. Canola oil is high in monounsaturated fat.

   c. Olive oil is high in omega-3 fatty acids.

   d. Butter is high in omega-6 fatty acids.

   e. Avocados are high in saturated fat.

8. Which of the following is highest in omega-3 fatty acids?

   a. corn oil

   b. canola oil

   c. flax seed

   d. walnuts

   e. salmon

9. Which one of the following is associated with an increased risk of developing heart disease?

   a. a high concentration of HDL in the blood

b. daily exercise

c. a high-fibre, low-fat diet

d. a diet made up mostly of plant foods

e. a high concentration of LDL in the blood

10. Which of the following contribute to the lower heart disease risk associated with eating nuts?

a. They are high in monounsaturated fat and omega-3 fatty acids.

b. They are a good source of fibre and vegetable protein.

c. They provide antioxidants.

d. They contain plant sterols.

e. All of the above are correct.

11. The transport of cholesterol to the liver for elimination is accomplished by _____.

a. chylomicrons

b. VLDLs

c. HDLs

d. LDLs

12. Which of the following statements about *trans* fatty acids is false?

a. They have carbon–carbon double bonds, with the hydrogen atoms on the same side of the bond.

b. They have straighter carbon chains than a corresponding *cis* fatty acid.

c. They are formed during the hydrogenation of vegetable oils.

d. High levels in the diet increase the risk of heart disease.

13. Refer to the Nutrition Facts panel below and determine the approximate percentage of calories from saturated fat in this product.

a. 99%

b. 18%

c. 14%

d. 17%

e. 24%

Cheese sandwich crackers

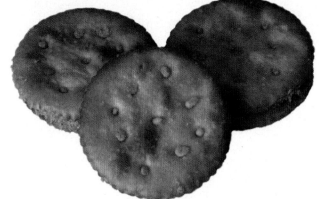

Luisa Begani

14. Which one of the following statements about micelles is true?

a. They help facilitate the absorption of lipids in the small intestine.

b. They help transport lipids in the bloodstream.

c. They are essential in the diet.

d. They break the bonds that hold fatty acids to glycerol.

e. They are transformed into chylomicrons in the blood.

15. Identify the molecule in the animal cell membrane labelled A in the diagram below.

a. cholesterol

b. protein

c. starch

d. phospholipid

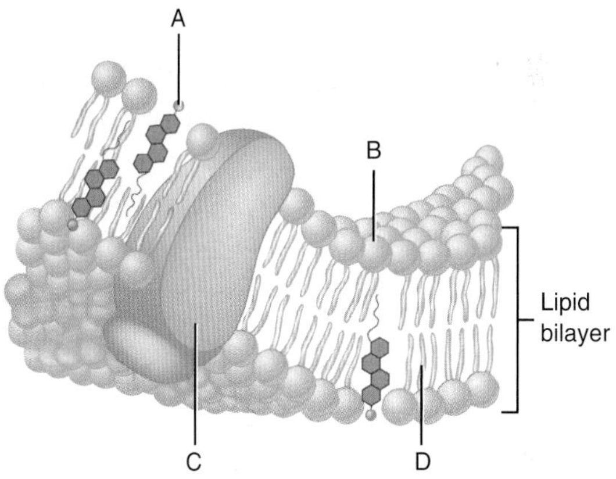

Cell exterior
(aqueous environment)

A

B

Lipid bilayer

C

D

Cytoplasm
(aqueous environment)

THE PLANNER ✓

Review your Chapter Planner on the chapter opener and check off your completed work.

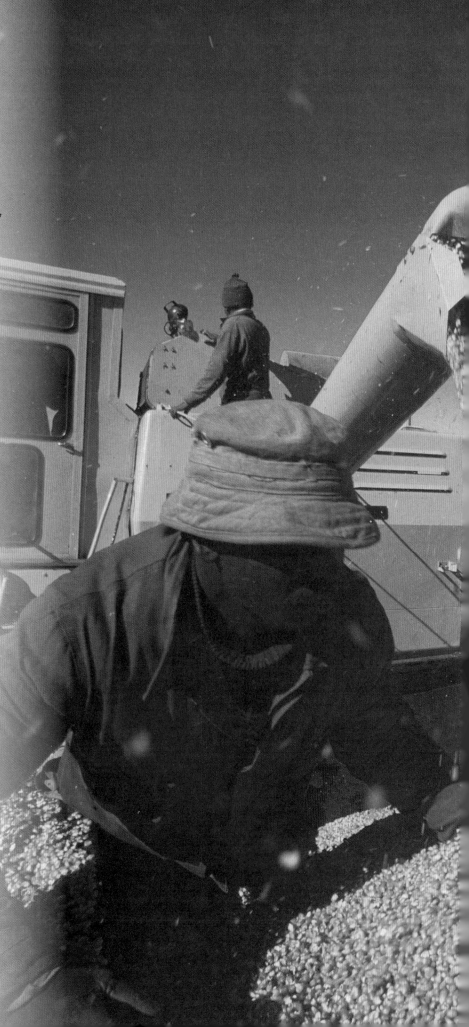

Proteins and Amino Acids

The word *protein* comes from the Greek *proteios*, meaning "of primary importance." This name is apt because proteins are essential to every process that takes place in our cells. Proteins catalyze chemical reactions, are fundamental components of muscular and skeletal tissue, and are vital in the body's immune response. Because of this primary importance, the generation, development, processing, and renewal of protein resources are major human activities.

Although protein is found in both plants and animals, people in Western culture fulfill most of their protein needs from animal products. As affluence has increased in non-Western societies, many non-Westerners have adopted Western habits, including increasing the amount of beef in their diets. This trend places greater demands on agriculture to provide grain to feed to cattle, which will then convert it to the preferred beef protein. This increase in beef consumption also leads to a larger environmental footprint, as an inefficient amount of land resources are used to raise the cattle, and the cattle themselves produce a significant amount of greenhouse emissions.

Agricultural production now faces a challenge from another front: biofuels. In Canada today, more and more grain crops are being grown not as food but to be converted into biofuel. Some argue that it is inefficient to feed grain protein to cattle so that the cattle will produce protein that we will consume, but at least this process is a nutrition cycle. Corn that is converted into ethanol to fuel an automobile feeds neither cattle nor humans. The challenge of obtaining enough protein and maintaining an adequate balance of plant and animal protein for the world's population is, like protein itself, clearly of primary importance.

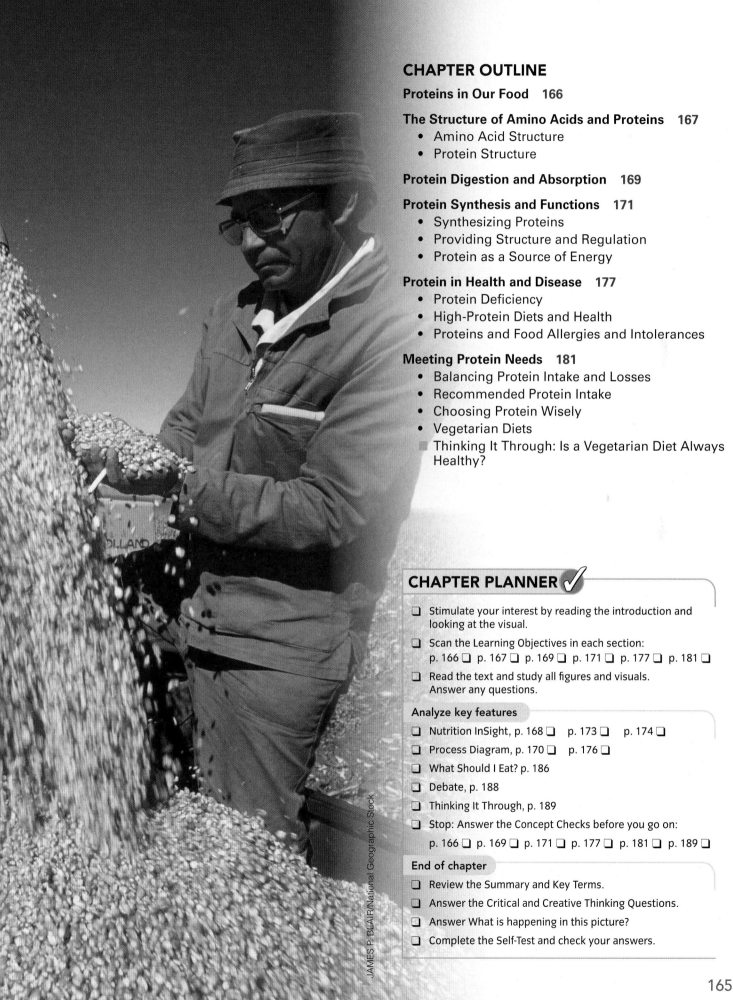

CHAPTER OUTLINE

CHAPTER PLANNER ✓

- ❏ Stimulate your interest by reading the introduction and looking at the visual.
- ❏ Scan the Learning Objectives in each section:
  p. 166 ❏ p. 167 ❏ p. 169 ❏ p. 171 ❏ p. 177 ❏ p. 181 ❏
- ❏ Read the text and study all figures and visuals. Answer any questions.

Analyze key features

- ❏ Nutrition InSight, p. 168 ❏   p. 173 ❏   p. 174 ❏
- ❏ Process Diagram, p. 170 ❏   p. 176 ❏
- ❏ What Should I Eat? p. 186
- ❏ Debate, p. 188
- ❏ Thinking It Through, p. 189
- ❏ Stop: Answer the Concept Checks before you go on:
  p. 166 ❏ p. 169 ❏ p. 171 ❏ p. 177 ❏ p. 181 ❏ p. 189 ❏

End of chapter

- ❏ Review the Summary and Key Terms.
- ❏ Answer the Critical and Creative Thinking Questions.
- ❏ Answer What is happening in this picture?
- ❏ Complete the Self-Test and check your answers.

JAMES P. BLAIR/National Geographic Stock

Proteins in Our Food

LEARNING OBJECTIVES

1. **Describe** which types of foods provide the most concentrated sources of protein.

2. **Compare** the nutrients in plant sources of protein with those in animal sources of protein.

When we think of protein, we usually think of a steak, a plate of scrambled eggs, or a glass of milk. These animal foods provide the most concentrated sources of protein in our diet, but plant foods such as grains, nuts, and **legumes** are also important sources of dietary protein. The proteins found in plants are made up of different combinations of **amino acids** than the proteins found in animals. Because of this difference, most plant proteins are not used as efficiently as animal proteins to build proteins in the human body. Nevertheless, a diet that includes a variety of plant proteins can easily meet most people's protein needs.

> **legumes** The starchy seeds of plants that produce bean pods, including peas, peanuts, beans, soybeans, and lentils.
>
> **amino acids** The building blocks of proteins. Each contains an amino group, an acid group, and a unique side chain.

The sources of protein in your diet have an impact not only on the amount of protein and variety of amino acids available to your body but also on the other nutrients that are consumed in the diet and on your overall health (**Figure 6.1**). Animal products provide B vitamins and readily absorbable sources of minerals such as iron, zinc, and calcium. They are low in fibre, however, and are often high in saturated fat and cholesterol—a nutrient mix that increases the risk of heart disease.

Plant sources of protein provide most, but not all, B vitamins and also supply iron, zinc, and calcium, but in less absorbable forms. Plant foods are generally excellent sources of fibre, phytochemicals, and unsaturated fats—nutrients that should be increased in our diets to promote health. *Eating Well with Canada's Food Guide* recommends that our diets be based on whole-grain products, vegetables, and fruits and include smaller amounts of meats and dairy products. Following these guidelines will provide plenty of protein from a mixture of plant and animal sources and minimize risk of disease.

CONCEPT CHECK STOP

1. **Which** is higher in protein, an egg or a 250-g serving of rice?

2. **What** nutrients are plentiful in meat and milk? In grains and legumes?

Animal versus plant proteins • Figure 6.1

a. Animal products are high in protein, iron, zinc, and calcium but add saturated fat and cholesterol to the diet.

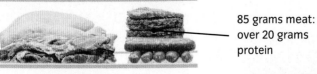

© iStockphoto.com/Cristian Baitg

250 mL milk: 8 grams protein

1 egg: 7 grams protein

85 grams meat: over 20 grams protein

b. Plant sources of protein are rich in fibre, phytochemicals, and monounsaturated and polyunsaturated fats.

Michael Newman/PhotoEdit

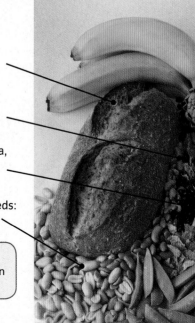

1 slice bread: about 2 grams protein

125 grams legumes: 6–10 grams protein

125 grams rice, pasta, or cereal: 2–3 grams protein

60 grams nuts or seeds: 5–10 grams protein

Ask Yourself

Why might a diet high in animal protein increase the risk of heart disease?

The Structure of Amino Acids and Proteins

LEARNING OBJECTIVES

1. **Describe** the general structure of an amino acid and of a protein.

2. **Distinguish** between essential and nonessential amino acids.

3. **Discuss** how the order of amino acids in a polypeptide chain affects protein structure.

4. **Explain** how a protein's structure is related to its function.

What do the proteins in a lamb chop, a kidney bean, and your thigh muscle have in common? They are all constructed of amino acids linked together to form one or more folded, chain-like strands. Twenty amino acids are commonly found in proteins. Each kind of protein contains a different number, combination, and sequence of these amino acids. These differences give specific proteins their unique functions in living organisms and their unique characteristics in foods.

Amino Acid Structure

Each amino acid consists of a carbon atom that is bound to a hydrogen atom; an amino group, which contains nitrogen; an acid group; and a side chain (**Figure 6.3a**). The nitrogen in amino acids distinguishes protein from carbohydrates and lipids; all three contain carbon, hydrogen, and oxygen, but only protein contains nitrogen. This quality also makes it inefficient for the body to use protein for

energy, as the body first needs to eliminate the nitrogen-containing group before the protein can be metabolized. The side chains of amino acids vary in size and structure; they give the different amino acids their unique properties.

Nine of the amino acids needed by the adult human body must be consumed in the diet because they cannot be made in the body (**Figure 6.3b**). If the diet is deficient in one or more of these essential amino acids (also called indispensable amino acids), the body cannot make new proteins without breaking down existing proteins to provide the needed amino acids. The other 11 amino acids that are commonly found in protein are **nonessential**, or **dispensable amino acids**, because they can be made in the body.

Under certain conditions, some of the nonessential amino acids cannot be synthesized in sufficient amounts to meet the body's needs. These are therefore referred to as **conditionally essential amino acids**. For example, the amino acid tyrosine can be made in the body from the essential amino acid phenylalanine. In individuals who have the inherited disease phenylketonuria (PKU), phenylalanine cannot be converted into tyrosine; for these individuals, tyrosine is an essential amino acid (**Figure 6.2**).

essential amino acids (also called **indispensable amino acids**) Amino acids that cannot be synthesized by the body in sufficient amounts to meet its needs and therefore must be included in the diet.

phenylketonuria (PKU) A genetic disease in which the amino acid phenylalanine cannot be metabolized normally, causing it to build up in the blood. If untreated, the condition results in brain damage.

Phenylketonuria • Figure 6.2

This warning on a can of diet pop probably doesn't mean much unless you have the genetic disease phenylketonuria (PKU). Individuals with PKU must limit their intake of the amino acid phenylalanine, which usually means limiting their consumption of high-protein foods. When a scientist looks at this label, she or he recognizes that the artificial sweetener aspartame in this pop is the source of the phenylalanine. The breakdown of aspartame in the digestive tract releases phenylalanine, which

cannot be properly metabolized by individuals with PKU. If they consume large amounts of this amino acid, compounds called phenylketones build up in their blood. In infants and young children, phenylketones interfere with brain development; and in pregnant women, they cause birth defects in the baby. To prevent these effects, individuals with PKU must consume a diet that provides just enough phenylalanine to meet the body's needs but not so much that phenylketones build up in their blood.

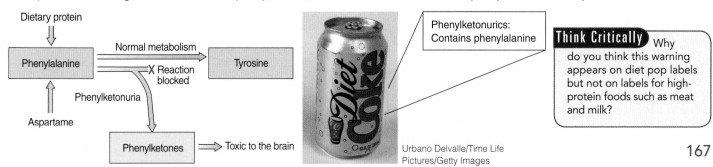

Phenylketonurics: Contains phenylalanine

Think Critically Why do you think this warning appears on diet pop labels but not on labels for high-protein foods such as meat and milk?

Urbano Delvalle/Time Life Pictures/Getty Images

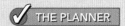

a. The general structure of an amino acid.

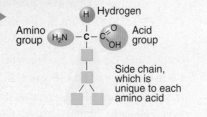

H Hydrogen

Amino group H₂N

Acid group

Side chain, which is unique to each amino acid

b. Twenty amino acids are commonly found in proteins. The table shown here lists them based on whether they are essential or nonessential and indicates those that are conditionally essential.

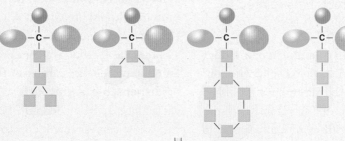

Amino acids bond to form polypeptides

Essential Amino Acids	Nonessential Amino Acids
Histidine	Alanine
Isoleucine	Arginine*
Leucine	Asparagine
Lysine	Aspartic acid
Methionine	Cysteine*
Phenylalanine	Glutamic acid
Threonine	Glutamine*
Tryptophan	Glycine*
Valine	Proline*
	Serine
	Tyrosine*

*Considered conditionally essential

c. Amino acids linked by peptide bonds are called **peptides**. When two amino acids are linked, they form a **dipeptide**; three form a **tripeptide**. Many amino acids bonded together constitute a polypeptide. Polypeptide chains may contain hundreds of amino acids. The sequence of amino acids is referred to as the **primary structure** of the protein.

Peptide bond

Polypeptide chains fold to form 3-dimensional shapes

d. The order and chemical properties of the amino acids in a polypeptide chain determine how the polypeptide folds. Hydrogen bonds between side chain causes the protein to fold into its **secondary structure**, consisting of coiled helices and folded sheets.

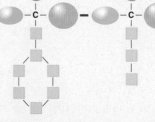

β pleated sheet

alpha helix

e. The **tertiary structure** of a protein is formed when the secondary structure folds further. This is due to weak interactions between amino acids, bonds between side chains, and interactions with the watery environment.

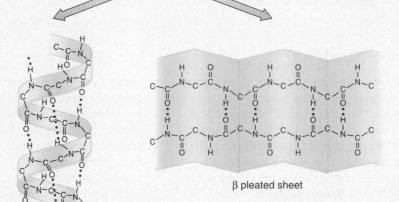

f. The **quaternary structure** of a protein molecule consists of several folded polypeptide chains.

Protein Structure

To form proteins, amino acids are linked together by **peptide bonds**, which join the acid group of one amino acid to the amino group of another amino acid (**Figure 6.3c**). Many amino acids bonded together constitute a polypeptide. A protein is formed when one or more polypeptide chains are folded into very specific three-dimensional shapes. Accordingly, all proteins are polypeptides, but not all polypeptides are proteins. The order and chemical properties of the amino acids in a polypeptide chain determine its final shape. The folding of the chain occurs in response to forces in the specific amino acid side chains that attract or repel amino acids from one another or from water (**Figure 6.3d, e**). The folded polypeptide chain may constitute the final protein, or it may join with several other folded polypeptide chains to form the final, fully functioning protein (**Figure 6.3f**).

> **polypeptide**
> A chain of amino acids linked by peptide bonds that is part of the structure of a protein.

The shape of a protein is essential to its function. For example, the elongated shape of the proteins collagen and alpha-keratin, found in connective tissue, helps them give strength to the skin, tendons, and ligaments. The spherical shape of the protein hemoglobin helps red blood cells carry and transport oxygen, and the long shape of muscle proteins allows them to overlap and shorten muscles during contraction.

When the shape of a protein is altered, the protein no longer functions normally. For example, when salivary amylase, which is an enzyme protein, enters the stomach, the acid causes the structure of the protein to change, and it no longer functions in the digestion of starch. This change in structure is called denaturation, referring to a change from a protein's natural tertiary or quaternary

> **denaturation**
> Alteration of a protein's three-dimensional structure.

Protein denaturation • Figure 6.4

When an egg is cooked, the heat denatures the protein. The protein in a raw egg white forms a clear, viscous liquid, but when cooking denatures it, the egg white becomes white and firm and cannot be restored to its original form. Other factors that denature the proteins in food include mechanical agitation, such as when cream is whipped to make whipped cream, and the addition of acid, such as when milk is curdled by the addition of an acid such as lemon juice.

© Can Stock Photo Inc. / glorcza

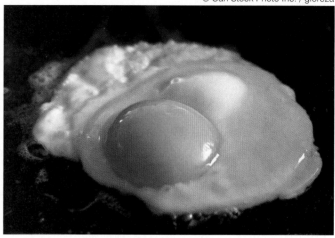

structure. Proteins in food are often denatured during processing and cooking (**Figure 6.4**).

CONCEPT CHECK

1. **Which** chemical element is found in protein but not in carbohydrate or lipid?

2. **Why** do we need to consume only some of the 20 amino acids that the body needs to make proteins?

3. **What** determines the shape of a protein?

4. **How** does denaturation affect the function of proteins?

Protein Digestion and Absorption

LEARNING OBJECTIVES

1. **Describe** the process of protein digestion.

2. **Discuss** how amino acids are absorbed.

P roteins must be digested before their amino acids can be absorbed into the body (**Figure 6.5**). Protein digestion begins in the mouth with the mechanical action of chewing, but the mouth has no protein-specific enzymes to chemically digest protein.

Protein digestion and absorption • Figure 6.5

 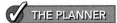
Protein must be broken down into small peptides and amino acids to be absorbed into the mucosal cells.

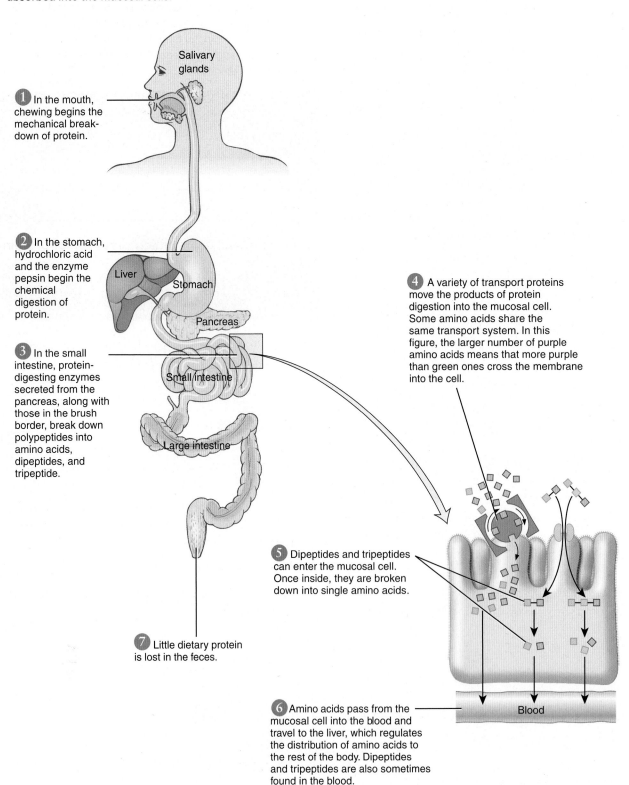

1 In the mouth, chewing begins the mechanical break-down of protein.

2 In the stomach, hydrochloric acid and the enzyme pepsin begin the chemical digestion of protein.

3 In the small intestine, protein-digesting enzymes secreted from the pancreas, along with those in the brush border, break down polypeptides into amino acids, dipeptides, and tripeptide.

Salivary glands

Liver
Stomach
Pancreas
Small intestine
Large intestine

4 A variety of transport proteins move the products of protein digestion into the mucosal cell. Some amino acids share the same transport system. In this figure, the larger number of purple amino acids means that more purple than green ones cross the membrane into the cell.

5 Dipeptides and tripeptides can enter the mucosal cell. Once inside, they are broken down into single amino acids.

7 Little dietary protein is lost in the feces.

6 Amino acids pass from the mucosal cell into the blood and travel to the liver, which regulates the distribution of amino acids to the rest of the body. Dipeptides and tripeptides are also sometimes found in the blood.

Blood

The chemical digestion of protein begins in the acidic environment of the stomach. Here, hydrochloric acid denatures proteins, opening up their folded tertiary or quaternary structure to make the polypeptide chains more accessible for enzymatic breakdown. Stomach acid also activates the protein-digesting enzyme *pepsin*, which breaks certain peptide bonds in the polypeptide chains, leaving shorter polypeptides. Most protein digestion occurs in the small intestine, where polypeptides are broken into even smaller peptides and amino acids by protein-digesting enzymes produced in the pancreas and small intestine. Single amino acids, dipeptides, and tripeptides are absorbed into the mucosal cells of the small intestine.

Amino acids enter your body by crossing from the lumen of the small intestine into the mucosal cells and then into the blood. This process involves one of several energy-requiring amino acid transport systems. Amino acids with similar structures use the same transport system (see Figure 6.5). As a result, amino acids may compete with one another for absorption. If there is an excess of any one of the amino acids sharing a transport system, more of it will be absorbed, slowing the absorption of competing amino acids. This competition for absorption is usually not a problem because foods contain a variety of amino acids, none of which are present in excessive amounts. However, when people consume amino acid supplements, especially single isolated amino acids, the supplemented amino acid may clog the transport system, reducing the absorption of other amino acids that share the same transport system. For example, weightlifters often take supplements of the amino acid arginine. Because arginine shares a transport system with lysine, large doses of arginine can inhibit the absorption of lysine, upsetting the balance of amino acids in the body.

CONCEPT CHECK

1. **Where** does the chemical digestion of protein begin?

2. **Why** might supplementing one amino acid reduce the absorption of other amino acids?

Protein Synthesis and Functions

LEARNING OBJECTIVES

1. **Explain** what is meant by the term *limiting amino acid*.

2. **Discuss** the steps involved in synthesizing proteins.

3. **Name** four functions of body proteins.

4. **Describe** the conditions under which the body uses protein to produce energy.

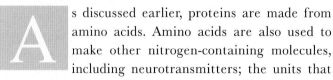 s discussed earlier, proteins are made from amino acids. Amino acids are also used to make other nitrogen-containing molecules, including neurotransmitters; the units that make up DNA and RNA; the skin pigment melanin; the vitamin niacin; creatine, which is used to fuel muscle contraction; and histamine, which causes blood vessels to dilate. The amino acids from proteins can also be metabolized to provide energy, or can be used to synthesize glucose or fatty acids.

The amino acids available for these functions come from the proteins consumed in the diet and from the breakdown of body proteins. These amino acids are referred to collectively as the **amino acid pool** (**Figure 6.6**). There is not actually a "pool" in the body containing a collection of amino acids, but these molecules are available in body fluids and cells to provide the raw materials needed to synthesize proteins and other molecules.

> **amino acid pool** All the amino acids in body tissues and fluids that are available for use by the body.

Synthesizing Proteins

The instructions for making proteins are contained in the nucleus of the cell in stretches of DNA called

Amino acid pool • Figure 6.6

Amino acids enter the available pool from the diet and from the breakdown of body proteins. Of the approximately 300 grams of protein synthesized by the body each day, only about 100 grams are made from amino acids consumed in the diet. The other 200 grams are produced by the recycling of amino acids from protein broken down in the body. Amino acids in the pool can be used to synthesize body proteins and other nitrogen-containing molecules, to provide energy, or to synthesize glucose or fatty acids.

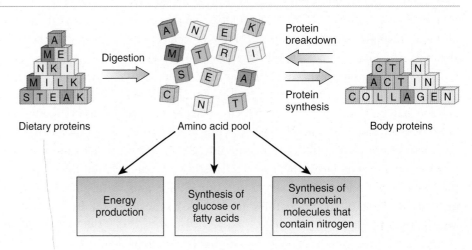

Dietary proteins   Amino acid pool   Body proteins

Energy production

Synthesis of glucose or fatty acids

Synthesis of nonprotein molecules that contain nitrogen

---

gene A length of DNA that contains the information needed to synthesize a specific polypeptide chain.

genes. When a protein is needed, the process of protein synthesis is turned on, and the information contained in the gene is used to make the necessary protein from the available amino acid pool (**Figure 6.7**).

Regulating protein synthesis The types of proteins made and when they are made are carefully regulated by the turning on and off of the genes that code for each protein. When a gene is turned on, the protein is made, and the gene is said to be *expressed*. Not all genes are expressed in all cells or at all times; only the proteins that are needed are made at any given time, which allows the body to save energy and resources. For example, when your diet is high in iron, the gene that codes for the protein ferritin, which stores iron, is turned on. Turning on this gene causes ferritin to be made and allows the body to hold on to the iron by storing it in this protein. When the diet is low in iron, the production of ferritin is turned off so that our body doesn't waste amino acids and energy making a protein that isn't needed.

Limiting amino acids During the synthesis of a protein, a shortage of one amino acid can stop the process. Just as on an assembly line, if one part is missing, the line stops—because a different part cannot be substituted.

transamination The process by which an amino group from one amino acid is transferred to a carbon compound to form a new amino acid.

If the missing amino acid is a nonessential amino acid, it can be made in the body, and protein synthesis can continue. Most nonessential amino acids are made through a process called **transamination**, which involves

transferring the amino group from one amino acid to a carbon-containing molecule to form the needed amino acid (**Figure 6.7a**). If the missing amino acid is an essential amino acid, the body can break down its own protein to obtain it. If an amino acid cannot be supplied, protein synthesis will stop, and that specific protein cannot be made.

The essential amino acid that is present in shortest supply relative to the body's need for it is called the **limiting amino acid**. It is so named because lack of this amino acid limits the ability to synthesize the desired protein (**Figure 6.7c**). Different food sources of protein provide different combinations of amino acids. The limiting amino acid in a food is the one supplied in the lowest amount relative to the body's need. For example, the limiting amino acid in wheat is lysine, whereas the limiting amino acid in peanut butter is methionine. When the diet provides adequate amounts of all the essential amino acids needed to synthesize a specific protein, synthesis of the polypeptide chains that make up the protein can be completed.

limiting amino acid The essential amino acid that is available in the lowest concentration relative to the body's needs.

Providing Structure and Regulation

When you think of the protein in your body, you probably think of muscle, but muscle contains only a few of the many types of proteins found in your body. The human body has more than 500,000 proteins, each with a unique function. Some perform important structural roles, and others help regulate specific body processes.

a. Amino acids can be thought of as building blocks. Protein consumed in the diet and body proteins that are broken down supply these building blocks to the amino acid pool. Most nonessential amino acids can be made from carbon compounds by adding an amino group through transamination.

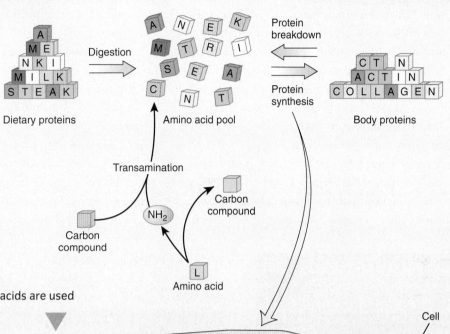

Dietary proteins

Digestion

Amino acid pool

Protein breakdown

Protein synthesis

Body proteins

Transamination

Carbon compound

NH₂

Carbon compound

Amino acid

b. Essential and nonessential amino acids are used to synthesize body proteins.

1. The first step in protein synthesis occurs inside the nucleus. It involves transferring, or transcribing, the blueprint or code for the protein from the DNA gene into a molecule of messenger RNA (mRNA). This process is called **transcription**.

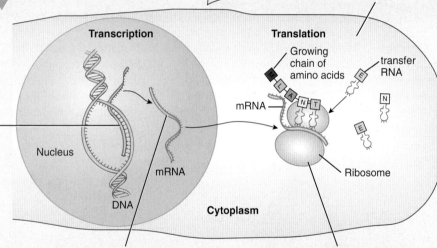

Cell

Transcription

Translation

Growing chain of amino acids

transfer RNA

mRNA

Nucleus

mRNA

DNA

Ribosome

Cytoplasm

2. The mRNA takes the genetic information from the nucleus of the cell to structures called ribosomes in the cytoplasm of the cell, where proteins are made.

3. Transfer RNA reads the genetic code and delivers the needed amino acids to the ribosome to form a polypeptide chain. This process is called **translation**.

c. The amino acids needed for protein synthesis come from the amino acid pool. If the protein to be made requires more of a particular amino acid than is available, that amino acid limits protein synthesis and is referred to as the *limiting amino acid*.

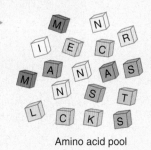

Amino acid pool

A shortage of the amino acid represented by the orange blocks limits the ability to synthesize a protein that is high in this amino acid.

Protein

Structural proteins are found in skin, hair, ligaments, and tendons (**Figure 6.8a**). Proteins also provide structure to individual cells, where they are an integral part of the cell membrane, cytoplasm, and organelles. Proteins such as enzymes, which speed up biochemical reactions (**Figure 6.8b**) and transport proteins that travel in the blood or help materials cross membranes, regulate processes throughout the body (**Figure 6.8c**).

Proteins are an important part of the body's defence mechanisms. Skin, which is made up primarily of protein, is the first barrier against infection and injury. Foreign particles such as dirt or bacteria that are on the skin cannot enter the body and can be washed away. If the skin is broken and blood vessels are injured, blood-clotting proteins help prevent too much blood from being lost. If a foreign material does get into the body, *antibodies*, which are immune system proteins, help destroy it (**Figure 6.8d**).

Some proteins have contractile properties, which allow muscles to move various parts of the body (**Figure 6.8e**). Others are hormones, which regulate biological processes. The hormones insulin, growth hormone, and glucagon are made from amino acids. These protein hormones act rapidly because they affect the activity of proteins that are already present in the cell.

Proteins also help regulate fluid balance (**Figure 6.8f**) and prevent the level of acidity in body fluids from deviating from the normal range. The chemical reactions of

Nutrition InSight　Protein functions • Figure 6.8

a. Structure: Collagen, which is the most abundant protein in the body, plays important structural roles. It is the major protein in ligaments, which hold our bones together, and in tendons, which attach muscles to bones, and it forms the protein framework of bones and teeth. ▼

b. Catalyzing reactions: Enzymes, such as this one that speeds up the breakdown of starch, are protein molecules. All chemical reactions occurring within the body require the help of enzymes. The specific structure or shape of each enzyme allows it to interact with the molecules in the specific reaction it accelerates. Without enzymes, metabolic reactions would occur too slowly to support life. ▼

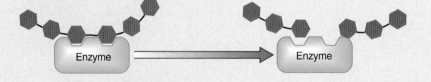

© Can Stock Photo Inc. / Eraxion

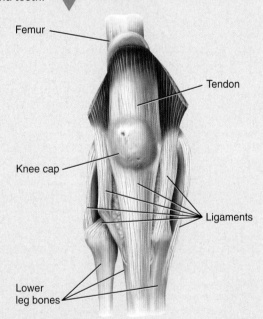

Femur

Tendon

Knee cap

Ligaments

Lower
leg bones

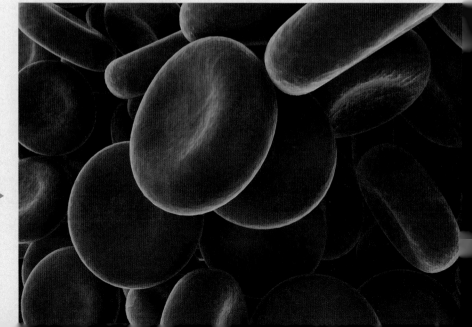

c. Transport: Proteins help transport materials throughout the body and into and out of cells. The protein hemoglobin, which gives these red blood cells their colour, shuttles oxygen to body cells and carries away carbon dioxide. ▶

metabolism require a specific level of acidity, or pH, to function properly. Inside the body, pH must be maintained at a relatively neutral level to allow metabolic reactions to proceed normally. If the pH changes, these reactions will slow or stop. Proteins both within cells and in the blood help prevent large changes in acidity.

Protein as a Source of Energy

In addition to all the essential functions performed by body proteins, proteins can be broken down and their amino acids used to provide energy or synthesize glucose or fatty acids (**Figure 6.9**). Each gram of dietary protein can provide 4 kilocalories of energy. Under typical circumstances, only

a small amount of the energy used to fuel body processes comes from protein. When the diet does not provide enough energy to meet the body's needs, such as during starvation or when consuming a weight-loss diet, body protein is used to provide energy. Because our bodies do not store protein, functional body proteins, such as enzymes and muscle proteins, must be broken down to yield amino acids, which can then be used as fuel or to make glucose. This use of body protein ensures that cells have a constant energy supply but also robs the body of the functions performed by these proteins.

Amino acids are also used for energy when the amount of protein consumed in the diet is greater than the amount needed to make body proteins and other molecules. This

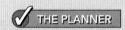

THE PLANNER

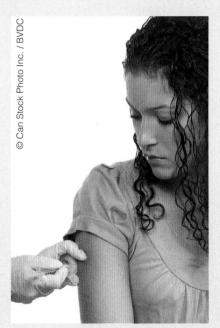

© Can Stock Photo Inc. / BVDC

▲ **d. Protection from disease:** Young women can now be immunized against the human papilloma virus (HPV). The vaccine contains a small amount of dead or inactivated HPV virus. It does not make a person sick, but it does stimulate the immune system to make proteins called *antibodies*, which specifically attack the virus and prevent HPV from being contracted.

e. Movement: The proteins actin and myosin in the arm and leg muscles of this rock climber are able to slide past each other to contract the muscles. A similar process causes contraction in the heart muscle and in the muscles of the digestive tract, blood vessels, and body glands. ▼

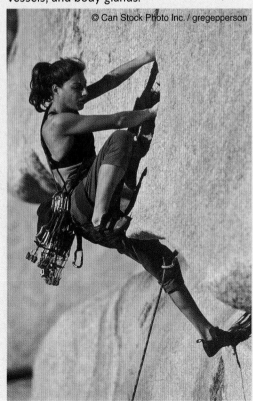

© Can Stock Photo Inc. / gregepperson

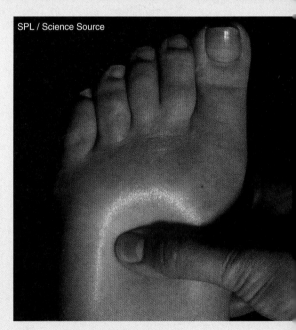

SPL / Science Source

▲ **f. Fluid balance:** Blood proteins contribute to the number of dissolved particles in the blood. Since proteins are charged particles, they help attract water to keep it in the blood. If protein levels in the blood fall too low, osmosis causes fluid to leak out of the blood vessels and accumulate in the tissues, causing swelling known as **edema**, shown here. Proteins also regulate fluid balance because some are membrane transporters, which pump dissolved substances from one side of a membrane to the other.

Producing ATP from amino acids • Figure 6.9

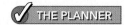

The compounds remaining after the amino group (NH_2) has been removed through a process called **deamination** are composed of carbon, hydrogen, and oxygen and can be broken down to produce adenosine tryphosphate (ATP) or used to make glucose or fatty acids.

1. The amino group is removed by deamination and converted into the waste product **urea**: urea is removed from the blood by the kidneys and excreted in the urine.

2. Deamination of some amino acids results in three-carbon molecules that can be used to synthesize glucose.

3. Deamination of other amino acids results in the formation of acetyl CoA that enters the citric acid cycle to yield two molecules of carbon dioxide.

4. Deamination of other amino acids forms molecules that enter the citric acid cycle directly.

5. When excess calories are consumed, the acetyl CoA derived from the breakdown of amino acids can be used to synthesize fatty acids, which may then be stored as adipose tissue.

6. In the electron transport chain, the final step of aerobic metabolism, the energy from the amino acid molecules is trapped and used to produce ATP and water.

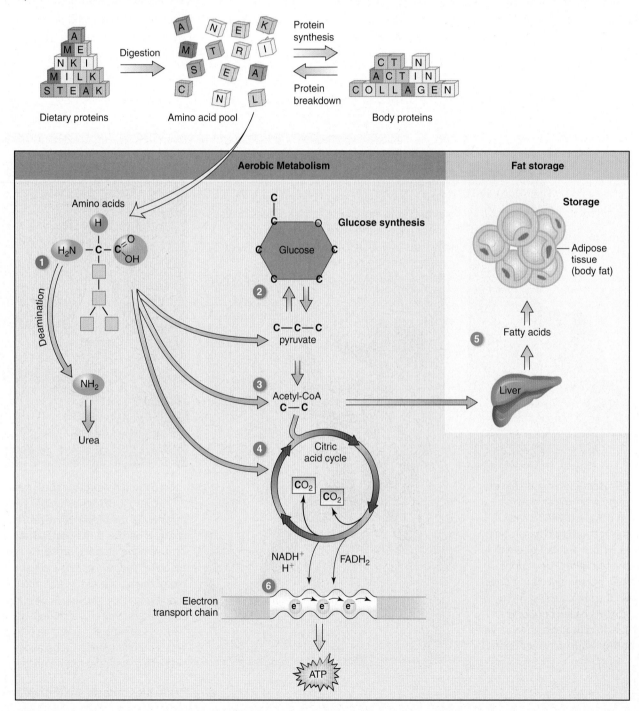

situation occurs in many Canadians every day because our typical diet contains more protein than we need. The body first uses amino acids from the diet to make body proteins and other nitrogen-containing molecules. Then, because extra amino acids can't be stored, they are metabolized to provide energy. When your diet includes more calories than you need, amino acids can be converted into fatty acids, which are stored as triglycerides in adipose tissue, thus contributing to weight gain.

Protein in Health and Disease

LEARNING OBJECTIVES

1. **Distinguish** kwashiorkor from marasmus.

2. **Explain** why protein-energy malnutrition is more common in children than in adults.

3. **Discuss** the potential risks associated with high-protein diets.

4. **Explain** how a dietary protein can trigger a food allergy.

We need to eat protein to stay healthy. If we don't eat enough of it, less-essential body proteins are broken down, and their amino acids are used to synthesize the proteins critical for survival. For example, when the diet is deficient in protein, muscle protein is broken down to provide amino acids to make hormones and enzymes, which have an immediate need. If protein deficiency continues, eventually so much body protein is lost that all life-sustaining functions cannot be supported. Conversely, too much protein or the wrong proteins can also contribute to health problems.

Protein Deficiency

Protein deficiency is a great concern in the developing world but is generally not a problem in economically developed societies like Canada, where plant and animal sources of protein are abundant. Usually, protein deficiency accompanies a general lack of food and other nutrients. The term **protein-energy malnutrition (PEM)** refers to a continuum of conditions ranging from pure protein deficiency, called

> **protein-energy malnutrition (PEM)** A condition characterized by loss of muscle and fat mass and an increased susceptibility to infection that results from the long-term consumption of insufficient amounts of energy and/or protein to meet the body's needs.

kwashiorkor, to an overall energy deficiency, called **marasmus** (**Figure 6.10**).

A pure protein deficiency occurs when the diet is extremely limited or when protein needs are high, as they are in young children. Hence, kwashiorkor is typically a disease found in children (**Figure 6.10a**). The word *kwashiorkor* comes from the Ga tribe of the African Gold Coast. It means "the disease that the first child gets when a second child is born."[1] When the new baby is born, the older child is no longer breastfed. Rather than receiving protein-rich breast milk, the young child is fed a watered-down version of the diet eaten by the rest of the family. This diet is low in protein and often high in fibre and, thus, difficult to digest. Even if a child is able to consume adequate calories from diet, he or she may not be able to eat a large enough quantity to obtain adequate protein. Because children are growing, their protein needs per unit of body weight are higher than those of adults, which leads to a deficiency occurring more quickly.

At the other end of the continuum of protein-energy malnutrition is marasmus, meaning "to waste away" (**Figure 6.10b**). Marasmus is caused by starvation; the diet doesn't supply enough calories or nutrients to meet the body's needs. Marasmus may have some of the same

> **kwashiorkor** A form of protein-energy malnutrition in which only protein is deficient.
>
> **marasmus** A form of protein-energy malnutrition in which a deficiency of energy and protein in the diet causes severe body wasting.

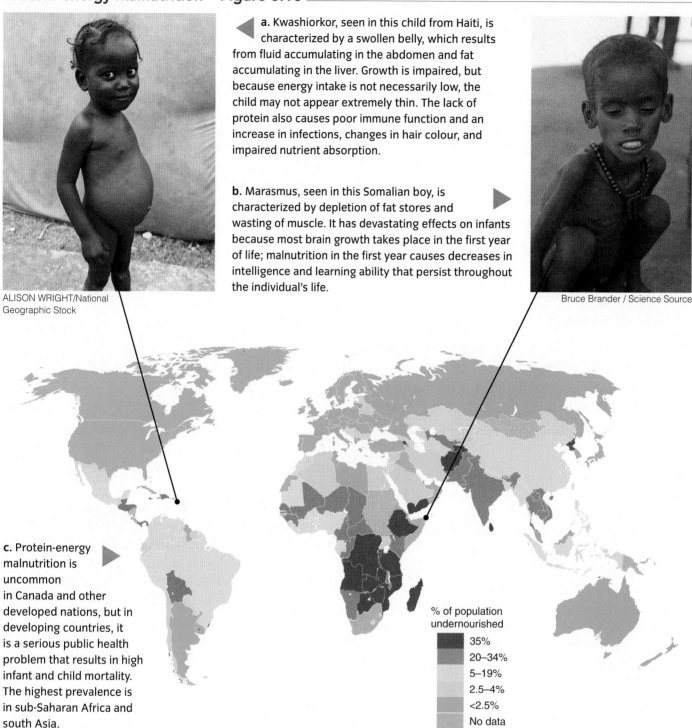

a. Kwashiorkor, seen in this child from Haiti, is characterized by a swollen belly, which results from fluid accumulating in the abdomen and fat accumulating in the liver. Growth is impaired, but because energy intake is not necessarily low, the child may not appear extremely thin. The lack of protein also causes poor immune function and an increase in infections, changes in hair colour, and impaired nutrient absorption.

b. Marasmus, seen in this Somalian boy, is characterized by depletion of fat stores and wasting of muscle. It has devastating effects on infants because most brain growth takes place in the first year of life; malnutrition in the first year causes decreases in intelligence and learning ability that persist throughout the individual's life.

ALISON WRIGHT/National Geographic Stock

Bruce Brander / Science Source

c. Protein-energy malnutrition is uncommon in Canada and other developed nations, but in developing countries, it is a serious public health problem that results in high infant and child mortality. The highest prevalence is in sub-Saharan Africa and south Asia.

% of population undernourished

- 35%
- 20–34%
- 5–19%
- 2.5–4%
- <2.5%
- No data

symptoms as kwashiorkor, but there are differences. In kwashiorkor, some fat stores are retained because energy intake is adequate. In marasmus, individuals appear emaciated because their stores of body fat have been depleted to provide energy. Although marasmus and kwashiorkor are most common in children, both can occur in individuals of all ages.

High-Protein Diets and Health

The recent popularity of high-protein, low-carbohydrate diets has raised questions about whether consuming too much protein can be harmful. As protein intake increases, so does the production of protein-breakdown products, such as urea, which must be eliminated from the body by the kidneys. To excrete more waste, more water must be lost in the urine. High-protein diets therefore increase water loss. Although not a concern for most people, it can be a problem if the kidneys are not able to concentrate urine, as is the case for infants. Feeding a newborn an infant formula that is too high in protein increases the amount of fluid lost in the urine and can lead to dehydration. High protein intake may also be detrimental for people with kidney disease; the increased wastes produced by a high-protein diet may speed the progression of renal failure.[2] However, there is little evidence that a high-protein diet will precipitate kidney disease in a healthy person.[3]

It has also been suggested that the amount and source of protein in the diet affect calcium status and bone health.[4] For healthy bones, intakes of both calcium and protein must be adequate. There is general agreement that diets that are moderate in protein (1.0 to 1.5 g/kg/day) are associated with normal calcium metabolism and do not alter bone metabolism.[4,5] However, a high protein intake may increase the amount of calcium lost in the urine. Some studies suggest that the amount of calcium lost in the urine is greater when protein comes from animal rather than vegetable sources.[6] These findings have contributed to a widely held belief that high-protein diets (especially diets that are high in animal protein) result in bone loss. However, clinical studies do not support the idea that animal protein has a detrimental effect on bone health or that vegetable-based proteins are better for bone health.[5] In fact, when calcium intake is adequate, high-protein diets are associated with greater bone mass and fewer fractures.[4] This effect is likely the case because in healthy adults, a high protein intake increases both intestinal calcium absorption and urinary excretion, so the increase in the amount of calcium lost in the urine does not cause an overall loss of body calcium.

The increase in urinary calcium excretion associated with high-protein diets has led to speculation that a high protein intake may increase the risk of kidney stones. Kidney stones are deposits of calcium and other substances in the kidneys and urinary tract. Higher concentrations of calcium and acid in the urine increase the likelihood that the calcium will be deposited, forming these stones. Epidemiological studies suggest that diets that are rich in animal protein and low in fluid contribute to the formation of kidney stones.[7]

The best-documented concern with high-protein diets is related more to the rest of the diet than to the amount of protein consumed. Typically, high-protein diets are also high in animal products; this dietary pattern is high in saturated fat and cholesterol and low in fibre, and it therefore may increase the risk of heart disease. The low-fibre content of these diets may also contribute to diverticulitis, or diverticulosis (**Figure 6.11**). High-protein diets are also

High-protein diets and diverticulosis • Figure 6.11

The former mixed martial arts champion Brock Lesnar attributes his chronic intestinal discomfort and decreased performance during the winter of 2009–2010 to a diet based primarily on proteins, which led to a severe case of diverticulosis. Diverticulosis is associated with low-fibre diets and results in outpouching of the colon, which can lead to severe abdominal pain and fever. Brock was forced to stop training, missed several competitions, and almost gave up his professional fighting career. He said of his former diet: "I'm a member of the NRA [National Rifle Association] and whatever I kill, I eat. And basically, I was just, for years, surviving on meat and potatoes and when the greens came by, I just kept passing them."[9] He has now changed his diet to include more grains and vegetables and fruits and has improved his condition significantly.

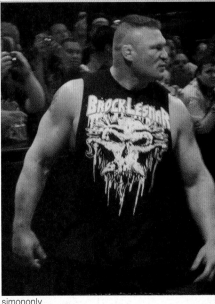

simononly

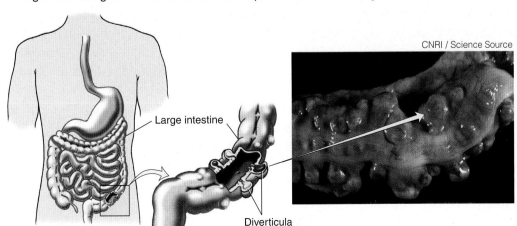

CNRI / Science Source

Large intestine

Diverticula

Food allergy labelling • Figure 6.12

For individuals with food allergies, food labels provide life-saving information. A label must indicate whether the product contains any of the 10 major food allergens: milk, eggs, peanuts, tree nuts, sesame seeds, fish, shellfish, crustaceans, soy, or wheat. Sometimes these food allergens are included in the ingredient list, but often, as on this label, they are also highlighted at the end of the list in a statement such as "Contains soy ingredients." Warnings such as "manufactured in a facility that processes peanuts" are included on products that may have been cross-contaminated with these allergens. Health Canada is constantly updating the list of potential allergens and the food labelling guidelines to ensure that consumers are informed of potential risks from from allergy-inducing ingredients or ingredient components (ingredients of ingredients).[10]

The ingredient list includes sources of protein in food as well as sources of **hydrolyzed protein** or **protein hydrolysates**. These are proteins that have been treated with acid or enzymes to break them down into amino acids and small peptides. They are added as flavourings, flavour enhancers, stabilizers, and thickening agents.

INGREDIENTS: CHICKEN BROTH, CARROTS, COOKED WHITE CHICKEN MEAT (WHITE CHICKEN MEAT, WATER, SALT, SODIUM PHOSPHATE, ISOLATED SOY PROTEIN, MODIFIED CORN STARCH, CORN STARCH, CARRAGEENAN), TOMATOES, WILD RICE, RICE, CELERY. LESS THAN 2% OF: SALT, MONOSODIUM GLUTAMATE, HYDROLYZED CORN PROTEIN, CHICKEN FAT, ONION POWDER, AUTOLYZED YEAST EXTRACT, PARSLEY FLAKES, NATURAL FLAVOUR. **CONTAINS SOY INGREDIENTS.**

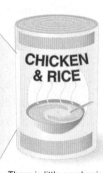

CHICKEN & RICE

Nutrition Facts Valeur nutritive		
Per 1 cup (239 g)/par 1 tasse (239g)		
Amount Teneur	% Daily Value % valeur quotidienne	
Calories / Calories 100		
Fat / Lipides 1.5 g		2 %
Saturated / saturés 2 g + Trans / trans 0 g		10 %
Cholesterol / Cholestérol 15 mg		5 %
Sodium / Sodium 850 mg		35 %
Carbohydrate / Glucides 15 g		5 %
Fibre / Fibres 1 g		4 %
Sugars / Sucres 1 g		
Protein / Protéines 7 g		
Vitamin A / Vitamine A		25 %
Vitamin C / Vitamine C		0 %
Calcium / Calcium		0 %
Iron / Fer		2 %

There is little emphasis on protein in the Nutrition Facts panel, where the grams of protein are given without any % Daily Value. A % Daily Value for protein is required only on products that make a claim about the product's protein content.

---

typically low in grains, vegetables, and fruits, a pattern associated with an increased risk of cancer.[8] Such diets are also usually high in energy and total fat, which may promote excess weight gain.

Proteins and Food Allergies and Intolerances

When a protein from the diet is absorbed without being completely digested, it can trigger a food allergy. Common

> **food allergy** An adverse immune response to a specific food protein.

causes of food allergies include the proteins from milk, eggs, peanuts, tree nuts, wheat, soy, fish, and shellfish (**Figure 6.12**). The first time the protein is consumed and a piece of it is absorbed intact, it stimulates the immune system. When the same protein is consumed again, the immune system sees it as a foreign substance and mounts an attack, causing an allergic reaction (see Chapter 3). Allergic reactions can cause symptoms such as a tingling mouth, nausea, vomiting, diarrhea, hives, and swelling. They can also lead to

> **food intolerance** or **food sensitivity** An adverse reaction to a food that typically does not involve the production of antibodies by the immune system.

a potentially life-threatening condition called anaphylaxis, which results in compromised breathing and dangerously low blood pressure.

Not all adverse reactions to proteins and amino acids are due to allergies; some are due to food intolerances, also called food

sensitivities. These reactions do not typically involve the immune system. The symptoms of a food intolerance can range from minor discomfort, such as the abdominal distress some people feel after eating raw onions, to more severe reactions. For example, some people report having a reaction after consuming **monosodium glutamate (MSG)**. MSG is a flavour enhancer made up of the amino acid glutamic acid bound to sodium. It is used in meat tenderizers and commonly added to Chinese food. In sensitive individuals, the glutamate in MSG causes a collection of symptoms, such as flushed face, tingling or burning sensations, headache, rapid heartbeat, chest pain, and general weakness, which are collectively referred to as **MSG symptom complex**, sometimes called Chinese restaurant syndrome.[11] Sensitive individuals should ask for food to be prepared without added MSG and should check ingredient lists for monosodium glutamate or potassium glutamate before consuming packaged foods. Although Health Canada currently requires explicit MSG labelling on foods, other potential sources of free glutamate may be less explicit, such as hydrolyzed vegetable protein, hydrolyzed plant protein, hydrolyzed soy protein, soy sauce, and autolysed yeast extracts. Sensitive individuals should also look for these ingredients, but for the general public, MSG is not considered a health hazard.[12]

Gluten intolerance, also called celiac disease, celiac sprue, or gluten-sensitive enteropathy, is

> **celiac disease** A disorder that causes damage to the intestines when the protein gluten is eaten.

another form of food intolerance. Individuals with celiac disease cannot tolerate gluten, a protein found in wheat, rye, and barley. Celiac disease is an autoimmune disease in which gluten causes the body to attack the villi in the small intestine, causing the intestinal wall to break down. Though it does involve the immune system, it is considered to be a food intolerance and not a food allergy mainly because the symptoms are gastrointestinal in nature and it is not life-threatening. Symptoms of celiac disease range from minor abdominal discomfort to headache, diarrhea, vomiting, abdominal bloating and cramps, abdominal pain, weight loss or gain, and anemia. Once thought to be a rare childhood disease, it is now believed to affect 1 in 133 Canadians, although it is difficult to know how many people actually have the disease because many remain undiagnosed.[13] The only current treatment option is to avoid gluten by eliminating from the diet all products containing wheat, rye, or barley or proteins isolated from these foods. These ingredients are abundant in such foods as breads, pastries, pastas, and cakes. Luckily, more and more gluten-free varieties of these foods are now available in many Canadian grocery stores and restaurants.

High-Protein Diets and Energy Balance

One of the reasons high protein diets have risen in popularity, is for their potential association with weight loss. In fact, high protein diets often show a more favorable rate of weight loss compared to other diets, such as those higher in carbohydrates.[14,15]

It is believed that one of the main reason high protein diets afford this benefit is for their potential to be more satiating, leading to a lower consumption of total calories, the main dietary predictor of energy balance.[15] The type of protein source may also predict tendency for weight loss. Canadian researcher Harvey Anderson from the University of Toronto has shown that whey protein (found in dairy products) tends to reduce short-term food intake compared to controls, carbohydrates and other proteins and is particularly satiating, promoting this reduction in appetite.[16] While it is unclear if these benefits are afforded from typical dairy intake patterns, these finding reinforce the fact that certain high protein diets may reduce energy intake, and as such, the tendency for fat deposition.

| CONCEPT CHECK | STOP |

1. **Why** do children with marasmus appear more emaciated than those with kwashiorkor?

2. **Why** is protein-energy malnutrition more common in children than in adults?

3. **Who** should be concerned about excessive protein intake?

4. **How** can allergic reactions to food be avoided?

Meeting Protein Needs
LEARNING OBJECTIVES

1. **Describe** how protein needs are determined.

2. **Explain** what is meant by protein quality.

3. **Review** a diet and replace the animal proteins with complementary plant proteins.

4. **Discuss** the benefits and risks of vegetarian diets.

To stay healthy, you need to eat enough protein to replace the protein you lose every day. Most Canadians get plenty of protein, and healthy diets can contain a wide range of intakes from both plant and animal sources. Individual protein needs may increase because of growth, injury, illness, and some types of physical activity.

Balancing Protein Intake and Losses

Current protein intake recommendations are based on **nitrogen balance** studies. These studies compare the amount of nitrogen consumed with the amount excreted. Studying nitrogen balance allows researchers to evaluate protein balance because protein is the only macronutrient that contains nitrogen. Most of the nitrogen we consume comes from dietary protein. Most of the nitrogen we lose is excreted in urine. Smaller amounts are lost in feces, skin, sweat, menstrual fluids, hair, and nails. When your body is in nitrogen balance, your nitrogen intake equals your nitrogen

nitrogen balance The amount of nitrogen consumed in the diet compared with the amount excreted over a given period.

Nitrogen balance • Figure 6.13

a. Nitrogen balance: Nitrogen intake = nitrogen output. The amount of protein being synthesized is equal to the amount being broken down, so the total amount of protein in the body is not changing. Healthy adults who consume adequate amounts of protein and are maintaining a constant body weight are in nitrogen balance.

Nitrogen intake

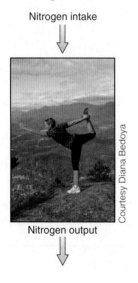

Nitrogen output

b. Negative nitrogen balance: Nitrogen intake < nitrogen output. More protein is being broken down than is being synthesized, so body protein is decreasing. Negative nitrogen balance can occur because of injury, illness, or a diet that is too low in protein or calories.

Nitrogen intake

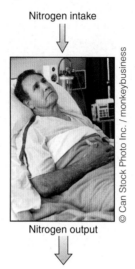

© Can Stock Photo Inc. / monkeybusiness

Nitrogen output

c. Positive nitrogen balance: Nitrogen intake > nitrogen output. More protein is being synthesized than is being degraded, so the body is gaining protein. Positive nitrogen balance occurs when the body is growing, during pregnancy, and when individuals are increasing their muscle mass, such as by lifting weights.

Nitrogen intake

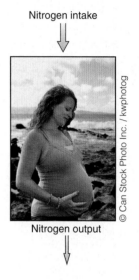

© Can Stock Photo Inc. / kwphotog

Nitrogen output

losses; in other words, you are consuming enough protein to replace losses. You are not gaining or losing body protein; you are maintaining it at a constant level. Nitrogen balance is negative if you're losing body protein and positive if the amount of body protein is increasing (**Figure 6.13**).

Recommended Protein Intake

Most of us eat more protein than we need: It is estimated that the typical Canadian adult consumes just less than 80 g of protein/day.[17] The RDA for protein for adults is 0.8 g/kilogram of body weight. For a person weighing 70 kg (154 lb.), the RDA is 56 g of protein/day. This recommendation is expressed per unit of body weight because protein is needed to maintain and repair the body. The more a person weighs, the more protein he or she needs for these purposes. Because children are small, they need less total protein than adults do, but because new protein must be synthesized for growth to occur, protein requirements per unit of body weight are much greater for infants and children than for adults. During the first year of life, growth is rapid, so a large amount of protein is required. As growth rate slows, requirements per unit of body weight decrease but continue to be greater than adult requirements until age 19 (**Table 6.1**). To calculate your protein needs per day,

multiply your weight in kilograms (which equals weight in pounds × 0.45) by the recommended amount for your age.

Protein needs are also increased during pregnancy and lactation. Additional protein is needed during pregnancy to support the expansion of maternal blood volume, the growth of the uterus and breasts, the formation of the placenta, and the growth and development of the fetus. The RDA for pregnant women is 25 g of protein/day higher than the recommendation for non-pregnant women. An extra 25 g/day is also needed during lactation to provide protein for the production of breast milk.

Protein requirements	Table 6.1
Age	**RDA (g/kg/day)**
0–6 months	1.52
7–12 months	1.50
13 months–3 years	1.10
4–13 years	0.95
14–18 years	0.85
≥19 years	0.80

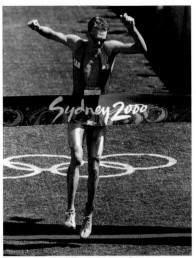

a. Endurance athletes, like triathlete Simon Whitfield, need more protein than others because some protein is used for energy and to maintain blood glucose during endurance events, such as triathlons. Endurance athletes may benefit from the daily consumption of 1.2 to 1.4 g of protein/kilogram of body weight.

Andy Lyons/Staff/Getty Images Sport

b. Strength athletes, such as weight lifter Marie-Eve Beauchemin-Nadeau, need extra protein to provide the raw materials needed for muscle growth; 1.2 to 1.7 g/kilogram/day is recommended.

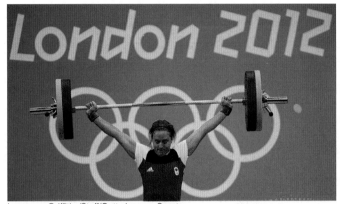

Laurence Griffiths/Staff/Getty Images Sport

Extreme stresses on the body, such as infections, fevers, burns, or surgery, increase the amount of protein that is broken down. For the body to heal and rebuild, the amount of protein lost must be replaced. The extra amount needed for healing depends on the injury. A severe infection may increase the body's protein needs by about 30%, whereas a serious burn can increase protein requirements by 200 to 400%.

Although most athletes can meet their protein needs by consuming the RDA of 0.8 g/kg of body weight, endurance athletes and strength athletes benefit from higher protein intakes (**Figure 6.14**).[18] Athletes often think they need supplements to meet their higher protein needs. However, because they typically also consume more calories, which increase the amount of dietary protein they consume, they can easily meet their protein needs through diet alone.

RDAs have also been developed for each of the essential amino acids;[3] these are not a concern in typical diet planning but are important when developing solutions for intravenous feeding. Protein and amino acid supplements are rarely needed to meet individuals' protein needs (**Figure 6.15**).

In addition to the RDA, the DRIs include a recommendation for protein intake as a percentage of calories: The Acceptable Macronutrient Distribution Range for protein is 10 to 35% of calories.[3] This range allows for different food preferences and eating patterns. A protein intake in this range will meet protein needs and allow sufficient intakes of other nutrients to promote health. A diet that provides 10% of calories from protein will meet the RDA but is a relatively low-protein diet compared with typical eating patterns in Canada. The upper end of this healthy range—35% of calories—is a relatively high-protein diet, about three times as much protein as the average Canadian eats. This amount of protein is not harmful, but diets that are this high in protein are probably high in animal products, which tend to be high in saturated fat and cholesterol. Therefore, unless protein sources are chosen carefully, a diet that contains 35% protein may include more saturated fat and cholesterol than a diet with the same number of calories but containing only 10% protein.

Protein and amino acid supplements • Figure 6.15

Supplements are marketed to boost total protein intake, to add individual amino acids, and to provide enzyme activity.

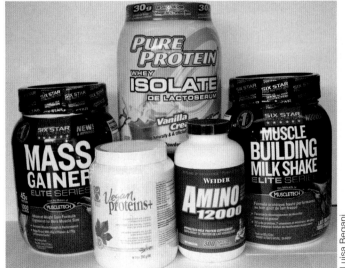

Luisa Begani

Choosing Protein Wisely

To evaluate protein intake, it is important to consider both the amount and the quality of protein in the diet. **Protein quality** is a measure of how good the protein in a food is at providing the essential amino acids the body needs to synthesize proteins. The **protein digestibility corrected amino acid score (PDCAAS)** is the most commonly used method for determining protein quality.[18] It takes into account the digestibility of a protein and its blend of essential amino acids and compares it with the amino acid needs of humans. Because we are animals, it makes sense that the mixtures of amino acids in animal proteins are generally more similar to what we need than the mixtures of amino acids found in plant proteins.

Thus, animal proteins generally score higher than proteins from plant sources. Animal proteins also tend to be digested more easily than plant proteins; only protein that is digested can contribute amino acids to meet the body's requirements.[19] Because foods of animal origin are easily digested and supply essential amino acids in the proper proportions for human use, these foods are sources of **high-quality protein**, or **complete dietary protein**, and have a higher PDCAAS. When your diet contains high-quality protein, you don't need to eat as much total protein to meet your needs. High-quality protein provides more of the essential amino acids in the proportions needed by the body than can be provided by the same amount of low-quality protein.

Compared with animal proteins, plant proteins are usually more difficult to digest and are lower in one or more of the essential amino acids. They are therefore referred to as **incomplete dietary protein** and have a lower PDCAAS. Exceptions are soy, quinoa, and chia seeds, which are high-quality plant sources of protein—as high or almost as high as egg or milk protein.

Complementary proteins If you get your protein from a single source and that source is an incomplete protein, it will be difficult to meet your body's protein needs. However, combining proteins that are limited in different amino acids can supply a complete mixture of essential amino acids. For example, legumes are limited in methionine but high in lysine. When legumes are consumed with grains, which are high in methionine and low in lysine, the combination provides all the needed amino acids (**Figure 6.16**). Vegetarian diets rely on this technique, called **protein complementation**, to meet protein needs. Eating plant

> **protein complementation**
> The process of combining proteins from different sources so that they collectively provide the proportions of amino acids required to meet the body's needs.

Protein complementation • Figure 6.16

a. The amino acids that are most often limited in plant proteins are lysine (lys), methionine (met), and cysteine (cys). As a general rule, legumes are deficient in methionine and cysteine but high in lysine. Grains, nuts, and seeds are deficient in lysine but high in methionine and cysteine.

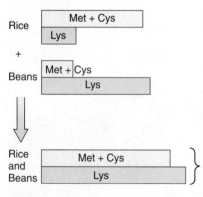

Rice
| Met + Cys |
| Lys |

+

Beans
| Met + | Cys |
| Lys |

↓

Rice and Beans
| Met + Cys |
| Lys |

When rice, which is limited in lys but high in met and cys, is eaten with beans, which are high in lys but limited in met and cys, the combination provides all the amino acids needed by the body.

Grains, Nuts, or Seeds + Legumes = Complete Protein

© Melanie Acevedo/FoodPix, Getty Images, Inc.

b. Many traditional diets take advantage of complementary plant proteins, such as lentils and rice or chickpeas and rice in India, rice and beans in Mexico and South America, hummus (chickpeas and sesame seeds) in the Middle East, and bread and peanut butter (peanuts are a legume) in Canada. Complementary proteins do not need to be consumed in the same meal, so eating an assortment of plant foods throughout the day can provide enough of all the essential amino acids.[27]

proteins that have complementary amino acid patterns can meet an individual's essential amino acid requirements without consuming any animal proteins.

Canada's Food Guide recommendations

Choose a diet that includes a variety of foods, which will provide enough protein and enough of each of the essential amino acids to meet the body's needs. If you follow the food guide recommendations, your diet will include both animal and plant sources of protein (**Figure 6.17**). A 250-mL glass of milk provides about 8 g of protein, and a serving of meats and alternatives can add another 7 to 10 g of protein. These two food groups contain the foods that are the highest in protein. Each serving from the grains group and a serving of vegetables provides 1 to 3 g, but because we eat a larger number of servings from these groups, they make an important contribution to our protein intake. However, just getting enough protein does not ensure a healthy diet. The sources of your dietary proteins also affect the healthfulness of your diet, particularly how well it meets the recommendations for fat and fibre intake (see *What Should I Eat?*).

Vegetarian Diets

In many parts of the world, diets based on plant proteins, called **vegetarian diets**, have evolved mostly out of necessity because people are living in areas where animal sources of protein are limited, either physically or economically. Compared with raising plants, raising animals requires more land and resources, and purchasing animals is more expensive than purchasing plants. The developing world relies on plant foods to meet protein needs. For example, in rural Mexico, most dietary protein comes from beans, rice, and tortillas (corn); in India, most dietary protein comes from lentils and rice. As a population's economic prosperity rises, the proportion of animal foods in its diet typically increases, but in developed countries, vegetarian diets are often followed for reasons other than economics, such as health, religion, personal ethics, or environmental awareness. **Vegan diets** eliminate all animal

> **vegetarian diets** Diets that include plant-based foods and eliminate some or all foods of animal origin.

> **vegan diets** Plant-based diets that eliminate all animal products.

Choosing healthy protein sources • Figure 6.17

The meat and meat alternatives and the milk and milk alternatives groups of *Eating Well with Canada's Food Guide* provide the most concentrated sources of protein. Dry beans and peas are the most concentrated sources of plant protein. These may be included in either the fruit and vegetables group or the meat and meat alternatives group. Fruit offers very little protein. Grain products are concentrated sources of carbohydrates, but may also contain protein, especially if they contain nuts or seeds.

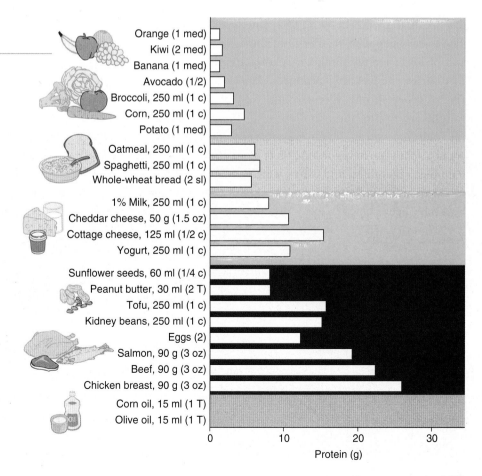

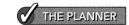

WHAT SHOULD I EAT?
Protein Sources

Get protein without too much saturated fat
- Plan on poultry or fish.
- Choose lean cuts of red meat.
- Grill, roast, or broil so that the fat will end up in the pan or the fire.

Eat both animal and plant proteins
- Have your beef or chicken in a stir-fry with lots of vegetables.
- Serve a small portion of meat over noodles.

- Add nuts and seeds to snacks and salads.
- Have a meatless meal or a meatless day at least once a week.

Go with beans
- Try hummus—made from ground chickpeas and sesame seeds.
- Add kidney beans or chickpeas to soups.
- Snack on edamame.
- Enjoy homemade tacos or burritos stuffed with pinto beans or black beans.

> Use iProfile to look up the protein content of your favourite vegetarian entree.

products, but other types of vegetarian diets are less restrictive (**Table 6.2**).

Benefits of vegetarian diets A vegetarian diet can be a healthy, low-cost alternative to a meat-and-potatoes diet. Vegetarians have been shown to have not only lower body weight but also a reduced incidence of obesity and of other chronic diseases, such as diabetes, cardiovascular disease, high blood pressure, and some types of cancer.[28,29] The lower body weight of vegetarians is most likely a result of lower energy intake, as plants are generally lower in calories than animal products. The reductions in the risk of other chronic diseases may be due to lower body weight and to consuming a diet that is lower in saturated fat and cholesterol, which may increase disease risk. It could also be due to vegetarian diets being higher in grains, legumes, vegetables, and fruits, which add fibre, vitamins, minerals, antioxidants, and phytochemicals—substances that have been shown to lower disease risk. It is likely that

the total dietary pattern, rather than any single factor alone, is responsible for the health-promoting effects of vegetarian diets.

In addition to reducing disease risks, diets that rely more heavily on plant protein than on animal protein are more economical. For example, a vegetarian stir-fry over rice costs about half as much as a meal of steak and potatoes, yet both meals provide a significant portion of the day's protein requirement. A meal comprising a 170-g (6-oz) steak, a baked potato with sour cream, and a tossed salad provides about 50 of protein, whereas a dish of rice with tofu and vegetables provides about 30 g.

Risks of vegetarian diets Despite the health and economic benefits of vegetarian diets, a poorly planned vegetarian diet can cause nutrient deficiencies. Protein deficiency is a risk when vegan diets that contain little high-quality protein are consumed by small children or

Types of vegetarian diets   Table 6.2

Diet	Exclusions and inclusions
Semivegetarian	Excludes red meat but may include fish, poultry, dairy products, and eggs.
Pescetarian	Excludes all animal flesh except fish.
Lacto-ovo vegetarian	Excludes all animal flesh but does include eggs and dairy products such as milk and cheese.
Lacto vegetarian	Excludes animal flesh and eggs but does include dairy products.
Vegan	Excludes all food of animal origin.

by adults with increased protein needs, such as pregnant women and those recovering from illness or injury. Most people can easily meet their protein needs with a well-planned lacto and lacto-ovo vegetarian diets. These diets contain high-quality animal proteins from eggs or milk, which complement the limiting amino acids in the plant proteins.

Vitamin and mineral deficiencies are a greater concern for vegetarians than is protein deficiency. Of primary concern to vegans is vitamin B_{12}. Because this B vitamin is found almost exclusively in animal products, vegans must take vitamin B_{12} supplements or consume foods fortified with vitamin B_{12} to meet their needs for this nutrient. Another nutrient of concern is calcium. Dairy products are the major source of calcium in the North American diet, so diets that eliminate these foods must rely on plant sources of calcium. Likewise, because most dietary vitamin D comes from fortified milk, this vitamin must be made in the body from exposure to sunlight or consumed in other sources or from supplements. Iron and zinc may be deficient in vegetarian diets because red meat is an excellent source of these minerals, and they are poorly absorbed from plant sources. Because dairy products are low in iron and zinc, lacto-ovo vegetarians, lacto vegetarians, and vegans are at risk for deficiencies of these minerals. Omega-3 fatty acids, including EPA and DHA (see Chapter 5), are also a concern in vegan diets.[27] **Table 6.3**

provides suggestions for how to meet the need for the nutrients just discussed.

Planning vegetarian diets Well-planned vegetarian diets, including vegan diets, can meet nutrient needs at all stages of the life cycle, from infancy, childhood, and adolescence to early, middle, and late adulthood, and during pregnancy and lactation.[27] One way to plan a healthy vegetarian diet is to modify the selections from *Eating Well with Canada's Food Guide*. The food choices and recommended amounts from the grain products and vegetables and fruits groups should stay the same for vegetarians. Vegetarians who do not consume milk or meat can also rely on the "alternatives" found in the milk and milk alternatives and meat and meat alternatives groups to meet their protein needs. Those who avoid all animal foods can choose dry beans, nuts, and seeds from the meat and meat alternatives group. Soy products provide high-quality plant protein, but their consumption is controversial (see *Debate: Is Soy Protein a Healthy Alternative to Animal Protein?*). Fortified soymilk, almond milk, or rice milk can be substituted for dairy foods. To obtain adequate vitamin B_{12}, vegans must take supplements or use products fortified with vitamin B_{12}. Obtaining plenty of omega-3 fatty acids from foods such as canola oil, nuts, and ground flaxseed ensures adequate synthesis of the long-chain omega-3 fatty acids DHA and EPA (see *Thinking It Through*).

Meeting nutrient needs with a vegan diet[24]   Table 6.3

Nutrient at risk	Sources in vegan diets
Calcium	Tofu processed with calcium; broccoli, kale, bok choy, and legumes; products fortified with calcium, such as soy beverages, grain products, and orange juice
Iodine	Iodized salt, sea vegetables (seaweed), and foods grown near the sea
Iron	Legumes, tofu, dark green leafy vegetables, dried fruit, whole grains, iron-fortified grain products (absorption is improved when iron-containing foods are consumed with vitamin C found in citrus fruit, tomatoes, strawberries, and dark green vegetables)
Omega-3 fatty acids	Canola oil, ground flaxseed and flaxseed oil, soybean oil, walnuts, sea vegetables (seaweed), and DHA-rich microalgae
Protein	Soy-based products, legumes, seeds, nuts, grains, and vegetables
Vitamin B_{12}	Products fortified with vitamin B_{12}, such as soy beverages and breakfast cereals; nutritional yeast; dietary supplements
Vitamin D	Sunshine; products fortified with vitamin D, such as soy beverages, breakfast cereals, and margarine
Zinc	Whole grains, wheat germ, legumes, nuts, tofu, and fortified breakfast cereals

Debate   Is Soy Protein a Healthy Alternative to Animal Protein?

The Issue: Many people have switched from cow's milk to soymilk and snack on edamame (boiled green soybeans), soy nuts, and soy-based protein bars. Will increasing your intake of soy benefit your health or cause health problems?

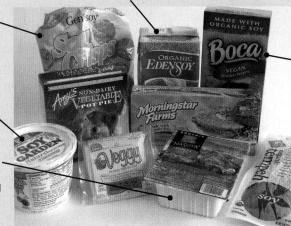

Soy flour can be incorporated into baked goods.

Soy milk is a substitute for cow's milk.

Soy butter is similar to peanut butter and can be spread on crackers and sandwiches.

Tofu, also known as bean curd, is added to soups, salads, and stir-fries.

Texturized soy protein (TSP), also known as texturized vegetable protein (TVP), is formed into chunks, woven or spun into fibres, or otherwise shaped and flavoured to produce vegetarian versions of burgers, hotdogs, meatballs, and chicken.

Teri Stratford

Soy is found in many traditional Asian foods, such as tofu and miso, and it is used as a meat substitute in various vegetarian products. A high intake of soy has been linked to a lower incidence of heart disease, type-2 diabetes, osteoporosis, and certain types of cancer.[20] This association has contributed to a dramatic rise in the number of available soy products in North America. Between 2000 and 2007, more than 2,700 new foods with soy as an ingredient were introduced.[21] Since 1981, Canada has had a 7-fold increase in the amount of soybean crops. The versatility of soybean as a crop makes it an important component of our agricultural output.[22]

But many are also concerned about the safety of soy for certain segments of the population. Should we be opting for, or out of, soy consumption?

Soy provides high-quality protein—comparable with the protein in eggs and milk. Soy products are also high in healthy polyunsaturated fat, fibre, vitamins, and minerals, and they are low in unhealthy saturated fat. Soy protein is also believed to have a positive effect on cholesterol in the body.[20]

Furthermore, soy provides phytochemicals called isoflavones, which have estrogen-like effects. Some speculate that consuming soy isoflavones will reduce the symptoms of menopause (including hot flashes), reduce bone loss, and lead to preventive effects in terms of certain forms of cancer, including breast cancer.

It sounds like we should all switch to soy. However, a more careful look at the research on soy suggests that it may not be as beneficial as initially hoped, and many are now concerned that soy might not be safe for everyone. A review of the effect of soy on blood cholesterol concluded that it has only a small effect in lowering LDL cholesterol, and this effect occurs only when large amounts, about 50 g/day, are consumed.[23] But, because soy contains substances that may interfere with thyroid gland function, overconsumption has been accused of contributing to low levels of thyroid hormones in individuals with compromised thyroid function and/or whose iodine intake is marginal.[24] The health effects of those estrogen-like soy isoflavones are also confusing. Clinical trials support a role of isoflavones

in the prevention of bone loss, but results are inconsistent.[25] Research has not consistently shown soy to reduce the symptoms of menopause.[25] Isoflavones have been found to promote the growth of breast tumours in animals, and therefore women who have breast cancer are typically advised to avoid soy.[25] In women who do not have breast cancer, soy appears to be protective if it is consumed in moderate amounts throughout life, but switching to soy milk after menopause may have no effect.[26] Other arguments against soy include the fact that phytates found in soy can block the absorption of certain micronutrients, increasing the chance for deficiency. Also, soy is listed by Health Canada as one of the nine most common allergens. Lastly, those who are against genetic modification argue that soy is one of the most commonly bioengineered crops and that we do not know the potential long-term outcomes of the consumption of genetically modified foods.

So, is soy good for you? Choosing soy products, such as those shown in the photo, will provide plant protein equivalent in quality to animal proteins, and can help you meet your protein needs without much saturated fat. High intakes of soy may help reduce the risk of heart disease. But it is not clear what effect these amounts will have on breast cancer risk or thyroid function. Studies in Asian populations that typically consume soy support its benefits, but there is little evidence that switching to soy will have the same effect as a moderate soy intake throughout life.

Good sources of soy		
Food	Serving	Protein (g)
Soy milk, regular	250 mL (1 cup)	7
Tofu, regular	28 g (1 oz)	2.5
Miso	15 mL (1 Tbsp)	2
Tempeh	15 mL (1 Tbsp)	2
Roasted soybeans	60 mL (¼ cup)	15
Soybean sprouts	250 mL (1 cup)	9
Texturized soy protein (TSP)	28 g (1 oz)	14
Veggie hotdog	1	13
Soy veggie burger	85 g (3 oz)	12
Tofutti frozen dessert, regular	125 mL (½ cup)	2
Soy flour, regular	15 mL (1 Tbsp)	2
Soy butter	30 mL (2 Tbsp)	7

Think Critically An intake of about 50 g of soy protein per day has been shown to lower blood cholesterol in some people. Based on the protein content of foods in the table, is consuming more soy products a reasonable way for Canadians to lower cholesterol? Why or why not?

THINKING IT THROUGH

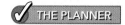
✓ THE PLANNER

Is a Vegetarian Diet Always Healthy?

Jeremy is 26 years old and weighs 70 kg (154 lb.). A year ago, he decided to stop eating meat for health reasons. Now that he is studying protein in his nutrition class, he has become concerned that his lacto vegetarian diet isn't meeting his needs.

What is the RDA for protein for someone of Jeremy's age and weight?
▼

Your answer: _____

_____

Jeremy records his food intake for one day and then uses iProfile to assess his nutrient intake. He is pleased to discover that his diet provides 65.7 g of protein, which exceeds his RDA, but he is shocked to discover that his diet is high in saturated fat.

This is a photo of Jeremy's typical lunch. Why is it high in saturated fat?
▼

Your answer: _____

_____

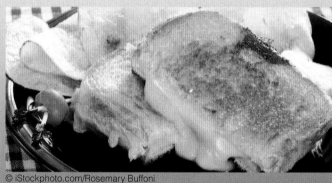
© iStockphoto.com/Rosemary Buffoni

For breakfast, Jeremy typically has cereal with milk, and for dinner he has cheese pizza or cheese lasagna. He snacks on chips and ice cream.

Is this diet providing all the health benefits of a vegetarian diet?
▼

Your answer: _____

_____

When he sees his diet analysis, Jeremy decides to try a vegan diet.

What could be included in Jeremy's vegan diet to meet his needs for calcium and vitamin D?
▼

Your answer: _____

_____

Suggest a sandwich Jeremy could have for lunch that makes use of complementary plant proteins.
▼

Your answer: _____

_____

(Check your answers in Appendix I.)

CONCEPT CHECK STOP

1. **What** circumstances result in a positive nitrogen balance?

2. **Why** is the quality of animal protein considered to be higher than that of plant protein?

3. **What** protein source could you serve with pasta that would complement the wheat protein in the pasta?

4. **Why** are vegans at risk for vitamin B_{12} deficiency?

Summary

 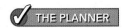

1 Proteins in Our Food 166

• Dietary protein comes from both animal and plant sources. Animal sources of protein are generally good sources of iron, zinc, and calcium but are high in saturated fat and cholesterol. Plant sources of protein, such as **legumes**, are higher in unsaturated fat, fibre, and phytochemicals. **Amino acids** are the building blocks from which proteins are made. Each amino acid contains an amino group, an acid group, and a unique side chain.

Animal versus plant proteins • Figure 6.1

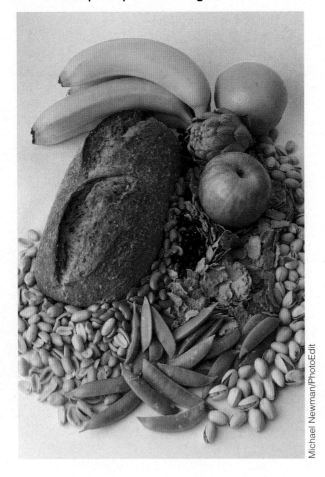

Michael Newman/PhotoEdit

sufficient amounts are called **essential**, or **indispensable**, **amino acids** and must be consumed in the diet. **Conditionally essential amino acids** are nonessential amino acids that become essential ones when the body cannot synthesize enough to meet needs. An example is the nonessential amino acid tryosine, which becomes an essential amino acid in people with the genetic disease, **phenylketonuria (PKU)**.

• Protein synthesis is a complex process that involves several levels of structure. The primary structure of a protein consists of a chain of amino acids, held together by **peptide bonds** to form a peptide. **Peptides** exist as **dipeptides**, **tripeptides**, and **polypeptides**. Polypeptides can become proteins once they fold to create unique three-dimensional structures. Alpha-helices and beta-pleated sheets are found in the **secondary structure** of a protein. The **tertiary structure** involves further folding of the polypeptide to perhaps form a fully functioning protein. Some proteins have a **quaternary structure**, where several folded polypeptides join to form a final arrangement. The shape of a protein is critical to its function. When proteins are cooked or processed, the **denaturation**, which refers to the change in structure from the original three-dimensional shape of the protein, changes its original function.

Amino acid and protein structure • Figure 6.3

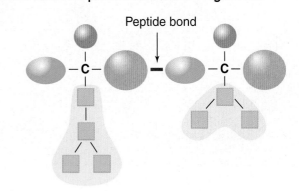

Peptide bond

2 The Structure of Amino Acids and Proteins 167

• Of the 20 amino acids required for protein synthesis, 11 are **nonessential**, or **dispensable amino acids**, meaning the body can synthesize them when they are absent in the diet. The amino acids that the body is unable to make in

3 Protein Digestion and Absorption 169

• Digestion breaks dietary protein into small peptides and amino acids that can be absorbed. Because amino acids that share the same transport system compete for absorption, an excess of one can inhibit the absorption of another.

Protein digestion and absorption • Figure 6.5

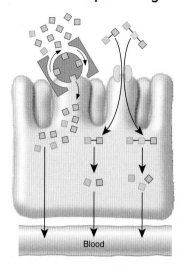

Blood

Protein functions • Figure 6.8

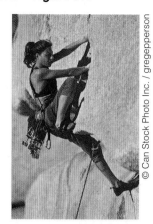

© Can Stock Photo Inc. / gregepperson

4 Protein Synthesis and Functions 171

- Amino acids are used to synthesize proteins and other nitrogen-containing molecules. Dietary proteins and body protein can be broken down to contribute to the **amino acid pool**, from which the body draws to synthesize new proteins.

- **Genes**, which are located in the nucleus of the cell, code for the order of amino acids in the polypeptide chains that make up proteins. During **transcription**, the first stage of protein synthesis, a copy of the genetic code is made. Next, during **translation**, this copy is used to synthesize the primary structure of a protein. **Regulatory** mechanisms ensure that proteins are made only when they are needed. For a protein to be synthesized, all the amino acids it contains must be available. If a non-essential amino acid is missing from the diet, it can be synthesized from another amino acid through the process of **transamination**. If an essential amino acid is missing, protein synthesis cannot continue and the protein will not be made. The amino acid present in shortest supply relative to need is called the **limiting amino acid**.

- In the body, protein molecules form structures, regulate body functions, transport molecules through the blood and in and out of cells, function in the immune system, and aid in muscle contraction and acid balance. Their role in fluid balance also helps protect against **edema**, an accumulation of fluid in the body. Amino acids also can provide energy, but are less efficient fuel sources than carbohydrates or fats. Before amino acids can be used for energy, the amino group must be removed via **deamination**. This amino group forms **urea** and is excreted in urine.

- When the diet is deficient in energy or when the diet contains more protein than needed, amino acids are used as an energy source and to synthesize glucose or fatty acids.

5 Protein in Health and Disease 177

- **Protein-energy malnutrition (PEM)** is a health concern primarily in developing countries. **Kwashiorkor** occurs when the protein content of the diet is deficient but energy is adequate. It is most common in children. **Marasmus** occurs when total energy intake is deficient.

- High-protein diets increase the production of urea and other waste products that must be excreted in the urine and therefore can increase water losses. High protein intakes increase urinary calcium losses, but when calcium intake is adequate, high-protein diets are associated with greater bone mass and fewer fractures. Diets high in animal proteins and low in fluid are associated with an increased risk of kidney stones. High-protein diets can be high in saturated fat and cholesterol.

- If proteins are absorbed without being completely digested, they can trigger an immune system reaction, resulting in a **food allergy**, which can be fatal in some cases. Some amino acids and proteins can also cause **food intolerances**. **MSG symptom complex** is an example of a food intolerance to the flavour enhancer, **monosodium glutamate**. **Celiac disease** is a food intolerance to the protein gluten. Although this disease involves the immune system, it is classified as a food intolerance because its symptoms are mostly gastrointestinal and are not as severe as those evidenced in food allergies.

Protein-energy malnutrition • Figure 6.10

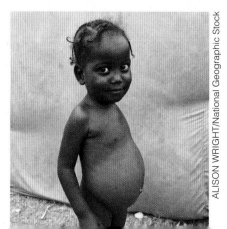

ALISON WRIGHT/National Geographic Stock

6 Meeting Protein Needs 181

- Protein requirements are determined by looking at **nitrogen balance**, the amount of nitrogen consumed as dietary protein compared with the amount excreted as protein waste products.

- For healthy adults, the RDA for protein is 0.8 g/kilogram of body weight. Growth, pregnancy, lactation, illness, injury, and certain types of physical exercise increase protein requirements. Recommendations for a healthy diet are to ingest 10 to 35% of calories from protein.

- Animal proteins, such as eggs and beef, are considered **high-quality proteins**, or **complete dietary proteins**. These proteins have a high **protein digestibility corrected amino acid score (PDCAAS)**, which means that they are well digested and have the correct blend of amino acids to meet the body's needs. Most plant proteins are limited in one or more of the amino acids needed to make body protein; therefore, they are considered **incomplete proteins**. The **protein quality** of plant sources can be increased by **protein complementation**, which combines proteins with different limiting amino acids to supply enough of all the essential amino acids.

- Compared with meat-based diets, **vegetarian diets** are lower in saturated fat and cholesterol and higher in fibre, certain vitamins and minerals, antioxidants, and phytochemicals. People consuming **vegan diets** must plan their diets carefully to meet their needs for vitamin B$_{12}$, calcium, vitamin D, iron, zinc, and omega-3 fatty acids.

Protein complementation • Figure 6.16

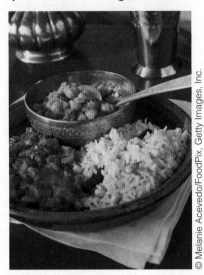

© Melanie Acevedo/FoodPix, Getty Images, Inc.

Key Terms

- amino acid pool 171
- amino acids 166
- celiac disease 180
- conditionally essential amino acids 167
- corrected amino acid score (PDCAAS) 184
- deamination 176
- denaturation 169
- dipeptide 168
- edema 175
- essential, or indispensable, amino acids 167

- food allergy 180
- food intolerance or food sensitivity 180
- gene 172
- high-quality protein or complete dietary protein 184
- incomplete dietary protein 184
- kwashiorkor 177
- legumes 166
- limiting amino acid 172
- marasmus 177
- monosodium glutamate (MSG) 180

- MSG symptom complex 180
- nitrogen balance 181
- nonessential, or dispensable, amino acids 167
- peptide bonds 169
- peptides 168
- phenylketonuria (PKU) 167
- polypeptide 169
- primary structure 168
- protein complementation 184
- protein digestibility protein-energy malnutrition (PEM) 177

- protein quality 184
- quaternary structure 168
- secondary structure 168
- tertiary structure 168
- transamination 172
- transcription 173
- translation 173
- tripeptide 168
- urea 176
- vegan diets 185
- vegetarian diets 185

Critical and Creative Thinking Questions

1. Children with the genetic disease phenylketonuria must consume a low-phenylalanine diet to prevent the accumulation of damaging phenylketones. Why can they not simply eliminate phenylalanine from their diet altogether?

2. Suraj consumes about 120 grams of protein/day. Of this, about 30 grams is broken down and used to make ATP, and 30 grams is used to synthesize body fat. What does this information tell you about Suraj's protein and energy intake?

3. Vladamir is a bodybuilder. He is concerned about his protein intake. If Vladamir weighs 9 kg (200 lb.) and consumes about 3,600 kilocalories/day, 15% of which comes from protein, will his diet supply enough protein to meet the daily recommendation for strength athletes, which is 1.6 to 1.7 grams of protein/kilogram of body weight per day? How about if he consumed only 2,500 kilocalories/day?

4. Fluid accumulates in the bellies of children with kwashiorkor. Use your understanding of how protein helps regulate fluid balance to explain why this occurs.

5. Suggest a breakfast, lunch, and dinner menu that supplies complementary sources of plant proteins.

6. At a recent physical examination, a blood test indicated that Taliah's blood urea concentration is elevated. What might be the cause of the elevation? What can she do to reduce the amount of urea produced?

7. Make a vegetarian meal plan for yourself for one day. Use iProfile to ensure the meal plan meets your calorie and protein needs. Next, plan a meal plan for one day that includes meat. Go to the grocery store and calculate how much each day's meals will cost. Use this information to explain the economic benefits or pitfalls of these two eating plans.

What is happening in this picture?

Sickle cell anemia is caused by an abnormality in the gene for the protein hemoglobin. It causes red blood cells to take on a sickle shape.

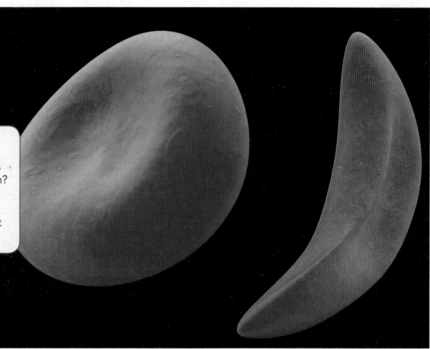

Think Critically

1. Sickle cell hemoglobin differs from normal hemoglobin by one amino acid. Why might this difference change the shape of the hemoglobin?
2. Do you think sickle-shaped red blood cells can travel easily through narrow capillaries?
3. How might this disorder affect the ability to get oxygen to the body's cells?

Self-Test

(Check your answers in Appendix J.)

1. Which part of this amino acid will differ, depending on the particular amino acid?
   a. A
   b. B
   c. C
   d. D

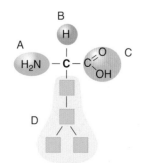

2. Amino acids that cannot be made by the adult human body in sufficient amounts are called _____.
   a. essential amino acids
   b. complete proteins
   c. incomplete amino acids
   d. hydrolyzed proteins
   e. nonessential amino acids

3. Based on the diagram, which letters label the parts of the digestive tract where chemical digestion of protein occurs?

   a. A and B

   b. A and C

   c. B and C

   d. B and D

   e. C and D

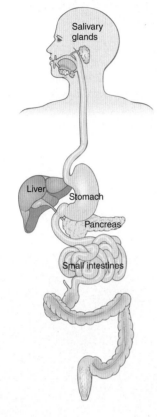

4. Which one of the following is made from amino acids?

   a. triglycerides

   b. glycogen

   c. lecithin

   d. cholesterol

   e. enzymes

5. Which of the following letters best labels transcription?

   a. A   b. B   c. C   d. D

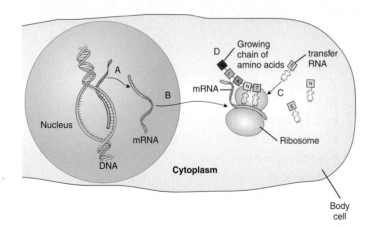

6. _____ is the process of transferring an amino group from an amino acid to another molecule to form a second amino acid.

   a. Deamination

   b. Transamination

   c. Denaturation

   d. Hydrogenation

7. Which colour amino acid is considered the most limiting for the synthesis of this specific protein?

   a. yellow

   b. green

   c. orange

   d. red

   e. blue

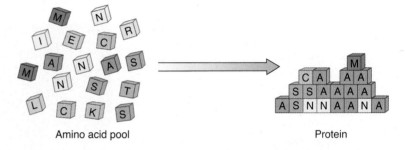

Amino acid pool   Protein

8. Which of the following groups of people requires the least protein per kilogram of body weight?

   a. adult men

   b. pregnant women

   c. infants

   d. young children

9. What element is found in proteins but not in carbohydrates and lipids?

   a. carbon

   b. nitrogen

   c. phosphorous

   d. oxygen

   e. hydrogen

10. Which of the following is least likely to be low in a vegan diet?

   a. calcium

   b. vitamin D

   c. iron

   d. fibre

   e. vitamin B$_{12}$

11. Which of the following values for nitrogen intake and output are most likely to belong to a healthy 9-year-old boy?

    a. nitrogen in = 14 g, nitrogen out = 16 g

    b. nitrogen in = 15 g, nitrogen out = 15 g

    c. nitrogen in = 14 g, nitrogen out = 10 g

    d. nitrogen in = 20 g, nitrogen out = 22 g

12. When amino acids are broken down to generate energy or synthesize glucose, the amino group must be removed. What waste product is generated from it?

    a. ketones

    b. urea

    c. free fatty acids

    d. carbon dioxide

    e. oxygen

13. Which of the following is *not* a good example of protein complementation?

    a. sunflower seeds and peanuts

    b. rice and beans

    c. chickpeas and sesame seeds

    d. corn and rice

    e. lentils and rice

14. When extra protein is consumed, it is stored in the muscle for later use.

    a. True

    b. False

15. Which one of the following statements about children with kwashiorkor is false?

    a. Their fat stores are completely depleted.

    b. They are more susceptible to infections than healthy children.

    c. They have swollen bellies.

    d. They have hair colour changes.

    e. They do not grow well.

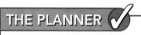

THE PLANNER

Review your Chapter Planner on the chapter opener and check off your completed work.

7 Vitamins

The British have long been referred to as "Limeys." If you eat a lot of carrots, your night vision will improve. Mom says to go outside and get some sunshine.

All three statements are related to an alphabet soup of essential compounds known as *vitamins*. British sailors on long voyages developed a debilitating disease called scurvy due to a lack of vitamin C. Consumption of adequate amounts of citrus fruits—such as limes—prevented them from developing this condition, and thus a nickname was born. Carrots are high in vitamin A, which is critical to the perception of light. And when exposed to sunlight, our bodies make the vitamin D we need; without vitamin D, we can't absorb enough calcium to build strong bones.

Northern Canadians enduring sunless Arctic winters have long acquired adequate amounts of vitamin D from a traditional diet of fish, bird eggs, seal, walrus, and whale blubber. But as their diet has changed over time—consumption of walrus and whale has been declining over the past 30 years—vitamin D deficiencies are increasing in these populations. If those of us who live in more temperate regions do not get enough sunlight, we must also obtain vitamin D from our diet, most often by consuming fortified milk.

As the British Royal Navy discovered—and diverse cultures, such as the Canadian Inuit, have appreciated for thousands of years—some foods can counteract certain ailments. Only relatively recently have the agents in these foods been isolated and recognized for the significant role they play in preventing or alleviating illness and ensuring good health.

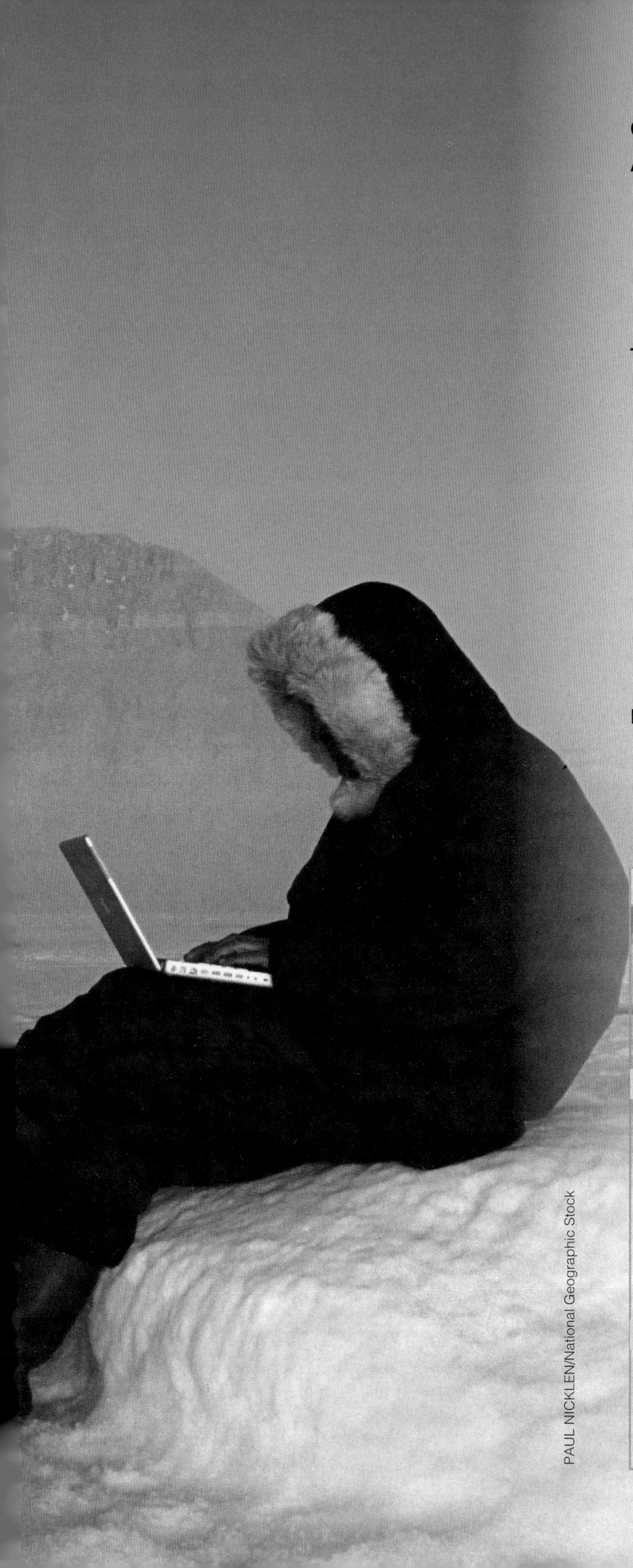

CHAPTER OUTLINE

CHAPTER PLANNER ✓

- ☐ Stimulate your interest by reading the introduction and looking at the visual.

- ☐ Scan the Learning Objectives in each section:
  p. 198 ☐   p. 205 ☐   p. 222 ☐   p. 237 ☐

- ☐ Read the text and study all figures and visuals. Answer any questions.

Analyze key features

- ☐ Hot Topic, p. 199 ☐   p. 241 ☐

- ☐ Process Diagram, p. 201 ☐   p. 203 ☐   p. 217 ☐   p. 225 ☐   p. 228 ☐

- ☐ Nutrition InSight, p. 202 ☐   p. 212 ☐   p. 226 ☐   p. 230 ☐

- ☐ Thinking It Through, p. 224

- ☐ What Should I Eat?, p. 233

- ☐ Stop: Answer the Concept Checks before you go on:
  p. 205 ☐   p. 222 ☐   p. 236 ☐   p. 241 ☐

End of chapter

- ☐ Review the Summary and Key Terms.

- ☐ Answer the Critical and Creative Thinking Questions.

- ☐ Answer What is happening in this picture?

- ☐ Complete the Self-Test and check your answers.

PAUL NICKLEN/National Geographic Stock

A Vitamin Primer

LEARNING OBJECTIVES

1. **Discuss** the dietary sources of vitamins.

2. **Describe** how bioavailability affects vitamin requirements.

3. **Explain** the function of coenzymes.

4. **Explain** the function of antioxidants.

V**itamins** are organic compounds that are essential in small amounts to promote and regulate body processes necessary for growth, reproduction, and the maintenance of health. When a vitamin is lacking in the diet, deficiency symptoms occur. When the vitamin is restored to the diet, the symptoms resolve.

Vitamins have traditionally been assigned to two groups, based on their solubility in water or fat. This chemical characteristic allows generalizations to be made about how the vitamins are absorbed, transported, excreted, and stored in the body. The **water-soluble vitamins** include the B vitamins and vitamin C. The **fat-soluble vitamins** include vitamins A, D, E, and K (**Table 7.1**). The vitamins were initially named alphabetically, in approximately the order in which they were identified. The B vitamins were first thought to be a single chemical substance but were later found to be many different substances. Vitamins B_6 and B_{12} are the only ones that are still routinely referred to by their numbers.

Vitamins in Our Food

Almost all foods contain some vitamins, and all the food groups contain foods that are good sources of a variety of vitamins (**Figure 7.1**). The amount of a vitamin in a food depends on the amount that is naturally present in the

The vitamins   Table 7.1

Water-soluble vitamins	Fat-soluble vitamins
B vitamins	Vitamin A
• Thiamin (B_1)	Vitamin D
• Riboflavin (B_2)	Vitamin E
• Niacin (B_3)	Vitamin K
• Biotin	
• Pantothenic acid	
• Vitamin B_6 (pyridoxine)	
• Folate (folic acid)	
• Vitamin B_{12} (cobalamin)	
Vitamin C (ascorbic acid)	

food, what is added to it, and how the food is processed, cooked, and stored.

Fortification adds nutrients to foods. Nutrients are sometimes added to foods to comply with government fortification programs that mandate additions to prevent vitamin or mineral deficiencies and to promote health in the population (see *Hot Topic: Should the Government Regulate Food Fortification?*). For example, grains are *enriched* with

GRAIN PRODUCTS	VEGETABLES & FRUIT	OILS	MILK & ALTERNATIVES	MEAT & ALTERNATIVES
Thiamin	Riboflavin	Vitamin E	Riboflavin	Thiamin
Riboflavin	Niacin		Vitamin A	Riboflavin
Niacin	Vitamin B_6		Vitamin D	Niacin
Pantothenic acid	Folate		Vitamin B_{12}	Biotin
Vitamin B_6	Vitamin C			Pantothenic acid
Folate	Vitamin A			Folate
	Vitamin E			Vitamin B_{12}
	Vitamin K			Vitamin A
				Vitamin D
				Vitamin K
				Vitamin B_6

Vitamins in the food guide
• Figure 7.1 _____

Vitamins are found in all the food groups and in oils, but some food groups lack specific vitamins. For example, grain products and fruits and vegetables lack vitamin B_{12}, and grain products and meat and meat alternatives are low in vitamin C. These shortfalls stress the importance of eating a balanced diet inclusive of all the food groups.

HOT TOPIC

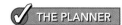

Should the government regulate food fortification?

The Nutrition Facts panel on a box of breakfast cereal shows an abundance of vitamins and minerals, many of which have been added through fortification. Adding micronutrients to food can help minimize symptoms of deficiency in a population, but it is not without its risks.

Neural tube defects are one of the most common birth defects and often lead to miscarriages. These defects are associated with low intakes of folate. In 1998, it became mandatory to fortify certain grain products with folate in Canada and the United States. Since then, the incidence of neural tube defects in newborns has decreased by almost 50% in Canada and 25% in the United States.[1,2] In the early 1900s, the niacin deficiency disease *pellagra* caused more than 3,000 deaths annually in the southern United States. In 1938, American bakers voluntarily began enriching flour with B vitamins, a move that led to a decline in mortality from pellagra (see graph).[3] In Canada, the fortification of foods has historically followed the recommendations outlined by the World Health Organization (WHO) and is meant to reduce micronutrient deficiencies. In 2005, Health Canada proposed its own discretionary fortification policy aimed at improving the nutritional quality of food and treating or preventing nutritional problems.[4] In one study, these proposed changes to the acceptable fortification ranges of foods were modelled against the typical Canadian intake pattern, and a decrease in nutrient deficiencies was noticed in various age and sex groups for several micronutrients, including vitamin A, vitamin C, folate, and calcium.[5] While the fortification of foods has advantages, it is not without its criticisms.

Nutritional scientists recognize that indiscriminate fortification of many foods, such as breakfast cereals, can increase the risk of nutrient toxicities. In the aforementioned study, fortification decreased the incidence of deficiency in some groups; however, it also led to nutrient intakes above the upper limit (UL) in other age–sex groups for nutrients such as vitamin A, folate, and calcium.[5] This trend was most frequently evidenced in younger age groups. The possibility of excessive consumption has also been evidenced in the United States, where almost 20% of toddlers who take vitamin supplements have folate intakes that exceed the UL, and more than half of infants and children up to age 3 exceed the UL for zinc.[6,7]

Another argument against food fortification is that it may give people a false sense of security about the healthfulness of their food. Just because a food has been fortified with vitamins and minerals, it does not mean it is necessarily good for you.

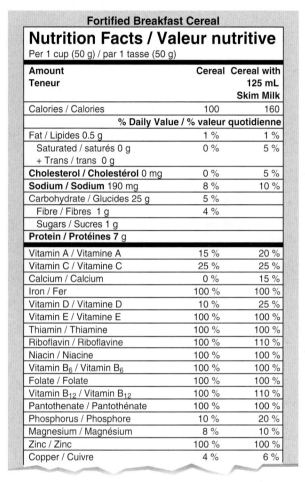

Fortified Breakfast Cereal		
Nutrition Facts / Valeur nutritive		
Per 1 cup (50 g) / par 1 tasse (50 g)		
Amount / Teneur	**Cereal**	**Cereal with 125 mL Skim Milk**
Calories / Calories	100	160
% Daily Value / % valeur quotidienne		
Fat / Lipides 0.5 g	1 %	1 %
Saturated / saturés 0 g + Trans / trans 0 g	0 %	5 %
Cholesterol / Cholestérol 0 mg	0 %	5 %
Sodium / Sodium 190 mg	8 %	10 %
Carbohydrate / Glucides 25 g	5 %	
Fibre / Fibres 1 g	4 %	
Sugars / Sucres 1 g		
Protein / Protéines 7 g		
Vitamin A / Vitamine A	15 %	20 %
Vitamin C / Vitamine C	25 %	25 %
Calcium / Calcium	0 %	15 %
Iron / Fer	100 %	100 %
Vitamin D / Vitamine D	10 %	25 %
Vitamin E / Vitamine E	100 %	100 %
Thiamin / Thiamine	100 %	100 %
Riboflavin / Riboflavine	100 %	110 %
Niacin / Niacine	100 %	100 %
Vitamin B_6 / Vitamin B_6	100 %	100 %
Folate / Folate	100 %	100 %
Vitamin B_{12} / Vitamin B_{12}	100 %	110 %
Pantothenate / Pantothénate	100 %	100 %
Phosphorus / Phosphore	10 %	20 %
Magnesium / Magnésium	8 %	10 %
Zinc / Zinc	100 %	100 %
Copper / Cuivre	4 %	6 %

Ask Yourself

In view of these risks, how should the Canadian government regulate the fortification of food?

Number of U.S. deaths from pellagra

- Voluntary flour enrichment
- Mandatory enrichment for some states
- Mandatory enrichment in 22 states

Year

Because heat, light, air, and the passage of time all cause foods to lose nutrients, most of us try to purchase fresh produce, but is fresh always best?

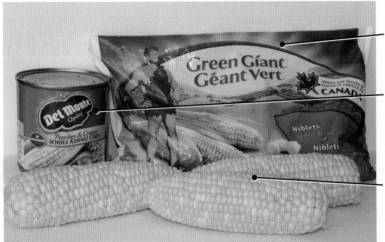

Frozen foods are often frozen in the field at the peak of freshness in order to minimize nutrient losses. Thus, frozen fruits and vegetables may supply more vitamins than "fresh" ones.

The high temperatures used in canning reduce nutrient content. However, because canned foods keep for a long time, do not require refrigeration, and are often less expensive than fresh or frozen foods, they provide an available, affordable source of nutrients that may be the best choice in some situations.

Sometimes "fresh" produce is lower in nutrients than you would expect because it is picked before it is mature and it has spent a week in a truck travelling to the store, several days on a shelf, and maybe another week in your refrigerator.

Luisa Begani

B vitamins and iron to prevent deficiencies, and milk is fortified with vitamin D to promote bone health. In other cases, manufacturers add nutrients with the goal of increasing product sales.

The vitamins in foods can be damaged by exposure to light or oxygen, washed away during preparation, or destroyed by cooking. Thus, the processing steps used by food producers can lead to nutrient losses, as can the cooking and storage methods used at home (**Figure 7.2**). Vitamin losses can be minimized through food preparation methods that reduce exposure to heat and light, which destroy some vitamins, and to water, which washes away water-soluble vitamins (**Table 7.2**).

Tips for preserving the vitamins in your food   Table 7.2

- Store food away from heat and light, and eat food soon after purchasing it.
- Cut fruits and vegetables as close as possible to the time when they will be cooked or served.
- Don't soak vegetables before you cook them.
- Cook vegetables using as little water as possible by microwaving, pressure-cooking, roasting, grilling, stir-frying, or baking rather than boiling.
- If foods are cooked in water, use the cooking water to make soups and sauces so that you can retrieve some of the nutrients.
- Don't rinse rice before cooking, to avoid washing away water-soluble vitamins.

Vitamin Bioavailability

About 40 to 90% of the vitamins in food are absorbed, primarily in the small intestine (**Figure 7.3**). The composition of the diet and conditions in the digestive tract and the rest of the body influence vitamin **bioavailability**. For example, fat-soluble vitamins are absorbed along with dietary fat. If the diet is very low in fat, absorption of these vitamins is impaired.

> **bioavailability** The extent to which the body can absorb and use a nutrient.

After vitamins have been absorbed into the blood, they must be transported to the cells. Most of the water-soluble vitamins are bound to blood proteins for transport. Fat-soluble vitamins are incorporated into chylomicrons for transport from the intestine. The bioavailability of a vitamin depends on the availability of these transport systems.

Some vitamins are absorbed in an inactive form called either a **provitamin** or a **vitamin precursor**. To perform vitamin functions, provitamins must be converted into active vitamin forms once they are inside the body. How much of each provitamin can be converted into the active vitamin and the rate at which this process occurs affect the amount of a vitamin available to function inside the body.

> **provitamin** or **vitamin precursor** A compound that can be converted into the active form of a vitamin in the body.

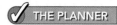

Vitamin absorption • Figure 7.3

THE PLANNER

Most vitamin absorption takes place in the small intestine. The mechanism by which vitamins are absorbed and transported affects their bioavailability.

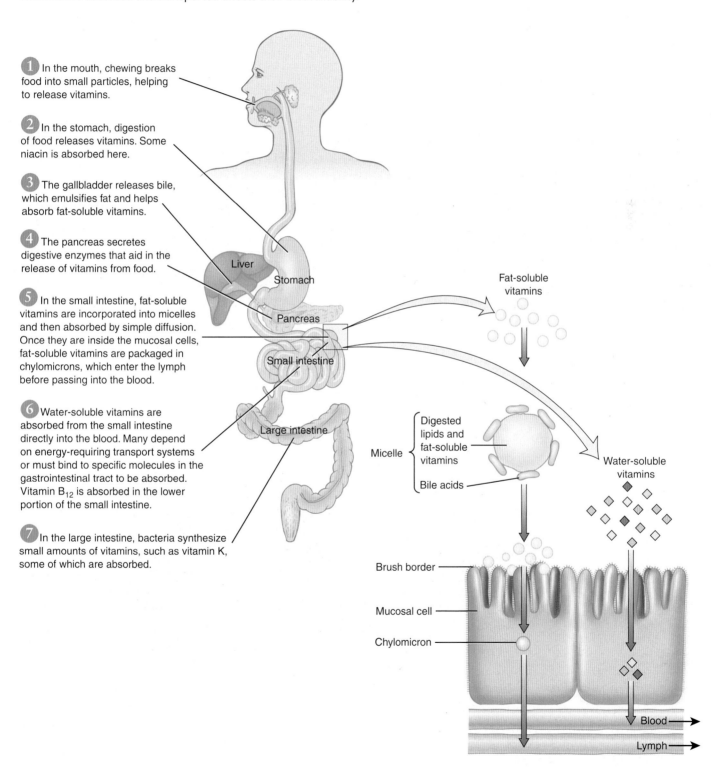

1 In the mouth, chewing breaks food into small particles, helping to release vitamins.

2 In the stomach, digestion of food releases vitamins. Some niacin is absorbed here.

3 The gallbladder releases bile, which emulsifies fat and helps absorb fat-soluble vitamins.

4 The pancreas secretes digestive enzymes that aid in the release of vitamins from food.

5 In the small intestine, fat-soluble vitamins are incorporated into micelles and then absorbed by simple diffusion. Once they are inside the mucosal cells, fat-soluble vitamins are packaged in chylomicrons, which enter the lymph before passing into the blood.

6 Water-soluble vitamins are absorbed from the small intestine directly into the blood. Many depend on energy-requiring transport systems or must bind to specific molecules in the gastrointestinal tract to be absorbed. Vitamin B_{12} is absorbed in the lower portion of the small intestine.

7 In the large intestine, bacteria synthesize small amounts of vitamins, such as vitamin K, some of which are absorbed.

Liver
Stomach
Pancreas
Small intestine
Large intestine

Fat-soluble vitamins

Micelle
Digested lipids and fat-soluble vitamins
Bile acids

Water-soluble vitamins

Brush border
Mucosal cell
Chylomicron

Blood
Lymph

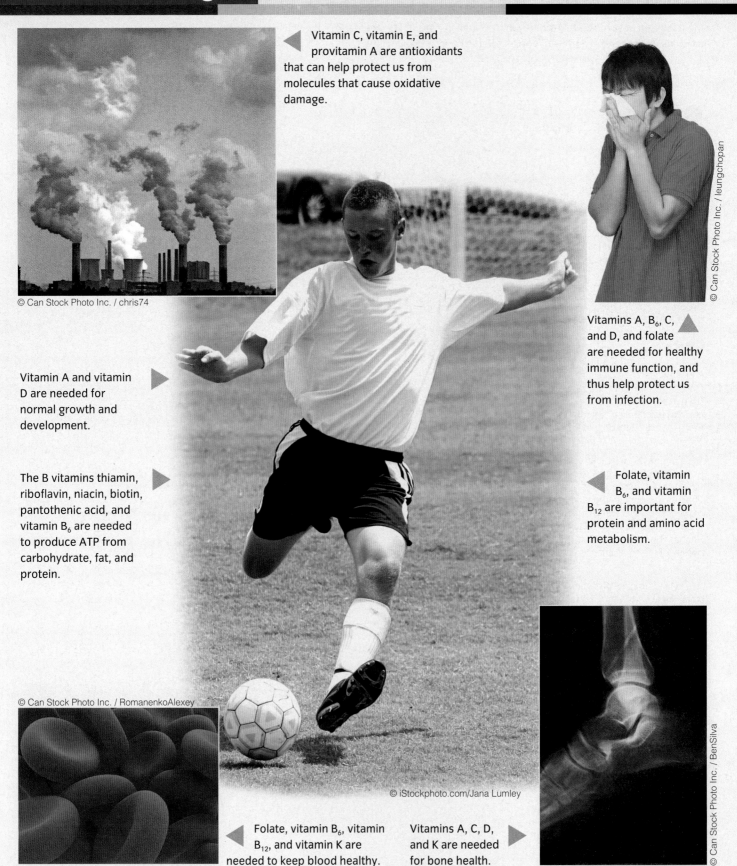

Vitamin C, vitamin E, and provitamin A are antioxidants that can help protect us from molecules that cause oxidative damage.

© Can Stock Photo Inc. / chris74

Vitamins A, B_6, C, and D, and folate are needed for healthy immune function, and thus help protect us from infection.

© Can Stock Photo Inc. / leungchopan

Vitamin A and vitamin D are needed for normal growth and development.

The B vitamins thiamin, riboflavin, niacin, biotin, pantothenic acid, and vitamin B_6 are needed to produce ATP from carbohydrate, fat, and protein.

Folate, vitamin B_6, and vitamin B_{12} are important for protein and amino acid metabolism.

© Can Stock Photo Inc. / RomanenkoAlexey

© iStockphoto.com/Jana Lumley

Folate, vitamin B_6, vitamin B_{12}, and vitamin K are needed to keep blood healthy.

Vitamins A, C, D, and K are needed for bone health.

© Can Stock Photo Inc. / BenSilva

Coenzymes • Figure 7.5

Coenzymes bind to enzymes to promote their activity. They act as carriers of electrons, atoms, or chemical groups that participate in the reaction. All the B vitamins are coenzymes, but some coenzymes are not dietary essentials and therefore are not vitamins. Coenzymes are essential for the proper functioning of numerous enzymes involved in metabolism.

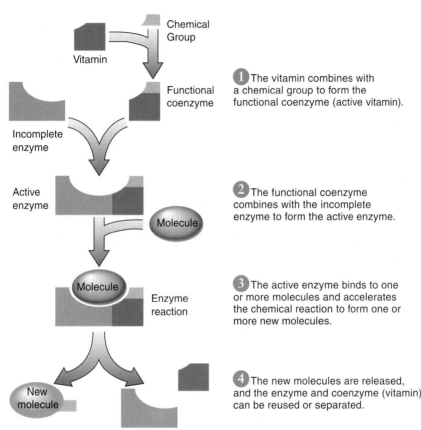

1 The vitamin combines with a chemical group to form the functional coenzyme (active vitamin).

2 The functional coenzyme combines with the incomplete enzyme to form the active enzyme.

3 The active enzyme binds to one or more molecules and accelerates the chemical reaction to form one or more new molecules.

4 The new molecules are released, and the enzyme and coenzyme (vitamin) can be reused or separated.

Vitamin Functions

Vitamins promote and regulate the body's activities. Each vitamin has one or more important functions (**Figure 7.4**). For example, vitamin A is needed for vision and for normal growth and development. Vitamin K is needed for blood clotting and bone health. Often, more than one vitamin is needed to ensure the health of a particular organ or system. Some vitamins act in a similar manner to do their jobs. For example, all the B vitamins act as coenzymes (**Figure 7.5**).

A few vitamins function as **antioxidants**, substances that

coenzymes
Organic non-protein substances that bind to enzymes to promote their activity.

antioxidant
A substance that is able to neutralize reactive oxygen molecules and thereby prevent cell damage.

protect against **oxidative damage**. Oxidative damage is caused when reactive oxygen molecules steal electrons from, or *oxidize*, other compounds, causing changes in their structure and function. Reactive oxygen molecules such as **free radicals** can be generated by normal oxygen-requiring reactions inside the body, such as cellular respiration, or can result from environmental sources, such as air pollution or cigarette smoke. Free radicals cause damage by snatching electrons from DNA, proteins, carbohydrates, or unsaturated fatty acids. This loss of electrons results in changes in the structure and function of these molecules. Antioxidants act by destroying free radicals and other reactive oxygen molecules before they can do

free radicals One type of highly reactive atom or molecule that causes oxidative damage.

A Vitamin Primer **203**

How antioxidants work • Figure 7.6

Antioxidants, such as vitamin C, function by donating electrons to free radicals. A donated electron stabilizes the free radical so that it is no longer reactive and cannot steal electrons from important molecules in and around cells.

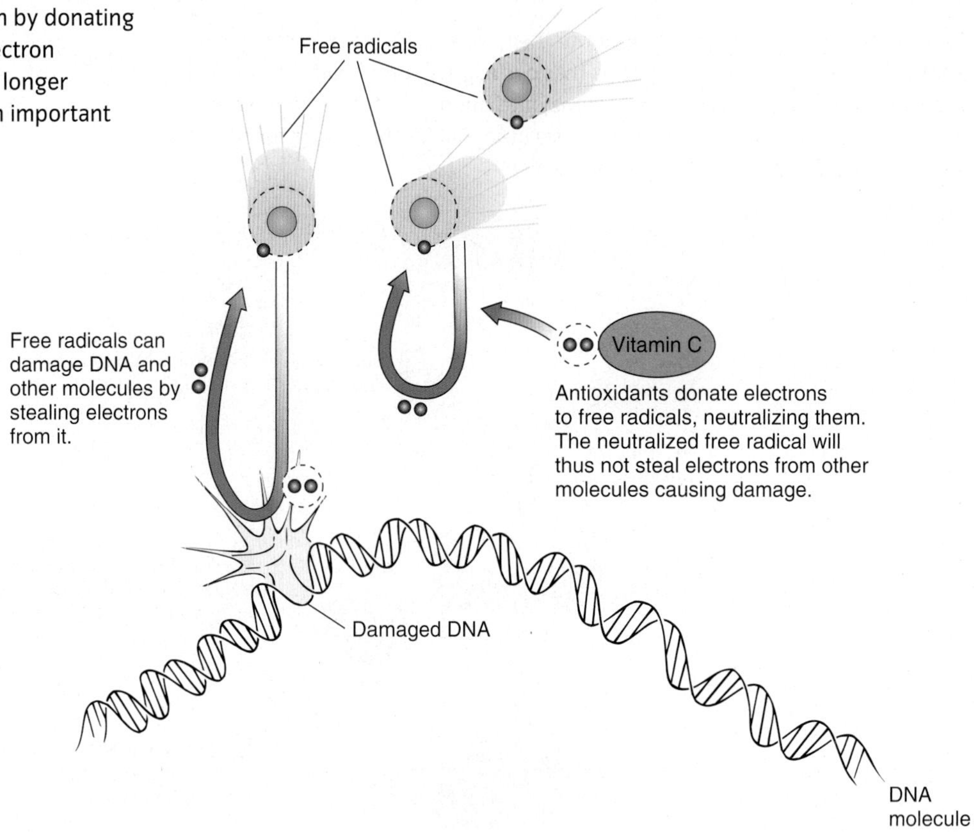

Free radicals

Free radicals can damage DNA and other molecules by stealing electrons from it.

Vitamin C

Antioxidants donate electrons to free radicals, neutralizing them. The neutralized free radical will thus not steal electrons from other molecules causing damage.

Damaged DNA

DNA molecule

damage (**Figure 7.6**). Some antioxidants are produced in the body; others, such as vitamin C, vitamin E, and the mineral selenium, are consumed in the diet.[8] Oxidative damage is implicated in the pathophysiology of cancer, diabetes, and cardiovascular disease, and may be linked to Alzheimer's disease and Parkinson's disease. A diet rich in antioxidants may accordingly minimize the risk of these chronic diseases in the Canadian population; however, the effects of antioxidant treatment are not yet conclusive.[9,10]

Meeting Vitamin Needs

The right amounts and combinations of vitamins and other nutrients are essential to health. Despite our knowledge of what vitamins do and how much of each we need, not everyone consumes the recommended amounts. In developing countries, vitamin deficiencies remain a major public health problem. In Canada and other industrialized countries, thanks to a more varied food supply and food fortification, vitamin-deficiency diseases have been almost eliminated. In these countries,

concern now focuses on meeting the needs of high-risk groups, such as children and pregnant women; determining the consequences of marginal deficiencies, such as the effect of low B vitamin intake on heart disease risk; and evaluating the risk of consuming large amounts of certain vitamins.

The Recommended Daily Allowances (RDAs) and Adequate Intakes (AIs) of the Dietary Reference Intakes (DRIs) recommend amounts that provide enough of each of the vitamins to prevent a deficiency and promote health (see Chapter 2). Because more is not always better when it comes to nutrient intake, the DRIs have also established Upper Intake Levels (ULs) as a guide to amounts that avoid the risk of toxicity (see Appendix A).

Food labels can help identify packaged foods that are good sources of vitamins. Labels are required to list the amounts of vitamin A and vitamin C in foods as a percentage of the Daily Values (**Figure 7.7**). Daily Values of other vitamins are often provided voluntarily. Fresh fruits, vegetables, fish, meat, and poultry, which are excellent sources of many vitamins, do not carry food labels.

Vitamins on food labels • Figure 7.7

As a general guideline, if the % Daily Value is 5% or less, the food is a poor source of that nutrient; if it is 10 to 19%, the food is a good source; and if the % Daily Value is 20% or more, the food is an excellent source.

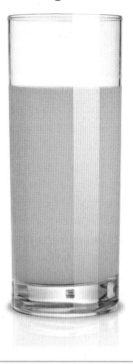

Orange Juice

Nutrition Facts Valeur nutritive		
Per 250 mL / par 250 mL		
Amount Teneur		% Daily Value % valeur quotidienne
Calories / Calories 110		
Fat / Lipides 0 g		0 %
Saturated / saturés 0 g + Trans / trans 0 g		0 %
Cholesterol / Cholestérol 0 mg		
Sodium / Sodium 0 mg		0 %
Potassium/ Potassium 470 mg		13 %
Carbohydrate/ Glucides 27 g		9 %
Sugars / Sucres 23 g		
Protein/ Protéines 2 g		
Vitamin A / Vitamine A		0 %
Vitamin C / Vitamine C		120 %
Calcium / Calcium		2 %
Iron / Fer		0 %
Folate / Folate		25 %

To determine the exact amount of a vitamin in a food, look up the Daily Value and multiply it by the % Daily Value on the label.

CONCEPT CHECK STOP

1. **What** food groups contain the greatest variety of vitamins?

2. **Why** might a low-fat diet affect the bioavailability of fat-soluble vitamins?

3. **What** is the principal function of coenzymes?

4. **How** do antioxidants protect our cells?

The Water-Soluble Vitamins

LEARNING OBJECTIVES

1. **Discuss** the role of thiamin, riboflavin, and niacin in producing ATP.

2. **Explain** why vitamin B_6 is so important for protein metabolism.

3. **Compare** the functions of folate and vitamin B_{12}.

4. **Relate** the role of vitamin C in the body to the symptoms of scurvy.

The water-soluble vitamins include the B vitamins and vitamin C. The B vitamins are directly involved in converting the energy in carbohydrate, fat, and protein into adenosine triphosphate (ATP), the form of energy that is used to run the body. The B vitamins are not, however, sources of energy themselves. Vitamin C is needed to synthesize connective tissue and to protect us from damage by oxidation.

Because water-soluble vitamins are not stored to any great extent, supplies of most of these vitamins are rapidly depleted. For this reason, water-soluble vitamins must be consumed regularly. Nevertheless, it takes more than a few days to develop deficiency symptoms, even when one of these vitamins is completely eliminated from the diet. For years, we thought that because most water-soluble vitamins are not stored in the body and are excreted in the urine, high doses were not harmful. However, we now recognize that high doses of some of these vitamins can be toxic.

Thiamin

Thiamin, the first of the B vitamins to be discovered, is sometimes called vitamin B₁. **Beriberi**, the neurological disease that results from a deficiency of this vitamin, came to the attention of Western medicine in colonial Asia in the 19th century. It became such a problem that the Dutch East India Company sent a team of scientists to determine its cause. A young physician named Christian Eijkman worked on this problem for more than 10 years. His success came as a result of a twist of fate. He ran out of food for his experimental chickens and, instead of the usual brown rice, fed them white rice. Shortly thereafter, the chickens displayed beriberi-like symptoms. When he fed them brown rice again, their health was restored. These results provided evidence that the cause of beriberi was not a poison or a microorganism as previously thought, but rather something that was missing from the diet.

Eijkman's studies enabled the prevention and cure of beriberi through feeding people a diet that was adequate in thiamin, but the vitamin itself was not isolated until 1926. We now know that refining grains by polishing the bran layer off rice kernels to make white rice removes the thiamin-rich portion of the grain. Therefore, in populations where white rice was the staple of the diet, beriberi became a common health problem. The incidence of beriberi in eastern Asia increased dramatically in the late 1800s due to the rising popularity of polished rice.

Thiamin is part of a coenzyme that is needed to convert pyruvate into acetyl CoA, an essential intermediate in the process of extracting energy from glucose. It is particularly important for nerve function because glucose is the energy source for nerve cells. In addition to thiamin's role in energy production, it is needed for the synthesis of **neurotransmitters**, the metabolism of other sugars and certain amino acids, and the synthesis of ribose, a sugar that is part of the structure of RNA (ribonucleic acid).

In addition to being found in the bran layer of brown rice and other whole grains, thiamin is added to enriched grains and is particularly abundant in pork, legumes, and seeds (**Figure 7.8**). When inadequate amounts of thiamin

> **beriberi** A thiamin deficiency disease that causes weakness, nerve degeneration, and, in some cases, heart changes.

> **neurotransmitter** A chemical substance produced by a nerve cell that can stimulate or inhibit another cell.

Meeting thiamin needs • Figure 7.8

A large proportion of the thiamin consumed in Canada comes from enriched grains used to make foods that we consume in abundance, such as sandwiches, pizza, pasta, baked goods, and breakfast cereals. The dashed lines indicate the RDAs for adult men and women, which are 1.2 mg/day and 1.1 mg/day, respectively.

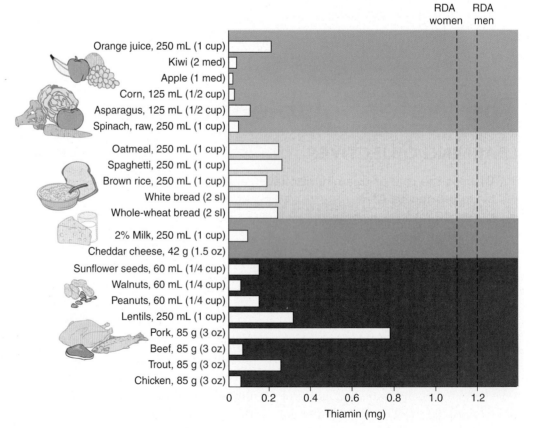

How thiamin functions • Figure 7.9

a. The active thiamin coenzyme, thiamin pyrophosphate, is needed to convert pyruvate into acetyl CoA, which can continue through cellular respiration to produce larger amounts of ATP. Acetyl CoA is also needed to synthesize the neurotransmitter acetylcholine. Without thiamin, glucose, which is the primary fuel for the brain and nerve cells, cannot be used normally, and acetylcholine cannot be synthesized.

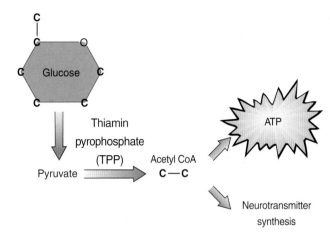

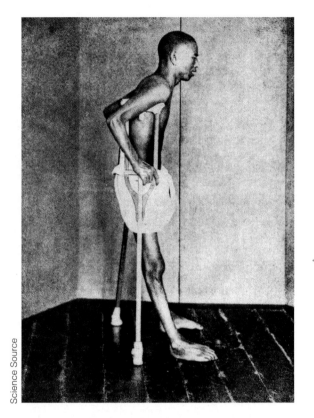

b. For more than 1,000 years, beriberi flourished in East Asian countries. In Sri Lanka, the word *beriberi* means "I cannot, I cannot" referring to the extreme weakness and depression that are the earliest symptoms of the disease. These symptoms may be caused by the inability of nerve cells to produce energy from glucose. Other neurological symptoms, such as poor coordination, tingling sensations, and paralysis, may be related to the body's inability to synthesize certain neurotransmitters when thiamin is deficient.

are consumed, the deficiency affects the nervous and cardiovascular systems. The neurological symptoms of beriberi can be related to the functions of thiamin (**Figure 7.9**). Beriberi can also cause cardiovascular symptoms such as rapid heartbeat and enlargement of the heart, but it is not clear from the functions of thiamin why these cardiovascular symptoms occur.[11]

Beriberi is rare in North America today, but a form of thiamin deficiency called **Wernicke-Korsakoff syndrome** occurs more frequently in alcoholics. People with this condition experience mental confusion, psychosis, memory disturbances, and eventually coma. Alcoholics are particularly vulnerable because alcohol decreases thiamin absorption in the gastrointestinal tract. In addition, their thiamin intake is low because alcohol contributes calories to the diet but brings with it almost no nutrients.

Although thiamin is needed to provide energy, unless the diet is deficient in thiamin, increasing thiamin intake does not increase the ability to produce ATP. There is no UL for thiamin because no toxicity has been reported when an excess of this vitamin is consumed from either food or supplements.[11]

Riboflavin

Riboflavin is a water-soluble vitamin that provides a visible indicator of excessive consumption; the excess is excreted in the urine, turning it a bright fluorescent yellow. The colour may surprise you, but it is harmless. No adverse effects of high doses of riboflavin from either foods or supplements have been reported.

Riboflavin forms two active coenzymes that act as electron carriers, flavin adenine dinucleotide (FAD) and

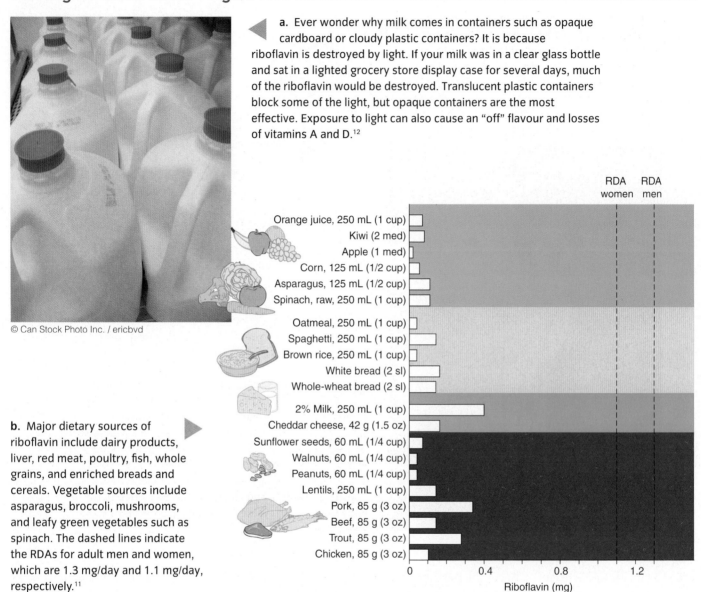

© Can Stock Photo Inc. / ericbvd

a. Ever wonder why milk comes in containers such as opaque cardboard or cloudy plastic containers? It is because riboflavin is destroyed by light. If your milk was in a clear glass bottle and sat in a lighted grocery store display case for several days, much of the riboflavin would be destroyed. Translucent plastic containers block some of the light, but opaque containers are the most effective. Exposure to light can also cause an "off" flavour and losses of vitamins A and D.[12]

b. Major dietary sources of riboflavin include dairy products, liver, red meat, poultry, fish, whole grains, and enriched breads and cereals. Vegetable sources include asparagus, broccoli, mushrooms, and leafy green vegetables such as spinach. The dashed lines indicate the RDAs for adult men and women, which are 1.3 mg/day and 1.1 mg/day, respectively.[11]

flavin mononucleotide (FMN). They function in deamination reactions as well as in the citric acid cycle and beta-oxidation, all of which help produce ATP from carbohydrate, fat, and protein. Riboflavin is also involved directly or indirectly in converting several other vitamins, including folate, niacin, vitamin B_6, and vitamin K, into their active forms.

One of the best sources of riboflavin in the diet is milk (**Figure 7.10**). When riboflavin is deficient, injuries heal poorly because new cells cannot grow to replace the damaged ones. This deficiency often occurs in combination with protein energy malnutrition and/or alcoholism and is known as ariboflavinosis. The tissues that grow most

rapidly, such as the skin and the linings of the eyes, mouth, and tongue, are the first to be affected. These tissues show symptoms such as cracking of the lips and at the corners of the mouth; increased sensitivity to light; burning, tearing, and itching of the eyes; and flaking of the skin around the nose, eyebrows, and earlobes.

A deficiency of riboflavin usually occurs in conjunction with deficiencies of other B vitamins because the same foods are also sources of those vitamins and because riboflavin is needed to convert other vitamins into their active forms. Some of the symptoms seen in cases of riboflavin deficiency therefore also reflect deficiencies of these other nutrients.

Niacin

In the early 1900s, psychiatric hospitals in the southeastern United States were filled with patients with the niacin-deficiency disease **pellagra** (**Figure 7.11**). **Niacin**, also known as nicotinic acid, is part of the coenzyme NAD, the electron carrier that functions in glucose metabolism. It also participates in reactions that synthesize fatty acids

> **pellagra** A disease resulting from niacin deficiency, which causes dermatitis, diarrhea, dementia, and, if not treated, death.

and cholesterol. The need for niacin is so widespread in metabolism that a deficiency causes major changes throughout the body. The early symptoms of pellagra include fatigue, decreased appetite, and indigestion. These are followed by symptoms that can be remembered as the three Ds: dermatitis, diarrhea, and dementia. If left untreated, niacin deficiency may result in a fourth D—death.

Tracking down the cause of pellagra • Figure 7.11

In 1914, Dr. Joseph Goldberger was appointed to investigate the pellagra epidemic in the Southern United States. He unravelled the mystery of its cause by using the scientific method. He observed that individuals in institutions such as hospitals, orphanages, and prisons suffered from pellagra, but the staff did not. If pellagra were an infectious disease, both populations would have been equally affected. He therefore hypothesized that pellagra was due to a deficiency in the diet. He conducted some experiments, and the results supported his hypothesis. In 1937, the deficient dietary component was identified as the water-soluble B vitamin niacin.

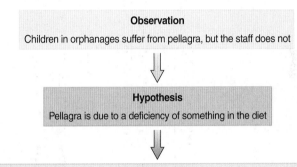

Observation
Children in orphanages suffer from pellagra, but the staff does not

Hypothesis
Pellagra is due to a deficiency of something in the diet

Experiments

Experimental design: Nutritious foods including meat, milk, and vegetables are added to the diets of children in two orphanages.

Results: Those consuming the healthier diets recover from pellagra. Those without the disease who eat the new diet do not contract pellagra, supporting the hypothesis that it is caused by dietary deficiency.

Experimental design: Eleven volunteers are fed a diet believed to be lacking in the dietary substance that prevents pellagra.

Results: Six of the eleven develop symptoms of pellagra after 5 months of consuming the experimental diet, supporting the hypothesis that it is caused by a dietary deficiency.

Continued experiments: Various studies involving both animals and humans eventually reveal that nicotinic acid, better known as the B vitamin niacin, cures pellagra.

Theory
Pellagra is caused by a deficiency of the B vitamin niacin.

This photograph illustrates the cracked, inflamed skin that is characteristic of pellagra. The rash most commonly appears on areas of the skin that are exposed to sunlight or other stresses.

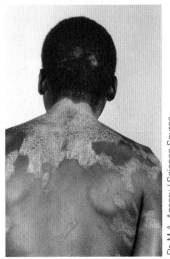

Dr. M.A. Ansary / Science Source

Meeting niacin needs • Figure 7.12

Meat, fish, peanuts, and whole and enriched grains are the best sources of niacin. Other sources include legumes and wheat bran. Food composition tables and databases do not include the amount of niacin that could be made from the tryptophan in a food. The dashed lines indicate the RDAs for adult men and women, which are 16 mg NE/day and 14 mg NE/day, respectively.

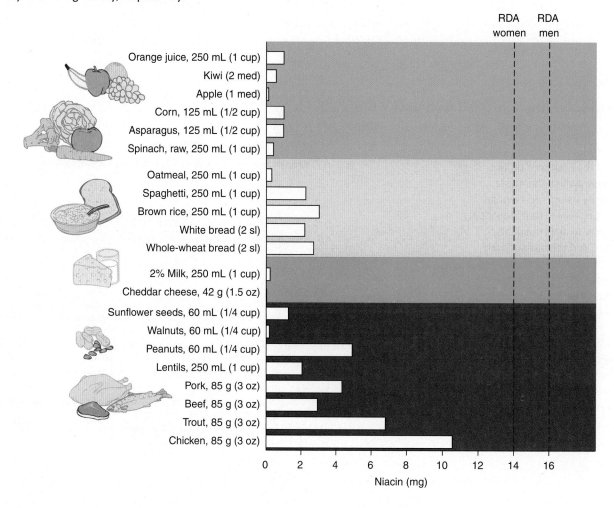

Meats and grains are good sources of niacin (**Figure 7.12**). Niacin can also be synthesized in the body from the essential amino acid tryptophan; however, tryptophan is only used to make niacin if enough is available to first meet the needs of protein synthesis. When the diet is low in tryptophan, it is not used to synthesize niacin. Because some of the requirement for niacin can be met through the synthesis of niacin from tryptophan, the RDA is expressed as niacin equivalents (NEs). One NE is equal to 1 mg of niacin or 60 mg of tryptophan, the amount needed to make 1 mg of niacin.[11]

The reason niacin deficiency was so prevalent in the U.S. South in the early 1900s is that corn formed the basis of the local diet of the people living in poverty. Corn is low in tryptophan, and the niacin found naturally in corn is bound to other molecules and is therefore not well absorbed. Today, as a result of the enrichment of grains with an available form of niacin, pellagra is rare in North America, but remains a problem in areas of Africa where the diet is based on corn.[13] Despite the corn-based diet in Mexico and Central American countries, pellagra is uncommon in those countries, in part because the treatment of corn with limewater, as is done during the making of tortillas, enhances the availability of niacin. The diet in these regions also includes legumes, which provide both niacin and a source of tryptophan for the synthesis of niacin.

Supplemental doses of niacin are sometimes provided to patients to lower cholesterol, either alone or in combination with other lipid-improving drugs and strategies. It is believed to work by slowing the production of LDL by the liver and by increasing HDL. Supplemental niacin should only be taken under a doctor's prescription and people should not self-medicate.[14,15]

There is no evidence of any adverse effects due to the consumption of niacin that occurs naturally in foods, but niacin supplements can be toxic. Excess niacin supplementation can cause flushing of the skin, a tingling sensation in the hands and feet, a red skin rash, nausea, vomiting, diarrhea, high blood sugar levels, abnormalities in liver function, and blurred vision. The UL for adults is 35 mg per day. Daily doses of 50 mg or greater of a form of niacin are used as a drug to treat elevated blood cholesterol; this amount should be consumed only when prescribed by a physician.

Biotin

Biotin is part of the coenzyme that replenishes the oxaloacetate stores needed for the citric acid cycle to occur. Biotin is essential for energy production and glucose synthesis and is also important in the metabolism of fatty acids and amino acids. Good sources of biotin in the diet include cooked eggs, liver, yogurt, and nuts. Fruit and meat are poor sources. Bacteria in the gastrointestinal tract synthesize biotin, and some of this biotin is absorbed into the body to help meet our biotin needs. An AI of 30 μg/day has been established for adults.[11]

Although biotin deficiency is uncommon, it has been observed in people with malabsorption or malnutrition and those taking certain medications for long periods.[11] Eating raw eggs can also cause biotin deficiency because raw egg whites contain a protein called avidin that tightly binds biotin and prevents its absorption. (Raw eggs should never be eaten anyway because they can contain harmful bacteria.) Thoroughly cooking eggs kills bacteria and denatures avidin so that it cannot bind biotin. Biotin deficiency in humans causes nausea, thinning hair, loss of hair colour, a red skin rash, depression, lethargy, hallucinations, and

tingling of the extremities. High doses of biotin have not resulted in toxicity symptoms; there is no UL for biotin.

Pantothenic Acid

Pantothenic acid, which gets its name from the Greek word *pantothen* (meaning "from everywhere"), is widely distributed in foods. It is particularly abundant in meat, eggs, whole grains, and legumes, and it is found in lesser amounts in milk, vegetables, and fruits.

In addition to being "from everywhere" in the diet, pantothenic acid seems to be needed everywhere in the body. It is part of coenzyme A (CoA), which is needed for the breakdown of carbohydrates, fatty acids, and amino acids, and for the modification of proteins and the synthesis of neurotransmitters, steroid hormones, and hemoglobin. Pantothenic acid is also needed to form a molecule that is essential for the synthesis of cholesterol and fatty acids.

The wide distribution of pantothenic acid in foods makes deficiency rare in humans. The AI is 5 mg/day for adults. Pantothenic acid is relatively nontoxic, and there are insufficient data to establish a UL.[11]

Vitamin B$_6$

Vitamin B$_6$ is particularly important for amino acid and protein metabolism. It is needed to synthesize nonessential amino acids, make neurotransmitters, synthesize hemoglobin, convert tryptophan into niacin, and break down glycogen to release glucose into the blood.

There are three forms of vitamin B$_6$: pyridoxal, pyridoxine, and pyridoxamine. These can be converted into the active coenzyme pyridoxal phosphate, which is needed for the activity of more than 100 enzymes involved in the metabolism of carbohydrate, fat, and protein.

Vitamin B$_6$ deficiency leads to poor growth, skin lesions, decreased immune function, anemia, and neurological symptoms. Because vitamin B$_6$ is needed for amino acid metabolism, the onset of a deficiency can be hastened by a diet that is low in vitamin B$_6$ but high in protein.

Many of the symptoms can be linked to the chemical reactions that depend on this vitamin coenzyme (**Figure 7.13**). For example, poor growth, skin lesions, and decreased antibody formation may result from a diet that is low in vitamin B$_6$ because of its central role in protein and energy metabolism.

a. Vitamin B_6 is needed for *transamination* reactions, which synthesize nonessential amino acids by transferring an amino group to a carbon compound, and for *deamination* reactions, which remove the amino group from amino acids so that the remaining carbon compound can be used to provide energy or synthesize glucose. Vitamin B_6 is also needed to remove the acid group from amino acids so that the remaining molecule can be used to synthesize neurotransmitters.

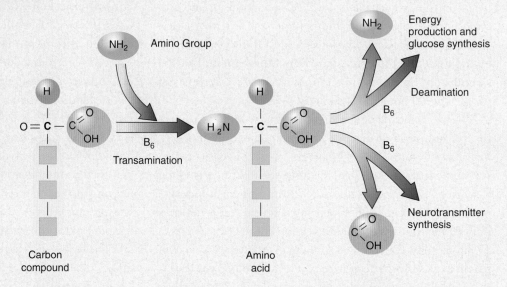

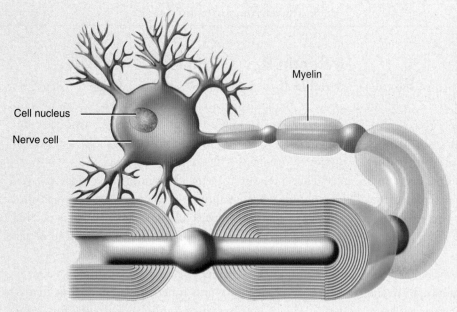

Cell nucleus

Nerve cell

Myelin

b. Vitamin B_6 is needed for the synthesis of lipids that are part of the myelin coating on nerves. Myelin is essential for nerve transmission. The role of vitamin B_6 in myelin formation and neurotransmitter synthesis may explain the neurological symptoms that occur with deficiency, such as numbness and tingling in the hands and feet, depression, headaches, confusion, and seizures.

Meat and fish are excellent sources of vitamin B_6, and whole grains and legumes are good plant sources (**Figure 7.14**). Refined grain products such as white rice and white bread are not good sources of vitamin B_6 because the vitamin is lost during refining and is not added back through enrichment. Vitamin B_6 is, however, added to many fortified breakfast cereals, which make an important contribution to vitamin B_6 intake. Vitamin B_6 is destroyed by heat and light, so it can easily be lost during processing.

No adverse effects have been associated with high intake of vitamin B_6 from foods, but large doses found in supplements can cause severe nerve impairment. To prevent nerve damage, the UL for adults is set at 100 mg/day

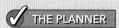
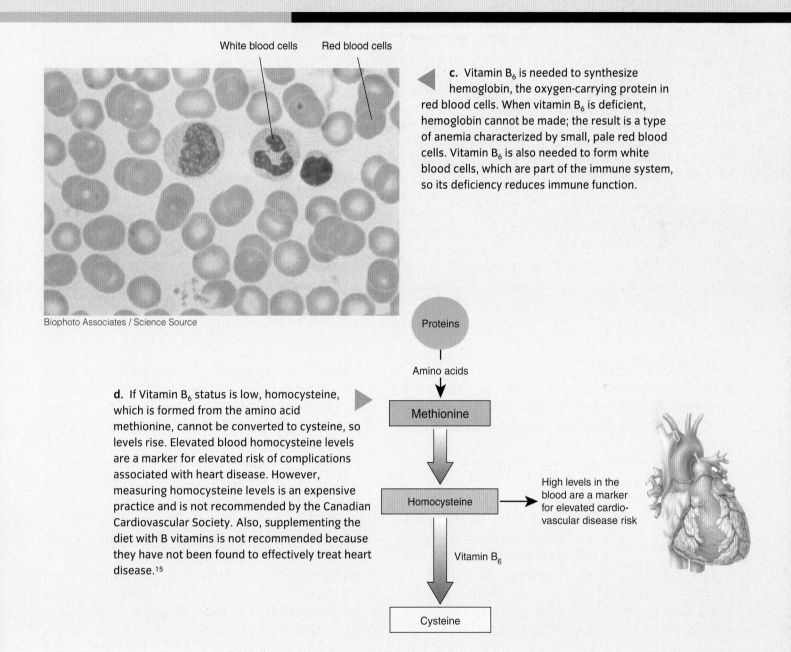

White blood cells   Red blood cells

Biophoto Associates / Science Source

c. Vitamin B$_6$ is needed to synthesize hemoglobin, the oxygen-carrying protein in red blood cells. When vitamin B$_6$ is deficient, hemoglobin cannot be made; the result is a type of anemia characterized by small, pale red blood cells. Vitamin B$_6$ is also needed to form white blood cells, which are part of the immune system, so its deficiency reduces immune function.

d. If Vitamin B$_6$ status is low, homocysteine, which is formed from the amino acid methionine, cannot be converted to cysteine, so levels rise. Elevated blood homocysteine levels are a marker for elevated risk of complications associated with heart disease. However, measuring homocysteine levels is an expensive practice and is not recommended by the Canadian Cardiovascular Society. Also, supplementing the diet with B vitamins is not recommended because they have not been found to effectively treat heart disease.[15]

Proteins

Amino acids

Methionine

Homocysteine → High levels in the blood are a marker for elevated cardiovascular disease risk

Vitamin B$_6$

Cysteine

from food and supplements.[11] Despite the potential for toxicity, high-dose supplements of vitamin B$_6$ are available over the counter, making it easy to obtain a dose that exceeds the UL. People take vitamin B$_6$ supplements to reduce the symptoms of premenstrual syndrome (PMS), treat carpal tunnel syndrome, and strengthen immune function. There is little evidence that supplements consistently relieve the symptoms of carpal tunnel syndrome or provide significant benefit for women with PMS.[16,17] Vitamin B$_6$ supplements have been found to improve immune function in older adults.[11] However, because elderly people frequently have low intakes of vitamin B$_6$, it is unclear whether the beneficial effects of supplements are due to an improvement in vitamin B$_6$ status or to stimulation of the immune system.

The Water-Soluble Vitamins **213**

Meeting vitamin B₆ needs
• Figure 7.14 _____

Animal sources of vitamin B₆ include chicken, fish, pork, and organ meats. Good plant sources include whole-wheat products, brown rice, soybeans, sunflower seeds, and some fruits and vegetables, such as bananas, broccoli, and spinach. The dashed line indicates the RDA for adult men and women ages 19 to 50, which is 1.3 mg/day.[11] The RDA increases with age: Men over 50 years old should consume 1.7 mg/day, and women over 50 years old should consume 1.5 mg/day.

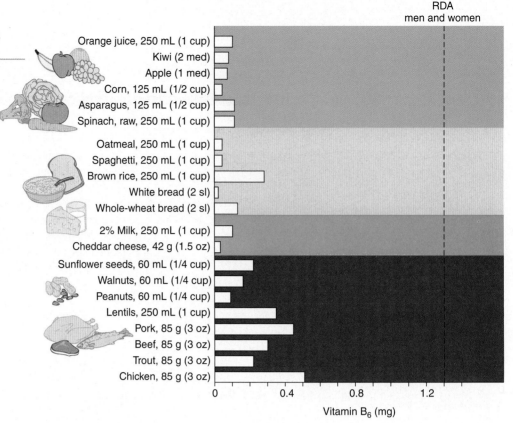

Folate (Folic Acid)

Folate is a B vitamin that is especially important during embryonic development. Low folate intake during pregnancy increases the risk of birth defects called **neural tube defects** (**Figure 7.15**). The formation of the neural tube, which later develops into the brain and spinal cord, occurs very early during pregnancy. Therefore, to reduce the risk of neural tube defects, a woman's folate status must be adequate before she becomes pregnant and during the critical early days of pregnancy. In 1998, to help ensure adequate folate intake in women of childbearing age, the U.S. Food and Drug Administration (FDA) mandated that the **folic acid** form of the vitamin be added to all enriched grains and cereal products. Canada soon followed suit and implemented mandatory fortification at equivalent levels to those set by the FDA. Since then, the incidence of neural tube defects in Canada has decreased by almost 50%, and a 25% reduction has been observed in the United States.[4,5]

Folate and *folacin* are general terms for compounds whose chemical structures and nutritional properties are similar to those of folic acid. The folic acid form, which is added to enriched grains and other fortified products and used in dietary supplements, is more easily absorbed, so its bioavailability is about twice that of folate found naturally in foods. The RDA for folate is expressed in dietary folate equivalents (DFEs). This measure corrects for differences in the bioavailability of different forms of folate. One DFE is equal to 1 microgram (µg) of food folate, 0.6 µg of synthetic folic acid from fortified food or supplements consumed with food, or 0.5 µg of synthetic folic acid consumed on an empty stomach.

Folate-derived coenzymes are needed for the synthesis of DNA and the metabolism of some amino acids. Cells must synthesize DNA in order to replicate, so folate is particularly important in tissues in which cells divide rapidly, such as the intestines, skin, embryonic and fetal tissues, and bone marrow, where red blood cells are made. When folate is deficient, cells cannot divide normally. One of the most notable symptoms of folate deficiency is a type of anemia called **macrocytic anemia**, or **megaloblastic anemia** (**Figure 7.16**). Other symptoms of folate deficiency include poor growth, problems with nerve

neural tube defects Abnormalities in the brain or spinal cord that result from errors that occur during prenatal development.

folic acid An easily absorbed form of the vitamin folate that is used in dietary supplements and fortified foods.

macrocytic anemia or **megaloblastic anemia** A reduction in the blood's capacity to carry oxygen that is characterized by abnormally large immature and mature red blood cells.

Neural tube defects • Figure 7.15

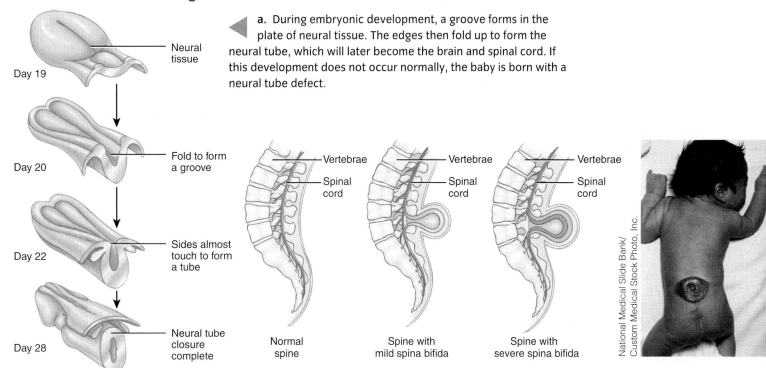

a. During embryonic development, a groove forms in the plate of neural tissue. The edges then fold up to form the neural tube, which will later become the brain and spinal cord. If this development does not occur normally, the baby is born with a neural tube defect.

Day 19 — Neural tissue

Day 20 — Fold to form a groove

Day 22 — Sides almost touch to form a tube

Day 28 — Neural tube closure complete

Vertebrae
Spinal cord

Vertebrae
Spinal cord

Vertebrae
Spinal cord

Normal spine

Spine with mild spina bifida

Spine with severe spina bifida

National Medical Slide Bank/ Custom Medical Stock Photo, Inc.

b. If a lower portion of the neural tube does not close normally, the result is **spina bifida**, a condition in which the spinal cord forms abnormally. Many babies with spina bifida have learning disabilities and nerve damage that causes varying degrees of paralysis of the lower limbs. If the head end of the neural tube does not close properly, the brain doesn't form completely; the result is anencephaly (partial or total absence of the brain). Babies with anencephaly are usually blind, deaf, and unconscious, and they die soon after birth.

Folate deficiency and anemia • Figure 7.16

Folate is needed for DNA replication. Without folate, developing red blood cells cannot divide. Instead, they just grow bigger. The abnormally large immature red blood cells, called megaloblasts, then mature into abnormally large red blood cells called macrocytes. Because fewer mature red cells are produced when folate is deficient, the blood's oxygen-carrying capacity is reduced.

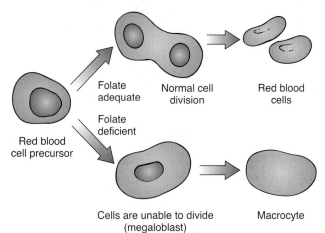

Red blood cell precursor

Folate adequate — Normal cell division — Red blood cells

Folate deficient — Cells are unable to divide (megaloblast) — Macrocyte

development and function, diarrhea, and inflammation of the tongue.

Low folate status may also increase the risk of developing heart disease and cancer of the ovary, pancreas, breast, and colon.[18-20] Folate's connection with heart disease may relate the metabolism of homocysteine. Elevated levels of homocysteine are a predictor of adverse effects associated with heart disease. Adequate intake of folate, vitamin B_{12}, and vitamin B_6 may prevent homocysteine levels from rising, but supplementation with these vitamins does not show a consistent pronounced reduction in disease risk (**Figure 7.17**).[15]

Population groups most at risk of folate deficiency include pregnant women and premature infants (because of their rapid rates of cell division and growth), the elderly (because of their limited intake of foods high in folate), alcoholics (because alcohol inhibits the absorption of folate), and tobacco smokers (because smoke inactivates folate in the cells lining the lungs).[11]

The relationship between folate and vitamin B₁₂ • Figure 7.17

Vitamin B_{12} deficiency prevents folate from being converted into one of its active forms. This interrelationship has raised concerns that our folate-fortified food supply will prevent folate-deficiency symptoms and allow B_{12} deficiencies to go unnoticed. The UL for adults, set at 1000 μg/day of folic acid from supplements and/or fortified foods, is based on an amount that will not mask the macrocytic anemia caused by vitamin B_{12} deficiency.

Supplemental folic acid can prevent macrocytic anemia, thus "hiding" vitamin B_{12} deficiency. Untreated vitamin B_{12} deficiency can cause irreversible nerve damage.

Folic acid from food and supplements

Proteins

Amino acids

Active folate

Inactive folate

Methionine

B_{12}

Homocysteine → High levels in the blood are a marker for elevated cardiovascular disease risk

This form of folate, needed for the synthesis of DNA, cannot be made if vitamin B_{12} is deficient. The resulting folate deficiency causes macrocytic anemia.

Folate and vitamin B_{12} are both needed to convert homocysteine to methionine. When either is deficient, homocysteine levels rise.

Vitamin B_6

Cysteine

Meeting folate needs • Figure 7.18

Folate is named after the Latin word for *foliage* because leafy greens such as spinach are good sources of this vitamin. Fair sources include grains, corn, snap beans, mustard greens, broccoli, and some nuts. Only small amounts of folate are found in meats, cheese, milk, fruits, and other vegetables. The dashed line indicates the RDA for adult men and women, which is 400 μg/day.

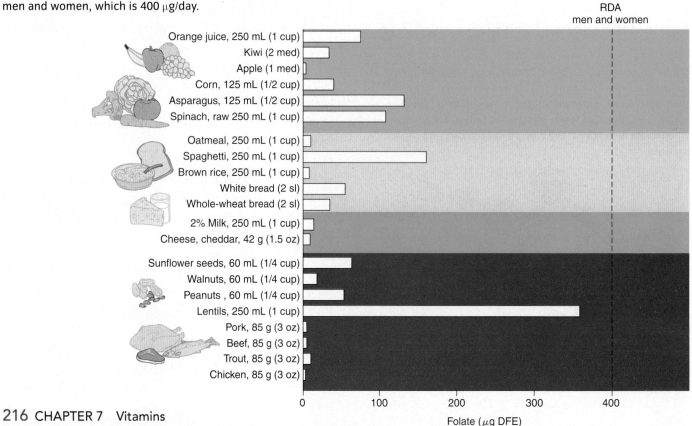

RDA men and women

Orange juice, 250 mL (1 cup)
Kiwi (2 med)
Apple (1 med)
Corn, 125 mL (1/2 cup)
Asparagus, 125 mL (1/2 cup)
Spinach, raw 250 mL (1 cup)

Oatmeal, 250 mL (1 cup)
Spaghetti, 250 mL (1 cup)
Brown rice, 250 mL (1 cup)
White bread (2 sl)
Whole-wheat bread (2 sl)

2% Milk, 250 mL (1 cup)
Cheese, cheddar, 42 g (1.5 oz)

Sunflower seeds, 60 mL (1/4 cup)
Walnuts, 60 mL (1/4 cup)
Peanuts , 60 mL (1/4 cup)
Lentils, 250 mL (1 cup)
Pork, 85 g (3 oz)
Beef, 85 g (3 oz)
Trout, 85 g (3 oz)
Chicken, 85 g (3 oz)

0   100   200   300   400

Folate (μg DFE)

Asparagus, oranges, legumes, liver, and yeast are excellent food sources of folate (**Figure 7.18**). Whole grains are a fair source, and, as discussed earlier, folic acid is added to enriched grain products, including enriched breads, flours, corn meal, pasta, and rice. Because supplementing folic acid early in pregnancy has been shown to reduce neural tube defects in the fetus, *Eating Well with Canada's Food Guide* recommends that women of childbearing age consume a multivitamin that contains folic acid each day.[21]

Vitamin B$_{12}$

In the early 1900s, **pernicious anemia** amounted to a death sentence. There was no cure. In the 1920s, researchers George Minot and William

> **pernicious anemia** A macrocytic anemia resulting from vitamin B$_{12}$ deficiency that occurs when dietary vitamin B$_{12}$ cannot be absorbed due to a lack of intrinsic factor.
>
> **intrinsic factor** A protein produced in the stomach that is needed for the absorption of adequate amounts of vitamin B$_{12}$.

Murphy pursued their belief that pernicious anemia could be cured by adjusting the diet. They discovered that they could restore patients' health by feeding them about 113 to 226 g (4 to 8 oz) of slightly cooked liver at every meal. Today we know that eating liver cured pernicious anemia because liver is a concentrated source of **vitamin B$_{12}$**. Individuals with pernicious anemia lack a protein produced in the stomach called **intrinsic factor** that enhances vitamin B$_{12}$ absorption (**Figure 7.19**). Today, pernicious anemia is treated with injections of vitamin B$_{12}$ rather than with plates full of liver.

Vitamin B$_{12}$, also known as **cobalamin**, is necessary for the production of ATP from certain fatty acids, to convert homocysteine to methionine (see Figure 7.17), and to maintain

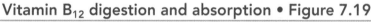

Vitamin B$_{12}$ digestion and absorption • Figure 7.19

✓ THE PLANNER

The body stores and reuses vitamin B$_{12}$ more efficiently than it does most other water-soluble vitamins, so deficiency is typically caused by poor absorption rather than by low intake alone. Absorption of adequate amounts of vitamin B$_{12}$ depends on the presence of stomach acid, protein-digesting enzymes, and intrinsic factor.

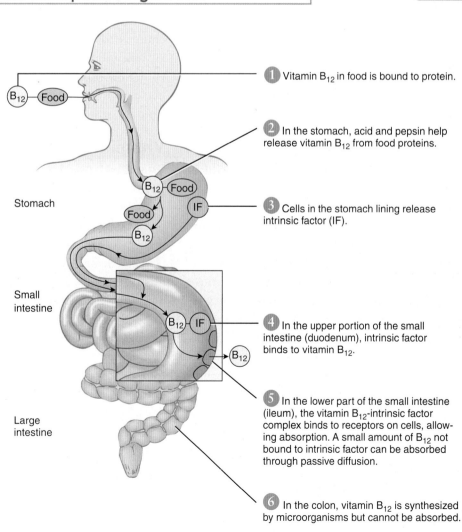

1. Vitamin B$_{12}$ in food is bound to protein.

2. In the stomach, acid and pepsin help release vitamin B$_{12}$ from food proteins.

3. Cells in the stomach lining release intrinsic factor (IF).

4. In the upper portion of the small intestine (duodenum), intrinsic factor binds to vitamin B$_{12}$.

5. In the lower part of the small intestine (ileum), the vitamin B$_{12}$-intrinsic factor complex binds to receptors on cells, allowing absorption. A small amount of B$_{12}$ not bound to intrinsic factor can be absorbed through passive diffusion.

6. In the colon, vitamin B$_{12}$ is synthesized by microorganisms but cannot be absorbed.

217

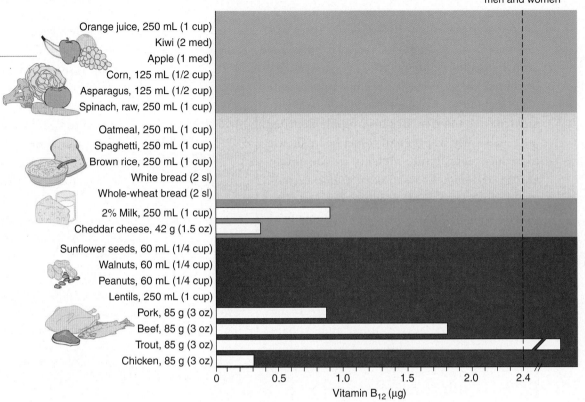

Meeting vitamin B₁₂ needs • Figure 7.20

Animal foods provide vitamin B₁₂, but plant foods do not unless they have been fortified with it or contaminated by bacteria, soil, insects, or other sources of B₁₂. The dashed line indicates the RDA for adult men and women of all ages, which is 2.4 μg/day. No toxic effects have been reported for vitamin B₁₂ intakes of up to 100 μg/day from food or supplements. Insufficient data are available to establish a UL for vitamin B₁₂.[11]

Orange juice, 250 mL (1 cup)
Kiwi (2 med)
Apple (1 med)
Corn, 125 mL (1/2 cup)
Asparagus, 125 mL (1/2 cup)
Spinach, raw, 250 mL (1 cup)

Oatmeal, 250 mL (1 cup)
Spaghetti, 250 mL (1 cup)
Brown rice, 250 mL (1 cup)
White bread (2 sl)
Whole-wheat bread (2 sl)

2% Milk, 250 mL (1 cup)
Cheddar cheese, 42 g (1.5 oz)

Sunflower seeds, 60 mL (1/4 cup)
Walnuts, 60 mL (1/4 cup)
Peanuts, 60 mL (1/4 cup)
Lentils, 250 mL (1 cup)

Pork, 85 g (3 oz)
Beef, 85 g (3 oz)
Trout, 85 g (3 oz)
Chicken, 85 g (3 oz)

RDA men and women

Vitamin B₁₂ (μg)

the myelin coating on nerves (see Figure 7.13B). When vitamin B₁₂ is deficient, homocysteine levels rise, and folate cannot be converted into its active form. The lack of folate causes macrocytic anemia. Lack of vitamin B₁₂ also leads to degeneration of the myelin that coats the nerves in the spinal cord and brain, resulting in symptoms such as numbness and tingling, abnormalities in gait, memory loss, and disorientation. If not treated, vitamin B₁₂ deficiency eventually causes paralysis and death.

Vitamin B₁₂ is found naturally only in animal products (**Figure 7.20**). Therefore, meeting vitamin B₁₂ needs is a concern among vegans—those who consume no animal products. To meet their needs for this vitamin, vegans must consume supplements or foods fortified with vitamin B₁₂.[22] Vitamin B₁₂ deficiency is also a concern in older adults because of a condition called **atrophic gastritis**, which reduces the secretion of stomach acid. Without sufficient stomach acid, the enzymes that release the vitamin B₁₂ bound to proteins in food cannot function properly, so vitamin B₁₂ remains bound to the food proteins and cannot be absorbed (see Figure 7.19). In addition, lack of stomach acid allows large numbers of microbes to grow in the gut and compete for available vitamin B₁₂, reducing

atrophic gastritis An inflammation of the stomach lining that results in reduced secretion of stomach acid, microbial overgrowth, and, in severe cases, a reduction in the production of intrinsic factor.

absorption. Atrophic gastritis affects 10 to 30% of adults over age 50. To ensure adequate B₁₂ absorption, it is recommended that individuals over age 50 meet their RDA by consuming foods fortified with vitamin B₁₂ or taking vitamin B₁₂ supplements.[11] The vitamin B₁₂ in these products is not bound to proteins, so it is absorbed even when stomach acid levels are low.

Vitamin C

Vitamin C, also known as **ascorbic acid**, is best known for its role in the synthesis and maintenance of **collagen** (**Figure 7.21**). Collagen, the most abundant protein in the body, can be thought of as the glue that holds the body together. It forms the base of all connective tissue. It is the framework for bones and teeth; the main component of ligaments, tendons, and the scars that bind a wound together; and it gives structure to the walls of blood vessels. When vitamin C is lacking, collagen cannot be formed and maintained, and the symptoms of **scurvy** appear. In the 17th and 18th centuries, sailors were far more likely to die of scurvy than to be killed in shipwrecks or battles.

scurvy A vitamin C deficiency disease characterized by bleeding gums, tooth loss, joint pain, bleeding into the skin and mucous membranes, and fatigue.

In addition to its role in the synthesis and maintenance of collagen, vitamin C is needed in reactions that synthesize neurotransmitters, hormones, bile acids, and carnitine,

Vitamin C, collagen synthesis, and scurvy
• Figure 7.21

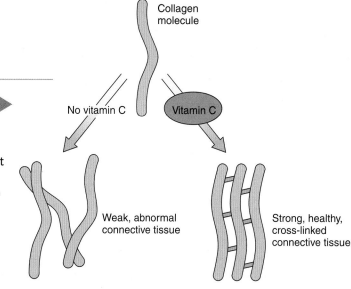

Collagen molecule

No vitamin C

Vitamin C

Weak, abnormal connective tissue

Strong, healthy, cross-linked connective tissue

a. A reaction requiring vitamin C is essential for the formation of bonds that hold adjacent collagen strands together and give the protein strength. Like all other body proteins, collagen is continuously being broken down and reformed. Without vitamin C, the bonds holding adjacent collagen molecules together cannot be formed and maintained, so the collagen that is broken down cannot be replaced. The inability to form healthy collagen causes the symptoms of scurvy.

© Medical-on-Line / Alamy

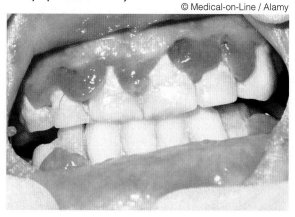

b. When vitamin C intake is below 10 mg/day, the symptoms of scurvy begin to appear. The gums become inflamed, swell, and bleed. The teeth loosen and eventually fall out. The capillary walls weaken and rupture, causing bleeding under the skin and into the joints. This causes raised red spots on the skin, joint pain and weakness, and easy bruising. Wounds do not heal, old wounds may reopen, and bones fracture. People with scurvy become tired and depressed, and they suffer from hysteria.

which is needed for breakdown of fatty acids. It is also an antioxidant that acts in the blood and other body fluids. Because its antioxidant properties help maintain the immune system, the ability to fight infection is decreased when this vitamin is deficient. Vitamin C's antioxidant action also regenerates the active antioxidant form of vitamin E and enhances iron absorption in the small intestine by keeping iron in its more readily absorbed form.

Citrus fruits are an excellent source of vitamin C. A large orange contains enough vitamin C to meet the RDA of 90 mg/day for men and 75 mg/day for women.[4] Other fruits and vegetables are also good sources of this vitamin (**Figure 7.22**).

Vitamin C is destroyed by oxygen, light, and heat, so it is readily lost in cooking. This loss is accelerated in low-acid foods and by the use of copper or iron cooking utensils. Although most Canadians consume enough vitamin C to prevent severe deficiency, marginal vitamin C deficiency is a concern for individuals who consume few fruits and vegetables. Cigarette smoking increases the requirement for vitamin C because the vitamin is used to break down compounds in cigarette smoke. It is recommended that cigarette smokers consume an extra 35 mg of vitamin C daily—an amount that can easily be supplied by 125 g (1/2 cup) of broccoli.[8]

One-third of the population of Canada takes vitamin C supplements,[23] usually in the hope that they will prevent the common cold. Although vitamin C does not prevent colds, it may help reduce the duration and severity of cold symptoms.[24] It has also been suggested that vitamin C supplements reduce the risk of cardiovascular disease and cancer, but there is insufficient evidence to support this claim.[8]

Excessive vitamin C supplementation can cause diarrhea, nausea, and abdominal cramps, and it may increase the risk of kidney stone formation. In individuals who are unable to regulate iron absorption, excess vitamin C can increase absorption, allowing amounts of iron in the body to reach toxic levels. For those with sickle cell anemia, excess vitamin C can worsen symptoms. And doses greater than 3 g/day may interfere with drugs prescribed to slow blood clotting. In chewable form, large doses of vitamin C can dissolve tooth enamel. The UL for vitamin C has been set at 2000 mg/day from food and supplements.[8]

Choline

Choline is a water-soluble substance that you may see included in supplements called "vitamin B complex." It is needed to synthesize several important molecules in the body, including the neurotransmitter acetylcholine, but because choline can be synthesized to a limited extent by humans, it is not currently classified as a vitamin. There is evidence that choline is essential in healthy men and women, but not yet clear is whether choline is also essential in the diets of infants and children.[11,25] The DRIs have set an AI for this compound: 550 mg/day for men, and 425 mg/day for women.[11]

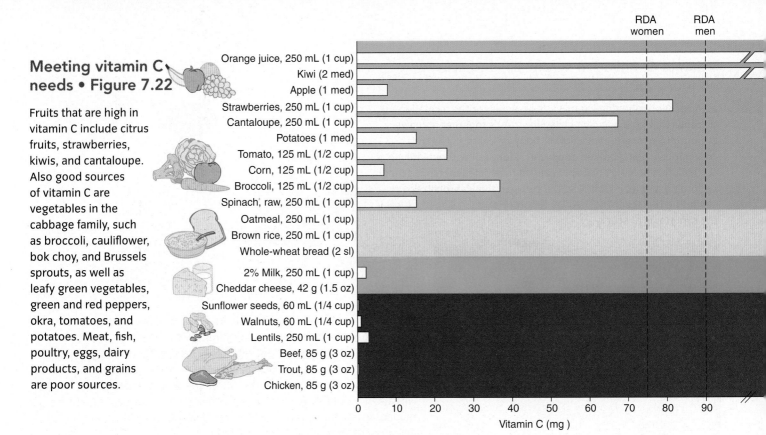

Meeting vitamin C needs • Figure 7.22

Fruits that are high in vitamin C include citrus fruits, strawberries, kiwis, and cantaloupe. Also good sources of vitamin C are vegetables in the cabbage family, such as broccoli, cauliflower, bok choy, and Brussels sprouts, as well as leafy green vegetables, green and red peppers, okra, tomatoes, and potatoes. Meat, fish, poultry, eggs, dairy products, and grains are poor sources.

Orange juice, 250 mL (1 cup)
Kiwi (2 med)
Apple (1 med)
Strawberries, 250 mL (1 cup)
Cantaloupe, 250 mL (1 cup)
Potatoes (1 med)
Tomato, 125 mL (1/2 cup)
Corn, 125 mL (1/2 cup)
Broccoli, 125 mL (1/2 cup)
Spinach, raw, 250 mL (1 cup)
Oatmeal, 250 mL (1 cup)
Brown rice, 250 mL (1 cup)
Whole-wheat bread (2 sl)
2% Milk, 250 mL (1 cup)
Cheddar cheese, 42 g (1.5 oz)
Sunflower seeds, 60 mL (1/4 cup)
Walnuts, 60 mL (1/4 cup)
Lentils, 250 mL (1 cup)
Beef, 85 g (3 oz)
Trout, 85 g (3 oz)
Chicken, 85 g (3 oz)

RDA women   RDA men

Vitamin C (mg)

Choline is found in many foods, including large amounts in egg yolks, broccoli, nuts, and wheat germ. Because the average daily choline intake in Canada exceeds the recommendation, a deficiency is unlikely in healthy Canadians.[11] Excess choline intake can cause a fishy body odour, sweating, reduced growth rate, low blood pressure, and liver damage. The amounts needed to cause these symptoms are much higher than can be obtained from foods. The UL for choline for adults is 3.5 g/day.[11]

Table 7.3 lists the water-soluble vitamins and choline.

A summary of the water-soluble vitamins and choline Table 7.3

Vitamin	Sources	Recommended intake for adults	Major functions	Deficiency diseases and symptoms	Groups at risk of deficiency	Toxicity	UL
Thiamin (vitamin B$_1$, thiamin mononitrate)	Pork, whole and enriched grains, seeds, nuts, legumes	1.1–1.2 mg/day	Part of coenzyme TPP required for glucose and energy metabolism; needed for neurotransmitter synthesis and normal nerve function	Beriberi: weakness, apathy, irritability, nerve tingling, poor coordination, paralysis, heart changes	Alcoholics, those living in poverty	None reported	ND
Riboflavin (vitamin B$_2$)	Dairy products, whole and enriched grains, leafy green vegetables, meats	1.1–1.3 mg/day	Part of coenzymes FAD and FMN required for energy and lipid metabolism	Inflammation of the mouth and tongue, cracks at corners of the mouth	None	None reported	ND
Niacin (nicotinamide, nicotinic acid, vitamin B$_3$)	Beef, chicken, fish, peanuts, legumes, whole and enriched grains; can be made from tryptophan	14–16 mg NE/day	Part of coenzyme NAD required for energy metabolism and lipid synthesis and breakdown	Pellagra: diarrhea, dermatitis on areas exposed to sun, dementia and possibly death	Those consuming a limited diet based on corn; alcoholics	Flushing nausea, rash, tingling extremities	35 mg/day from fortified foods and supplements

Vitamin	Sources	Recommended intake for adults	Major functions	Deficiency diseases and symptoms	Groups at risk of deficiency	Toxicity	UL
Biotin	Liver, egg yolks; synthesized in the gut	30 μg/day	Part of the coenzyme required for replenishing oxaloacetate in the citric acid cycle; required for lipid synthesis	Dermatitis, nausea, depression, hallucinations	Those consuming large amounts of raw egg whites; alcoholics	None reported	ND
Pantothenic acid (calcium pantothenate)	Meat, legumes, whole grains; widespread in foods	5 mg/day	Coenzyme in energy metabolism and lipid synthesis and breakdown	Fatigue, rash	Alcoholics	None reported	ND
Vitamin B$_6$ (pyridoxine, pyridoxal phosphate, pyridoxamine)	Meat, fish, poultry, legumes, whole grains, nuts and seeds	1.3–1.7 mg/day	Part of coenzyme pyridoxal phosphate required for protein and amino acid metabolism, neurotransmitter symptoms, and hemoglobin synthesis, many other reactions	Headache, convulsions, other neurological symptoms, nausea, poor growth, anemia	Women, alcoholics	Numbness, nerve damage	100 mg/day
Folate (folic acid, folacin, pteroylglutamic acid)	Leafy green vegetables, legumes, seeds, enriched grains, orange juice	400 μg DFE/day	Coenzyme in DNA synthesis and amino acid metabolism	Macrocytic anemia, inflammation of tongue, diarrhea, poor growth, neural tube defects	Pregnant women, alcoholics	Masks B$_{12}$ deficiency	1000 μg/day from fortified food and supplements
Vitamin B$_{12}$ (cobalamin, cyano-cobalamin)	Animal products	2.4 μg/day	Coenzyme in folate metabolism; nerve function	Pernicious anemia, macrocytic anemia, nerve damage	Vegans, elderly, people with stomach or intestinal disease	None reported	ND
Vitamin C (ascorbic acid, ascorbate)	Citrus fruit, broccoli, strawberries, greens, peppers	75–90 mg/day	Coenzyme in collagen (connective tissue) synthesis; hormone and neurotransmitter joint synthesis; antioxidant	Scurvy: poor wound healing, bleeding gums, loose teeth, bone fragility, pain, pinpoint hemorrhages	Alcoholics, elderly men	GI distress, diarrhea	2000 mg/day
Choline*	Egg yolks, organ meats, leafy greens, nuts, synthesis in the body	425–550 mg/day	Synthesis of cell membranes and neuro-transmitters	Liver dysfunction	None	Sweating, low blood pressure, liver damage	3500 mg/day

*Choline is technically not a vitamin, but recommendations have been made for its intake.

Note: UL, Tolerable Upper Intake Level; NE, niacin equivalent; DFE, dietary folate equivalent; ND, not determined due to insufficient data.

1. **Why** do people think B vitamin supplements give them energy?

2. **What** is the role of vitamin B_6 in amino acid metabolism?

3. **How** can folate and vitamin B_{12} deficiency both cause macrocytic anemia?

4. **What** is the role of vitamin C in collagen formation?

The Fat-Soluble Vitamins

LEARNING OBJECTIVES

1. **Explain** the role of vitamin A in maintaining healthy eyes.

2. **Relate** the functions of vitamin D to the symptoms that occur when it is deficient in the body.

3. **Describe** the function of vitamin E.

4. **Discuss** how vitamin K is involved in blood clotting.

The fat-soluble vitamins—A, D, E, and K—are found along with fats in foods. They require special handling for absorption into and transport through the body. Because excesses of these vitamins can be stored in the liver and fatty tissues, intakes can vary without a risk of deficiency as long as the average intake over a period of weeks or months meets the body's needs. However, the solubility of these vitamins in fat limits their routes of excretion and therefore increases the risk of toxicity.

Vitamin A

Did you ever hear that eating carrots would help you see in the dark? It turns out to be true. Carrots are a good source of **beta-carotene**, a provitamin that can be converted into vitamin A in your body. **Vitamin A** is needed for vision and healthy eyes.

Vitamin A in the diet Vitamin A is found in our diet both preformed and in provitamin form. Preformed vitamin A compounds, known as retinoids, are derived from animal sources. Three retinoids are active in the body: retinal, retinol, and retinoic acid. **Carotenoids** are yellow-orange pigments found in plants, some of which are vitamin A precursors; once inside the body, they can be converted into retinoids (**Figure 7.23a**). Beta-carotene is the most potent vitamin A precursor. Alpha-carotene and beta-cryptoxanthin are also provitamin A carotenoids, but are not converted into retinoids as efficiently as beta-carotene. Carotenoids that are not converted into retinoids may function as antioxidants and thus may play a role in protecting against cancer and heart disease.

You can meet your needs for vitamin A by eating animal products that are sources of retinoids, such as eggs and dairy products, and by eating fruits and vegetables that are sources of provitamin A carotenoids (**Figure 7.23b**) (see *Thinking It Through: How Much Vitamin A Is in Your Fast-Food Meal?*). Because carotenoids are not absorbed as well as retinoids are and are not completely converted into vitamin A in the body, this form of vitamin A provides less functional vitamin A. To account for this difference, a correction factor, referred to as retinol activity equivalents (RAE), is used to express the amount of usable vitamin A in foods; 1 RAE is the amount of retinol, beta-carotene, alpha-carotene, or beta-cryptoxanthin that provides vitamin A activity equal to 1 μg of retinol (see Appendix H).[26]

Because carotenoids and retinoids must combine with bile acids and other dietary fats in order to be absorbed, vitamin A absorption is impaired when dietary fat intake is very low (less than 10 g/day). However, low fat intake is rarely a problem in Canada and other industrialized countries, where typical fat intake is greater than 50 g/day. In developing countries, vitamin A deficiency may occur not only because the diet is low in vitamin A but also because the diet is too low in fat for the vitamin to be absorbed efficiently. Diseases that cause fat

retinoids The chemical forms of preformed vitamin A: retinol, retinal, and retinoic acid.

carotenoids Natural pigments synthesized by plants and many microorganisms. They give yellow and red-orange fruits and vegetables their colour.

Meeting vitamin A needs • Figure 7.23

a. Provitamin A is found in fruits and vegetables. Beta-carotene is plentiful in carrots, squash, apricots, and other orange and yellow vegetables and fruits. It is also found in leafy green vegetables such as spinach and broccoli, in which the yellow-orange pigment is masked by green chlorophyll. Other carotenoids that provide some provitamin A activity include alpha-carotene, which is found in leafy green vegetables, carrots, and squash, and beta-cryptoxanthin, which is found in papaya, sweet red peppers, and winter squash. To prevent vitamin A deficiency, *Eating Well with Canada's Food Guide* recommends consuming at least one orange and one dark green vegetable a day to help meet your requirements.[21]

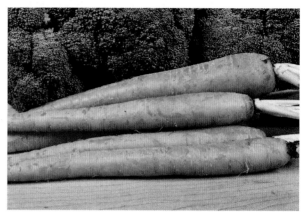

© Can Stock Photo Inc. / miromiro

b. Grains and meats are generally poor sources of vitamin A. The dashed lines indicate the RDA for adult men and women, which are 900 μg/day and 700 μg/day, respectively. No specific recommendations have been made for intakes of carotenoids; their intake is considered only with regard to the amount of retinol they provide.

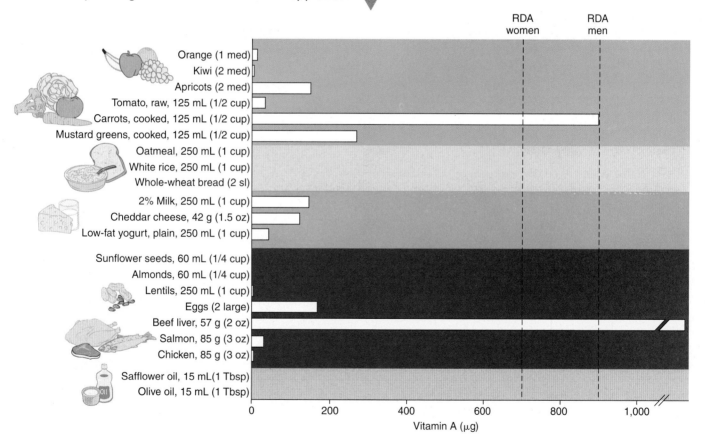

malabsorption can also interfere with vitamin A absorption and cause a deficiency.

Protein and zinc status are also important in preventing vitamin A deficiency. To move from liver stores to other body tissues, vitamin A must be bound to a protein called retinol-binding protein. When protein is deficient, inadequate amounts of retinol-binding protein are made, and vitamin A cannot be transported to the tissues where it is needed. Likewise, when zinc is deficient, a vitamin A deficiency may occur because zinc is needed to make the proteins needed for vitamin A transport and metabolism.

THINKING IT THROUGH 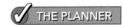 THE PLANNER

How Much Vitamin A Is in Your Fast-Food Meal?

John lives on his own, goes to school, and works part-time. He eats breakfast at home and usually takes a sandwich for lunch; dinner is always fast food. He recently heard that fast food is low in some vitamins, particularly vitamin A. To check on his vitamin A intake, John uses iProfile to look up the nutrient compositions of his favourite fast-food meals.

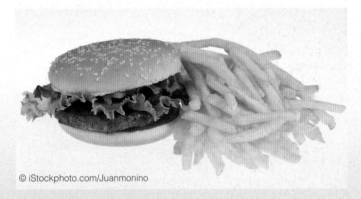

© iStockphoto.com/Juanmonino

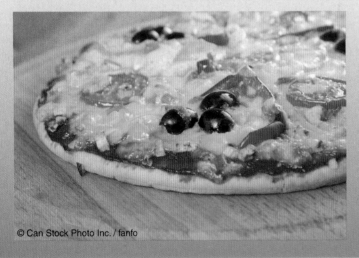

© Can Stock Photo Inc. / fanfo

Which of the meals shown here is higher in vitamin A? Which ingredients are sources of the vitamin?
▼

Your answer: _____

_____

John doesn't want to give up his fast food, so he looks at his other meals to make sure they provide plenty of vitamin A. For breakfast, he has Cheerios with milk, toast with jam, and coffee; for lunch, he packs a ham-and-cheese sandwich on whole-wheat bread, potato chips, an apple, and a pop.

Which foods in John's breakfast and lunch are good sources of vitamin A?
▼

The cereal is fortified with vitamin A, and the milk and cheese also contain vitamin A. The bread, meat, and chips contain little or none. Together, these foods provide only about 20% of the vitamin A John should consume on an average day.

What can John add to his breakfast and lunch to provide some good sources of vitamin A? What can he swap out of his meals for these foods so he does not overconsume?
▼

Your answer: _____

_____

John's meals are also low in vitamin C. What can he add to his breakfast and lunch to increase his intake of vitamin C?
▼

Your answer: _____

_____

(Check your answers in Appendix I.)

Vitamin A functions and deficiency Vitamin A is needed for vision and eye health because it is involved in the perception of light and because it is needed for normal **cell differentiation**, the process whereby immature cells change in structure and function to become specialized.

Vitamin A helps us see because retinal is part of **rhodopsin**, a visual pigment in the eye. When light strikes rhodopsin, it initiates a series of events that result in a nerve signal being sent to the brain, which allows us to see (**Figure 7.24**). After the light stimulus has passed,

rhodopsin is re-formed. Because some retinal is lost in these reactions, it must be replaced by vitamin A from the blood. If blood levels of vitamin A are low, as they are in someone who is vitamin A deficient, the regeneration of rhodopsin is delayed. This delay causes difficulty seeing in dim light, a condition called **night blindness**. Night blindness is one of the first and most easily reversible symptoms of vitamin A deficiency. If the deficiency progresses, more serious and less reversible symptoms can occur.

The visual cycle • Figure 7.24

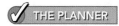

Looking into the bright headlights of an approaching car at night can lead to temporary blindness in all of us, but for someone with vitamin A deficiency, the blindness lasts longer. This blindness occurs because of the role of vitamin A in the visual cycle.

1. Light strikes the visual pigment rhodopsin, which is formed by combining retinal with the protein opsin.

2. The retinal molecule changes from a bent to a straight configuration.

3. A nerve signal is sent to the brain, telling us that there is light, and retinal is released from opsin.

4. Some retinal is lost from the cycle.

5. Some retinal returns to its original configuration and binds opsin to begin the cycle again.

6. When vitamin A status is normal, vitamin A from the blood replaces any retinal lost from the cycle.

7. When vitamin A is deficient, not enough vitamin A is available in the blood, and the regeneration of rhodopsin is delayed. Until it is reformed, light cannot be perceived.

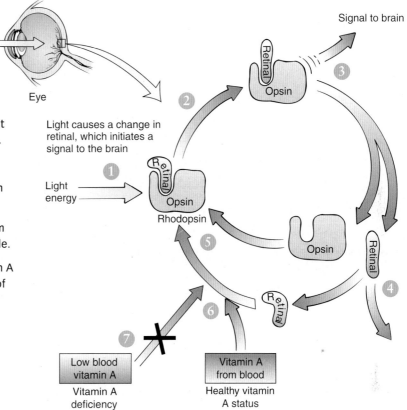

Vitamin A affects cell differentiation through its role in **gene expression**: It can turn certain genes on or off. When a specific gene is turned on, it instructs the cell to make a particular protein. Proteins have structural and regulatory functions within cells and throughout the body. This turning on (or off) of specific genes increases (or decreases) the production of certain proteins and thereby affects various cellular and body functions. By affecting gene expression, vitamin A can determine what type of cell an immature cell will become.

gene expression The events of protein synthesis in which the information coded in a gene is used to synthesize a protein.

The carotenoid form of vitamin A can act as an antioxidant in the body. Like other antioxidants, it is implicated in the reduction in risk of cancer, heart disease, and type-2 diabetes.

Vitamin A is necessary for the maintenance of epithelial tissue, which makes up the skin, and the tissues that line the eyes, intestines, lungs, vagina, and bladder. When vitamin A is deficient, epithelial cells do not differentiate normally because vitamin A is not available to turn on or off the production of particular proteins. All epithelial tissues are affected by vitamin A deficiency, but the eye is particularly susceptible (**Figure 7.25**). Eye disorders that are associated with vitamin A deficiency are collectively known as **xerophthalmia**. Night blindness is an early stage of xerophthalmia and can be treated by increasing vitamin A intake. If left untreated, xerophthalmia affects the epithelial lining of the eye and can result in permanent blindness.

xerophthalmia A spectrum of eye conditions resulting from vitamin A deficiency that may lead to blindness.

The ability of vitamin A to regulate the growth and differentiation of cells makes it essential throughout life for normal reproduction, growth, and immune function. In reproduction, vitamin A is needed to direct cells to differentiate and to form the shapes and patterns needed

The Fat-Soluble Vitamins **225**

The lining of the eye normally contains cells that secrete mucus, which lubricates the eye. When these cells die, immature cells differentiate to become new mucus-secreting cells that replace the dead cells. Without vitamin A, the immature cells can't differentiate normally, and instead of becoming mucus-secreting cells, they become cells that produce a hard protein called keratin.

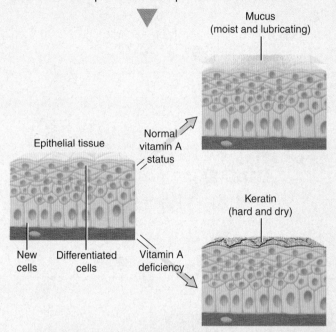

Mucus
(moist and lubricating)

Epithelial tissue

New cells

Differentiated cells

Normal vitamin A status

Keratin
(hard and dry)

Vitamin A deficiency

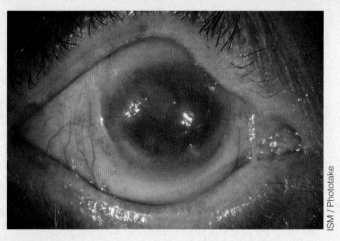

ISM / Phototake

When mucus-secreting cells are replaced by keratin-producing cells, the surface of the eye becomes dry and cloudy. As xerophthalmia progresses, the drying of the cornea results in ulceration and infection. If left untreated, the damage is irreversible and causes permanent blindness.

Ask Yourself

On which continents is clinical vitamin A deficiency most prevalent?

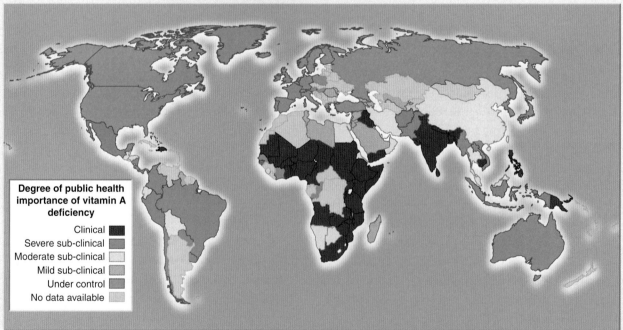

Degree of public health importance of vitamin A deficiency

- Clinical
- Severe sub-clinical
- Moderate sub-clinical
- Mild sub-clinical
- Under control
- No data available

Vitamin A deficiency is a threat to the health, sight, and lives of millions of children in the developing world. Clinical cases of deficiency where the individual shows noticeable symptoms such as night-blindness are easier to detect. Many individuals who currently aren't showing symptoms are still moderately or severely deficient in the vitamin and are at high risk for developing clinical signs of deficiency in the future. It is estimated that more than 250 million preschool children worldwide have vitamin A deficiency, and that 250,000 to 500,000 children go blind annually due to vitamin A deficiency. Children who are deficient in vitamin A have poor appetites, are anemic, are more susceptible to infections, and are more likely to die in childhood.[27]

Vitamin A and carotenoid toxicity • Figure 7.26

a. Foods generally do not naturally contain large enough amounts of nutrients to be toxic. Polar bear liver is an exception. It contains about 100,000 μg of vitamin A in just 28 g (1 oz) and can cause vitamin A toxicity. In Canada, the hunting of polar bears is restricted to Aboriginal people or sport hunters under the direction of Aboriginal people, in accordance with conservation practices. Aboriginal people are typically aware of the toxicity from polar bear liver, and it is rarely consumed. Although polar bear liver is not a common dish at most dinner tables, supplements of preformed vitamin A also have the potential to deliver a toxic dose.

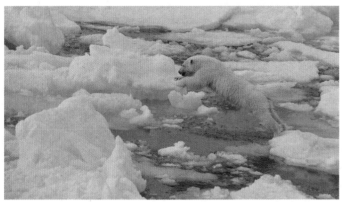

© Can Stock Photo Inc. / vlad2000

b. Because preformed vitamin A can be toxic, supplements typically contain beta-carotene. Carotenoids are not toxic because when they are consumed in high doses, their absorption from the diet decreases, and their conversion to active vitamin A is limited. Beta-carotene supplements or regular consumption of large amounts of carrot juice, however, can cause hypercarotenemia. This harmless buildup of carotenoids in the adipose tissue makes the skin look yellow-orange, particularly on the palms of the hands and the soles of the feet.

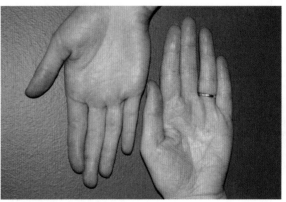

New Zealand Dermatological Society Incorporated. DermNetNZ.org

for the development of a complete organism. In growing children, vitamin A affects the activity of cells that form and break down bone; a deficiency early in life can cause abnormal jawbone growth, resulting in crooked teeth and poor dental health. In the immune system, vitamin A is needed for the differentiation that produces the different types of immune cells. When vitamin A is deficient, the activity of specific immune cells cannot be stimulated; the result is increased susceptibility to infections.

Vitamin A toxicity The retinoid form of vitamin A found in animal sources is toxic in large doses, causing symptoms such as nausea, vomiting, headache, dizziness, blurred vision, and a lack of muscle coordination (**Figure 7.26a**). Excess vitamin A is a particular concern for pregnant women because it may contribute to birth defects. Derivatives of vitamin A that are used to treat acne (Retin A and Accutane) should never be used by pregnant women because they cause birth defects. High intakes of vitamin A have also been found to increase the incidence of bone fractures.[28] The UL is set at 2800 μg/day of preformed vitamin A for 14- to 18-year-olds and 3000 μg/day for adults.[25]

Although plant-derived carotenoids are not considered toxic, large daily intakes can lead to a condition known as **hypercarotenemia** (**Figure 7.26b**). Beta-carotene supplements have also been associated with an increase in lung cancer in cigarette smokers.[29] Therefore, smokers are advised to avoid beta-carotene supplements and to instead rely on food sources to obtain carotenoids in their diet. There is no UL for carotenoids, and the small amounts found in standard-strength multivitamin supplements are not likely to be harmful for any group.

> **hypercarotenemia**
> A condition caused by the accumulation of carotenoids in the adipose tissue, causing the skin to appear yellow-orange.

Vitamin D

Vitamin D is known as the sunshine vitamin because it can be made in the skin with exposure to ultraviolet (UV) light. Because vitamin D can be made in the body, it is especially essential in the diet when exposure to sunlight is limited or the body's ability to synthesize it is reduced.

Vitamin D functions and deficiency Vitamin D, whether from the diet or from synthesis in the skin, is inactive until it is modified by biochemical reactions

Vitamin D activation and function • Figure 7.27

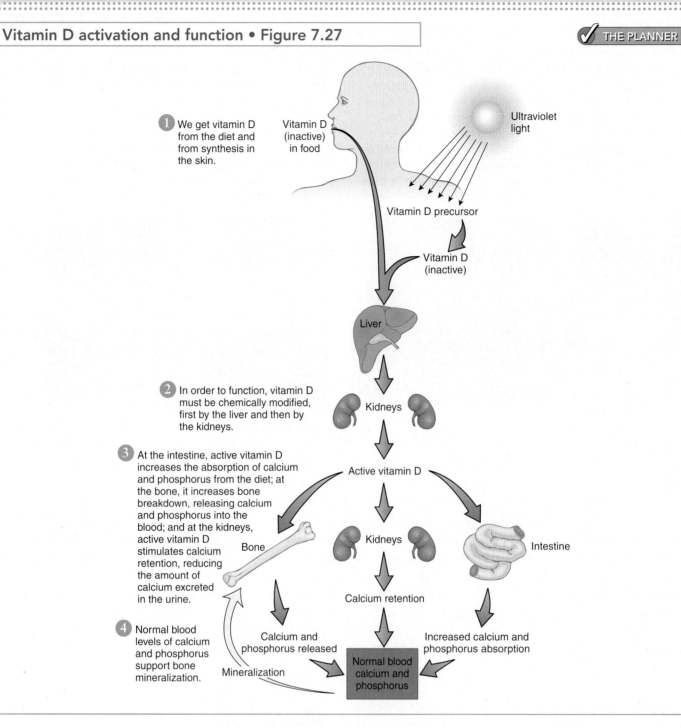

1 We get vitamin D from the diet and from synthesis in the skin.

Vitamin D (inactive) in food

Ultraviolet light

Vitamin D precursor

Vitamin D (inactive)

Liver

2 In order to function, vitamin D must be chemically modified, first by the liver and then by the kidneys.

Kidneys

3 At the intestine, active vitamin D increases the absorption of calcium and phosphorus from the diet; at the bone, it increases bone breakdown, releasing calcium and phosphorus into the blood; and at the kidneys, active vitamin D stimulates calcium retention, reducing the amount of calcium excreted in the urine.

Active vitamin D

Bone

Kidneys

Intestine

Calcium retention

4 Normal blood levels of calcium and phosphorus support bone mineralization.

Calcium and phosphorus released

Increased calcium and phosphorus absorption

Mineralization

Normal blood calcium and phosphorus

---

in both the liver and the kidney (**Figure 7.27**). Active vitamin D is needed to maintain normal levels of the minerals calcium and phosphorus in the blood. Calcium is important for bone health, but also has many additional critical functions in the body, such as nerve conduction, muscle contraction, and glandular secretion. Blood levels of calcium are regulated so that a steady supply of the mineral is available when and where it is needed.

When calcium levels in the blood drop too low, the body responds immediately to ensure the continuation of critical processes, such as heart contraction. The response starts with the release of **parathyroid hormone (PTH)**, which stimulates the activation of vitamin D by the kidney. Active vitamin D enters the blood and travels to its major target tissues—intestine and bone—where it acts to increase the blood's calcium and phosphorus levels (see Figure 7.27). Vitamin D, like vitamin A, acts through its role

parathyroid hormone (PTH)
A hormone released by the parathyroid gland that acts to increase blood calcium levels.

Vitamin D deficiency • Figure 7.28

The vitamin D deficiency disease rickets causes short stature and bone deformities. The characteristic bowed legs occur because the bones are too weak to support the body. It is seen in children with poor diets and little exposure to sunlight, in those who have disorders that affect fat absorption, and in some vegan children who do not receive adequate exposure to sunlight.[32]

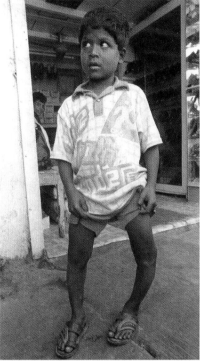

RAFIQUR RAHMAN/REUTERS /Landov

in gene expression. In the intestine, it turns on genes that make a protein that is needed for the absorption of calcium. In the bone, it turns on genes that are needed for the differentiation of cells that break down bone.

rickets A vitamin D deficiency disease in children, characterized by poor bone development resulting from inadequate calcium absorption.

osteomalacia A vitamin D deficiency disease in adults, characterized by loss of minerals from bone, bone pain, muscle aches, and an increase in bone fractures.

When vitamin D is deficient, only about 10 to 15% of the calcium in the diet can be absorbed. Since bone is broken down to maintain calcium levels, a lack of adequate calcium can compromise bone structure. In children, vitamin D deficiency is called **rickets**; it is characterized by narrow rib cages known as pigeon breasts and by bowed legs (**Figure 7.28**). In adults, vitamin D deficiency disease is called **osteomalacia**. It does not cause bone deformities because adults are no longer growing, but bones are weakened because not enough calcium is available to form bone-strengthening mineral deposits. Insufficient bone mineralization leads to fractures of the weight-bearing bones, such as those in the hips and spine. This lack of calcium in bones can precipitate or exacerbate **osteoporosis**, which is a loss of total bone mass, not just minerals (discussed

further in Chapter 8). Osteomalacia is common in adults with kidney failure because the conversion of vitamin D to the active form is reduced in these patients.

Vitamin D has recently garnered increasing attention for its potential ability to reduce chronic disease risk and promote health. Vitamin D deficiency has been hypothesized to contribute to an increased risk of cancer, cardiovascular disease, type-2 diabetes, and autoimmune disorders.[30] Recent evidence, however, is mixed and inconclusive; it is unclear whether vitamin D provides benefits beyond its role in bone health.[31]

Meeting vitamin D needs Vitamin D is not widespread in the diet. It is found naturally in liver, egg yolks, and oily fish such as salmon (**Figure 7.29a**). Foods fortified with vitamin D include milk, margarine, and some yogurts, and cheeses. The major source of vitamin D for most humans is exposure to sunlight.[33] Anything that interferes with the transmission of UV radiation to the earth's surface or its penetration into the skin will affect the synthesis of vitamin D. Therefore, individuals who do not spend time outdoors, or those who cover their skin when they are outdoors are at risk of vitamin D deficiency (**Figure 7.29b–d**).

The exposure to UV radiation is also affected by the time of year and the geographical location of the area. For instance, the high latitude at which Canada is located limits our year-round absorption of vitamin D. From October to March, vitamin D synthesis due to sunlight exposure is absent, and dietary intake or supplementation is recommended. At latitudes that are farther north, a longer supplementation period may be required over the winter months.

The recommended intake of vitamin D for men and women aged 9 to 70 is now 15 μg/day (up from 5 μg/day) to reflect its critical necessity in the human body.[33] This RDA has been set on the assumption that minimal vitamin D is synthesized in the skin. The recommended intake is increased for older adults: 20 μg/day for those over the age of 70.[33]

Too much vitamin D in the body is toxic as it can cause high calcium concentrations in the blood and urine, deposition of calcium in soft tissues such as the blood vessels and kidneys, and cardiovascular damage. Synthesis of vitamin D from exposure to sunlight does not produce toxic amounts because the body regulates vitamin D formation. The UL for adults for vitamin D is currently 100 μg (4000 IU)/day.[33]

The Fat-Soluble Vitamins **229**

a. Only a few foods are natural sources of vitamin D. Without adequate sun exposure, supplements, or fortified foods, it is difficult to meet the body's needs for this vitamin. The dashed line indicates the AI for children and adults ages 9 to 70, which is 15 µg/day. The requirement is expressed in µg, but the vitamin D content of foods and supplements may also be given as International Units (IUs); one IU is equal to 0.025 µg of vitamin D (40 IU = 1 µg of vitamin D; see Appendix H).

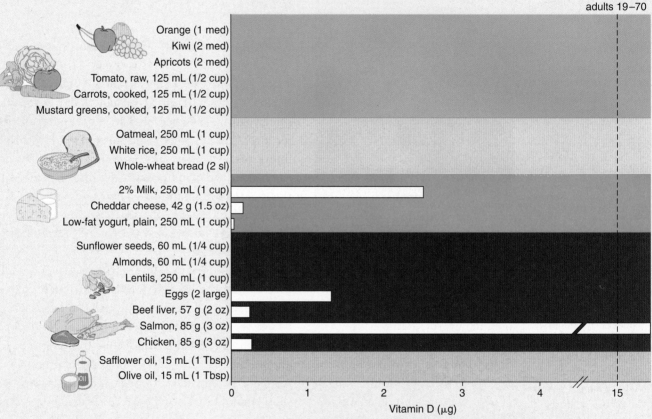

b. The angle at which the sun strikes the earth affects the body's ability to synthesize vitamin D in the skin. During the winter, at latitudes greater than about 40 degrees north or south, there is not enough UV radiation to synthesize adequate amounts. Since Canada is located entirely above 40 degrees north, Canadians are at risk for vitamin D deficiency between October and March. However, for the remaining months at 42 degrees latitude, as little as 5 to 10 minutes of midday sun exposure three times weekly can provide a light-skinned individual with adequate vitamin D.[34]

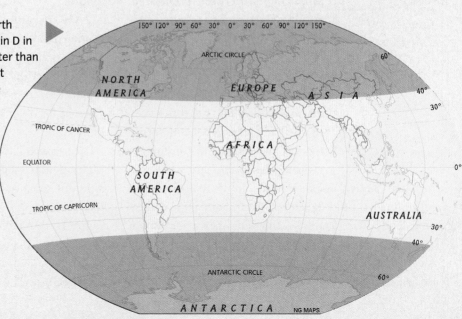

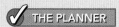

c. Sunscreen with an SPF of 15 will decrease vitamin D synthesis by 99%.[35] Sunscreen is important for reducing the risk of skin cancer, but some time in the sun without sunscreen may be needed to meet vitamin D needs. In the summer, children and active adults usually spend enough time outdoors without sunscreen to meet their vitamin D requirements. ▼

d. Dark skin pigmentation prevents UV light rays from penetrating into the layers of the skin where vitamin D is formed and reduces the body's ability to make vitamin D in the skin by as much as 99%. Dark-skinned individuals living in temperate climates have a higher rate of vitamin D deficiency than do those living near the equator. ▼

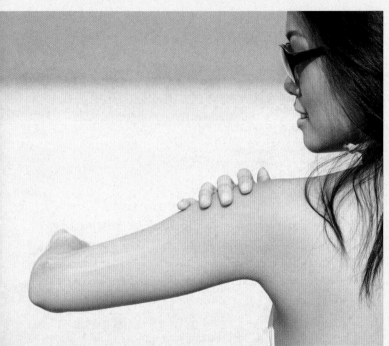

© Can Stock Photo Inc. / EastWestImaging

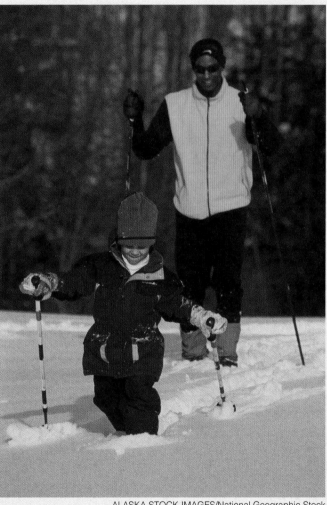

ALASKA STOCK IMAGES/National Geographic Stock

◄ **e.** Concealing clothing worn by certain cultural and religious groups prevents sunlight from striking the skin, which explains why vitamin D deficiency is common in women and children in some of the sunniest regions of the world. Elderly people also typically cover their skin with clothing when they are outdoors. Risk of vitamin D deficiency in elderly people is further compounded because they typically consume a diet that is low in vitamin D, and the ability to synthesize vitamin D in the skin declines with age. As a result, the new DRIs recommend that adults 70 years of age and older consume 5 μg per day more than younger adults.

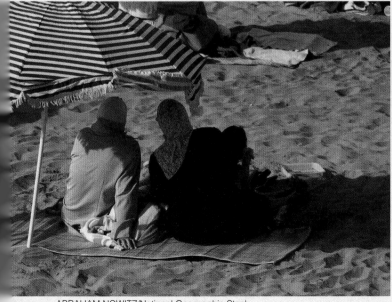

ABRAHAM NOWITZ/National Geographic Stock

The antioxidant role of vitamin E • Figure 7.30

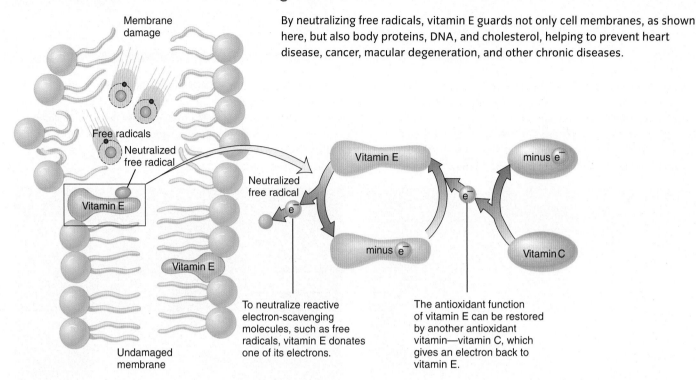

Membrane damage

By neutralizing free radicals, vitamin E guards not only cell membranes, as shown here, but also body proteins, DNA, and cholesterol, helping to prevent heart disease, cancer, macular degeneration, and other chronic diseases.

Free radicals

Neutralized free radical

Vitamin E

Neutralized free radical

Vitamin E

minus e⁻

e⁻

minus e⁻

Vitamin E

minus e⁻

Vitamin C

Vitamin E

Undamaged membrane

To neutralize reactive electron-scavenging molecules, such as free radicals, vitamin E donates one of its electrons.

The antioxidant function of vitamin E can be restored by another antioxidant vitamin—vitamin C, which gives an electron back to vitamin E.

Vitamin E

Vitamin E is an antioxidant that protects lipids throughout the body by neutralizing reactive oxygen compounds before they can cause damage (**Figure 7.30**). Vitamin E protects membranes in red blood cells, white blood cells, nerve cells, and lung cells, where it is particularly important because oxygen concentrations in lung cells are high.[36] Vitamin E can also defend cells against damage caused by heavy metals, such as lead and mercury, and toxins, such as carbon tetrachloride, benzene, and a variety of drugs.

Vitamin E deficiency Because vitamin E is needed to protect cell membranes, a deficiency causes those membranes to break down. Red blood cells and nerve tissue are particularly susceptible. As a result of a vitamin E deficiency, red blood cell membranes may rupture, causing a type of anemia called **hemolytic anemia**, which is most common in premature infants. All newborn infants have low blood levels of vitamin E because little of this vitamin is transferred from mother to fetus until the last weeks of pregnancy. The vitamin E levels are lower in premature infants because they are born before much vitamin E has been transferred from the mother. To prevent vitamin E deficiency in premature infants, special formulas for these infants contain higher amounts of vitamin E.

Vitamin E deficiency is rare in adults, occurring only when other health problems interfere with fat absorption, which reduces vitamin E absorption. In such cases, the vitamin E deficiency is usually characterized by symptoms associated with nerve degeneration, such as poor muscle coordination, weakness, and impaired vision.

The antioxidant role of vitamin E suggests that it may help reduce the risk of cancer, heart disease, Alzheimer's disease, macular degeneration, and a variety of other chronic diseases associated with oxidative damage. Particular attention has been paid to vitamin E's potential benefits in guarding against heart disease. In addition to its antioxidant function, vitamin E has anti-inflammatory properties, and may be involved in the immune response, help regulate genes that affect both cell growth and death, and help detoxify harmful sustances.[37] However, studies that have examined the association between vitamin E intake and cardiovascular disease have shown mixed results.[37,38] Also, no conclusive evidence has been found that supplementing with vitamin E promotes a reduced risk of cardiovascular disease or other chronic disease.[38] It seems that the best approach is to get plenty of dietary vitamin E (see *What Should I Eat?*).[38]

Meeting vitamin E needs Nuts, seeds, and plant oils are the best sources of vitamin E; fortified products such as breakfast cereals also make a significant contribution to our vitamin E intake (**Figure 7.31**). The need for vitamin E

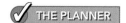

WHAT SHOULD I EAT?

Vitamins

Focus on foliage for folate, vitamin A, and vitamin K
- Have a heaping helping of leafy greens.
- Snack on an orange—you'll get some folate.
- Add lentils and kidney beans to soups and stews.
- Utilize a hidden source of beta-carotene by eating something dark green and leafy.

B (vitamin) sure
- Don't forget the whole grains to get vitamin B_6.
- Enrich your diet with some enriched grains.
- Start your day with a bowl of fortified breakfast cereal.

Get your antioxidants
- Go with nuts and seeds to increase your vitamin E.
- Think colour when choosing your fruits and veggies each day.
- Add carrot sticks to your lunch to increase your vitamin A intake.
- Savour some strawberries and kiwis for dessert—they are loaded with vitamin C.

Soak up some D
- Get outside to stay fit and make some vitamin D.
- Have three servings of dairy per day to ensure that you get enough vitamin D.

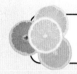

Use iProfile to calculate your vitamin C intake for a day.

Meeting vitamin E needs • Figure 7.31

Dietary sources of vitamin E include sunflower seeds, nuts, peanuts, and refined plant oils such as canola, safflower, and sunflower oils. Vitamin E is also found in leafy green vegetables, such as spinach and mustard greens, and in wheat germ. The dashed line represents the RDA for adults of 15 mg alpha-tocopherol/day.

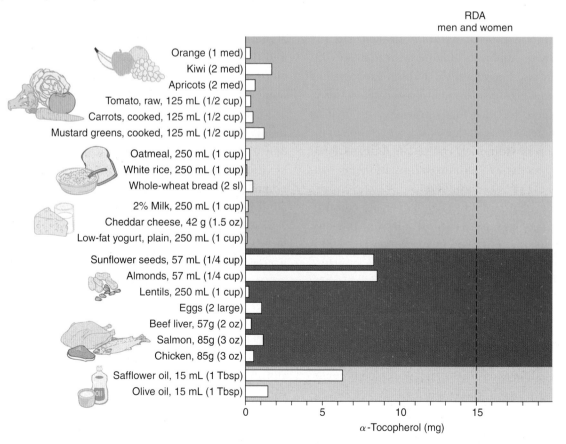

Vitamin K and blood clotting • Figure 7.32

Blood clotting requires a series of reactions that result in the formation of a fibrous protein called **fibrin**. Fibrin fibres form a net that traps platelets and blood cells and forms the structure of a blood clot. With a vitamin K deficiency, several of the clotting factors, including **prothrombin**, are not made correctly, and the blood will not clot.

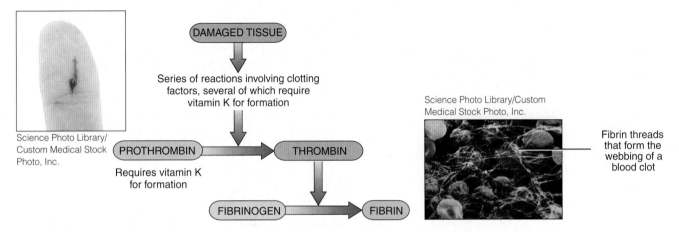

Science Photo Library/ Custom Medical Stock Photo, Inc.

DAMAGED TISSUE

Series of reactions involving clotting factors, several of which require vitamin K for formation

PROTHROMBIN → THROMBIN

Requires vitamin K for formation

FIBRINOGEN → FIBRIN

Science Photo Library/Custom Medical Stock Photo, Inc.

Fibrin threads that form the webbing of a blood clot

increases as polyunsaturated fat intake increases because polyunsaturated fats are particularly susceptible to oxidative damage; fortunately, polyunsaturated oils are one of the best sources of dietary vitamin E. However, vitamin E is sensitive to destruction by oxygen, metals, light, and heat, so when vegetable oils are repeatedly used for deep-fat frying, most of their vitamin E is destroyed.

The chemical name for vitamin E is **tocopherol**. Several forms of vitamin E occur naturally in food, but the body can use only the alpha-tocopherol form to meet vitamin E requirements. Therefore, the RDA is expressed as mg of alpha-tocopherol. Synthetic alpha-tocopherol used in supplements and fortified foods provides only half as much vitamin E activity as the natural form. Supplement labels often express vitamin E content in International Units (IUs). Appendix H contains information for converting IUs into mg of beta-tocopherol.

There is no evidence of adverse effects from consuming large amounts of vitamin E naturally present in foods. The amounts typically contained in supplements are also safe for most people; however, large doses can interfere with blood clotting, so individuals taking blood-thinning medications should not take vitamin E supplements. The UL is 1000 mg/day from supplemental sources.

Vitamin K

Blood is a fluid that flows easily through your blood vessels, but when you cut yourself, blood must solidify, or clot, to stop the bleeding. **Vitamin K** is needed for the production of several blood proteins called clotting factors that cause blood to clot (**Figure 7.32**). The *K* in vitamin K comes from the Danish word for coagulation, *koagulation*, which means "blood clotting." Abnormal blood coagulation is the major symptom of vitamin K deficiency. Without vitamin K, even a bruise or small scratch could cause you to bleed to death (**Figure 7.33**).

Vitamin K is also needed for the synthesis of several proteins involved in bone formation and breakdown. With a vitamin K deficiency, bone mineral density is reduced, and the risk of fractures increases.[39] Therefore, adequate vitamin K may be important for the prevention or treatment of osteoporosis.[40]

Unlike other fat-soluble vitamins, the body uses vitamin K rapidly, so a constant supply is necessary. Although only a small number of foods provide a significant amount of vitamin K, typical intakes in North America meet recommendations, and deficiency is very rare in the healthy adult population (**Figure 7.34**) Another source of vitamin K is synthesis by bacteria in the intestine. Deficiency can be precipitated by long-term antibiotic use, which kills the bacteria in the gastrointestinal tract that synthesize the vitamin. Newborns are at risk of deficiency because when a baby is born, no bacteria are present in the gut to synthesize vitamin K. Also, little vitamin K is transferred to the baby from the mother before birth, and breast milk is a poor source of this vitamin. To ensure normal blood clotting, infants are typically given a vitamin K injection within six hours of birth.

A summary of the fat-soluble vitamins is provided in **Table 7.4.**

The benefits and risks of anticoagulation agents • Figure 7.33

Warfarin is a potent compound used to eliminate some unwanted houseguests. Interestingly, this same rat poison can also be used to save lives. In 1941, Dr. Frank Schofield, working out of the Ontario Veterinary College, noticed that cattle that were ingesting mouldy clover hay were bleeding excessively. This critical discovery later led to the discovery of the vitamin K inhibitor warfarin and its derivative, dicoumarol. Warfarin is an anticoagulant, which means it prevents blood from clotting. When rats eat warfarin, minor bumps and scrapes cause them to bleed to death.

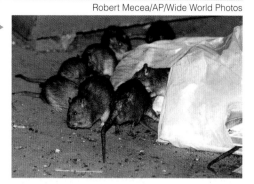
Robert Mecea/AP/Wide World Photos

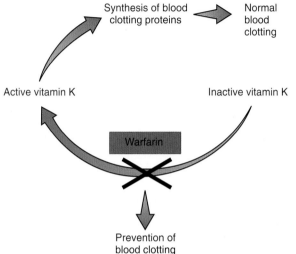

Think Critically Why might patients taking warfarin need to avoid vitamin K supplements?

Blood clot formation is essential to survival, but blood clots in the arteries cause heart attacks and strokes, which kill approximately 30,000 Canadians annually.[41] Scientists have taken advantage of what they learned about dicoumarol and vitamin K and have used this knowledge to save human lives. Dicoumarol was the first anticoagulant used in humans that could be taken orally rather than by injection. In the 1950s, the more potent anticoagulant, warfarin, also known by the brand name Coumadin, was developed and is still used today to treat heart attack patients.

Meeting vitamin K needs • Figure 7.34

Leafy green vegetables, such as spinach, broccoli, Brussels sprouts, kale, and turnip greens, and some vegetable oils are good sources of vitamin K. The dashed lines indicate the AI for adult men and women, which are 120 µg/day and 90 µg/day, respectively.

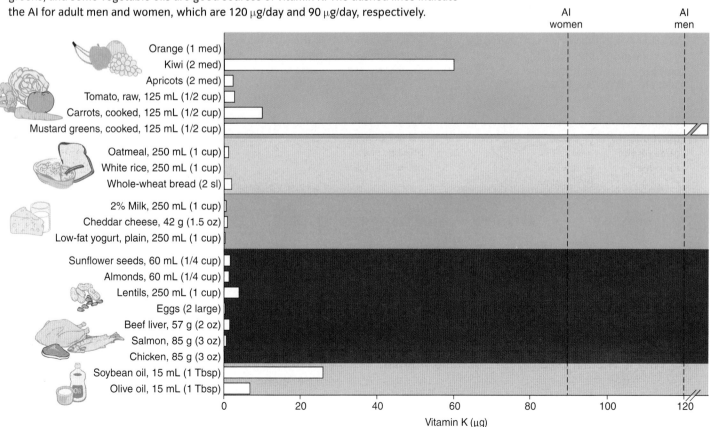

A summary of the fat-soluble vitamins   Table 7.4

Vitamin	Sources	Recommended intake for adults	Major functions	Deficiency diseases and symptoms	Groups at risk of deficiency	Toxicity	UL
Vitamin A (retinol, retinal, retinoic acid, vitamin A acetate, vitamin A palmitate, retinyl palmitate, provitamin A, carotene, beta-carotene, carotenoids)	Retinol: liver, fish, fortified milk and margarine, butter, eggs; carotenoids: carrots, leafy greens, sweet potatoes, broccoli, apricots, cantaloupe	700–900 µg/day	Vision, health of cornea and other epithelial tissue, cell differentiation, reproduction, immune function	Night blindness, xerophthalmia, poor growth, dry skin, impaired immune function	People living in poverty (particularly children and pregnant women), people who consume very low-fat or low-protein diets	Headache, vomiting, hair loss, liver damage, skin changes, bone pain, fractures, birth defects	3000 µg/day of preformed vitamin A
Vitamin D (calciferol, chole-calciferol, calcitriol, ergo-calciferol, dihydroxy vitamin D)	Egg yolk, liver, fish oils, tuna, salmon, fortified milk, synthesis from sunlight	15 µg/day	Absorption of calcium and phosphorus, maintenance of bone	Rickets in children: abnormal growth, misshapen bones, bowed legs, soft bones; osteomalacia in adults: weak bones and one and muscle pain	Some breast-fed infants; children and elderly people (especially those with dark skin and little exposure to sunlight); people with kidney disease	Calcium deposits in soft tissues, growth retardation, kidney damage	100 µg/day
Vitamin E (tocopherol, alpha-tocopherol)	Vegetable oils, leafy greens, seeds, nuts, peanuts	15 mg/day	Antioxidant, protects cell membranes	Broken red blood cells, nerve damage	People with poor fat absorption, premature infants	Inhibition of vitamin K activity	1000 mg/day from supplemental sources
Vitamin K (phylloquin-ones, mena-quinone)	Vegetable oils, leafy greens, synthesis by intestinal bacteria	90–120 µg/day	Synthesis of blood-clotting proteins and proteins in bone	Hemorrhage	Newborns (especially premature), people on long-term antibiotics	Anemia, brain damage	ND

Note: UL, Tolerable Upper Intake Level; ND, not determined due to insufficient evidence.

CONCEPT CHECK

1. **How** does vitamin A help us see in the dark?

2. **Why** is vitamin D called the sunshine vitamin?

3. **How** does vitamin E protect membranes?

4. **What** is the main symptom of vitamin K deficiency?

Meeting Needs with Dietary Supplements

LEARNING OBJECTIVES

1. **List** some population groups that may benefit from vitamin and mineral supplements.

2. **Discuss** the benefits and risks of herbal supplements.

3. **Explain** how the safety of dietary supplements is monitored.

Approximately 40% of Canadians take dietary supplements, a large proportion of which are vitamin and mineral supplements.[42] We take them for a variety of reasons—to energize ourselves, to protect ourselves from disease, to cure illnesses, to lose weight, to enhance what we obtain from the foods we eat, and to simply ensure against deficiencies. For some people, these products may be beneficial and, under some circumstances, even necessary, but supplements also have the potential to cause harm.

Some dietary supplements contain vitamins and minerals, some contain herbs and other plant-derived substances, and some contain compounds that are found in the body but are not essential in the diet.[43] Although supplements can help us to obtain adequate amounts of specific nutrients, they do not provide all the benefits of foods. A pill that meets a person's vitamin needs does not provide the energy, protein, minerals (discussed in detail in Chapter 8), fibre, or phytochemicals supplied by food sources of these vitamins.

Who Needs Vitamin/Mineral Supplements?

Eating a variety of foods is the best way to meet nutrient needs, and most healthy adults who consume a reasonably good diet do not need supplements. In fact, an argument against the use of supplements is that supplement use gives people a false sense of security, leading them to pay less attention to the nutrient content of the foods they choose. For some people, however, taking supplements may be the only way to meet certain nutrient needs because of low intakes, increased needs, or excess losses (**Table 7.5**).

Groups for whom dietary supplements are recommended[44] Table 7.5	
Group	**Recommendation**
Dieters	People who consume fewer than 1,600 kilocalories/day should take a multivitamin/multimineral supplement.
Vegans and those who eliminate all dairy foods	To obtain adequate vitamin B_{12}, people who do not eat animal products need to take supplements or consume foods fortified with vitamin B_{12}. Because dairy products are an important source of calcium and vitamin D, vegetarians and others who do not consume dairy products (due to lactose intolerance, milk allergies, or for other reasons) may benefit from taking supplements that provide calcium and vitamin D.
Infants and children	Supplemental fluoride, vitamin D, and iron are recommended under certain circumstances.
Young women and pregnant women	Women of childbearing age should consume 400 µg of folic acid daily from either fortified foods or supplements. Supplements of iron and folic acid are recommended for pregnant women, and multivitamin/multimineral supplements are usually prescribed during pregnancy.
Older adults	Because of the high incidence of atrophic gastritis in adults over the age of 50, vitamin B_{12} supplements or fortified foods are recommended. Because older adults may find it difficult to meet the AI for vitamin D and calcium, supplements of these nutrients are often recommended. Health Canada recommends that adults over the age of 70 supplement their diet with extra vitamin D.
Individuals with dark skin pigmentation	People with dark skin may be unable to synthesize enough vitamin D to meet their needs and may therefore benefit from supplementation.
Individuals with restricted diets	Individuals with health conditions that limit the foods they eat or how nutrients are used may require vitamin and mineral supplements.
People taking medications	Medications may interfere with the body's use of certain nutrients.
Cigarette smokers and alcohol users	People who smoke heavily require more vitamin C and possibly vitamin E than do nonsmokers.[8,45] Alcohol consumption inhibits the absorption of B vitamins and may interfere with B vitamin metabolism.

Herbal Supplements

Technically, an herb is a nonwoody, seed-producing plant that dies at the end of the growing season. However, the term *herb* is generally used to refer to any botanical or plant-derived substance. Throughout history, folk medicine has used herbs to prevent and treat disease. Today, herbs and herbal supplements are still popular (**Figure 7.35**). They are readily available and relatively inexpensive, and they can be purchased without a trip to the doctor or a prescription. Although these features are appealing to consumers

Popular herbal supplements • Figure 7.35

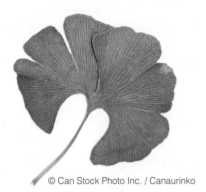

© Can Stock Photo Inc. / Canaurinko

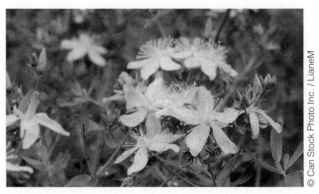

© Can Stock Photo Inc. / LianeM

▲ *Ginkgo biloba*, also called "maidenhair," is a popular herbal medicinal supplement in Canada. It is marketed to enhance memory and to treat a variety of circulatory ailments,[47] but supplements have not been found to benefit memory or other aspects of cognitive function in healthy adults.[48] Taking Ginkgo biloba may cause side effects that include headaches and gastrointestinal symptoms.[46] Ginkgo biloba also interacts with a number of medications. It can cause bleeding when combined with warfarin or aspirin, elevated blood pressure when combined with a thiazide diuretic, and coma when combined with the antidepressant trazodone.[49]

▲ St. John's wort, taken to promote mental well-being, contains low doses of the chemical found in the antidepressant drug fluoxetine (Prozac). The results of some clinical trials suggest that it is effective for the treatment of depression. Side effects include nausea and allergic reactions. St. John's wort should not be used in conjunction with prescription antidepressant drugs, and it has been found to interact with anticoagulants, heart medications, birth control pills, and medications used to treat HIV infection.[46,50,51]

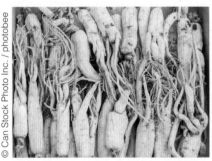

© Can Stock Photo Inc. / photobee

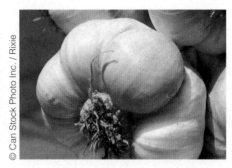

© Can Stock Photo Inc. / Rixie

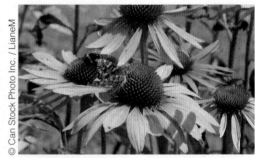

© Can Stock Photo Inc. / LianeM

▲ Ginseng has been used in Asia for centuries for its energizing, stress-reducing, and aphrodisiac properties. Today, ginseng is added to many beverages such as juice for its believed effects on cardiovascular, central nervous system, endocrine, and sexual functions. Despite claims, there is little evidence that ginseng benefits health, and it may not be safe for everyone.[52,53] It can cause diarrhea, headache, insomnia, and changes in blood pressure and interacts with other medications.[46,49,53]

▲ Hippocrates recommended garlic for treating pneumonia and other infections, as well as for cancer and digestive disorders. Although it is no longer recommended for those purposes, recent research has shown that garlic may lower blood cholesterol.[54] Although we often season our food with garlic, garlic supplements are not safe for everyone. They can be harmful for people undergoing treatment for HIV infection,51 and can lead to bleeding in those taking the anticoagulant drug warfarin.[49]

▲ Aboriginal people used petals of the echinacea plant as a treatment for colds, flu, and infections. Today, the plant's root is typically used, and it is a popular herbal cold remedy. Echinacea is believed to act as an immune system stimulant, but there is little evidence that it is beneficial in either preventing or treating the common cold.[55] Although side effects have not been reported, allergies are possible.

who want to manage their own health, herbs and herbal supplements may also cause problems.

When a drug is prescribed by a physician, we are assured that it is an established treatment for our ailment, that each dose will contain the same amount of the drug, that the physician or pharmacist has considered other medications we are taking and other medical conditions that may alter the effectiveness of the drug, and that the drug itself will not cause a severe side effect. These assumptions cannot be made with herbs. Some herbs may be toxic, either alone or in combination with other drugs and herbs (**Table 7.6**). Some herbs may contain bacteria or other contaminants. And it is difficult to know what dose of an herb you are taking. Even herbs that have been pressed and packaged

Potential benefits and side effects of common herbal ingredients   Table 7.6

Product	Suggested benefit	Side effects
Astragalus (Huang ch')	Immune stimulant	Low blood pressure, dizziness, fatigue
Cat's Claw (uña de gato)	Relieves arthritis and indigestion, immune stimulant	Headache, dizziness, vomiting. Should not be taken by pregnant women
Chamomile	Aids indigestion, promotes relaxation	Allergy possible
Chaparral*	Cancer cure, acne treatment, antioxidant	Liver damage, possibly irreversible
Comfrey (borage)*	As a poultice for wounds and sore joints, as a tea for digestive disorders	Do not take orally, even as tea; obstruction of blood flow to liver resulting in liver failure and possibly death
Dong Quai	Increases energy	May cause birth defects
Echinacea (purple coneflower, snake root, Indian head)	Topically for wound healing, internally as an immune stimulant, cold remedy	Allergy possible, adverse effects in pregnant women and people with autoimmune disorders
Ephedra (Ma Huang, Chinese ephedra, epitonin)*	Relieves cold symptoms, weight loss	High blood pressure, irregular heartbeat, heart attack, stroke, death; recalled from store shelves by Health Canada in 2002
Ginger	Relieves motion sickness and nausea	Irregular heartbeat with large doses
Ginkgo biloba (maidenhair)	Improves memory and mental function, improves circulation	Gastrointestinal (GI) distress, headache, allergic skin reactions
Ginseng	Enhances immunity, improves sexual function	Diarrhea, headache, insomnia, low or high blood pressure
Germander	Weight loss	Liver disease, possibly death
Kava	Relieves anxiety and stress	Visual disturbances, dizziness, GI discomfort, hepatitis
Kombucha tea (mushroom tea, kvass tea, kwassan, kargasck)	General well-being	GI upset, liver damage, possibly death
Lobelia (Indian tobacco)*	Relaxation, respiratory remedy	Breathing problems, rapid heartbeat, low blood pressure, convulsions, coma, death
Milk thistle	Protects against liver disease	May decrease effectiveness of some medications
Saw palmetto	Improves urinary flow with enlarged prostate	Constipation, diarrhea, headache, high blood pressure, nausea, urine retention, decreased libido
St. John's wort (hypericum)	Promotes mental well-being	Allergic reactions possible; contains similar ingredients as the antidepressant drug fluoxetine (Prozac) and should not be used by people taking antidepressants
Stephania (magnolia)*	Weight loss	Kidney damage, including kidney failure resulting in transplant or dialysis
Valerian	Mild sedative	GI upset, headache, restlessness
Willow bark*	Pain and fever relief	Reye's syndrome, allergies
Wormwood*	Relieves digestive ailments	Numbness or paralysis of legs, delirium, paralysis
Yohimbe	Aphrodisiac	Tremors, anxiety, high blood pressure, rapid heartbeat, psychosis, paralysis

*Has been shown to have serious side effects and should be avoided.

into pills may not provide the same dose in each pill. Also, because consumers decide what conditions to treat with herbal remedies, these remedies can be used inappropriately or instead of necessary medical intervention.[46]

Choosing Supplements with Care

Using dietary supplements can be part of an effective strategy to promote good health, but supplements are not a substitute for a healthy diet, and they are not without risks of their own.

In 2004, the National Health Products Regulations came into effect regulating the sale of natural health products (NHP) in Canada. NHPs include vitamins and minerals, herbal remedies, homeopathic medicine, traditional medicine, probiotics, and such products as amino acids and essential fatty acids.[56] Before manufacturers are able to sell an NHP, they must apply for and receive a licence from Health Canada. They must provide a detailed description of the product, including its medicinal and non-medicinal ingredients, the source, dose, and recommended usage. An NHP that has been fully evaluated and approved will be labelled with an eight-digit licence number. Some NHPs on the market are still being reviewed by Health Canada but may nonetheless appear on store shelves in the meantime. These products will have completed an initial assessment of safety and be awarded a product label in the form EN-XXXXXX, until they receive full approval.

Because supplements are not regulated as strictly as are drugs, consumers need to use care and caution when choosing dietary supplements (see *Hot Topic: Vitamin Enhanced Beverages*). If you choose to use dietary supplements, a safe option is a multivitamin/multimineral supplement that does not exceed 100% of the RDAs. Although there is little evidence that the average person benefits from such a supplement, there is also little evidence of harm. Here are some suggestions to help you when choosing or using dietary supplements:

- **Consider why you want it.** If you are taking it to ensure good health, does it provide both vitamins and minerals? If you want to supplement specific nutrients, are they contained in the product?
- **Compare product costs.** Just as more isn't always better, more expensive is not always better either, especially when the more expensive supplements include the exact same ingredients and doses.
- **Read the label.** Does the supplement contain potentially toxic levels of any nutrient? Are you taking the amount recommended on the label? For any nutrients that exceed 100% of the Daily Value, check to see whether they exceed the UL (see Appendix A) (**Figure 7.36**). Does the supplement contain any non-vitamin/non-mineral ingredients? If so, have any of them been shown to be toxic to someone in your situation?

Check the supplement facts • Figure 7.36

This Supplement Facts panel is from a supplement marketed to reduce appetite and therefore promote weight loss. Would you recommend it? Why or why not?

- **Check the expiration date.** Some nutrients degrade over time. Expired products will have a lower nutrient content than is shown on the label. The nutrient value is also lower when the product has not been stored properly.
- **Consider your medical history.** Do you have a medical condition that recommends the consumption or avoidance of certain nutrients? Are you taking prescription medication that an ingredient in the supplement may interact with? Check with a physician, dietitian, or pharmacist to help identify any possible interactions.
- **Approach herbal supplements with caution.** If you are ill or taking medications, consult your physician before taking herbs. Do not take herbs if you are pregnant, and do not give herbal supplements to children. Do not take combinations of herbs. Do not use herbs for long periods. Stop taking any product that causes side effects.
- **Report harmful effects.** If you suffer a harmful effect or an illness that you believe is related to the use of a supplement, seek medical attention and report it to the proper authorities.

Supplement Facts / Renseignements sur le produit	
Serving Size: 2 capsules	Servings Per Container: 30
Dose: 2 gélules	Portions Par Contenant: 30
Nutrition Information Information alimentaire	
Medicinal Ingredients (per dose unit) **Ingrédients médicinaux (Oral/Orale):**	
Green tea extract..500 mg	
L-GLUTAMINE..500 mg	
Vitamin B$_6$..8 mg	
Panax ginseng (Root)...200 mg	
Maca (Lepidummeyenii, Root)...175 mg	
**Daily Value not established/Apport quotidien non établi	

HOT TOPIC

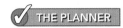

Vitamin-enhanced beverages

In Canada, any trip to a convenience store or university cafeteria will most likely lead to an encounter with a vitamin-enhanced beverage. Because of aggressive marketing campaigns and the widespread availability of vitamin-enhanced drinks, these beverages have become a billion-dollar industry. Names such as "Revive," "Energy," "Endurance," and "Focus" help market these products as beneficial nutritional supplements. But are these products really as healthy as they are portrayed?

Typically, if you want to know the nutritional content of a pre-packaged food or beverage you can check the Nutrients Facts box on the label. It may surprise you to find that in Canada, vitamin-enhanced beverages contain no such label because they are registered as Natural Health Products *not* as foods. They accordingly need to include a Supplement Facts Panel, which lists its vitamin content but does not list the amount of calories, carbohydrates, and sugars, which must be included on all Nutrient Facts boxes. This omission may lead a consumer to be misinformed about the quality of the product. For example, a bottle of vitamin-enhanced water typically contains more than 120 kilocalories and more than 125 g (1/2 cup) of sugar, but this information is not found on the label. Also, the vitamins found in many of these beverages, such as many of the B vitamins, are rarely deficient in the Canadian diet. Conversely, if too many of these beverages are consumed in a day, it may put an individual above their upper limits for certain vitamins. There is also speculation as to how available these vitamins are when taken into the body. For instance, the fat soluble vitamins require fat for their absorption, so if the beverage isn't consumed with a fat source, it cannot be effectively absorbed.

Another argument against these beverages is the false sense of security they give to consumers. Supplementing your diet with vitamins does not make you healthy; all the vitamins can possibly do is to prevent deficiencies. If you consume a varied diet and eat adequate amounts of fruits vegetables, whole grains, and lean meats, consuming vitamin-enhanced beverages will not make you any healthier. They can, however, increase the number of calories and the amount of sugar in your diet—and decrease the amount of money in your wallet.

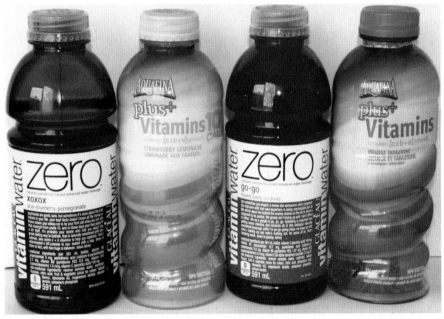

Luisa Begani

CONCEPT CHECK

 STOP

1. **Why** is it recommended that vegans and older adults take vitamin B$_{12}$ supplements?

2. **Why** is it important to tell your physician if you are taking an herbal supplement?

3. **How** does Health Canada influence the safety of dietary supplements?

Summary

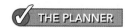

1 A Vitamin Primer 198

- **Vitamins** are essential organic nutrients that do not provide energy and are required in small quantities in the diet to maintain health. They are classified as either **water-soluble vitamins** or **fat-soluble vitamins** based on their solubility in either water or fat. Vitamins are present naturally in foods and added through fortification and enrichment.

- Vitamin **bioavailability** is affected by the composition of the diet, conditions in the digestive tract, and the ability to transport and activate the vitamin once it has been absorbed. Also, some vitamins are absorbed as inactive **provitamins**, or **vitamin precursors**, and must be activated before they can function.

- Vitamins promote and regulate body activities. The B vitamins act as **coenzymes**. Some vitamins are **antioxidants**, which protect the body from **oxidative damage** by **free radicals**.

- In developing countries, vitamin deficiencies remain a major public health problem. Vitamin deficiencies are less common in industrialized countries due to fortification and a more varied food supply.

Vitamin absorption • Figure 7.3

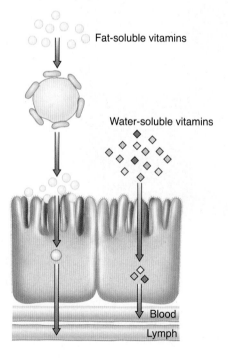

Fat-soluble vitamins

Water-soluble vitamins

Blood

Lymph

2 The Water-Soluble Vitamins 205

- **Thiamin** is a coenzyme that is particularly important for glucose metabolism and **neurotransmitter** synthesis; a deficiency of thiamin, called **beriberi**, is associated with numerous cases of nervous system abnormalities found in the developing world. In the developed world, thiamin deficiency is typically caused by alcohol abuse, and results in **Wernicke-Korsakoff syndrome**, which also negatively affects the nervous system. Thiamin is found in whole and enriched grains.

- **Riboflavin** coenzymes are needed for ATP production and for the utilization of several other vitamins. Milk is one of the best food sources of riboflavin.

- **Niacin** coenzymes are needed for the breakdown of carbohydrate, fat, and protein and for the synthesis of fatty acids and cholesterol. A deficiency of niacin results in **pellagra**, which is characterized by dermatitis, diarrhea, and dementia. The amino acid tryptophan can be converted into niacin. High doses of niacin will lower blood cholesterol but can cause toxicity symptoms.

- **Biotin** is needed for the synthesis of glucose and fatty acids and for the metabolism of certain amino acids. Some of our biotin need is met by bacterial synthesis in the gastrointestinal tract.

- **Pantothenic acid** is part of coenzyme A, required for the production of ATP from carbohydrate, fat, and protein and the synthesis of cholesterol and fat. It is widespread in the food supply.

- **Vitamin B$_6$** is particularly important for amino acid and protein metabolism. Deficiency causes numbness and tingling and may increase homocysteine levels in the blood. Food sources include meats and whole grains. Large doses of vitamin B$_6$ can cause nervous system abnormalities.

- **Folate** or **folic acid** is necessary for the synthesis of DNA, so it is especially important for rapidly dividing cells. Folate deficiency results in **macrocytic anemia**. Low levels of folate before and during early pregnancy are associated with an increased incidence of **neural tube defects** such as **spina bifida**. Food sources include liver, legumes, oranges, leafy green vegetables, and fortified grains. A high intake of folate can mask some of the symptoms of vitamin B$_{12}$ deficiency.

- Absorption of **vitamin B$_{12}$** (also known as **cobalamin**) requires stomach acid and **intrinsic factor**. Without intrinsic factor, only tiny amounts are absorbed, and **pernicious anemia** occurs. Vitamin B$_{12}$ is needed for the metabolism of folate and fatty acids and to maintain myelin. Deficiency results in macrocytic anemia and nerve damage. Vitamin B_{12} is found almost exclusively in animal products. Deficiency is a concern in vegans and in older individuals with **atrophic gastritis**.

- **Vitamin C** (also known as **ascorbic acid**) is necessary for the synthesis of **collagen**, hormones, and neurotransmitters. Vitamin C deficiency, called **scurvy**, is characterized by poor wound healing, bleeding, and other symptoms related to the improper formation and maintenance of collagen. Vitamin C is also a water-soluble antioxidant. The best food sources are citrus fruits.

- **Choline** is a water-soluble substance needed to synthesize several important molecules, including the neurotransmitter acetylcholine. Although choline is necessary for humans, because the body can synthesize choline itself, it is not currently classified as a vitamin.

Folate deficiency and anemia • Figure 7.16

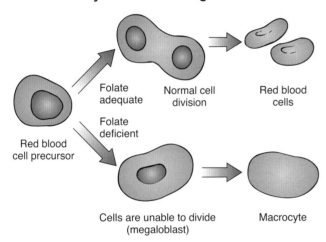

Red blood cell precursor

Folate adequate → Normal cell division → Red blood cells

Folate deficient → Cells are unable to divide (megaloblast) → Macrocyte

3 The Fat-Soluble Vitamins 222

- **Vitamin A** is a fat-soluble vitamin needed for growth and **cell differentiation**. It also helps form **rhodopsin**, a visual pigment necessary for the perception of light. Its role in **gene expression** makes it essential for maintenance of epithelial tissue, reproduction, and immune function. Vitamin A deficiency can lead to blindness and death. Vision problems associated with vitamin A deficiency are collectively known as **xeropthlamia**. An early sign of xeropthalmia is **night blindness**. Preformed vitamin A **retinoids** are found in liver, eggs, fish, and fortified dairy products. High intakes are toxic and have been linked to birth defects and bone loss. Provitamin A **carotenoids**, such as **beta-carotene**, are found in leafy greens and in yellow-orange fruits and vegetables such as mangoes, carrots, and apricots. Some carotenoids are antioxidants. Carotenoids are not toxic, but high levels in the blood, a condition called **hypercarotenemia**, can give the skin a yellow-orange appearance.

- **Vitamin D** can be made in the skin by exposure to sunlight, so dietary needs vary depending on the amount synthesized. **Parathyroid hormone (PTH)** helps regulate vitamin D levels by helping to activate it at the kidneys. Vitamin D is found in fish oils and fortified milk. It is essential for maintaining proper levels of calcium and phosphorus in the body. A deficiency in children results in **rickets**; in adults, vitamin D deficiency causes **osteomalacia** and **osteoporosis**. Adequate vitamin D is associated with reduced incidence of certain cancers.

- **Vitamin E** (also known as **tocopherol**) functions primarily as a fat-soluble antioxidant. It is necessary for reproduction and protects cell membranes from oxidative damage. Deficiency of vitamin E can lead to **hemolytic anemia**, whereby red blood cells rupture and are no longer able to carry oxygen. Vitamin E is found in nuts, plant oils, green vegetables, and fortified cereals.

- **Vitamin K** is essential for blood clotting because it helps activate the proteins **fibrin** and **prothrombin**. Because vitamin K deficiency is a problem in newborns, they are routinely given vitamin K injections at birth. Warfarin, a substance that inhibits vitamin K activity, is used medically as an anticoagulant. Vitamin K is found in plants and is synthesized by bacteria in the gastrointestinal tract.

Vitamin D activation and function • Figure 7.27

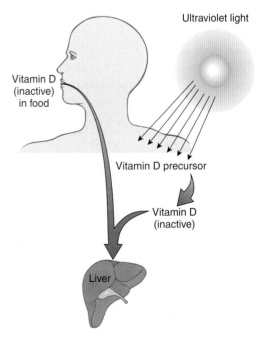

Ultraviolet light

Vitamin D (inactive) in food

Vitamin D precursor

Vitamin D (inactive)

Liver

4 Meeting Needs with Dietary Supplements 237

- Approximately 40% of Canadians take some type of dietary supplement. Vitamin and mineral supplements are recommended for dieters, vegetarians, pregnant women and women of childbearing age, older adults, and other nutritionally vulnerable groups.

- Herbal supplements are currently popular. These products may have beneficial physiological actions, but their dosage is not regulated, and they can be toxic either on their own or in combination with other herbs, medications, or medical conditions.

- Manufacturers are responsible for the consistency and safety of supplements before they are marketed. Health Canada regulates dietary supplement labelling and can monitor their safety once they are on the market. When choosing a dietary supplement, consumers need to carefully consider both the potential risks and benefits of the product.

Popular herbal supplements • Figure 7.35

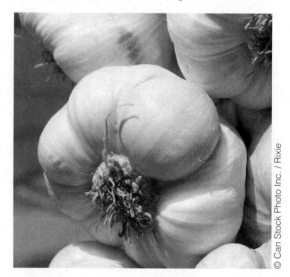

© Can Stock Photo Inc. / Rixie

Key Terms

- antioxidant 203
- ascorbic acid 218
- atrophic gastritis 218
- beriberi 206
- beta-carotene 222
- bioavailability 200
- biotin 211
- carotenoids 222
- cell differentiation 224
- choline 219
- cobalamin 217
- coenzymes 203
- collagen 218
- fat-soluble vitamins 198
- fibrin 234

- folate 214
- folic acid 214
- free radicals 203
- gene expression 225
- hemolytic anemia 232
- hypercarotenemia 227
- intrinsic factor 217
- macrocytic anemia or megaloblastic anemia 214
- neural tube defects 214
- neurotransmitters 206
- niacin 209
- night blindness 224
- osteomalacia 229
- osteoporosis 229

- oxidative damage 203
- pantothenic acid 211
- parathyroid hormone (PTH) 228
- pellagra 209
- pernicious anemia 217
- prothrombin 234
- provitamin or vitamin precursor 200
- retinoids 222
- rhodopsin 224
- riboflavin 207
- rickets 229
- scurvy 218
- spina bifida 215

- thiamin 206
- tocopherol 234
- vitamin A 222
- vitamin B_{12} 217
- vitamin B_6 211
- vitamin C 218
- vitamin D 227
- vitamin E 232
- vitamin K 234
- vitamins 198
- water-soluble vitamins 198
- Wernicke-Korsakoff syndrome 207
- xerophthalmia 225

Critical and Creative Thinking Questions

1. Hatsumi is 28 years old. She and her husband plan to start a family soon. Because Hatsumi is overweight and knows she will put on more weight if she has a baby, she begins a low-carbohydrate diet to slim down before she gets pregnant. She eliminates breads, grains, legumes, starchy vegetables, and fruit from her diet. What nutrient that is important early in pregnancy is lacking in this diet? What can Hatsumi add to her diet to increase her intake of this nutrient? Will taking a prenatal vitamin supplement prescribed at her first prenatal visit be enough to reduce the risk of neural tube defects?

2. The following dietary supplement products are on sale at a local nutrition store:

   Pyridoxine: 100 mg

   Stress tabs: pyridoxine, 35 mg; thiamin, 1 mg; riboflavin, 1.1 mg; niacin, 30 mg; choline, 500 mg

   Folic acid: 800 µg

   Do any of these supplements pose a risk for toxicity at the dose listed above? Which ones and why? What would happen if a consumer took twice the recommended dose? Would you recommend them for everyone? For a specific group? Why or why not?

3. Suman is a fast-food fanatic. For breakfast, he stops for coffee and doughnuts. Lunch is an iced tea, a ham-and-cheese sub with lettuce and mayonnaise, and a cookie. Dinner is a soft drink, burger, and fries. Name two vitamins likely to be lacking in Suman's diet if he eats like this every day. Why are these vitamins likely to be deficient?

4. Why might someone with kidney failure develop a vitamin D deficiency?

5. Explain why a dark-skinned Nigerian exchange student living in Vancouver, British Columbia, is at risk for vitamin D deficiency.

6. Explain why a deficiency either of vitamin B_{12} or of folate causes red blood cells to be larger than normal.

7. Explain why infections are more common and immunization programs are less successful in regions where vitamin A deficiency is prevalent.

What is happening in this picture?

These children, who live in Russia, are being exposed to UV radiation to prevent vitamin D deficiency.

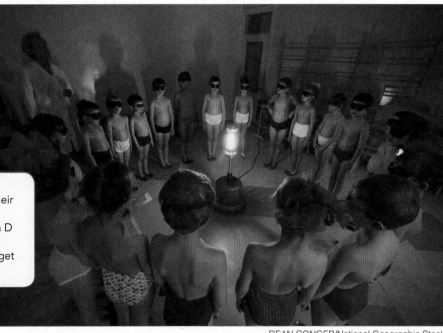

DEAN CONGER/National Geographic Stock

Think Critically

1. Why does this treatment help them meet their need for vitamin D?
2. Why are children in Russia at risk for vitamin D deficiency?
3. What else can be done to ensure that they get adequate amounts of vitamin D?

Self-Test

(Check your answers in Appendix J.)

1. Which of the following vitamins is *not* added to grains during enrichment?

   a. thiamin   d. vitamin B_6

   b. riboflavin   e. folate

   c. niacin

2. Which vitamin is needed for the reaction labelled with the letter A in the figure at right?

   a. thiamin   d. vitamin A

   b. vitamin C   e. vitamin K

   c. vitamin B_6

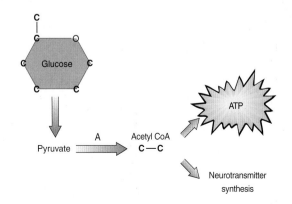

3. Which of the following descriptions of the water-soluble vitamins is false?

   a. niacin—a deficiency causes pellagra

   b. thiamin—can be synthesized from tryptophan

   c. pantothenic acid—found in most foods

   d. vitamin C—needed for the cross-linking of collagen

   e. vitamin B_6—needed for amino acid metabolism

4. Which of the following statements is true of all the B vitamins?

   a. They are all electron carriers.

   b. They are all needed for DNA synthesis.

   c. They are all coenzymes.

   d. They all contain energy that is used to fuel body activities.

   e. They are all fat soluble.

5. Which of the following nutrients is *not* essential in the diet when sun exposure is adequate?

   a. riboflavin

   b. vitamin E

   c. vitamin K

   d. vitamin D

6. Which of the following statements about folate is false?

   a. Adequate amounts decrease the incidence of neural tube defect–affected pregnancies.

   b. It is needed for DNA synthesis.

   c. A deficiency causes macrocytic anemia.

   d. It can be made in the body from methionine.

   e. Enriched grain products are fortified with folate.

7. The disease scurvy is due to a deficiency of _____.

   a. vitamin K

   b. vitamin D

   c. vitamin C

   d. vitamin A

   e. thiamin

8. A deficiency of vitamin K leads to _____.

   a. rickets

   b. blindness

   c. scurvy

   d. pellagra

   e. decreased blood clotting

9. Which of the following is a poor source of beta-carotene?

   a. milk

   b. carrots

   c. sweet potatoes

   d. spinach

   e. apricots

10. The food sources of _____ are illustrated by this graph.

   a. vitamin C

   b. folate

   c. vitamin B_{12}

   d. thiamin

   e. vitamin B_6

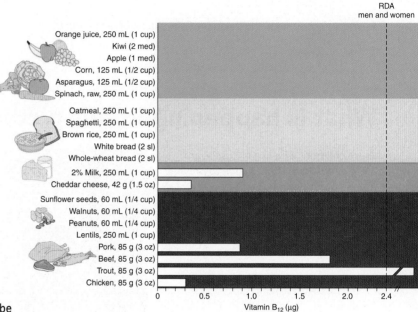

11. The actions of _____ are illustrated here.

   a. vitamin C

   b. vitamin D

   c. vitamin B_6

   d. vitamin K

   e. vitamin E

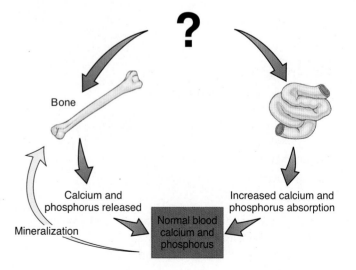

12. It is recommended that older adults get their vitamin B_{12} from fortified foods and supplements because _____.

    a. they eat a poor diet

    b. their requirement for B_{12} is higher than that of younger people

    c. many have atrophic gastritis and are not able to absorb the vitamin B_{12} found in foods

    d. they have higher vitamin B_{12} losses than other groups

13. Vitamin A deficiency causes the eye condition illustrated here because _____.

    a. the visual pigment rhodopsin cannot be synthesized

    b. collagen is not made correctly

    c. there is insufficient antioxidant protection

    d. bone development is abnormal

    e. mucus-secreting cells do not differentiate normally

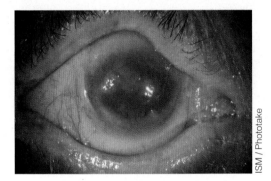

ISM / Phototake

14. Which of the following statements is true of vitamin E?

    a. It is needed in energy metabolism.

    b. It protects cell membranes from oxidative damage.

    c. Deficiency is a common problem in North America.

    d. Supplements increase fertility even in people with adequate vitamin E status.

    e. It is needed for night vision.

15. Elevated blood homocysteine has been associated with an increased risk of cardiovascular disease. Deficiencies of _____ may increase levels of homocysteine in the blood.

    a. pantothenic acid, riboflavin, and vitamin C

    b. biotin, thiamin, and vitamin B_6

    c. vitamin B_6, folate, and vitamin B_{12}

    d. thiamin, riboflavin, and niacin

THE PLANNER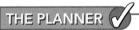

Review your Chapter Planner on the chapter opener and check off your completed work.

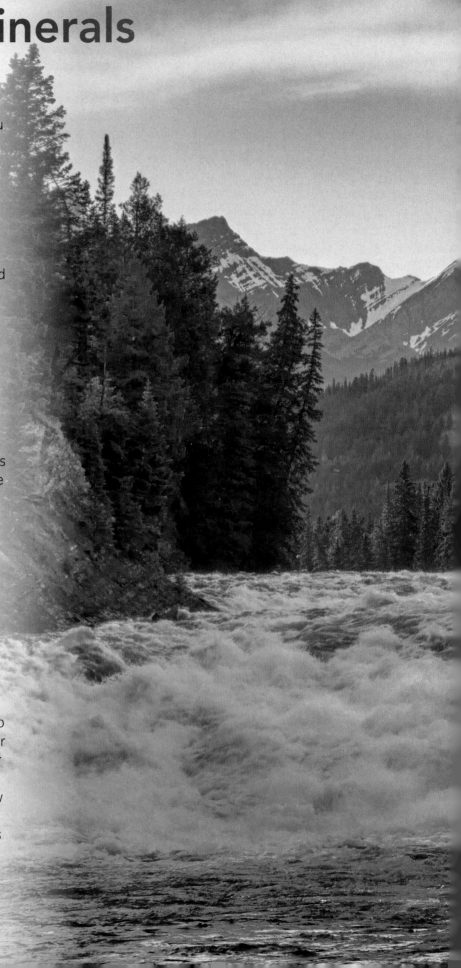

Water and Minerals

Water is an important part of the Canadian lifestyle and identity. We fish at Great Bear Lake, swim at Wasaga Beach, skate on the Rideau Canal, or play hockey on our local pond or backyard ice rink.

Water is not just a part of our recreation but an important part of our geography. We are bordered by three oceans, 2% of our land is covered by glaciers and icefields, and more than a million lakes are scattered throughout the nation. Water contributes billions of dollars to our economy and is one of our most highly regulated commodities.

Water is also the most critical nutrient in our body. In fact, the majority of the human body is composed of water. It can be found in every tissue and organ, both inside and outside of the cells.

Like water, minerals are also a critical component of both the Canadian landscape and economy. In Canada, mining accounts for billions in yearly revenue. Unlike water, however, minerals are needed in significantly smaller amounts in the human body, and the minerals mined in Canada aren't typically the ones we eat.

Getting the right amounts of minerals and water is essential to survival. Inadequate and excessive intakes of certain minerals are world health problems and contribute to high blood pressure, bone fractures, anemia, and increased risk of infection. Also, pollution and population growth are negatively affecting the water supply, and water access remains a large challenge to human survival.

Although Canada contains approximately 7% of the world's renewable fresh water,[1] we are also one of the world's largest consumers of water per capita, and we are polluting our waters with litter and contaminants. A future global water crisis would affect everyone, including Canadians. Now more than ever before, we need to protect our glaciers, reduce pollution, and conserve water as much as possible.

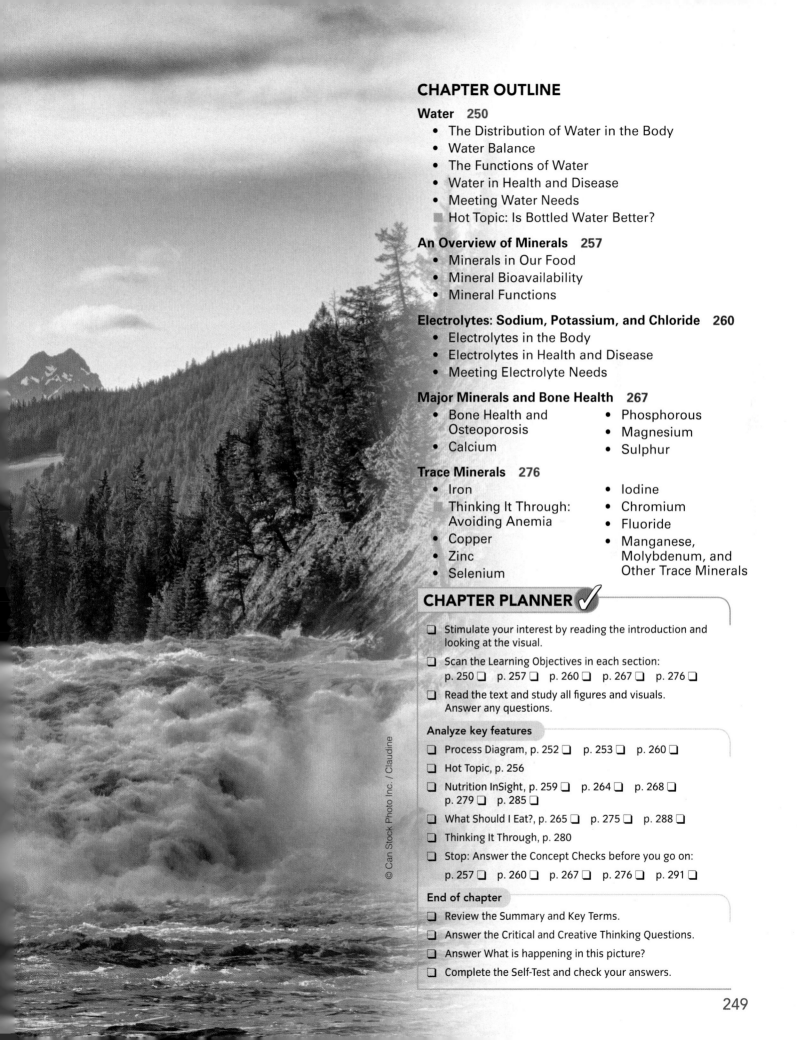

CHAPTER OUTLINE

CHAPTER PLANNER ✔

- ❏ Stimulate your interest by reading the introduction and looking at the visual.
- ❏ Scan the Learning Objectives in each section:
  p. 250 ❏   p. 257 ❏   p. 260 ❏   p. 267 ❏   p. 276 ❏
- ❏ Read the text and study all figures and visuals. Answer any questions.

Analyze key features

- ❏ Process Diagram, p. 252 ❏   p. 253 ❏   p. 260 ❏
- ❏ Hot Topic, p. 256
- ❏ Nutrition InSight, p. 259 ❏   p. 264 ❏   p. 268 ❏
  p. 279 ❏   p. 285 ❏
- ❏ What Should I Eat?, p. 265 ❏   p. 275 ❏   p. 288 ❏
- ❏ Thinking It Through, p. 280
- ❏ Stop: Answer the Concept Checks before you go on:
  p. 257 ❏   p. 260 ❏   p. 267 ❏   p. 276 ❏   p. 291 ❏

End of chapter

- ❏ Review the Summary and Key Terms.
- ❏ Answer the Critical and Creative Thinking Questions.
- ❏ Answer What is happening in this picture?
- ❏ Complete the Self-Test and check your answers.

© Can Stock Photo Inc. / Claudine

Water

LEARNING OBJECTIVES

1. **Explain** the forces that move water back and forth across cell membranes.

2. **Explain** the role of the kidneys in regulating the amount of water in the body.

3. **Describe** five functions of water in the body.

4. **Discuss** the effects of dehydration.

Have you ever felt nauseated, light-headed, or dizzy while exercising on a hot day? If so, you might have been suffering from **dehydration**. Lack of sufficient water in the body rapidly

> **dehydration**
> A state that occurs when not enough water is present to meet the body's needs.

causes deficiency symptoms. These symptoms can be alleviated almost as rapidly as they appeared by drinking enough water to restore your body's water balance.

The Distribution of Water in the Body

In adults, water accounts for about 60% of body weight, but water content varies in the body depending on the tissue. For instance, water makes up about 75% of muscle, but only about 25% of bone. Water is found both inside cells (intracellular) and outside cells (extracellular) in the blood, the lymph, and the spaces between cells (**Figure 8.1**). Water can also move freely between intracellular and extracellular spaces since the cell membranes that separate these areas are not watertight.

The distribution of water between various intra- and extracellular spaces depends on

Water distribution • Figure 8.1

About one-third of the water in the body is intracellular, located inside the cells. The other two-thirds is extracellular, located outside the cells. The extracellular portion includes the water in the blood and lymph, the water between cells, and the water in the digestive tract, eyes, joints, and spinal cord. The amount of water in blood, between cells, and inside cells is affected by blood pressure; and the force generated by osmosis and tissues is affected by blood pressure and the force generated by osmosis. In the capillaries, blood pressure pushes water out of the blood, while osmosis moves water into or out of the blood to equalize the concentration of dissolved particles, such as blood proteins.

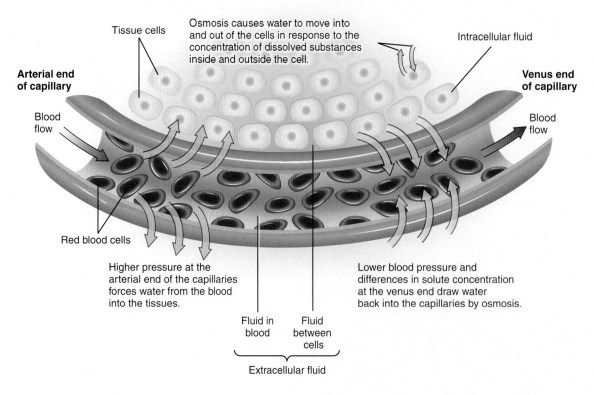

Tissue cells

Osmosis causes water to move into and out of the cells in response to the concentration of dissolved substances inside and outside the cell.

Intracellular fluid

Arterial end of capillary

Venus end of capillary

Blood flow

Blood flow

Red blood cells

Higher pressure at the arterial end of the capillaries forces water from the blood into the tissues.

Lower blood pressure and differences in solute concentration at the venus end draw water back into the capillaries by osmosis.

Fluid in blood

Fluid between cells

Extracellular fluid

differences in the concentrations of dissolved substances, or **solutes**, such as proteins, sodium, potassium, and other small molecules. These concentration differences drive *osmosis*, the diffusion of water in a direction that equalizes the concentration of dissolved substances on either side of a membrane (see Chapter 3). Also, some of these dissolved particles, like some proteins, carry electric charges. Since water has both a slightly positively charged pole and a slightly negatively charged pole, these particles further attract water into the bloodstream. Water is also moved by **blood pressure**, which forces water from the capillary blood vessels into the spaces between the cells of the surrounding tissues. When blood pressure is lower than the pressure created by osmosis, water is drawn back into the capillaries (see Figure 8.1).

> **blood pressure**
> The amount of force exerted by the blood against the walls of arteries.

The body regulates the amount of water in cells and in different extracellular spaces by adjusting the concentration of dissolved particles and relying on osmosis to move the water.

Water Balance

The amount of water in the body remains relatively constant over time. Because water cannot be stored in the body, water intake and output must be balanced to maintain the right amount. Most of the water we consume comes from the water and other liquids that we drink. Solid foods also provide water; most fruits and vegetables are more than 80% water, and even roast beef is about 50% water. A small amount of water is also produced in the body as a by-product of metabolic reactions. We lose water from our bodies in urine and feces, through evaporation from the lungs and skin, and in sweat (**Figure 8.2**).

Under most circumstances, the majority of water losses occur in the urine. In a healthy person, only a small amount of water is lost in the feces, usually less than 250 mL (1 cup) per day. This small amount is remarkable because every day about 9 L (almost 2½ gallons) of fluid enters the gastrointestinal tract, but more than 95% of this fluid is absorbed before the feces are eliminated. However, in cases of severe diarrhea, large amounts of water can be lost via this route. If the lost fluid is not replaced quickly, severe dehydration can occur.

We continuously lose water from the skin and respiratory tract due to evaporation. The amount of water lost through evaporation varies greatly, depending on activity,

Water balance • Figure 8.2

To maintain water balance, intake must equal output. A typical man who is in water balance loses and consumes almost 3 L (13 cups) of water daily. This figure approximates the amounts of water that enter the adult body from food, drink, and metabolism and the amounts lost in urine and feces, and through evaporation when not sweating. Increasing water consumption proportionately increases excretion of water in urine.

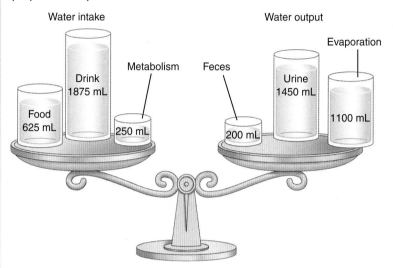

temperature, humidity, and body size. In a temperate climate, an inactive person loses about 1 L (4 cups) of water per day through evaporation; this amount increases when humidity is low and as a result of increases in activity, environmental temperature, and body size.

Water is also lost through sweat when you exercise or when the environment is hot. More sweat is produced as exercise intensity increases and as the environment becomes hotter and more humid. An individual doing light work at a temperature of 29°C will lose about 2 to 3 L (8 to 13 cups) of sweat per day. Strenuous exercise in a hot environment can increase this amount to 2 to 4 L (8 to 17 cups) in an hour.[2,3]

Regulating blood pressure and blood volume

A drop in blood pressure can lead to headaches and faintness, and it can compromise the blood's ability to effectively deliver its contents to the tissues. Our body therefore works very diligently to maintain blood pressure through three main mechanisms: thirst, water reabsorption at the kidneys, and vasoconstriction, or the narrowing of blood vessels.

When water losses increase, intake and retention of water must also increase to keep body water at a healthy level to maintain blood pressure. The need to consume water is signalled by the sensation of **thirst**. Thirst is caused

Stimulating water intake • Figure 8.3

The sensation of thirst motivates fluid intake in order to restore water balance.

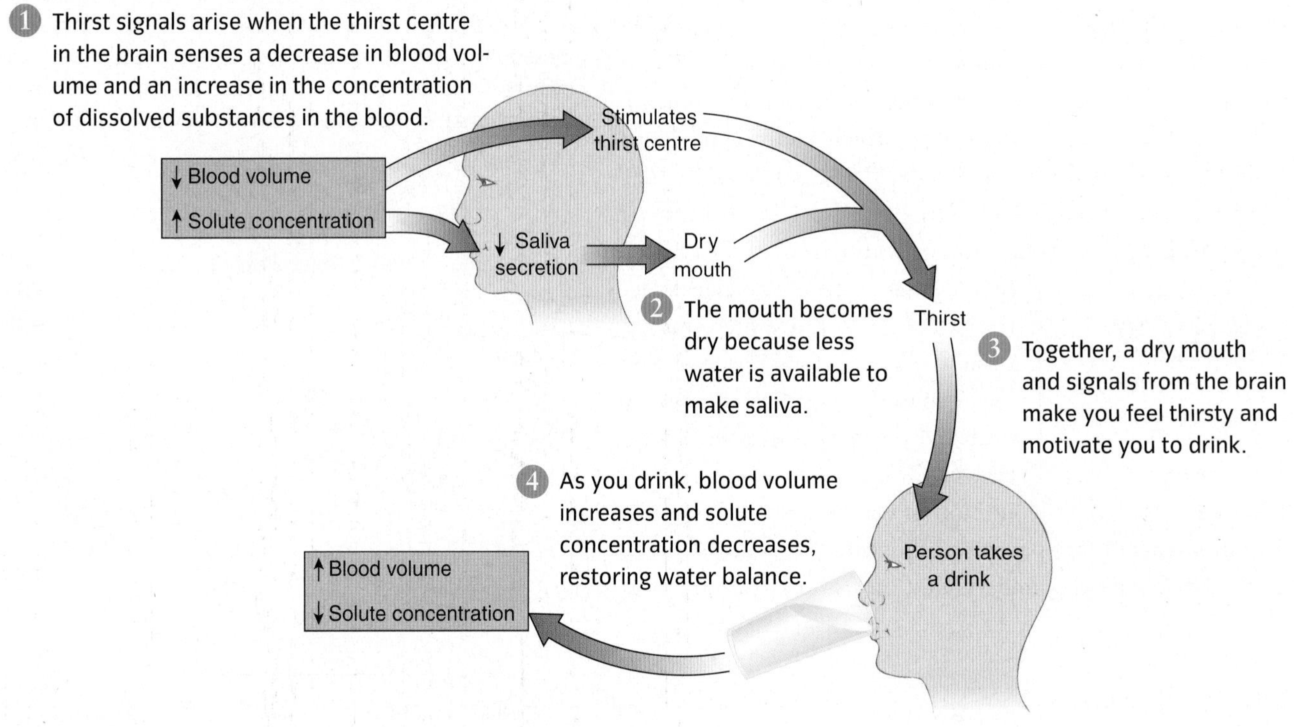

1 Thirst signals arise when the thirst centre in the brain senses a decrease in blood volume and an increase in the concentration of dissolved substances in the blood.

↓ Blood volume
↑ Solute concentration

Stimulates thirst centre

↓ Saliva secretion

Dry mouth

2 The mouth becomes dry because less water is available to make saliva.

Thirst

3 Together, a dry mouth and signals from the brain make you feel thirsty and motivate you to drink.

4 As you drink, blood volume increases and solute concentration decreases, restoring water balance.

↑ Blood volume
↓ Solute concentration

Person takes a drink

---

by dryness in the mouth and by signals from the brain (**Figure 8.3**). It is a powerful urge but often lags behind the need for water, and we don't always or can't always drink when we are thirsty. By the time you are thirsty, you may already be dehydrated; therefore, thirst alone cannot be relied on to maintain water balance.

Not drinking enough to replace water losses can be a problem for athletes exercising in hot weather. They lose water rapidly through sweat but do not feel thirsty until they have lost so much body water that their performance is compromised.[4] To maintain water balance, it is recommended that athletes drink at a rate that closely matches the rate of water loss due to sweating.[5]

The kidneys also play a vital role in the maintenance of blood volume and blood pressure by regulating water loss in urine. The kidneys typically produce about 1 to 2 L (4 to 8 cups) of urine/day, but urine production varies, depending on the amount of water consumed and the amount of waste that needs to be excreted.

The kidneys function like a blood filter. As blood flows through the kidneys, water molecules and other small molecules move through the filter and out of the blood, while blood cells and large molecules are retained in the blood. Some of the water and other molecules that are filtered out are reabsorbed into the blood, and the rest are excreted in the urine.

Even though the kidneys work to control how much water is lost, their ability to concentrate urine is limited because a minimum amount of water must be lost as dissolved wastes are excreted. If a lot of wastes need to be excreted, more water must be lost. Wastes that must be eliminated in the urine include urea and other nitrogen-containing molecules (produced by protein breakdown), ketones (from incomplete fat breakdown), sodium, and other minerals.

Vasoconstriction is another main mechanism by which blood pressure is maintained. Our blood vessels contain a type of muscle that is automatically regulated by the brain. A drop in blood pressure signals this muscle to contract, narrowing the blood vessel and increasing blood pressure accordingly.

Thirst, water conservation at the kidneys, and vasoconstriction are all controlled by hormones in the body that respond to changes in blood pressure, in blood volume, or in the solute concentration of the blood (**Figure 8.4**).

Hormonal regulation of blood volume and pressure • Figure 8.4

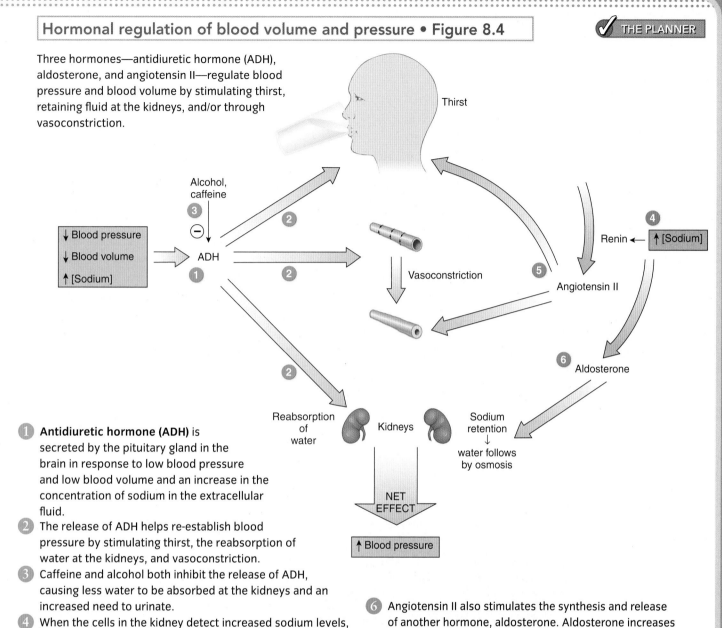

Three hormones—antidiuretic hormone (ADH), aldosterone, and angiotensin II—regulate blood pressure and blood volume by stimulating thirst, retaining fluid at the kidneys, and/or through vasoconstriction.

Thirst

Alcohol, caffeine

3 ⊖

↓ Blood pressure
↓ Blood volume
↑ [Sodium]

ADH **1**

2

2

2

Vasoconstriction

Renin ← ↑ [Sodium] **4**

5 Angiotensin II

6 Aldosterone

Reabsorption of water

Kidneys

Sodium retention
↓
water follows by osmosis

NET EFFECT

↑ Blood pressure

1 **Antidiuretic hormone (ADH)** is secreted by the pituitary gland in the brain in response to low blood pressure and low blood volume and an increase in the concentration of sodium in the extracellular fluid.

2 The release of ADH helps re-establish blood pressure by stimulating thirst, the reabsorption of water at the kidneys, and vasoconstriction.

3 Caffeine and alcohol both inhibit the release of ADH, causing less water to be absorbed at the kidneys and an increased need to urinate.

4 When the cells in the kidney detect increased sodium levels, the enzyme renin is released.

5 This enzyme activates the hormone angiotensin II, which then promotes thirst and vasoconstriction to increase blood pressure.

6 Angiotensin II also stimulates the synthesis and release of another hormone, aldosterone. Aldosterone increases blood volume and blood pressure by promoting the retention of sodium at the kidneys. When the kidneys retain sodium, water follows through the process of osmosis, and less water is excreted in urine.

The Functions of Water

Water doesn't provide energy, but it is essential to life. Water in the body serves as a medium for metabolic reactions, participates in metabolic reactions, helps regulate acid base balance, transports nutrients and wastes, provides protection, and helps regulate temperature.

Water in metabolism and transport Water is an excellent **solvent**. For example, it is used to dissolve many substances that are needed by the body, such as glucose, amino acids, minerals, and proteins. Also, the chemical reactions of metabolism that support life take place in water. Water also participates in several reactions, such as the dehydration reactions that join small molecules together and the hydrolysis reactions that break apart large molecules (see Figure 3.3). Some of the reactions that water participates in help to maintain the body's proper level of acidity. Moreover, water is the primary constituent

PROCESS DIAGRAM

of blood, which flows through our bodies, delivering oxygen and nutrients to cells and delivering waste products to the lungs and kidneys for excretion.

Water as protection Water bathes the cells of the body and lubricates and cleanses internal and external body surfaces. For example, the water in tears lubricates the eyes and washes away dirt; water in synovial fluid lubricates the joints; and water in saliva lubricates the mouth, helping us to chew and swallow food. Because water resists compression, it cushions the joints and other parts of the body against shock. In the amniotic sac, the cushioning effect of water protects the fetus as it grows inside the uterus.

Water and body temperature Because water holds heat and changes temperature slowly, it helps keep body temperature constant. Water actively regulates body temperature (**Figure 8.5**) by increasing or decreasing the amount of heat lost at the surface of the body. When body temperature starts to rise, the blood vessels in the skin dilate, causing more blood to flow close to the surface, where it can release some of the heat to the surrounding environment. Cooling is aided by the production and evaporation of sweat. When body temperature increases, the brain triggers the sweat glands in the skin to produce sweat, which is mostly water.

Sweat alone does not cool the body; it must also evaporate. But this evaporation is a problem in areas like Southern Ontario, where the summer months are not just hot, but can be extremely humid. Sweating cools the body because when it evaporates, a cooling sensation is left behind on the skin. When the weather is both hot *and* humid, sweat does not efficiently evaporate from the body, and people have a much more difficult time staying cool. When people say, "It's not the heat, it's the humidity," they capture the fact that experiencing heat combined with humidity is less bearable than a hot environment alone.

Clothing that permits the evaporation of sweat, such as microfibre-based fabrics and clothing made from

Water helps cool the body • Figure 8.5

Increased blood flow at the surface of the body causes the skin to become red in hot weather and during strenuous activity. Shunting blood to the skin allows heat to be transferred from the blood to the surroundings. Evaporation of sweat cools the skin and the blood near the surface of the skin.

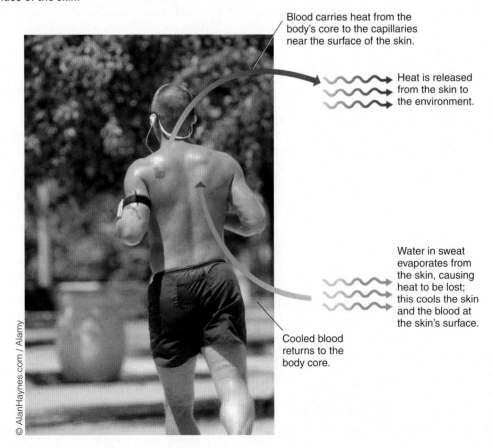

Blood carries heat from the body's core to the capillaries near the surface of the skin.

Heat is released from the skin to the environment.

Water in sweat evaporates from the skin, causing heat to be lost; this cools the skin and the blood at the skin's surface.

Cooled blood returns to the body core.

© AlanHaynes.com / Alamy

wicking material, such as polyester, can help to transfer moisture away from the skin, thereby helping to cool the body. Wearing loose, comfortable clothing may also help by allowing for more air flow. Regardless of how you decide to stay cool, remember that, if you are sweating, you are losing water, and you need to consume more fluids throughout the day to avoid dehydration.

Water in Health and Disease

Without food, you could probably survive for about eight weeks, but without water, you would last only a few days. Too much water can also be a problem if it changes the osmotic balance, disrupting the distribution of water within the body.

Dehydration Dehydration occurs when water loss exceeds water intake. Dehydration leads to a reduction in blood volume, which impairs the ability to deliver oxygen and nutrients to cells and remove waste products. Early symptoms of dehydration include thirst, headache, fatigue, loss of appetite, dry eyes and mouth, and dark-coloured urine (**Figure 8.6**). Dehydration affects both physical and cognitive performance. As dehydration worsens, it causes nausea, difficulty concentrating, confusion, disorientation, and may even lead to collapse. The milder symptoms of dehydration disappear quickly after water or some other beverage is consumed, but if left untreated, dehydration can become severe enough to require medical attention. A water loss of 10 to 20% of body weight can be fatal. Many

Are you at risk for dehydration? • Figure 8.6

Urine colour is an indication of whether you are drinking enough water. Pale yellow urine indicates you are well hydrated. The darker the urine, the greater the level of dehydration.

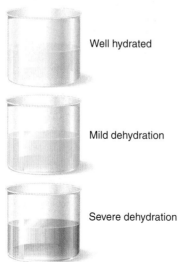

Well hydrated

Mild dehydration

Severe dehydration

people are at risk for dehydration. Athletes are at risk because they may lose large amounts of water in sweat. Older adults are at risk because the thirst mechanism becomes less sensitive with age. Infants are at risk because, relative to their weight, their body surface area is much greater than that of adults, so they lose proportionately more water through evaporation. Also, an infant's kidneys cannot concentrate urine efficiently, so, compared with adults, they can lose more water in their urine. In addition, they cannot tell us they are thirsty, so caregivers must ensure that infants get enough fluids to meet their needs.

Water intoxication Under normal circumstances, it is difficult to consume too much water. However, overhydration, or **water intoxication**, can occur under some conditions. When the body has too much water relative to the amount of sodium, the concentration of sodium in the blood drops, a condition called **hyponatremia**. When this condition occurs, osmosis moves water out of the blood vessels into the tissues, causing them to swell.

> **water intoxication** A condition that occurs when a person drinks enough water to significantly lower the concentration of sodium in the blood.

Swelling in the brain can cause disorientation, convulsions, coma, and death. The early symptoms of water intoxication may be similar to the symptoms of dehydration: nausea, muscle cramps, disorientation, slurred speech, and confusion. Thus, it is important to determine whether the symptoms are due to dehydration or water intoxication; drinking water will alleviate dehydration, but will worsen the symptoms of water intoxication.

Meeting Water Needs

You may have heard the old adage that you need to consume 8 cups, or two litres, of water each day; but the truth is that our water needs are typically even higher and also depend on our gender, activity level, and the nature of our diet. The Dietary Reference Intakes (DRIs) recommend water consumption of 3.7 L (3700 mL)/day for men and 2.7 L (2700 mL)/day for women, but every individual is different.[6] Activity increases water needs because it increases the amount of water lost in sweat; such losses are greater in a hot, humid environment. Diet affects water needs by changing the amount of waste that needs to be excreted in the urine or the amount of water lost in the feces. A low-calorie diet increases water needs because as body fat and protein are broken down to fuel the body, ketones and urea are produced and must be excreted in the urine. A high-salt diet

HOT TOPIC

 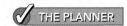

Is bottled water better?

The sale of bottled water in Canada is a growing industry; our per capita consumption of bottled water increased 40% from 1999 to 2004, and we spend hundreds of millions of dollars on bottled water each year.[7] Many people choose bottled water because they like the taste, it is convenient, and they claim that it is safer. But how good is this bottled water? Is it really safer and better than our tap water?

In 2000, the community of Walkerton, Ontario, was rocked by a water contamination scandal that led to thousands of cases of gastrointestinal discomfort and several deaths. Since then, some proponents of bottled water argue that tap water is not as safe as bottled water. The events that occurred at Walkerton were extremely unfortunate, but do not typically reflect the quality of Canadian drinking water. Issues with water contamination are extremely rare in urban communities in Canada, and tap water is extremely safe. However, in small, remote, rural communities, such as certain Aboriginal reserves, water quality is not always on par with the rest of the country. In these cases, extra care must be taken by community members to be aware of the quality of their water supply and to follow water advisories. In these specific communities, boiling water or using bottled water may be safer than consuming water from the tap.

That being said, the purity standards for bottled water set by Health Canada's Water Quality and Health Bureau are similar to those for municipal water systems. Also, a multi-barrier approach to safe tap water monitors and regulates water quality from the water source to the water treatment and distribution systems.[8] The bottled water industry, however, has fewer regulations and is often more self-monitored.

By definition, bottled water doesn't need to be anything special; it can be any water as long as it has no added ingredients except safe and suitable antimicrobial agents. Some of the bottled water sold in Canada is actually the same water that comes from municipal water supplies. Bottled water that comes from a tap must be clearly labelled as such. However, water that has been taken from a municipal water supply and then treated—for example, filtered or disinfected—need not indicate that it is tap water. "Distilled water" and "purified water" are examples of water that has been taken from municipal water supplies and then treated. For instance, Dasani water, which is owned by Coca-Cola, is sourced from Canadian municipal tap water in Calgary, Alberta, or Brantford, Ontario, and then filtered and sold for a markup of more than 3,000% of the original cost! Artesian water, spring water, well water, and mineral water come from underground sources rather than from municipal sources.

Two of the most significant arguments against bottled water are its cost and environmental impact.

Tap water costs as little as $0.002 per litre ($0.01/gallon), whereas bottled water can cost as much as $2.70 per litre ($10.00/gallon), making it significantly more expensive than gasoline. If you bought a 500-mL (16-oz) bottle of water each day for a toonie, then over one year, you will have spent more than $700 on water; you could have consumed the same amount of tap water for less than a loonie.

Bottled water generates 1.5 million tonnes of plastic waste per year, and consumes oil, which is used to produce the bottles. Recycling of these bottles is widely promoted, but nevertheless, many of these bottles end up in landfills where they can take hundreds, or even thousands of years to decompose.

So which is better? In Canada, bottled water and tap water are both generally great tasting, safe, and convenient. If you recycle your bottle, does it matter which you choose?

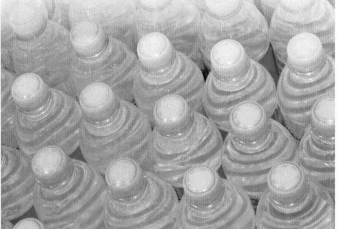

---

increases water losses because the excess must be excreted in the urine. A high-fibre diet increases water needs because more water is held in the intestines and excreted in the feces.

Most beverages, whether water, milk, juice, or pop, help to meet the overall need for water (see *Hot Topic: Is Bottled Water Better?*). Beverages containing caffeine, such as coffee, tea, and cola, increase water losses for a short period because caffeine inhibits antidiuretic hormone (ADH) and thus functions as a **diuretic**. Over the course of a day, however, the increase in water loss is small, so the net amount of water that caffeinated beverages add to the body is similar to the amount contributed by non-caffeinated beverages. Alcohol also inhibits ADH, by causing an increased urge to urinate; the overall effect it has on water balance depends on the relative amounts of water and alcohol in the beverages being consumed.[6]

> **diuretic** A substance that increases the amount of urine passed from the body.

1. **How** does osmosis affect the distribution of water in the body?

2. **What** is the role of the antidiuretic hormone?

3. **How** does water help cool the body?

4. **What** happens to the body if water losses exceed intake?

An Overview of Minerals

LEARNING OBJECTIVES

1. **Define** minerals in terms of nutrition.

2. **Describe** factors that affect mineral bioavailability.

3. **Discuss** the functions of minerals in the body.

Minerals are found in the ground on which we walk, the jewels we wear on our fingers, and even some of the makeup we wear on our faces, but perhaps their most significant impact on our lives comes from their importance in our diet. We need to consume more than 20 **minerals** in our diet to stay healthy. Some of these minerals make up a significant portion of our body weight; others are found in minute quantities. When we require more than 100 milligrams of a mineral per day in our diet, an amount equivalent in weight to about two drops of water, the mineral is considered a **major mineral**. Examples of major minerals include sodium, potassium, chloride, calcium, phosphorus, magnesium, and sulphur. Minerals needed in smaller amounts, referred to as **trace minerals**, include iron, copper, zinc, selenium, iodine, chromium, fluoride, manganese, molybdenum, and others. Just because we need more of the major minerals than of the trace minerals, it doesn't mean that the major minerals are more important. A deficiency of a trace mineral can be just as damaging to health as a deficiency of a major mineral.

minerals In nutrition, elements needed by the body in small amounts to maintain structure and regulate chemical reactions and body processes.

major minerals Minerals that are required in the diet in amounts greater than 100 mg/day or are present in the body in amounts greater than 0.01% of body weight.

trace minerals Minerals required in the diet in amounts of 100 mg or less/day or present in the body in amounts of 0.01% of body weight or less.

Minerals in Our Food

Minerals in the diet come from both plant and animal sources (**Figure 8.7**). Some minerals are functioning components of a plant or animal and are therefore present in consistent amounts. For instance, the iron content of beef is predictable because iron is part of the muscle protein that gives beef its red colour. In other foods, minerals are present as contaminants from the soil or from processing. For example, plants grown in an area where the soil is high in selenium are higher in selenium than plants grown in other areas. Similarly, milk is a source of iodine when it comes from dairies that use sterilizing solutions that contain iodine. Minerals are also intentionally added to food during processing. Sodium is added to soups and crackers as a flavour enhancer; iron is added to enriched grain products; and calcium, iron, and other minerals are sometimes added to fortified breakfast cereals.

Processing can also remove minerals from foods. For example, when vegetables are cooked, the cells are broken

Minerals in the food guide • Figure 8.7

Minerals are found in all the food groups, but some groups are particularly good sources of specific minerals. You can maximize your diet's mineral content by eating a variety of foods, including fresh fruits, vegetables, nuts, legumes, whole grains and cereals, milk, seafood, and lean meats.

VEGETABLES AND FRUIT	GRAIN PRODUCTS	MILK AND ALTERNATIVES	MEAT AND ALTERNATIVES
Iron, Calcium, Potassium, Magnesium, Molybdenum	Iron, Zinc, Selenium, Copper, Magnesium, Chromium, Sulphur, Manganese, Sodium, Potassium, Phosphorus	Calcium, Zinc, Phosphorus, Potassium, Iodine, Molybdenum	Iron, Zinc, Magnesium, Potassium, Chromium, Sulphur, Iodine, Selenium, Phosphorus, Copper, Manganese, Fluoride

down, and potassium is lost in the cooking water. When the skins of fruits and vegetables or the bran and germ of grains are detached during their refinement, magnesium, iron, selenium, zinc, and copper are lost.

Mineral Bioavailability

The *bioavailability* of minerals varies in the foods we consume. For some minerals, such as sodium, we absorb almost all that is present in our food, but for other minerals, we absorb only a small percentage. For example, calcium absorption is typically about 25%, and iron absorption may be as low as 5%. How much of a particular mineral is absorbed may vary from food to food, meal to meal, and person to person.

In general, the minerals in animal products are better absorbed than those in plant foods. The difference in absorption is due in part to the fact that plants contain substances such as phytic acid, tannins, oxalates, and fibre that bind minerals in the gastrointestinal tract and can reduce absorption (**Figure 8.8**). The North American diet generally does not contain enough of any of these components to cause a mineral deficiency, but diets in developing countries may. For example, in some populations, the phytate content of the diet is high enough to cause a zinc deficiency.

The presence of one mineral can also interfere with the absorption of another. For example, mineral **ions** that carry the same charge compete for absorption in the gastrointestinal tract. Calcium, magnesium, zinc, copper, and iron all carry a 2+ charge, so a high intake of one may reduce the absorption of another. Although this effect is generally not a problem when whole foods are consumed, a large dose of one mineral from a dietary supplement may interfere with the absorption of other minerals.

> **ions** Atoms or groups of atoms that carry an electrical charge.

The body's need for a particular mineral may also affect how much of that mineral is absorbed. For instance, if plenty of iron is stored in your body, you will absorb less of the iron you consume. Life stage can also affect absorption; for example, calcium absorption doubles during pregnancy, when the body's needs are high.

Mineral Functions

Minerals contribute to the body's structure and help to regulate body processes (**Figure 8.9**). Many minerals

---

Compounds that interfere with mineral absorption • Figure 8.8

Plant foods such as these contain substances that can reduce mineral absorption when consumed in large amounts.

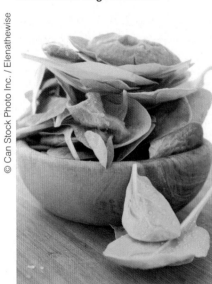

Oxalates, found in spinach, rhubarb, beet greens, and chocolate, have been found to interfere with the absorption of calcium and iron.

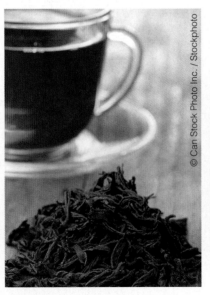

Tannins, found in tea, red wine, and some grains, can interfere with the absorption of iron.

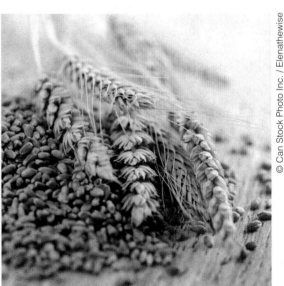

Phytates, found in whole grains, bran, and soy products, bind calcium, zinc, iron, and magnesium, limiting the absorption of these minerals. Phytates can be broken down by yeast, so the bioavailability of minerals is higher in yeast-leavened foods such as breads.

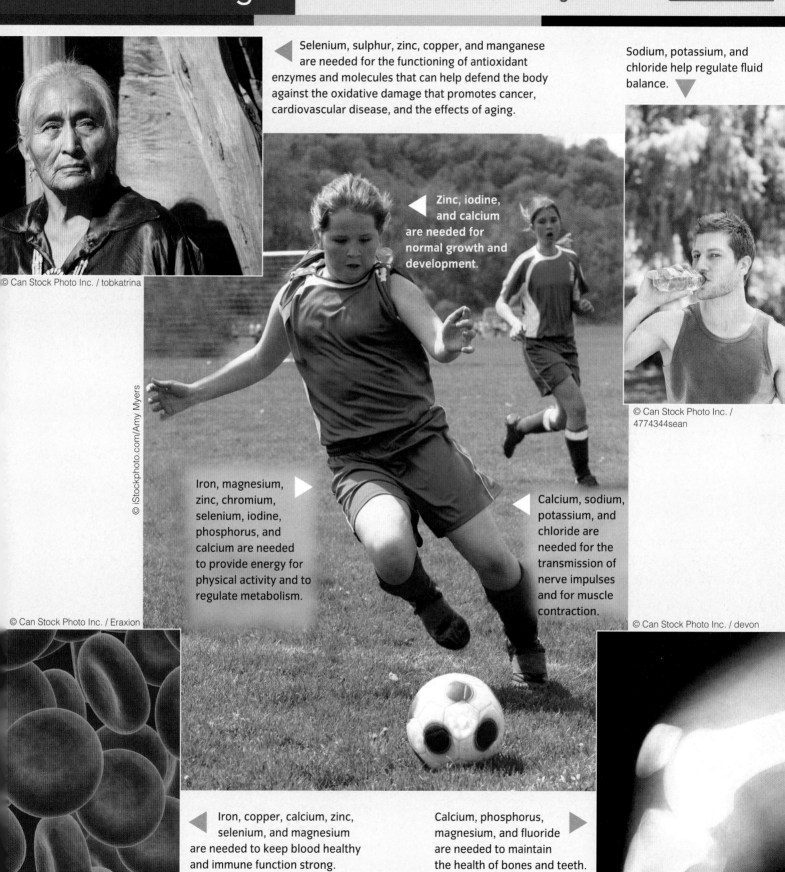

Selenium, sulphur, zinc, copper, and manganese are needed for the functioning of antioxidant enzymes and molecules that can help defend the body against the oxidative damage that promotes cancer, cardiovascular disease, and the effects of aging.

Sodium, potassium, and chloride help regulate fluid balance.

Zinc, iodine, and calcium are needed for normal growth and development.

Iron, magnesium, zinc, chromium, selenium, iodine, phosphorus, and calcium are needed to provide energy for physical activity and to regulate metabolism.

Calcium, sodium, potassium, and chloride are needed for the transmission of nerve impulses and for muscle contraction.

Iron, copper, calcium, zinc, selenium, and magnesium are needed to keep blood healthy and immune function strong.

Calcium, phosphorus, magnesium, and fluoride are needed to maintain the health of bones and teeth.

© Can Stock Photo Inc. / tobkatrina

© iStockphoto.com/Amy Myers

© Can Stock Photo Inc. / 4774344sean

© Can Stock Photo Inc. / Eraxion

© Can Stock Photo Inc. / devon

PROCESS DIAGRAM

Cofactors • Figure 8.10

The binding of a cofactor to an enzyme activates the enzyme. Coenzymes, discussed in Chapter 7, are a type of cofactor.

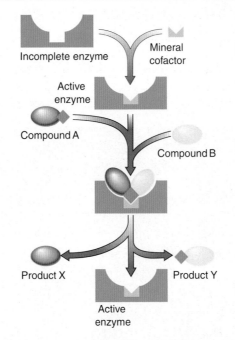

1 The mineral cofactor combines with the incomplete enzyme to form the active enzyme.

2 The active enzyme binds to the molecules involved in the chemical reaction (compounds A and B) and accelerates their transformation into the final products (products X and Y).

3 The final products are released, while the enzyme remains unchanged.

serve more than one function. For example, we need calcium not only to keep our bones strong but also to maintain normal blood pressure, allow muscles to contract, and transmit nerve signals from cell to cell. Some minerals help regulate water balance, others help regulate energy production, and some affect growth and development through their role in the expression of certain genes. Many minerals act as **cofactors** needed for enzyme activity (**Figure 8.10**). None of the minerals we require acts in

cofactors Inorganic ions or coenzymes that are required for enzyme activity.

isolation. Instead, they interact with each other and with other nutrients and other components of the diet.

CONCEPT CHECK **STOP**

1. **How** do minerals and vitamins differ?

2. **How** do phytates, oxalates, and tannins decrease mineral bioavailability?

3. **What** is the function of a cofactor?

Electrolytes: Sodium, Potassium, and Chloride

LEARNING OBJECTIVES

1. **Explain** how electrolytes function in the body.

2. **Define** hypertension and describe its symptoms and consequences.

3. **Discuss** how diet affects blood pressure.

4. **Contrast** the dietary sources of sodium and potassium.

We think of **electrolytes** as something we consume in a sports drink. But what exactly are they, and why do we need them? Electrolytes are negatively or positively charged ions that are important for the electrical activity of the body and for fluid balance. Although many substances in

electrolytes Positively and negatively charged ions that conduct an electrical current in solution. Commonly refers to sodium, potassium, and chloride.

the body are electrolytes, in nutrition and in sports drinks, *electrolytes* refer to the three principal electrolytes in body fluids: sodium, potassium, and chloride. These electrolytes help to transmit nerve signals, contract muscles, and promote water movement in the body.

Electrolytes in the Body

Sodium and potassium both carry a positive charge, and chloride carries a negative charge. Sodium is most commonly found combined with chloride as **sodium chloride**, commonly called "salt" or "table salt." The concentrations of sodium, potassium, and chloride inside a cell differ dramatically from their concentrations outside the cell. Potassium is the principal positively charged intracellular ion, sodium is the most abundant positively charged

extracellular ion, and chloride is the principal negatively charged extracellular ion.

Functions of electrolytes
Electrolytes help regulate fluid balance because the distribution of water throughout the body depends on the concentration of electrolytes and other solutes. Water moves by osmosis in response to differences in concentration. For example, if the concentration of sodium in the blood increases, water will move into the blood from intracellular and other extracellular spaces to equalize the concentration of sodium and other dissolved substances (**Figure 8.11a**).

Sodium and potassium are also essential for generating and conducting nerve impulses. Nerve impulses are created by the movement of sodium and potassium ions across the nerve cell membrane. When a nerve cell is

Electrolyte functions • Figure 8.11 _____

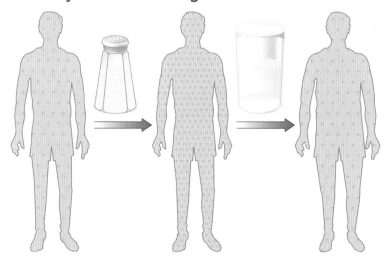

a. Have you ever noticed that you weigh more the morning after eating a salty dinner? The salt you consumed increased your blood sodium concentration and stimulated you to drink enough fluid to dilute it. The extra weight you see on the scale from one day to another typically reflects the extra water you have temporarily stowed away, not any extra fat.

b. You feel a pinprick because it stimulates nerves beneath the surface of the skin. This stimulation increases the permeability of the nerve cell membrane to sodium and then to potassium. The sodium rushes in (shown here), initiating a nerve impulse. Potassium then rushes out to restore the electrical charge across the membrane. The increase in sodium permeability at one spot triggers an increase on the adjacent patch of membrane, spreading the nerve impulse along the nerve to the brain. After the impulse has passed, the original ion concentrations inside and outside the membrane are restored by a sodium/potassium pump in the membrane so that a new nerve signal can be triggered.

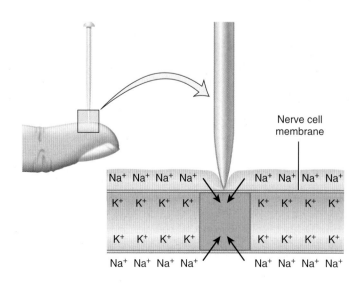

Electrolytes: Sodium, Potassium, and Chloride 261

at rest, potassium is concentrated inside the nerve cell, and sodium stays outside the cell. Sodium and potassium ions cannot pass freely across the cell membrane. But when a nerve is stimulated, the cell membrane becomes more permeable to sodium, allowing sodium ions to rush into the nerve cell, which initiates a nerve impulse (**Figure 8.11b**).

Regulating electrolyte balance Our bodies are efficient at regulating the concentration of electrolytes, even when dietary intake varies dramatically. Sodium and chloride balance is regulated to some extent by the intake of both salt and water. When salt intake is high, thirst is stimulated in order to increase water intake. Very low salt intake stimulates a "salt appetite" that causes you to crave salt. But this salt appetite isn't the same as the craving that triggers your desire to plunge into a bag of salty chips. Your craving for potato chips is a learned preference, not a physiological drive. If you cut back on your salt intake, your taste buds will become more sensitive to the presence of salt, and foods will taste saltier. You can reduce your salt intake in step-wise increments so the actual difference in taste isn't noticed as dramatically.

Thirst and salt appetite can help to ensure that the appropriate proportions of salt and water are taken in, but the kidneys are the primary regulator of the body's sodium, potassium, and chloride concentrations. Excretion of these electrolytes in the urine is decreased when intake is low and increased when intake is high.

Because water follows sodium by osmosis, the ability of the kidneys to conserve sodium provides a mechanism for conserving water in the body. This mechanism also helps to regulate blood pressure. When the concentration of sodium in the blood increases, water follows, causing an increase in blood volume. Any changes in blood volume can also change blood pressure. Changes in blood pressure, in turn, trigger the production and release of enzymes and hormones that affect the amount of sodium and, hence, the amount of water retained by the kidneys (see Figure 8.4).

Blood potassium levels also need to be regulated because even a small increase can be dangerous. When blood potassium levels begin to rise, body cells are stimulated to take up potassium. This short-term regulation prevents the amount of potassium in the extracellular fluid from becoming lethally high. Long-term regulation of potassium balance depends on the release of proteins such as **aldosterone** that cause the kidney to excrete potassium and retain sodium.

Electrolytes in Health and Disease

Electrolyte deficiencies are uncommon in healthy people because sodium, potassium, and chloride are plentiful in most diets, and the kidneys of healthy individuals are efficient at regulating the amounts of these electrolytes in the body. Acute deficiencies and excesses can occur due to illness or extreme conditions. The health problem most commonly associated with electrolyte imbalance is **hypertension**, or high blood pressure. Hypertension is a serious public health concern in Canada; more than one in five adult Canadians have hypertension, increasing their risk of a heart attack or stroke.[9]

> **hypertension** Blood pressure that is consistently elevated to 140/90 mm mercury or greater.

Electrolyte deficiency Deficiencies of any of the electrolytes can lead to electrolyte imbalance, which can cause disturbances in the acid–base balance, poor appetite, muscle cramps, confusion, apathy, constipation, and, eventually, irregular heartbeat. For example, the sudden death that can occur as a result of fasting, anorexia nervosa, or starvation may be due to heart failure caused by a potassium deficiency. Sodium, chloride, and potassium depletion can occur when losses of these electrolytes are increased by heavy and persistent sweating, chronic diarrhea or vomiting, or kidney disorders that lead to excessive excretion. Medications can also interfere with electrolyte balance. For example, certain diuretic medications that are used to treat high blood pressure cause potassium loss.

Electrolyte toxicity It is not possible for healthy people to consume too much potassium from foods. However, if supplements are consumed in excess or if kidney function is compromised, blood levels of potassium can increase and potentially lead to death due to an irregular heartbeat. A high oral dose of potassium generally causes vomiting, but if too much potassium enters the blood, it can cause the heart to stop.

Consuming more sodium than the body can handle is difficult because we are usually triggered to drink more water when we consume more sodium. Although elevation of blood sodium is rare, it can result from massive ingestion of salt, such as may occur from drinking seawater or consuming salt tablets. The most common cause of high blood sodium is dehydration, and the symptoms are similar to those of dehydration.

Hypertension Hypertension, or high blood pressure, has been called "the silent killer" because it has no outward symptoms but can lead to atherosclerosis, heart attack, stroke, kidney disease, and early death. Hypertension is caused by an increase in blood volume or a narrowing of the blood vessels. This complex disorder results from disturbances in one or more of the mechanisms that control body fluid and electrolyte balance.

Elevated blood pressure is treated with diet, exercise, and medication. To allow early treatment and to avoid the potentially lethal side effects blood pressure should be monitored regularly. A healthy blood pressure is 120/80 mm of mercury or less. Blood pressure between 120/80 and 139/89 is referred to as **prehypertension**, and blood pressure that is consistently 140/90 mm of mercury or greater indicates hypertension (see Appendix C).[10]

Risk of hypertension For most of the population, there is no identifiable cause of hypertension. Some of the risk of developing it is genetic; your risk is increased if you have a family history of the disease. Also, certain ethnic groups present significantly higher rates of the disease. A study by the Heart and Stroke Foundation of Canada found that, in Ontario, South Asians and Blacks had the highest rates of hypertension, approximately 50% higher than the rates of the mostly Caucasian general public.[11] Whether you are predisposed to hypertension or not, your risk of developing high blood pressure increases as you age and is higher if you are overweight, particularly if your excess fat is in your abdominal region. Blood pressure is also increased by lack of physical activity, heavy alcohol consumption, and stress.[12] Regular exercise can prevent or delay the onset of hypertension, and weight loss can help to reduce blood pressure in obese individuals. Your risk of developing high blood pressure can also be increased or decreased by your dietary choices.

Diet and blood pressure Dietary intake of sodium, chloride, potassium, calcium, and magnesium can affect your blood pressure and your risk of hypertension. Diets that are high in salt (sodium chloride) are associated with an increased incidence of hypertension, whereas diets that are high in potassium, calcium, and magnesium are associated with a lower average blood pressure.[13,14] Other components of the diet may also affect your risk, such as the amount of fibre and the type and amount of fat consumed. Although changing any one of these dietary factors will have only a minor impact on blood pressure, a dietary pattern that incorporates the recommended amounts of each of these dietary components can have a significant impact on blood pressure. The **DASH (Dietary Approaches to Stop Hypertension) diet** does just that.

The DASH diet provides moderate amounts of sodium and plenty of fibre, potassium, magnesium, and calcium; it is low in total fat, saturated fat, and cholesterol. Following the DASH diet has been found to lower blood pressure in individuals with elevated blood pressure, and reductions in blood pressure are even greater when the DASH diet is combined with a further reduction in sodium intake (**Figure 8.12**).[15,16]

Meeting Electrolyte Needs

Most people in Canada need to reduce their sodium intake and increase their potassium intake to meet recommendations for a healthy diet (see *What Should I Eat?*). Canadian adults between the ages of 14 and 50 should aim for an adequate intake of salt of 1500 mg/day, without exceeding an upper limit of 2300 mg/day. The needs of older adults and young children and infants are even lower. The typical daily intake of sodium in the Canadian diet is around 3400 mg, more than twice the recommended intake![18]

In 2007, the Canadian government assembled a working group to address the dangerously high levels of sodium in our diet. One of their main outcomes was a report that called for a daily sodium intake target of 2300 mg per person. To reach this target, the task force recommended the food industry reduce the amount of sodium in various food products and encouraged collaboration and investment across various industries and levels of government.[19] This task force was, however, abruptly disbanded in 2011 by the Canadian government, sparking criticism regarding the future of sodium reduction efforts and abilities.

The DRIs recommend a potassium intake of 4700 mg/day; the Daily Value is at least 3500 mg/day for adults, which is significantly higher than the typical 3400 mg/day consumed by most Canadians.

One of the reasons our diet is high in salt (sodium chloride) and low in potassium is that we eat a lot of processed foods, which are high in sodium and chloride, and too few fresh unprocessed foods, such as fruits, vegetables, whole grains, and fresh meats, which are high in potassium.

The effect of diet on blood pressure • Figure 8.12

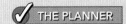

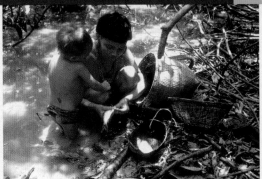

◄ This Yanomami Indian boy lives in the rainforests of Brazil. The Yanomami diet consists of locally grown crops, nuts, insects, fish, game, and less than a gram of salt a day, the lowest salt intake recorded for any population. The Yanomami have very low average blood pressure and no hypertension. Studying the salt intake and blood pressure of the Yanomami and 51 other populations around the world helped to establish a relationship between salt intake and hypertension; diets that are high in salt are associated with an increased incidence of hypertension.[13]

© Victor Englebert

A diet that is high in fruits and vegetables, which are good sources of potassium, magnesium, and fibre, reduces blood pressure more than a similar diet containing fewer fruits and vegetables. The amounts in the measuring cups shown here, about 500 g (2 cups) of fruit and 625 g (2 1/2 cups) of vegetables, represent the amount recommended for a 2,000-kilocalorie DASH diet.[17] ▶

Andy Washnik

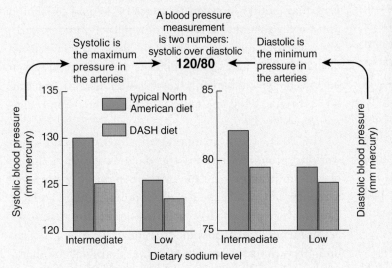

A blood pressure measurement is two numbers: systolic over diastolic
120/80

Systolic is the maximum pressure in the arteries

Diastolic is the minimum pressure in the arteries

Legend: typical North American diet / DASH diet

Left chart: Systolic blood pressure (mm mercury), y-axis 120–135, Dietary sodium level: Intermediate, Low

Right chart: Diastolic blood pressure (mm mercury), y-axis 75–85, Dietary sodium level: Intermediate, Low

The DASH diet (upper portion of the figure) is abundant in fruits and vegetables; includes low-fat dairy products, whole grains, legumes, and nuts; and incorporates moderate amounts of lean meat. These recommendations are similar to those of *Eating Well with Canada's Food Guide*. Choose whole grains; eat plenty of fruits and vegetables; consume beans, nuts, and seeds more often; and keep discretionary calories low by choosing lean meats and low-fat dairy products. ▼

The original DASH diet provided about 3000 mg of sodium/day, an amount only slightly less than the typical intake in Canada. When the sodium content of this diet was lowered, the result was an even greater reduction in blood pressure. Lowering sodium also reduced blood pressure in the group consuming a typical North American diet.[16]

Food Group	Sample Serving Size	Daily Servings per Kcalorie Level			
		1,600	2,000	2,600	3,100
Grains[a]	1 slice bread	6	7–8	10–11	12–13
Vegetables	250 mL (1 cup) raw, leafy vegetables	3–4	4–5	5–6	6
Fruits	1 medium fruit	4	4–5	5–6	6
Low-fat milk	250 mL (8 oz) milk	2–3	2–3	3	3–4
Meats, fish, poultry	90 g (3 oz) cooked meat, poultry, or fish	1–2	2 or less	2	2–3
Beans, nuts, and seeds	80 mL (1/3 cup) nuts	3 per week	4–5 per week	1	m
Fat and oils[b]	5 mL (1 tsp) vegetable oil	2	2–3	3	m
Sweets	15 mL (1 Tbsp) sugar	0	5 per week	2	2

[a]Whole grains are recommended for most servings to meet fibre recommendations.
[b]Fat content changes the number of servings for fats and oils; 15 mL (1 Tbsp) regular salad dressing equals one serving, 15 mL (1 Tbsp) low-fat dressing equals 1/2 serving, and 15 mL (1 Tbsp) of fat-free dressing equals 0 servings.

Source: Dietary Guidelines for Americans, 2005.

WHAT SHOULD I EAT?
Water and Electrolytes

Stay hydrated
- Drink before, during, and after you exercise.
- Chug two extra glasses of water when you are out on a hot day.
- Take a bottle of water with you in your car.

Boost your potassium intake
- Double your vegetable serving at dinner.
- Take two pieces of fruit for lunch.
- Drink orange juice instead of pop.

Reduce your sodium intake
- Choose more unprocessed foods.
- Do not add salt to the water when cooking rice, pasta, and cereals.
- Flavour foods with lemon juice, onions, garlic, pepper, curry, basil, oregano, or thyme rather than with salt.
- Limit salty snacks such as potato chips, salted nuts, salted popcorn, and crackers.
- Limit the use of high-sodium condiments such as soy sauce, barbecue sauce, ketchup, and mustard.

Use iProfile to compare the sodium content of fresh vegetables and canned vegetables.

A significant portion of the salt we eat is from foods that have had salt added during processing and manufacturing (**Figure 8.13**).

You can lower the amount of sodium in your diet by limiting your intake of processed foods and cutting down on the amount of salt added both during cooking and at the table. A diet that is high in fruits and vegetables will easily meet the potassium intake recommendations. Food labels can also help to identify low-sodium foods (**Figure 8.14**). Some medications contribute a significant amount of sodium, so check the drug facts labels on over-the-counter medications to identify those drugs that contain large amounts of sodium.

Table 8.1 summarizes information about water, sodium, chloride, and potassium.

Processing adds sodium • Figure 8.13

Just over three-quarters of our sodium intake comes from processed foods; these include both restaurant and fast foods.[18] Only 12% of our sodium intake comes from whole, unprocessed, unseasoned foods.[18] If we were to consume more foods in their natural states, our sodium intake would decrease dramatically.

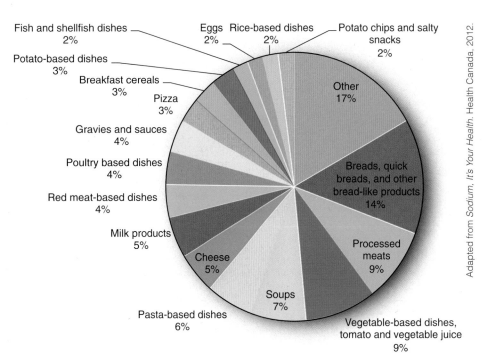

Fish and shellfish dishes 2%
Eggs 2%
Rice-based dishes 2%
Potato chips and salty snacks 2%
Potato-based dishes 3%
Breakfast cereals 3%
Pizza 3%
Gravies and sauces 4%
Poultry based dishes 4%
Red meat-based dishes 4%
Milk products 5%
Cheese 5%
Pasta-based dishes 6%
Soups 7%
Vegetable-based dishes, tomato and vegetable juice 9%
Processed meats 9%
Breads, quick breads, and other bread-like products 14%
Other 17%

Adapted from *Sodium, It's Your Health*. Health Canada, 2012.

Food labels are an important source of information on the sodium content of packaged foods. In addition to the information illustrated here, foods that meet the definition for low sodium may carry a health claim on their label stating that diets low in sodium may reduce the risk of high blood pressure. In order to have this label, the food must also provide 20% or less of the Daily Value for fat, saturated fat, and cholesterol per serving.

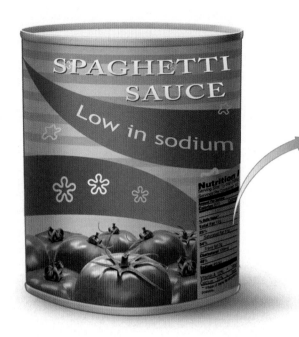

Nutrition Facts
Valeur nutritive
Per 125 mL / par 125 mL

Amount Teneur	% Daily Value % valeur quotidienne
Calories / Calories 50	
Fat / Lipides 1 g	2 %
Saturated / saturés 0 g + Trans / trans 0 g	0 %
Cholesterol / Cholestérol 0 mg	
Sodium / Sodium 120 mg	5 %
Potassium / Potassium 530 g	15 %
Carbohydrate / Glucides 9 g	3 %
Fibre / Fibres 1 g	4 %
Sugars / Sucres 7 g	
Protein / Protéines 3 g	
Vitamin A / Vitamine A	10 %
Vitamin C / Vitamine C	25 %
Calcium / Calcium	2 %
Iron / Fer	10 %

A summary of water and the electrolytes   Table 8.1

Nutrient	Sources	Recommended intake for adults	Major functions	Deficiency diseases and symptoms	Groups at risk of deficiency	Toxicity	UL
Water	Drinking water, other beverages, and food	2.7–3.7 L/day	Solvent, reactant, protector, transporter, regulator of temperature and pH	Thirst, weakness, poor endurance, confusion, disorientation, collapse	Infants, people with fever and diarrhea, elderly individuals, athletes	Confusion, coma, convulsions	ND
Sodium	Table salt, processed foods	<2300 mg; ideally 1500 mg/day	Major positive extracellular ion, nerve transmission, muscle contraction, fluid balance	Muscle cramps	People consuming a severely sodium-restricted diet, those who sweat excessively	High blood pressure in sensitive people	2300 mg/day
Potassium	Fresh fruits and vegetables, legumes, whole grains, milk, meat	4700 mg/day or more	Major positive intracellular ion, nerve transmission, muscle contraction, fluid balance	Irregular heartbeat, fatigue, muscle cramps	People consuming poor diets high in processed foods, those taking thiazide diuretics	Abnormal heartbeat	ND
Chloride	Table salt, processed foods	<3600 mg/day; ideally 2300 mg/day	Major negative extracellular ion, fluid balance	Unlikely	None	None likely	3600 mg/day

Note: UL, Tolerable Upper Intake Level; ND, not determined.

1. **Why** does eating a salty meal cause your weight to increase temporarily?

2. **Why** is hypertension called "the silent killer"?

3. **What** is the DASH diet?

4. **Which** types of foods contribute the most sodium to the Canadian diet?

Major Minerals and Bone Health

LEARNING OBJECTIVES

1. **Describe** factors that affect peak bone mass and the rate of bone loss.

2. **Explain** how blood calcium levels are regulated.

3. **List** foods that are good sources of calcium.

4. **Describe** the functions of calcium, phosphorus, and magnesium that are unrelated to their role in bone.

B ones are the hardest, strongest structures in the human body. They support our weight, whether we are stepping off a curb or jumping rope. Age, however, heralds a loss of bone strength. For many people, the loss is so great that the force of stepping off a curb is enough to cause their bones to fracture.

Bone is strong because it is composed of a protein framework, or matrix, consisting primarily of the protein collagen and is hardened by deposits of minerals. The mineral portion of bone is composed mainly of calcium associated with phosphorus, but it also contains magnesium, sodium, fluoride, and other minerals. Healthy bones require adequate dietary protein and vitamin C to maintain the collagen and a sufficient supply of calcium and other minerals to ensure solidity. Adequate vitamin D (discussed in Chapter 7) is needed to maintain appropriate levels of calcium and phosphorus. Growing evidence also supports the importance of vitamin K for bone health.[20] As important as proper nutrition is for healthy bones, strength training exercise throughout life is also a significant contributor to bone health.

Although many of us think of bone as a static structures that never changes, bone is constantly being broken down and re-formed through a process called **bone remodelling**. Bone remodelling involves bone-building cells called osteoblasts and bone-breaking cells called osteoclasts (**Figure 8.15**). When calcium levels are low in the blood, osteoclasts are activated to break down bone at its edge, which leads to the release of calcium from the bone matrix. Bone is again

bone remodelling A continuous process in which small amounts of bone are removed and replaced by new bone.

Bone remodelling • Figure 8.15

During bone remodelling, osteoclasts (pink) break down bone, and osteoblasts (blue) build bone.

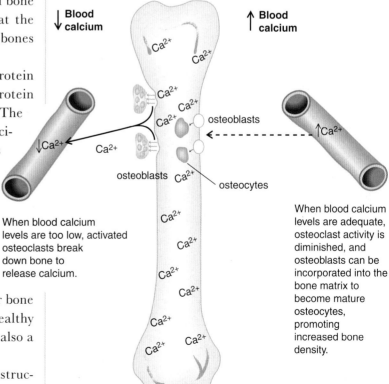

↓ Blood calcium

↑ Blood calcium

osteoblasts

osteoblasts

osteocytes

When blood calcium levels are too low, activated osteoclasts break down bone to release calcium.

When blood calcium levels are adequate, osteoclast activity is diminished, and osteoblasts can be incorporated into the bone matrix to become mature osteocytes, promoting increased bone density.

Bone mass and osteoporosis • Figure 8.16

a. Changes in the balance between bone formation and bone breakdown cause bone mass to increase in children and adolescents and decrease in adults as they grow older. ▼

Both men and women lose bone slowly after about age 35.

In growing children, total bone mass increases as the bones grow larger.

Men achieve a higher peak bone mass than do women.

In women, bone loss is accelerated for about 5 years after menopause.

— Males
— Females

During puberty, bone mass increases rapidly, and sex differences in bone mass appear.

Bone mass

Age (years)
0 10 20 30 40 50 60 70 80

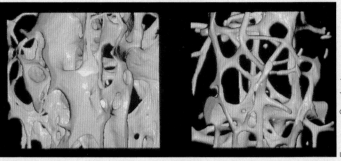

Normal bone   Bone weakened by osteoporosis

European Synchrotron Radiation Facility / CREATIS / Science Source

b. Osteoporosis, shown here compared with normal bone, is a major public health problem in Canada and elsewhere around the world. Approximately 2 million Canadians are living with osteoporosis; it affects 1 in 4 women and 1 in 8 men over the age of 50.[22]

Ask Yourself

During which age range can you have the most effect on increasing bone mass? How can you maximize your peak bone mass?

Normal spine

Osteoporotic spine

When weakened by osteoporosis, the front edge of the vertebrae collapses more than the back edge, so the spine bends forward.

c. Osteoporosis causes 70 to 90% of the 30,000 hip fractures that occur each year in Canada. Each fracture costs the health care system more than $20,000 in the first year alone.[22] Spinal compression fractures, shown here, are common and may result in loss of height and a stooped posture (called a "dowager's hump")

Larry Mulvehill / Science Source

rebuilt when osteoclast activity diminishes, and osteoblasts, which are immature bone cells, are incorporated into the edge of the bone. These bone cells will then develop into mature bone cells, called osteocytes, as calcium, phosphorus, and other components deposit into the bone matrix. The breakdown of bone can be prevented by consuming enough dietary calcium to maintain adequate blood levels of the mineral. When this is combined with ample weight-bearing activity, bone density is maximized.

Most bone is formed early in life. During childhood, bones grow larger; even after growth stops, bone mass continues to increase into young adulthood (**Figure 8.16a**). The maximum amount of bone that you have in your lifetime, called **peak bone mass**, is achieved between the ages of 16 and 30. Up to this point, bone formation occurs more rapidly than breakdown, so the total amount of bone increases. After about age 35 to 45, the amount of bone that is broken down begins to exceed the amount that is formed, so total bone mass decreases. Over time, if enough bone is lost, the skeleton is weakened, and fractures occur more easily, a condition referred to as **osteoporosis** (**Figure 8.16b, c**). It is estimated that osteoporosis cost Canada approximately $2.3 billion in 2010 alone: approximately 1.3% of health expenditures.[21]

peak bone mass The maximum bone density attained at any time in life, usually occurring in young adulthood.

osteoporosis A bone disorder characterized by reduced bone mass, increased bone fragility, and increased risk of fractures.

Bone Health and Osteoporosis

The risk of developing osteoporosis depends on the level of peak bone mass and the rate at which bone is lost. These variables are affected by genetics, gender, age, and hormone levels, and by such lifestyle factors as smoking, alcohol consumption, exercise, and diet (**Table 8.2**).

Women have a higher risk of osteoporosis because they have less bone than men and lose it faster as they age. **Age-related bone loss** occurs in both men and women, but women lose additional bone for about five years after **menopause**. This **postmenopausal bone loss** is related to the decline in estrogen level, which affects bone cells and decreases the amount of calcium absorbed in the intestines. A low calcium intake is the most significant dietary factor contributing to osteoporosis. The effect of diet on bone mass is discussed in more depth later in the chapter.

One factor associated with a reduced risk of osteoporosis is excess body weight.[23] Having greater body weight, whether that weight is due to an increase in muscle mass or to excess body fat, increases bone mass because it increases the amount of weight the bones must support. In other words, stressing the bones makes them grow stronger. A similar effect is seen in

age-related bone loss The bone loss that occurs in both men and women as they advance in age.

menopause The time in a woman's life when the menstrual cycle ends.

postmenopausal bone loss The accelerated bone loss that occurs in women for about five years after the menstrual cycle stops.

Factors affecting the risk of osteoporosis	Table 8.2
Risk factor	**How it affects risk**
Gender	Fractures due to osteoporosis are about twice as common in women as in men. Men are larger and heavier than women and therefore have a greater peak bone mass. Women lose more bone than men due to postmenopausal bone loss.
Age	Bone loss is a normal part of aging, and the risk of bone loss increases with age.
Race	Black Canadians have denser bones than do Caucasians and Southeast Asians, so their risk of osteoporosis is lower.[22]
Family history	Having a family member with osteoporosis increases risk.
Exercise	Weight-bearing exercise, such as walking and jogging, throughout life strengthens bone. Increasing weight-bearing exercise at any age can increase bone density.
Smoking	Tobacco use weakens bones.
Alcohol abuse	Long-term alcohol abuse reduces bone formation and interferes with the body's ability to absorb calcium.
Diet	A diet that is lacking in calcium and vitamin D plays a major role in the development of osteoporosis. Low calcium intake during the years of bone formation results in a lower peak bone mass, and low calcium intake in adulthood can accelerate bone loss.

people of all body weights who engage in weight-bearing exercise. In postmenopausal women, excess body fat may also reduce risk because adipose tissue is an important source of estrogen, which helps maintain bone mass and enhances calcium absorption.

Preventing and treating osteoporosis Osteoporosis is often called the "silent threat" because you can't feel your bones weakening. People with osteoporosis may not know that their bone mass is dangerously low until they are in their 50s or 60s and experience a bone fracture. Once osteoporosis has developed, it is difficult to restore lost bone. Therefore, the best treatment for osteoporosis is to prevent it by achieving a high peak bone mass and slowing the rate of bone loss. A life full of physical activity, specifically weight-bearing exercise, strengthens bones and is essential for achieving peak bone mass in youth. A diet containing adequate amounts of calcium and vitamin D will further produce greater peak bone mass and slow bone loss. Also associated with greater bone mass are higher intakes of zinc, magnesium, potassium, fibre, and vitamin C—nutrients that are plentiful in fruits and vegetables.[24] Bone density can be further increased and maintained by limiting smoking and alcohol consumption.

Risk of osteoporosis can be increased by high intakes of phytates, oxalates, and tannins, which reduce calcium absorption, and by high dietary sodium intake, which increases calcium loss in the urine.[25] High protein intake also increases urinary calcium losses, but when calcium intake is adequate, high levels of protein do not have a negative effect on bone mass.[26]

Osteoporosis is commonly treated in three ways: with medications called bisphosphonates to reduce bone breakdown, supplements of calcium and vitamin D, and regular weight-bearing exercise. Bisphosphonates inhibit the activity of cells that break down bone and have been shown to prevent postmenopausal bone loss, increase bone mineral density, and reduce the risk of fractures. Their effectiveness is enhanced by calcium supplementation.[27]

Calcium

In an average person, about 1.5% of body weight is due to calcium, and 99% of this calcium is found in the bones and teeth. The remaining calcium is located in body cells and fluids, where it is needed for muscle contraction, release of neurotransmitters, blood pressure regulation, cell communication, blood clotting, and other essential functions. Neurotransmitter release is critical to nerve function because neurotransmitters relay nerve impulses from one nerve to another and from nerves to other cells. Calcium in muscle cells is essential for muscle contraction because it allows the interaction of the muscle proteins actin and myosin. Calcium may help to regulate blood pressure by controlling the contraction of muscles in the blood vessel walls and signalling the secretion of substances that regulate blood pressure. It also is responsible for triggering glandular secretions throughout the body.

Calcium in health and disease The various roles of calcium are so vital to survival that powerful regulatory mechanisms maintain calcium concentrations both inside and outside cells. Slight changes in blood calcium levels trigger the release of hormones that work to keep calcium levels constant. For instance, when calcium levels drop, **parathyroid hormone (PTH)** is released (see Chapter 7). PTH acts in several tissues to increase blood calcium levels (**Figure 8.17**). When blood calcium levels are too high,

Raising blood calcium levels • Figure 8.17 ____

Low blood calcium triggers the secretion of parathyroid hormone (PTH) from the parathyroid gland. PTH stimulates osteoclast activity to release calcium from bone and causes the kidneys to reduce calcium loss in the urine and to activate vitamin D. Activated vitamin D increases the absorption of calcium from the gastrointestinal tract and acts with PTH to stimulate calcium release from the bone. The overall effect of PTH is to rapidly restore blood calcium levels to normal.

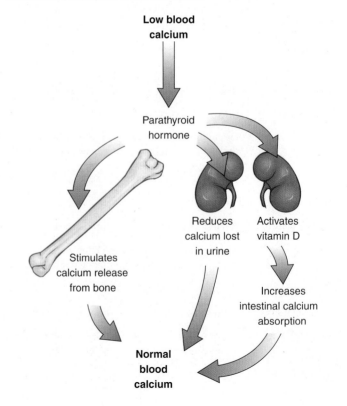

Low blood calcium

Parathyroid hormone

Stimulates calcium release from bone

Reduces calcium lost in urine

Activates vitamin D

Increases intestinal calcium absorption

Normal blood calcium

PTH secretion stops, and a hormone, **calcitonin**, is released, which acts primarily on bone to inhibit the release of calcium into the blood.

When too little calcium is consumed, the body maintains normal blood levels by stimulating osteoclasts to break down bone to release calcium, a process called **bone resorption**. This process provides a steady supply of calcium and causes no short-term symptoms. Over time, however, a calcium deficiency can reduce bone mass. Low calcium intake during the years of bone formation results in lower peak bone mass. If calcium intake is low after peak bone mass has been achieved, the rate of bone loss may be increased and, along with it, the risk of osteoporosis.

Too much calcium can also affect health. Elevated blood calcium levels can cause symptoms such as loss of appetite, nausea, vomiting, constipation, abdominal pain, thirst, and frequent urination. Severe elevation may cause confusion, delirium, coma, and even death. Because the level of calcium in the blood is finely regulated, elevated blood calcium is rare and is most often caused by cancer and by disorders that increase the secretion of PTH. It can also result from increases in intestinal calcium absorption due to excessive vitamin D intake or high intakes of calcium in combination with antacids.

High calcium intake from supplements can interfere with the availability of iron, zinc, magnesium, and phosphorus and may promote the formation of kidney stones in some individuals.[27] Based on the occurrence of kidney stones, elevated blood calcium, and the potential for decreased absorption of other essential minerals, the UL for calcium in adults has been set at 2500 mg/day.

Meeting calcium needs For adults ages 19 to 70, recommended calcium intake is 1000 mg/day. The recommended intake is 200 mg higher in adults over 70 because their calcium absorption is decreased due to lower blood levels of the active form of vitamin D and a decrease in responsiveness to vitamin D.[28] An additional drop in calcium absorption occurs in women after menopause due to the decrease in estrogen levels; Women over 50 years of age should therefore consume 1200 mg of calcium per day.[29] Calcium absorption is higher at times when the body's need for calcium is greater. In young adults, about 25% of dietary calcium is absorbed; during pregnancy, when the fetal skeleton is forming, the rate of absorption increases to over 50%; and during infancy, about 60% of dietary calcium is absorbed.

The main source of calcium in the North American diet is dairy products (**Figure 8.18**). Individuals who do

Food sources of calcium • Figure 8.18

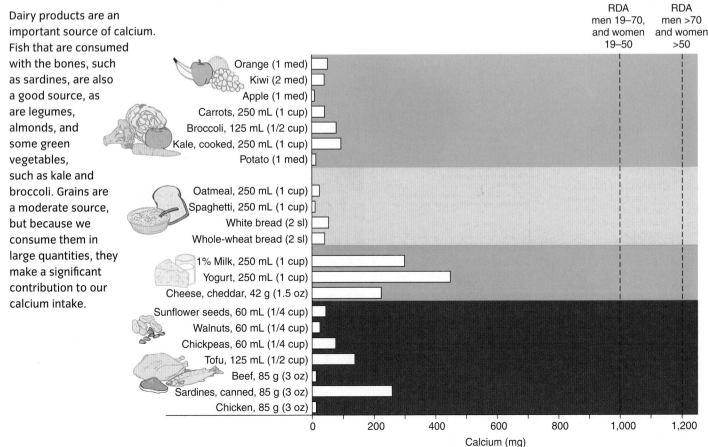

Dairy products are an important source of calcium. Fish that are consumed with the bones, such as sardines, are also a good source, as are legumes, almonds, and some green vegetables, such as kale and broccoli. Grains are a moderate source, but because we consume them in large quantities, they make a significant contribution to our calcium intake.

not consume dairy products can meet their calcium needs by consuming leafy dark green vegetables, fish consumed with bones, foods processed with calcium, and foods fortified with calcium, such as some juices.

Individuals who do not meet their calcium needs through their diet alone can benefit from calcium supplements (**Figure 8.19**). They may also provide additional benefits to some age groups. In young adults, supplemental calcium can increase peak bone mass, and in postmenopausal women, calcium supplements may reduce the rate of bone loss. Calcium is found in two main forms in supplements: as calcium carbonate or calcium citrate. The carbonate form is typically more accessible, inexpensive, and convenient. Since it requires stomach acid for absorption, this form of calcium should be consumed with foods. Citrate, on the other hand, can be absorbed well even when taken in the absence of food. This form may be more useful for those with absorptive or gastrointestinal disorders.

Whether your calcium comes from foods or from supplements, bioavailability must be considered. Vitamin D is the nutrient that has the most significant impact on calcium absorption. When calcium intake is high, calcium is absorbed by diffusion, but when intake is low to moderate, as it typically is, absorption depends on the active form of vitamin D. When vitamin D is deficient, less than 10% of dietary calcium may be absorbed, compared with the typical 25% absorption rate when vitamin D is present. Other dietary components that affect calcium absorption include acidic foods, lactose, and fat, which increase calcium absorption, and oxalates, phytates, tannins, and fibre, which inhibit calcium absorption. For example, spinach is a high-calcium vegetable, but only about 5% of its calcium is absorbed; the rest is bound by oxalates and excreted in the feces.[30] Vegetables such as kale, collard greens, turnip greens, mustard greens, and Chinese cabbage are low in oxalates, so their calcium is more readily absorbed. Chocolate also contains oxalates, but chocolate milk is still a good source of calcium because the amount of oxalates from the chocolate added to a glass of milk is small.

Phosphorus

Most of the phosphorus in your body is associated with calcium as part of the hard mineral crystals called hydroxyapatite, which are found in bones and teeth. The smaller

Calcium supplements • Figure 8.19

If you are not consuming enough calcium from foods, you can meet your calcium needs by taking a supplement that contains either a calcium compound alone or calcium with vitamin D. A multivitamin/multimineral supplement will provide only a small amount of the calcium you need. Read the label to make sure you choose an appropriate supplement.

Choose supplements that contain calcium carbonate or calcium citrate.

Choosing a supplement with vitamin D ensures that the vitamin will be available for calcium absorption.

Calcium Citrate with Vitamin D
Recommended Dose (Adults): Take 3 tablets daily or as directed by a health care practitioner.

Medicinal Ingredients:
Each tablet contains:
Calcium citrate .... 300 mg
Magnesium (citrate, oxide) .... 150 mg
Vitamin D (cholecalciferol) .... 100 IU
Non-medicinal ingredients:
Cellulose, Modified Cellulose Gum, Vegetable Stearic Acid, Silica, Vegetable Magnesium Stearate, Water-Soluble Cellulose, Titanium dioxide.
Note: For therapeutic use only.

Citrate de calcium avec vitamine D
Dose recommandé (adultes): Prendre 3 comprimés par jour ou selon l'avis d'un practicien de soins de santé.

Ingrédients médicin aux:
Chaque comprimé contient:
Calcium citrate .... 300 mg
Magnésium (citrate, oxyde) .... 150 mg
Vitamin D (cholécalciférol) .... 100 IU
Ingrédients non médicinaux: cellulose, gomme de cellulose modifiée,
acide stéarique végétal, silice, stéarate de magnésium végétal, cellulose hydrosoluble, dioxyde de titane.
Note: Pour usage thérapeutique seulement.

500 mg taken twice a day provides 100% of the AI for adults ages 19 to 50.

Calcium is absorbed best when taken in doses of 500 mg or less.

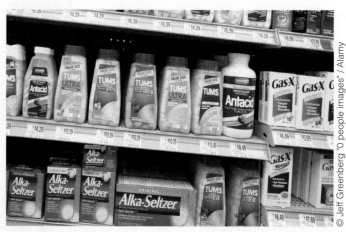

Some antacids are also sources of calcium. These are over-the-counter medications, so they carry a Drug Facts panel rather than a Supplement Facts panel.

© Jeff Greenberg "0 people images" / Alamy

Nonskeletal functions of phosphorus • Figure 8.20

Most of the phosphorus in the body helps form the structure of bones and teeth. Phosphorus also plays an important role in a host of cellular activities.

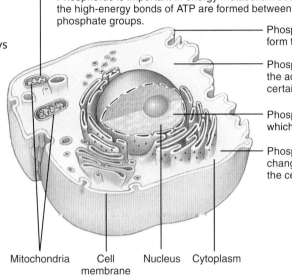

Phosphorus is important in energy metabolism because the high-energy bonds of ATP are formed between phosphate groups.

Phosphorus is a component of phospholipids, which form the structure of cell membranes.

Phosphorus is involved in regulating enzyme activity; the addition of a phosphorus-containing group to certain enzymes can activate or inactivate them.

Phosphorus is a major constituent of DNA and RNA, which orchestrate the synthesis of proteins.

Phosphorus is part of a compound that can prevent changes in acidity so that chemical reactions inside the cell can proceed normally.

Mitochondria   Cell membrane   Nucleus   Cytoplasm

amount of phosphorus in soft tissues performs an essential role as a structural component of phospholipids, DNA and RNA, and ATP. It is also important in regulating the activity of enzymes and maintaining the proper level of acidity in cells (**Figure 8.20**).

Phosphorus in health and disease Blood levels of phosphorus are not controlled as strictly as calcium levels, but the kidneys help to maintain phosphorus levels in a ratio with calcium that allows minerals to be deposited into bone. A deficiency of phosphorus can lead to bone loss, weakness, and loss of appetite. Inadequate phosphorus intake is rare because phosphorus is widely distributed in food. Marginal phosphorus status may be caused by losses due to chronic diarrhea or poor absorption due to overuse of aluminum-containing antacids.

Excessive phosphorus intake can lead to bone loss. Luckily, the current intake levels of Canadians are not believed to contribute to osteoporosis as long as calcium intake is adequate. Bone health may be affected by the increased use of food additives that contain phosphorus, particularly in pop, which often replaces milk.[31] The UL for phosphorus is 4000 mg/day for adults.[27]

Meeting phosphorus needs Good sources of phosphorus include dairy products, such as milk, yogurt, and cheese, and meat, cereals, bran, eggs, nuts, and fish. Phosphorous is also provided in the food additives used in baked goods, cheese, processed meats, and soft drinks. Most diets meet the RDA of 700 mg/day for adults.[27]

Magnesium

Magnesium is far less abundant in the body than are calcium and phosphorus, but it is still essential for healthy bones. About 50 to 60% of the magnesium in the body is in bone, where it helps maintain bone structure. The rest of the magnesium is found in cells and fluids throughout the body. Magnesium is involved in regulating calcium homeostasis and is needed for the action of vitamin D and many hormones, including PTH. Magnesium is important for the regulation of blood pressure and may play a role in maintaining cardiovascular health. In addition, magnesium forms a complex with ATP that stabilizes ATP's structure. Thus, magnesium is needed in every metabolic reaction that generates or uses ATP, including the reactions needed for the release of energy from carbohydrate, fat, and protein; the functioning of the nerves and muscles; and the synthesis of DNA, RNA, and protein. These roles make magnesium particularly important for dividing and growing cells.

Magnesium in health and disease Although overt magnesium deficiency is rare, the typical intake of magnesium in Canada is below the RDA. Low intakes of magnesium have been associated with chronic diseases, including osteoporosis.[32] Magnesium deficiency can cause nausea, muscle weakness and cramping, irritability, mental derangement, and changes in blood pressure and heartbeat. As discussed earlier, dietary patterns that are high in magnesium are associated with lower blood pressure, and epidemiological evidence suggests that the risk of atherosclerosis is lower for people with adequate magnesium intake than for those with less magnesium in their diet.[33] Areas with "hard" water, which is high in calcium and magnesium, tend to have lower rates of death from cardiovascular disease. Low blood magnesium levels affect levels of blood calcium and potassium; therefore, some of the symptoms of magnesium deficiency may be due to alterations in the levels of these other minerals.

No adverse effects have been observed from magnesium consumed in foods, but toxicity may occur from drugs containing magnesium, such as milk of magnesia and supplements that include magnesium. Kidney disease may also result in toxic levels of magnesium. Magnesium toxicity causes nausea, vomiting, low blood pressure, and other cardiovascular changes. The daily UL for adults and adolescents over age 9 is 350 mg of magnesium from supplements or medications.[27]

Meeting magnesium needs Magnesium is found in many foods but in small amounts, so you can't get all your magnesium needs from a single food (**Figure 8.21** and *What Should I Eat?*). Enriched grain products are poor sources because magnesium is lost in processing, and is not added back by enrichment. For example, removing the bran and germ from wheat kernels reduces the magnesium content of 250 g (1 cup) of white flour to only 28 mg, compared with the 166 mg in 250 g (1 cup) of whole-wheat flour. Magnesium absorption is enhanced by the active form of vitamin D and decreased by the presence of phytates and calcium.

Sulphur

Sulphur is part of the proteins in bones and other parts of the body because sulphur is contained in the amino acids methionine and cysteine, which are needed for protein synthesis. Cysteine is also part of glutathione, a molecule that plays an important role in detoxifying drugs and protecting cells from oxidative damage. The vitamins thiamin and biotin, which are essential for energy metabolism, also contain sulphur, and sulphur-containing ions are important in regulating acidity in the body.

We consume sulphur as a part of dietary proteins and sulphur-containing vitamins. Sulphur is also found in some food preservatives, such as sulphur dioxide, sodium sulphite, and sodium and potassium bisulphite. There is no recommended intake for sulphur, and no deficiencies are known when protein needs are met.

Table 8.3 provides a summary of the sources and functions of calcium, phosphorus, magnesium, and sulphur.

Sources of magnesium • Figure 8.21

Magnesium is a component of the green pigment chlorophyll, so leafy greens such as spinach and kale are good sources of this mineral. Also good sources of magnesium are nuts, seeds, legumes, bananas, and the germ and bran of whole grains. The dashed lines represent the RDAs of 420 and 320 mg/day for adult men and women over age 30, respectively.[27]

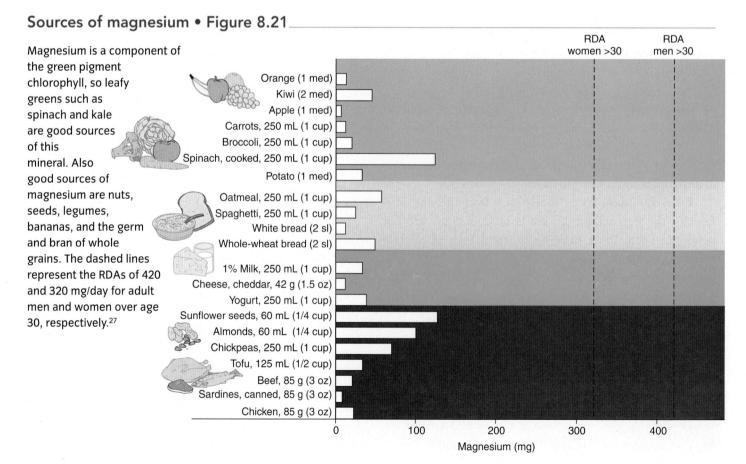

WHAT SHOULD I EAT?
Calcium, Phosphorus, and Magnesium

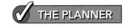 THE PLANNER

Get calcium into your body and your bones
- Have two servings of dairy a day: milk, yogurt, cottage cheese.
- Bone up on calcium by eating sardines or canned salmon, which are eaten with the bones.
- Choose leafy greens—they are a vegetable source of calcium.
- Walk, jog, lift weights, or do power yoga—weight-bearing exercises build up bone.

Don't fret about phosphorus—it's in almost everything you eat

Maximize your magnesium
- Choose whole grains.
- Sprinkle nuts and seeds on your salad, cereal, and stir-fry.
- Go for the green—whenever you eat green, you are eating magnesium; most greens also contain calcium.

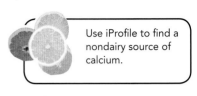

Use iProfile to find a nondairy source of calcium.

A summary of calcium, phosphorus, magnesium, and sulphur   Table 8.3

Mineral	Sources	Recommended intake for adults	Major functions	Deficiency diseases and symptoms	Groups at risk of deficiency	Toxicity	UL
Calcium	Dairy products, fish consumed with bones, leafy green vegetables, fortified foods	1000 mg/day; 1200 mg/day for women > 50 and men > 70	Bone and tooth structure, nerve transmission, muscle contraction, blood clotting, blood pressure regulation, hormone secretion	Increased risk of osteoporosis	Postmenopausal women; elderly people; those who consume a vegan diet, are lactose intolerant, or have kidney disease	Elevated blood calcium, kidney stones, and other problems in susceptible individuals	2500 mg/day for adults aged 19–50, 2000 mg/day for adults > 70
Phosphorus	Meat, dairy, cereals, baked goods	700 mg/day	Structure of bones and teeth, membranes, ATP, and DNA; acid–base balance	Bone loss, weakness, lack of appetite	Premature infants, alcoholics, elderly people	Calcium resorption from bone	4000 mg/day
Magnesium	Greens, whole grains, legumes, nuts, seeds	310 mg/day for women 19–30; 320 mg/day for women > 30; 400 mg/day for men 19–30; 420 mg/day for men > 30	Bone structure, ATP stabilization, enzyme activity, nerve and muscle function	Nausea, vomiting, weakness, muscle pain, heart changes	Alcoholics, individuals with kidney and gastrointestinal disease	Nausea, vomiting, low blood pressure	350 mg/day from nonfood sources
Sulphur	Protein foods, preservatives	None specified	Part of amino acids, vitamins, acid–base balance	None when protein needs are met	None	None likely	ND

Note: UL, Tolerable Upper Intake Level; ND, not determined.

Trace Minerals

LEARNING OBJECTIVES

1. **Relate** the primary function of iron to the effects of iron deficiency.

2. **Compare** the antioxidant functions of selenium and vitamin E.

3. **Explain** why iodine deficiency causes the thyroid gland to enlarge.

4. **Describe** the functions of copper, zinc, chromium, and fluoride.

J ust as the best cooks know that a pinch of this or a dash of that can enhance the flavour of a special dish, the presence of minute quantities of certain minerals can boost the nutritional impact of a person's diet. The trace minerals, so called because they are needed in extremely small amounts, are essential to health. For some trace minerals, the amount in food is affected by where the food is grown and/or how it is handled. When modern transportation systems increase the availability of foods produced in many locations, these variations balance each other and are unlikely to affect an individual's mineral status. In countries where the diet consists predominantly of locally grown foods, trace mineral deficiencies and excesses are more likely to occur.

Iron

In the 1800s, iron tablets were used to treat young women whose blood lacked "colouring matter." Today, we know that the "colouring matter" is the iron-containing protein **hemoglobin**. The hemoglobin in red blood cells transports oxygen to body cells and carries carbon dioxide away from body cells for elimination by the lungs. Most of the iron in the body is part of hemoglobin, but iron is also needed for the production of other iron-containing proteins. For example, iron is part of **myoglobin**, a protein found in muscle that enhances the amount of oxygen available for use in muscle contraction. Iron is essential for ATP production because it is a part of several proteins needed in the electron transport chain. Iron-containing proteins are also involved in drug metabolism and immune function. This mineral is so essential to the body that deficiency of iron may drive people to consume strange matter such as dirt in an effort to meet their needs (**Figure 8.22**).

Pica and mineral deficiencies • Figure 8.22

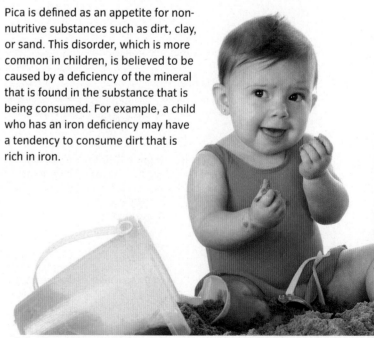

Pica is defined as an appetite for non-nutritive substances such as dirt, clay, or sand. This disorder, which is more common in children, is believed to be caused by a deficiency of the mineral that is found in the substance that is being consumed. For example, a child who has an iron deficiency may have a tendency to consume dirt that is rich in iron.

© Can Stock Photo Inc. / McIninch

Iron absorption and transport The amount of iron absorbed from the intestine depends on the form of the iron and on the dietary components consumed along with it. Much of the iron in meats is **heme iron**—iron that is part of a chemical complex found in proteins such as hemoglobin and myoglobin. Heme iron is absorbed more than twice as efficiently as the non-heme iron found in plant sources such as leafy green vegetables, legumes, and grains. The amount of non-heme iron absorbed can be enhanced or reduced by the foods and nutrients consumed in the same meal.

> **heme iron** A readily absorbable form of iron that is chemically associated with certain proteins and is found in meat, fish, and poultry.

Once iron is absorbed, the amount that is delivered to the cells of the body depends to some extent on the body's needs. When the body's iron status is high, less iron is transported in the blood for storage or delivery to cells and more is left in the mucosal cells of the intestine and lost when the cells die and are sloughed into the intestinal lumen. When iron status is low, more iron is transported out of the mucosal cells for use by the body (**Figure 8.23**). This regulation is important because iron that leaves the mucosal cells is not easily eliminated. Even when red blood cells die, the iron in their hemoglobin is not lost from the body; instead, it is recycled and can be incorporated into new red blood cells. Even in healthy individuals, most iron loss occurs through blood loss, including blood lost during menstruation and the small amounts lost from the gastrointestinal tract. Some iron is also lost through the shedding of cells from the intestine, skin, and urinary tract.

Iron absorption, uses, and loss • Figure 8.23

The amount of iron available to the body depends on both the amount absorbed into the mucosal cells of the small intestine and the amount transported to the rest of the body. The iron that is transported may be used to synthesize iron-containing proteins, such as hemoglobin needed for red blood cell formation, or increase iron stores in the liver or spleen.

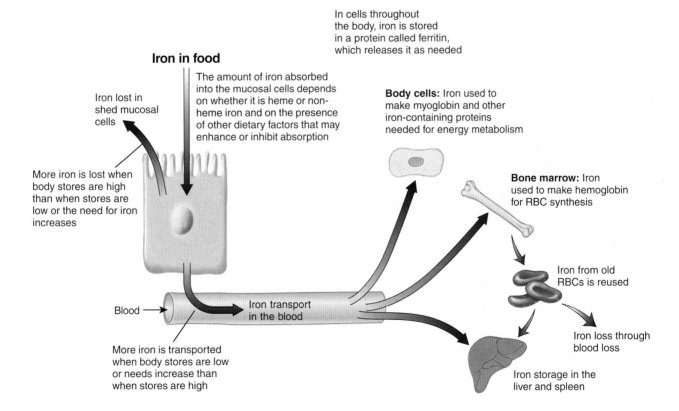

In cells throughout the body, iron is stored in a protein called ferritin, which releases it as needed

Iron in food

The amount of iron absorbed into the mucosal cells depends on whether it is heme or non-heme iron and on the presence of other dietary factors that may enhance or inhibit absorption

Iron lost in shed mucosal cells

More iron is lost when body stores are high than when stores are low or the need for iron increases

Body cells: Iron used to make myoglobin and other iron-containing proteins needed for energy metabolism

Bone marrow: Iron used to make hemoglobin for RBC synthesis

Iron from old RBCs is reused

Blood

Iron transport in the blood

More iron is transported when body stores are low or needs increase than when stores are high

Iron loss through blood loss

Iron storage in the liver and spleen

Sources of iron • Figure 8.24

The best sources of highly absorbable heme iron are red meats and organ meats such as liver and kidney. Legumes, leafy greens, and whole grains are good sources of non-heme iron; enriched grains are also good sources of non-heme iron because it is added during enrichment. The RDA for adult men and postmenopausal women is 8 mg/day. Due to menstrual losses, the RDA for women of childbearing age is set much higher, 15 mg/day for young women 14 to 18 years and 18 mg/day for women 19 to 50.

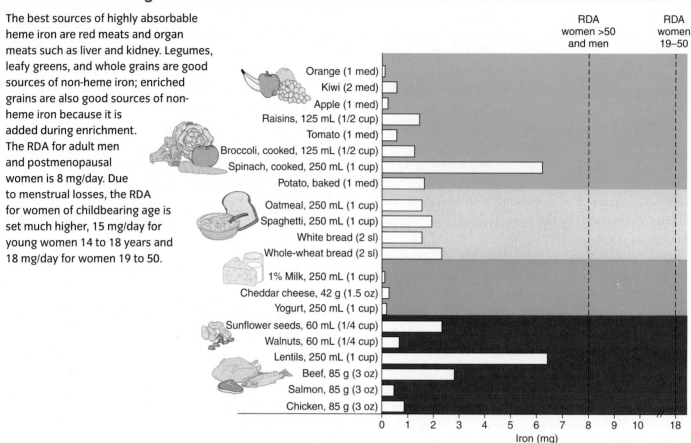

Meeting iron needs Iron in the diet comes from both plant and animal sources (**Figure 8.24**). Animal products provide both heme and non-heme iron, but only the less readily absorbed non-heme iron is found in plants. Non-heme iron absorption can be enhanced as much as sixfold if it is consumed with foods that are rich in vitamin C. For example, lentils, which are high in non-heme iron, can be combined in a meal with red peppers, which are high in vitamin C. Another way to increase iron absorption is to consume beef, fish, or poultry in the same meal that includes a source of non-heme iron. For example, a small amount of hamburger in a pot of chili will enhance the body's absorption of iron from the beans. The use of iron pots or pans can also increase iron intake, as some iron leaches into the food when cooked. Iron absorption is decreased by fibre, phytates, tannins, and oxalates, which bind iron in the gastrointestinal tract. The presence of other minerals with the same charge, such as calcium, may also decrease iron absorption.

The RDA for iron assumes that the diet contains both plant and animal sources of iron.[34] A separate RDA category has been created for vegetarians. These recommendations are higher, to take into account their lower iron absorption from plant sources. People who do not eat meat can increase their iron intake by consuming foods that have been fortified with iron and by using cookware made with iron.

In cases where iron intake from the diet is too low to satisfy the body's needs, an individual may require iron supplements. Iron supplements come in two forms: ferrous and ferric iron. The ferrous form is the better absorbed form and is the one typically prescribed by Canadian doctors. Since individual needs vary, doctors must carefully evaluate and monitor their patients to ensure the right amount and form of iron are prescribed for each individual. Because iron supplements can promote symptoms of toxicity in high amounts, they should be taken only on doctor's orders.

Iron in health and disease When the body has too little iron, hemoglobin cannot be produced. When sufficient hemoglobin is not available, the red blood cells that are formed are small and pale, and they are unable to deliver adequate oxygen to the tissues. This condition is known as **iron deficiency anemia (Figure 8.25)**. Symptoms of iron deficiency anemia include fatigue,

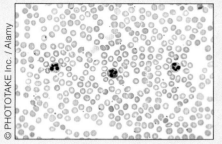

Normal red blood cells

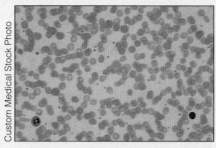

Iron deficiency anemia

Iron deficiency anemia is the final stage of iron deficiency. Inadequate iron intake first causes a decrease in the amount of stored iron, followed by low iron levels in the blood plasma. After plasma levels have dropped, insufficient iron is available to maintain hemoglobin in red blood cells.

Iron deficiency anemia occurs when too little iron is available to synthesize adequate amounts of hemoglobin. It is evidenced by red blood cells that are small and pale.

Iron stores

Iron in plasma

Iron in RBCs

| Adequate iron status | Low iron stores | Depleted iron stores | Low levels of circulating iron | Iron deficiency anemia |

Normal   Depletion   Deficiency

Iron Status

The risk of iron deficiency is highest among individuals with greater iron losses, those with greater needs due to growth and development, and those who are unable to obtain adequate dietary iron. In Canada, an estimated 3.5 to 10% of children suffer from iron-deficiency anemia.[35] These rates are even higher (14 to 50%) in certain Aboriginal populations.[36] The incidence is greatest among women and children who are living in poverty and are members of minority groups.[37]

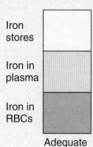
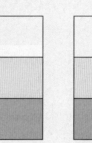

Courtesy Sprinkles Global Health Initiative

Dr. Stanley Zlotkin, working out of The Hospital for Sick Children (known commonly as "Sick Kids") in Toronto, has significantly addressed micronutrient deficiencies in Canada and across the world with his invention of Sprinkles, a tasteless dry powder that can be added to the meals of children and other individuals suffering from or at risk for nutrient deficiencies. The iron deficiency form of Sprinkles contains a mixture of vitamins A and C, folic acid, iron, and zinc. The multi-micronutrient formula combines 14 vitamins and minerals.[38]

Women of childbearing age lose iron due to menstruation. Pregnant women, infants, children, and teens have greater iron needs due to growth and development.

Demographic

Women of child-bearing age, pregnant women, infants, children, adolescents

Dietary

Low total iron, vegetarian diets, dieting

Social/medical

Poverty, intestinal parasites

Diets that are low in meat, which contains the most readily absorbed form of iron (heme iron), and high in phytates and fibre, which reduce iron absorption, increase the risk of deficiency. Low-calorie diets can also reduce iron intake.

Individuals living in poverty are less likely than others to consume adequate iron. Intestinal parasites cause blood loss, which increases iron losses.

Trace Minerals 279

weakness, headache, decreased work capacity, inability to maintain body temperature in a cold environment, changes in behaviour, decreased resistance to infection, impaired development in infants, and increased risk of lead poisoning in young children. Anemia is the last stage of iron deficiency. Earlier stages have no symptoms because

they do not affect the amount of iron in red blood cells, but levels of iron in the blood plasma and in body stores are low (see *Thinking It Through*). Iron deficiency anemia is the most common nutritional deficiency; more than 2 billion people, or more than 30% of the world's population, suffer from iron deficiency anemia.[39]

THINKING IT THROUGH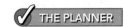

Avoiding Anemia

Jodie is a 26-year-old graduate student from Edmonton who has been a lacto-ovo vegetarian for the past six months. She has been working long hours and is always tired. She tries to eat a healthy diet but wonders why she always feels exhausted.

What puts Jodie at risk for iron deficiency anemia?
▼

Your answer: _____

_____

Jodie goes to the health centre to see whether a medical reason can explain her tiredness. A sample of blood is taken to check Jodie for anemia. The results of Jodie's blood work are summarized in the figure below.

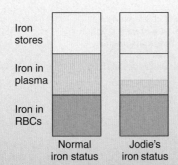

Iron
stores

Iron in
plasma

Iron in
RBCs

Normal
iron status

Jodie's
iron status

What does the blood test reveal about Jodie's iron status? Is her tiredness due to iron deficiency anemia? Why or why not?
▼

Your answer: _____

_____

Jodie meets with a dietitian. A diet analysis reveals that because she consumes no meat, most of her protein comes from dairy products. Each day, Jodie consumes about eight servings of whole grains, three fresh fruits, and about 250 g (1 cup) of cooked vegetables. She drinks four glasses of iced tea daily. Her average iron intake is about 12 mg/day.

Name three dietary factors that put Jodie at risk for iron deficiency.
▼

Your answer: _____

_____

How can Jodie increase her iron intake?
▼

She can switch to an iron-fortified breakfast cereal, eat more leafy greens, snack on dried fruits, and include more legumes in her diet. She can also exchange her stainless-steel cookware for an iron skillet.

What can Jodie do to increase the absorption of the non-heme iron in her diet?
▼

Your answer: _____

_____

(Check your answers in Appendix I.)

Iron toxicity • Figure 8.26

To protect children from mistaking iron pills for candy, the labels of iron-containing drugs and supplements often display a warning urging people to store them out of the reach of children or other individuals who might consume them in excess.

WARNING: CLOSE TIGHTLY AND KEEP OUT OF REACH OF CHILDREN. CONTAINS IRON, WHICH CAN BE HARMFUL OR FATAL TO CHILDREN IN LARGE DOSES. IN CASE OF ACCIDENTAL OVERDOSE, SEEK PROFESSIONAL ASSISTANCE OR CONTACT A POISON CONTROL CENTRE IMMEDIATELY.

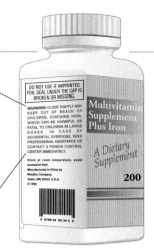

An UL of 45 mg/day from all sources has been set for iron.[34] It can cause health problems if too much is consumed. For example, one of the most common forms of poisoning among children under age 6 is acute iron toxicity caused by excessive consumption of iron-containing supplements. Iron poisoning can cause damage to the lining of the intestine, abnormalities in body acidity, shock, and liver failure. Even a single large dose can be fatal (**Figure 8.26**).

Accumulation of iron in the body over time, referred to as **iron overload**, is most commonly due to an inherited condition called **hemochromatosis**, which permits increased iron absorption.[40] Approximately 1 in 300 Canadians has hemochromatosis, and 1 in 9 Canadians is a carrier for the genetic mutation that causes it. Hemochromatosis is the most common genetic disorder in the Western world.[41] People who have hemochromatosis show no symptoms early in life, but, in middle age, they develop nonspecific symptoms such as weight loss, fatigue, weakness, and abdominal pain. If allowed to progress, the accumulation of excess iron can damage the heart and liver and increase the risk of diabetes and cancer. The treatment for hemochromatosis is simple: regular blood withdrawal. Iron loss through blood withdrawal will prevent the complications of iron overload, but to be effective, the treatment must be initiated before any organs have been damaged. Therefore, genetic screening is essential to identify and treat individuals before any damage occurs.

> **hemochromatosis** An inherited disorder that results in increased iron absorption.

Copper

Although it may seem logical that iron deficiency is caused by consuming too little iron, it is also caused by consuming too little copper. Iron status relies on copper status because a copper-containing protein is needed for iron to be transported from the intestinal cells. Even when iron intake is adequate, iron can't get to tissues if copper is not present. Thus, copper deficiency results in iron deficiency that may lead to anemia. Copper also functions as a component of several important proteins and enzymes that are involved in connective tissue synthesis, lipid metabolism, maintenance of heart muscle, and function of the immune and central nervous systems.[34]

We consume copper in seafood, nuts and seeds, whole-grain breads and cereals, and chocolate; the richest dietary sources of copper are organ meats such as liver and kidney. As with many other trace minerals, soil content affects the amount of copper in plant foods. The RDA for copper for adults is 900 micrograms (μg)/day.

When the body has too little copper, the protein collagen does not form normally, resulting in skeletal changes similar to those seen in vitamin C deficiency. Copper deficiency also causes elevated blood cholesterol, reflecting copper's role in cholesterol metabolism. Copper deficiency has been associated with impaired growth, degeneration of the heart muscle and the nervous system, and changes in hair colour and structure. Because copper is needed to maintain the immune system, a diet that is low in copper increases the incidence of infections. Also, because copper is an essential component of one form of the antioxidant enzyme superoxide dismutase (SOD), a copper deficiency will weaken the body's antioxidant defences.

Severe copper deficiency is relatively rare, although it may occur in premature infants. It can also occur when zinc intake is high because high dietary zinc interferes with the absorption of copper. Copper toxicity from dietary sources is also rare but can occur as a result of drinking from contaminated water supplies or consuming acidic foods or beverages that have been stored in copper containers. Toxicity is more likely to occur from supplements containing copper. Excessive copper intake causes abdominal pain, vomiting, and diarrhea. The UL has been set at 10 mg of copper/day.[34]

Zinc and gene expression • Figure 8.27

One of zinc's most important roles is in gene expression. Zinc-containing DNA-binding proteins allow vitamin A, vitamin D, and numerous hormones to interact with DNA. The zinc forms "fingers" in the protein structure. When a vitamin or hormone binds to the protein, the zinc fingers bind to DNA, turning on genes and, thus, the synthesis of the proteins for which they code. Without zinc, these vitamins and hormones cannot function properly.

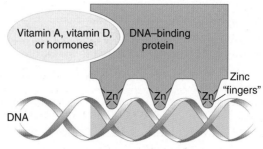

Zinc

Zinc, the most abundant intracellular trace mineral, is involved in the functioning of approximately 100 different enzymes, including zinc superoxide dismutase, an antioxidant which is vital for protecting cells from free-radical damage. Zinc maintains adequate levels of metal-binding proteins, which also scavenge free radicals.[42] Zinc is also needed by enzymes that function in the synthesis of DNA and RNA, in carbohydrate metabolism, in acid–base balance, and in a reaction needed for the absorption of folate from food. Zinc also plays a role in the storage and release of insulin, the mobilization of vitamin A from the liver, and the stabilization of cell membranes. It influences hormonal regulation of cell division and is therefore needed for the growth and repair of tissues, the activity of the immune system, and the development of sex organs and bone. Some of the functions of zinc can be traced to its role in gene expression (**Figure 8.27**).

Our bodies regulate the amount of zinc transported from the mucosal cells of the intestine into the blood. For example, when zinc intake is high, more zinc is held in the mucosal cells and lost in the feces when these cells die. When zinc intake is low, more dietary zinc passes into the blood for delivery to tissues.

Meeting zinc needs We consume zinc in red meat, liver, eggs, dairy products, vegetables, and seafood (**Figure 8.28**). Because many plant foods are high in substances that bind zinc, zinc is absorbed better from animal sources than from plant sources.

Food sources of zinc • Figure 8.28

Good sources of zinc include protein-rich foods, such as meat, seafood, shellfish, dairy products, legumes, and seeds. Refined grains are not good sources of zinc because zinc is lost in milling and not added back. Yeast-leavened grain products are better sources of zinc than are unleavened products because yeast leavening reduces phytate content. The dashed lines represent the RDA for adult men and women, which are 11 and 8 mg/day, respectively.

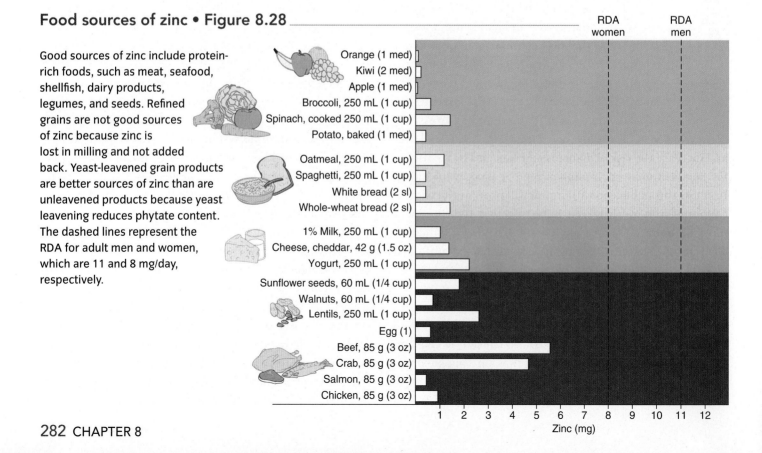

Zinc in health and disease Symptomatic zinc deficiency is relatively uncommon in North America, but in developing countries, it has important health and developmental consequences. Zinc deficiency interferes with growth and development, impairs immune function, and causes skin rashes and diarrhea. Diminished immune function is a concern even when zinc deficiency is mild. Because zinc is needed for the proper functioning of vitamins A and D and the activity of numerous enzymes, its deficiency symptoms can resemble the deficiency symptoms of other essential nutrients.

The risk of zinc deficiency is greater in areas where the diet is high in substances that limit zinc absorption, such as phytates, fibre, tannins, and oxalates. In the 1960s, a syndrome of growth depression and delayed sexual development was observed in Iranian and Egyptian men consuming a diet based on plant protein. The diet was not low in zinc, but it was high in grains containing phytates, which interfered with zinc absorption, thus causing the deficiency.

It is difficult to consume a toxic amount of zinc from food. However, high doses from supplements can cause toxicity symptoms. A single dose of 1 to 2 g can cause gastrointestinal irritation, vomiting, loss of appetite, diarrhea, abdominal cramps, and headaches. High intakes have been shown to decrease immune functions, interfere with the absorption of copper, and reduce blood concentrations of HDL cholesterol (i.e., "good cholesterol"). High doses of zinc can also interfere with iron absorption because iron and zinc are transported through the blood by the same protein. The converse is also true: Too much iron can limit the transport of zinc. Zinc and iron are often found together in foods, but food sources do not contain large enough amounts of either to cause imbalances.

Zinc supplements are marketed to improve the immune function, enhance fertility and sexual performance, and cure the common cold. For individuals consuming adequate zinc, there is no evidence that extra zinc is beneficial. Supplements have not been shown to improve sexual function, and little evidence supports the effectiveness of zinc lozenges in reducing the duration and severity of cold symptoms.[43] However, in individuals with a mild zinc deficiency,

supplementation may result in improved wound healing, immunity, and appetite; in children, it can result in improved growth and learning; and in older adults, it can improve the immune response.[44] A UL has been set at 40 mg/day from all sources.[34]

Selenium

The amount of selenium in food varies greatly, depending on the concentration of selenium in the soil where the food is produced. In regions of China with low soil selenium levels, a form of heart disease called **Keshan disease** occurs in children and young women. This disease can be prevented and cured with selenium supplements. In contrast, people living in regions of China with very high selenium in the soil may develop symptoms of selenium toxicity (**Figure 8.29**).

Selenium is incorporated into the structure of certain proteins, including the antioxidant enzyme **glutathione peroxidase**. Glutathione peroxidase neutralizes peroxides

> **glutathione peroxidase** A selenium-containing enzyme that protects cells from oxidative damage by neutralizing peroxides.

Soil selenium and health • Figure 8.29

The amount of selenium in the soil varies widely from one region of China to another. When the diet consists primarily of locally grown food, these differences affect selenium intake and, therefore, health. When the diet includes foods from many different locations, the high selenium content of foods grown in one geographic region is offset by the low selenium content of foods from other regions.

Hair and nail brittleness and loss occur in people living in regions of China with high selenium levels in the soil (intake of 5 mg/day). Other toxicity symptoms include nausea, diarrhea, abdominal pain, nervous system abnormalities, fatigue, and irritability.

Selenium deficiency causes muscular discomfort, weakness, and in some cases Keshan disease. However, Keshan disease is not caused entirely by selenium deficiency. It is believed to be due to a combination of selenium deficiency and a viral infection.[45]

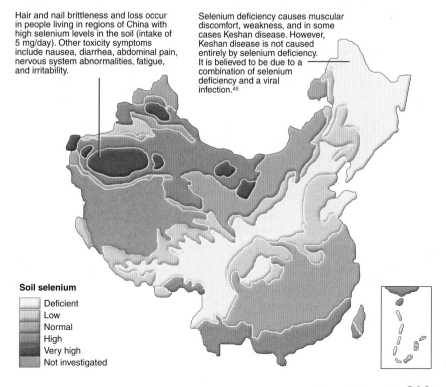

Soil selenium
- Deficient
- Low
- Normal
- High
- Very high
- Not investigated

before they can form free radicals, which cause oxidative damage (**Figure 8.30**). In addition to its antioxidant role in glutathione peroxidase, selenium is part of a protein needed for the synthesis of the **thyroid hormones**, which regulate metabolic rate.

Meeting selenium needs

Selenium deficiencies and excesses are not a concern in Canada because the foods we typically consume come from many different locations around the country and around the world. The RDA for selenium for adults is 55 μg/day.[46] The average intake in Canada meets, or nearly meets, this recommendation for all age groups. Seafood, kidney, liver, and eggs are excellent sources of selenium. Grains, nuts, and seeds can be good sources, depending on the selenium content of the soil in which they were grown. Fruits, vegetables, and drinking water are generally poor sources. The UL for adults is 400 μg/day from diet and supplements.[46]

Glutathione peroxidase • Figure 8.30

Glutathione peroxidase is a selenium-containing enzyme that neutralizes peroxides before they can form free radicals. Selenium therefore can reduce the body's need for vitamin E, which neutralizes free radicals.

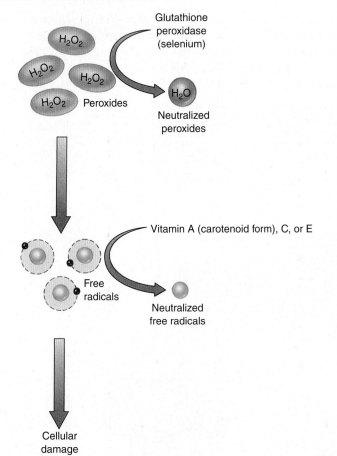

Selenium and cancer

An increased incidence of cancer has been observed in regions where selenium intake is low, suggesting that selenium plays a role in preventing cancer. In 1996, a study investigating the effect of selenium supplements on people with a history of skin cancer found that the supplement had no effect on the recurrence of skin cancer but that the incidence of lung, prostate, and colon cancer decreased in the selenium-supplemented group.[47] This result led to speculation that selenium supplements could reduce the risk of cancer. Continued study, however, has led to the conclusion that the reduction in the incidence of lung and prostate cancer seen in the 1996 study occurred primarily in people who began the study with low levels of selenium. It appears that an adequate level of selenium is necessary to prevent cancer, but the role of supplemental selenium in preventing cancer is still under investigation.[48]

Iodine

About three-fourths of the iodine in the body is found in a small gland in the neck called the **thyroid gland**. Iodine is concentrated in this gland because it is an essential component of the thyroid hormones, which are produced here. Thyroid hormones regulate metabolic rate, growth, and development, and promote protein synthesis.

Iodine in health and disease

Thyroid hormone levels are carefully regulated. If blood levels drop, **thyroid-stimulating hormone** is released to signal the thyroid gland to take up iodine and synthesize more thyroid hormones. When the supply of iodine is adequate, thyroid hormones can be produced, and the return of thyroid hormones to normal levels turns off the synthesis of thyroid-stimulating hormone. If iodine is deficient, thyroid hormones cannot be synthesized (**Figure 8.31**). Without sufficient thyroid hormones, metabolic rate slows, causing fatigue and weight gain.

When thyroid hormone levels in the blood drop but iodine levels are too low to synthesize more thyroid hormones, the thyroid gland increases in size, forming a **goiter**, as it tries to synthesize sufficient thyroid hormones, but is unable to do so because of the iodine deficiency. Because of the importance of the thyroid hormones for growth and development, iodine deficiency disorders other than goiter are also prevalent (see Figure 8.31).

goiter An enlargement of the thyroid gland caused by a deficiency of iodine.

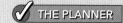
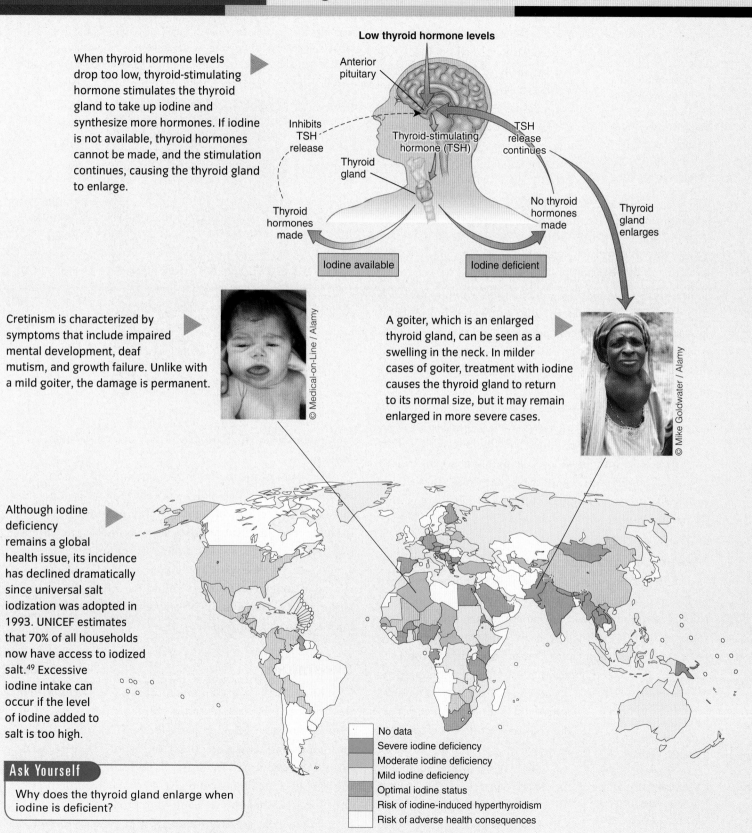

When thyroid hormone levels drop too low, thyroid-stimulating hormone stimulates the thyroid gland to take up iodine and synthesize more hormones. If iodine is not available, thyroid hormones cannot be made, and the stimulation continues, causing the thyroid gland to enlarge.

Low thyroid hormone levels

Anterior pituitary

Inhibits TSH release

Thyroid-stimulating hormone (TSH)

TSH release continues

Thyroid gland

Thyroid hormones made

No thyroid hormones made

Thyroid gland enlarges

Iodine available

Iodine deficient

© Medical-on-Line / Alamy

Cretinism is characterized by symptoms that include impaired mental development, deaf mutism, and growth failure. Unlike with a mild goiter, the damage is permanent.

A goiter, which is an enlarged thyroid gland, can be seen as a swelling in the neck. In milder cases of goiter, treatment with iodine causes the thyroid gland to return to its normal size, but it may remain enlarged in more severe cases.

© Mike Goldwater / Alamy

Although iodine deficiency remains a global health issue, its incidence has declined dramatically since universal salt iodization was adopted in 1993. UNICEF estimates that 70% of all households now have access to iodized salt.[49] Excessive iodine intake can occur if the level of iodine added to salt is too high.

No data
Severe iodine deficiency
Moderate iodine deficiency
Mild iodine deficiency
Optimal iodine status
Risk of iodine-induced hyperthyroidism
Risk of adverse health consequences

Ask Yourself

Why does the thyroid gland enlarge when iodine is deficient?

Source: de Benoist B et al., eds. Iodine status worldwide. WHO Global Database on Iodine Deficiency. Geneva, World Health Organization, 2004. Data was produced by WHO using the best available evidence and do not necessarily correspond to the official statistics of Member States.

For example, if iodine is deficient during pregnancy, the risk of stillbirth and spontaneous abortion increases; insufficient iodine during pregnancy can lead to a child being born with a condition called cretinism. Iodine deficiency impairs mental function and reduces intellectual capacity in children and adolescents. Although iodine deficiency can be easily prevented, it is the world's most prevalent cause of brain damage.[49]

> **cretinism** A condition resulting from poor maternal iodine intake during pregnancy that impairs mental development and growth in the offspring.

Iodine deficiency is most common in regions where the soil is low in iodine and fish and seafood access is low. The risk of iodine deficiency is also increased by the consumption of foods that contain **goitrogens**, substances that interfere with iodine utilization or thyroid function. Goitrogens are found in turnips, rutabaga, cabbage, millet, and cassava. When these foods are boiled, the goitrogen content is reduced because some of these compounds leach into the cooking water. Goitrogens are primarily a problem in African countries where cassava is a dietary staple. Goitrogens are not a problem in Canada because the typical diet does not include large amounts of goitrogen-containing foods.

Chronically high intakes of iodine or a sudden increase in iodine intake can also cause an enlargement of the thyroid gland. For example, in a person with a marginal intake, a large dose from supplements could cause thyroid enlargement even at levels that would not be toxic in a healthy person. The UL for adults is 1100 µg of iodine/day from all sources.[34]

Meeting iodine needs The iodine content of food varies, depending on the soil in which plants are grown and where animals graze. When Earth was formed, all soils were high in iodine, but mountainous areas and river valleys have little iodine left in the soil today because it has been washed out by glaciers, snow, rain, and floodwaters. The iodine washed from the soil has accumulated in the oceans. Therefore, the best sources of iodine are foods from the sea, such as fish, seafood, and seaweed.

> **iodized salt** Table salt to which a small amount of sodium iodide or potassium iodide has been added for the purpose of supplementing the iodine content of the diet.

Today, most of the iodine in the North American diet comes from iodized salt (**Figure 8.32**). Iodine deficiency is rare in North America, and typical iodine intake

Iodized salt • Figure 8.32

Iodized salt was first introduced in Switzerland in the 1920s as a way to combat iodine deficiency. Salt was chosen because it is readily available, inexpensive, and consumed in regular amounts throughout the year. It takes only about half a teaspoon of iodized salt to provide the recommended amount of iodine. Iodized salt should not be confused with sea salt, which is a poor source of iodine because its iodine is lost in the drying process.

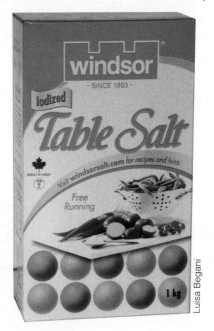

Luisa Begani

meets or exceeds the RDA of 150 µg/day for adult men and women.[34]

We also obtain iodine from contaminants and other additives in foods. The iodine content of dairy products is increased as a result of iodine-containing additives used in cattle feed and disinfectants used on milking machines and milk storage tanks. Iodine-containing sterilizing agents are also used in fast-food restaurants, and iodine is used in dough conditioners and in some food colourings. Despite our intake of iodine from iodized salt and contaminants, toxicity is rare in Canada.

Chromium

Chromium is the key component of what has been called the "glucose tolerance factor," a small peptide required to maintain normal blood glucose levels. It is believed that chromium enhances the effects of insulin,[50] which facilitates the entry of glucose into cells and stimulates the synthesis of proteins, lipids, and glycogen. When chromium is deficient, more insulin is required to produce the same effect. A deficiency of chromium therefore affects the body's ability to regulate blood glucose, causing diabetes-like symptoms such as elevated blood glucose levels and increased insulin levels.[50]

Dietary sources of chromium include liver, brewer's yeast, nuts, and whole grains. Milk, vegetables, and fruits are poor sources. Refined carbohydrates such as white breads, pasta, and white rice are also poor sources because chromium is lost in milling and not added back during the enrichment process. Chromium intake can be increased by cooking in stainless-steel cookware because chromium leaches from the steel into the food. The recommended intake for chromium is 35 µg/day for men aged 19 to 50 and 25 µg/day for women aged 19 to 50.[34]

Overt chromium deficiency is not a problem in Canada; nevertheless, chromium, in the form of chromium picolinate, is a common dietary supplement, and is especially popular with athletes and dieters because it is thought to reduce body fat and increase muscle mass (**Figure 8.33**). Toxicity is always a concern when consuming nutrient supplements, but in the case of chromium, there is little evidence of dietary toxicity in humans. The DRI committee concluded that there was insufficient data to establish a UL for chromium.[34]

Chromium picolinate supplements • Figure 8.33

Because chromium is needed for insulin action and insulin promotes protein synthesis, adequate chromium is necessary to increase lean body mass. However, studies of chromium picolinate and other chromium supplements in healthy human subjects have not found them to have beneficial effects on muscle strength, body composition, or weight loss.[51]

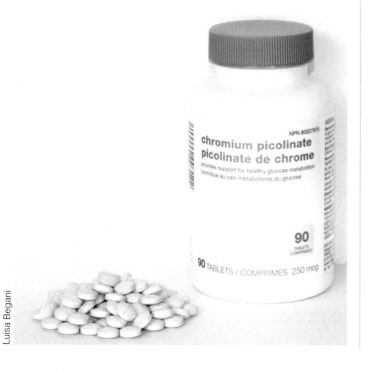

Luisa Begani

Fluoride

Fluoride helps prevent **dental caries** (cavities) in both children and adults. During tooth formation, fluoride is incorporated into fluorapatite crystals that make up tooth enamel. These fluoride-containing crystals are more resistant to acid than the crystals that form when fluoride is not present. Fluoride therefore helps protect the teeth from the cavity-causing acids produced by bacteria in the mouth. Adequate fluoride has its greatest effect during the period of maximum tooth development (up to age 13), but it continues to have benefits throughout life. In addition to making tooth enamel more acid resistant, fluoride in saliva prevents cavities by reducing the amount of acid produced by bacteria, inhibiting the dissolution of tooth enamel by acid, and increasing enamel re-mineralization after acid exposure. Fluoride is also incorporated into the mineral crystals in bone. Evidence suggests that fluoride stimulates bone formation and therefore may strengthen bones in adults who have osteoporosis. Slow-release fluoride supplements have been shown to increase bone mass and prevent new fractures.[52]

Meeting fluoride needs Fluoride is present in small amounts in almost all soil, water, plants, and animals. The richest dietary sources of fluoride are toothpaste, mouthwash, tea, marine fish consumed with their bones, and fluoridated water (see *What Should I Eat?*). Because food readily absorbs the fluoride in cooking water, the fluoride content of food can be significantly increased when it is handled and prepared using water that contains fluoride. Cooking utensils also affect the fluoride content of foods. For example, foods cooked with Teflon utensils can pick up fluoride from the Teflon, whereas using aluminum cookware can decrease the fluoride content of foods. Bottled water usually does not contain fluoride, so people who habitually drink bottled water need to obtain fluoride from other sources.

The recommended intake for fluoride for people 6 months of age and older is 0.05 mg/kg/day, which is equivalent to about 3.8 mg/day for a 76-kg (168-lb.) man and 3.1 mg/day for a 61-kg (135-lb.) woman. Fluoridated water provides about 0.7 to 1.2 mg of fluoride/litre.

Fluoridation of water To promote dental health, fluoride is added to public water supplies in many communities. However, fluoridated water is not found throughout the country equally. For example, in British Columbia and Quebec, most tap water in unfluorinated. When fluoride intake is low, tooth decay is more frequent (**Figure 8.34**).

WHAT SHOULD I EAT?
Trace Minerals

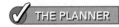

Use iProfile to find the trace element content of a cup of pinto beans.

THE PLANNER

Add more iron
- Eat red meat, poultry, or fish—they are all good sources of heme iron.
- Add raisins to your oatmeal.
- Fortify your breakfast by eating iron-fortified cereal.
- Dust off the iron skillet.
- Serve some beans or lentils—they are a good vegetarian source of iron.

Increase iron absorption
- Drink orange juice with your iron-fortified cereal.
- Don't take your calcium supplement with your iron sources.

Think zinc
- Scramble some eggs.
- Beef up your zinc by having a serving of meat.
- Eat whole grains, but make sure they are yeast leavened.

Trace down your minerals
- Check to see whether your water is fluoridated.
- See whether your salt is iodized.
- Replace refined grains with whole grains to increase your chromium intake.
- Prepare some seafood to add selenium to your diet.

Water fluoridation is a safe, inexpensive way to prevent dental caries, but some people still believe that the added fluoride increases the risk of cancer and other diseases. These beliefs are not supported by the scientific literature; the small amounts of fluoride consumed in drinking water promote dental health and do not pose a risk for health problems such as cancer, kidney failure, or bone disease.[53]

Although the levels of fluoride included in public water supplies are safe, too much fluoride can be toxic. In children, too much fluoride causes **fluorosis** (see Figure 8.34).

The fluoride in toothpaste is good for your teeth, but swallowing it can increase fluoride intake to dangerous levels. Swallowed toothpaste is estimated to contribute about 0.6 mg per day of fluoride in young children.

In adults, doses of 20 to 80 mg of fluoride/day can result in changes in bone health that may be crippling, changes in kidney function, and possibly changes in nerve and muscle

> **fluorosis** A condition caused by chronic overconsumption of fluoride, characterized by black and brown stains and cracking and pitting of the teeth.

Just the right amount of fluoride
• Figure 8.34

This graph illustrates that the incidence of dental caries in children increases when the concentration of fluoride in the water supply is lower. If the fluoride concentration of the water is too high, it increases the risk of fluorosis.

© Can Stock Photo Inc. / circotasu

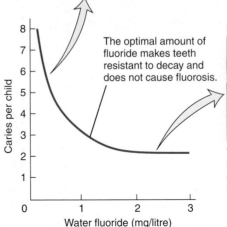

Too little fluoride makes teeth more susceptible to dental caries.

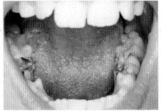

The optimal amount of fluoride makes teeth resistant to decay and does not cause fluorosis.

Dr. P. Marazzi / Science Source

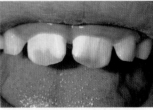

Too much fluoride (intakes of 2 to 8 mg/day or greater in children) causes teeth to appear mottled, a condition called fluorosis.

Interpreting Data

Based on this graph, what concentration of water fluoride will protect against dental caries but not cause fluorosis?

a. 2.5 mg/litre   c. 1 mg/litre
b. 2 mg/litre   d. 0.5 mg/litre

function. Death has been reported in cases involving an intake of 5 to 10 g/day. The UL for fluoride is set at 0.1 mg/kg/day for infants and children less than 9 years of age and at 10 mg/day for those between 9 and 70 years.[27]

Manganese, Molybdenum, and Other Trace Minerals

In addition to the seven trace minerals we have just examined, the human body has many other trace minerals. DRI recommendations have been set for two of them: manganese and molybdenum.[34]

Manganese is a constituent of some enzymes and an activator of others. Enzymes that require manganese are involved in carbohydrate and cholesterol metabolism, bone formation, and synthesis of urea. Manganese can also prevent oxidative damage because it is a component of a form of superoxide dismutase. The recommended intake for manganese is 2.3 mg/day for adult men and 1.8 mg/day for adult women. The best dietary sources of manganese are whole grains, nuts, legumes, and leafy green vegetables.

Molybdenum is also needed to activate enzymes. For example, it functions in the metabolism of sulphur-containing amino acids and nitrogen-containing compounds that are present in DNA and RNA, in the production of a waste product called uric acid, and in the oxidation and detoxification of various other compounds. The recommended intake for molybdenum is 45 µg/day for adult men and women. The molybdenum content of food varies depending on the molybdenum content of the soil in the regions where the food is produced. The most reliable sources include milk and milk products, organ meats, breads, cereals, and legumes. Molybdenum is readily absorbed from foods; the amount in the body is regulated by excretion in the urine and bile.

Some evidence suggests that other trace minerals, such as arsenic, boron, nickel, silicon, and vanadium, also play a role in human health. The DRI committee reviewed the need for and functions of these minerals, but insufficient data was available to establish recommended intakes for any of them. Other trace minerals that are believed to play a physiological role in human health include aluminum, bromine, cadmium, germanium, lead, lithium, rubidium, and tin. Their specific functions have not yet been defined, and they have not yet been evaluated by the DRI committee. All minerals, both those that are known to be essential and those that are still being assessed for their role in human health, can be obtained by choosing a variety of foods from each of the food guide food groups.

Table 8.4 provides a summary of the trace minerals.

A summary of the trace minerals Table 8.4							
Mineral	Sources	Recommended intake for adults	Major functions	Deficiency diseases and symptoms	Groups at risk of deficiency	Toxicity	UL
Iron	Red meats, leafy greens, dried fruit, legumes, whole and enriched grains	8–18 mg/day	Part of hemoglobin (which delivers oxygen to cells), myoglobin (which holds oxygen in muscle), and proteins needed for ATP production; needed for immune function	Iron deficiency anemia: fatigue; weakness; small, pale red blood cells; low hemoglobin levels; inability to maintain normal body temperature	Infants and preschool children, adolescents, women of childbearing age, pregnant women, athletes, vegetarians	Gastrointestinal	45 mg/day
Copper	Organ meats, nuts, seeds, whole grains, seafood, cocoa	900 µg/day	A component of proteins needed for iron absorption, lipid metabolism, collagen synthesis, nerve and immune function, and protection against oxidative damage	Anemia, poor growth, bone abnormalities	People who consume excessive amounts of zinc in supplements	Vomiting, abdominal pain, diarrhea, liver damage	10 mg/day

(Continues on next page)

A summary of the trace minerals   Table 8.4   (Continued)

Mineral	Sources	Recommended intake for adults	Major functions	Deficiency diseases and symptoms	Groups at risk of deficiency	Toxicity	UL
Zinc	Meat, seafood	8–11 mg/day	Regulates protein synthesis; functions in growth, development, wound healing, immunity, and antioxidant enzymes	Poor growth and development, skin rashes, decreased immune function	Vegetarians, low-income children, elderly people	Decreased copper absorption, depressed immune function	40 mg/day
Selenium	Meats, seafood, eggs, whole grains, nuts, seeds	55 μg/day	Antioxidant as part of glutathione peroxidase, synthesis of thyroid hormones; spares vitamin E	Muscle pain, weakness, Keshan disease	Populations in areas where the soil is low in selenium	Nausea, diarrhea, vomiting, fatigue, changes in hair and nails	400 μg/day
Iodine	Iodized salt, seafood, seaweed, dairy products	150 μg/day	Needed for synthesis of thyroid hormones	Goiter, cretinism, impaired brain function, growth and developmental abnormalities	Populations in areas where the soil is low in iodine and iodized salt is not used	Enlarged thyroid	1110 μg/day
Chromium	Brewer's yeast, nuts, whole grains, meat, mushrooms	25–35 μg/day	Enhances insulin action	High blood glucose	Malnourished children	None reported	ND
Fluoride	Fluoridated water, tea, fish, toothpaste	3–4 mg/day	Strengthens tooth enamel, enhances re-mineralization of tooth enamel, reduces acid production by bacteria in the mouth	Increased risk of dental caries	Populations in areas with unfluoridated water, those who drink mostly bottled water	Fluorosis: mottled teeth, kidney damage, bone abnormalities	10 mg/day
Manganese	Nuts, legumes, whole grains, tea, leafy vegetables	1.8–2.3 mg/day	Functions in carbohydrate and cholesterol metabolism and antioxidant enzymes	Growth retardation	None	Nerve damage	11 mg/day
Molybdenum	Milk, organ meats, grains, legumes	45 μg/day	Cofactor for a number of enzymes	Unknown in humans	None	Arthritis, joint inflammation	2 mg/day

Note: UL, Tolerable Upper Intake Level; ND, not determined.

1. **Why** does iron deficiency cause fatigue?

2. **How** does selenium reduce the body's need for vitamin E?

3. **What** is the function of iodine?

4. **How** does fluoride protect the teeth?

Summary

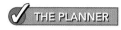

1 Water 250

- Water deficiency can quickly result in the symptoms of **dehydration**, which can typically be resolved by consuming water.

- Water, which is found both intracellularly and extracellularly, accounts for about 60% of adult body weight. The amount of water in the blood is a balance between the forces of **blood pressure** and osmosis. The kidneys regulate urinary water losses and the concentration of **solutes** within urine.

Water balance • Figure 8.2

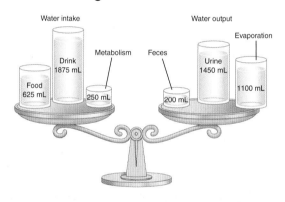

- Because water isn't stored in the body, intake from fluids and foods must replace water losses from evaporation and through urine, feces, and sweat. Water intake is stimulated by the sensation of **thirst**. Hormones such as **antidiuretic hormone**, angiotensin II, and aldosterone further help regulate water levels in the body.

- In the body, water is a **solvent** where chemical reactions occur; it also transports nutrients and wastes, provides protection, helps regulate temperature, and participates in chemical reactions and acid–base balance.

- Dehydration occurs when there is too little water in the body. Water **intoxication** causes **hyponatremia**, which can result in abnormal fluid accumulation in body tissues.

- The recommended intake of water is 2.7 L/day for women and 3.7 L/day for men; needs vary depending on environmental conditions and activity level. Many beverages are excellent sources of water. The exceptions are beverages such as coffee and alcohol, which provide water but also act as **diuretics**, promoting the excretion of water.

2 An Overview of Minerals 257

- **Major minerals** and **trace minerals** are distinguished by the amounts needed in the diet and found in the body. Both plant and animal foods are good sources of **minerals**.

- Mineral bioavailability is affected by the food source of the mineral, the body's need, and interactions with other minerals, vitamins, and dietary components, such as fibre, phytates, oxalates, and tannins. Minerals are often found as **ions** in the body, carrying either a positive or negative charge.

- Minerals are needed to provide structure and to regulate biochemical reactions, often as **cofactors**.

Compounds that interfere with mineral absorption • Figure 8.8

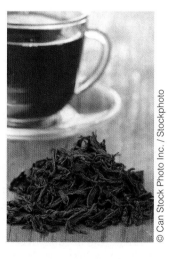

© Can Stock Photo Inc. / Stockphoto

3 Electrolytes: Sodium, Potassium, and Chloride 260

- The minerals sodium, potassium, and chloride are **electrolytes** that are important in the maintenance of fluid balance and the functioning of nerves and muscles. The kidneys are the primary regulator of electrolyte and fluid balance.

- Sodium, potassium and chloride are the main electrolytes in the body. Electrolytes are responsible for the electrical activity of the body and the maintenance of fluid balance. A major dietary source of sodium and chloride comes from our consumption of **sodium chloride**, more commonly referred to as table salt. Hormones such as **aldosterone** help regulate the levels of electrolytes in the body.

- Sodium, potassium, and chloride depletion can occur when losses are increased by heavy and persistent sweating, chronic diarrhea, or vomiting. Diets high in sodium and low in potassium are associated with an increased risk of **hypertension**. **Prehypertension** is defined as a blood pressure between 120/80 and 139/89 mm of mercury, while hypertension is blood pressure that is consistently 140/90 mm of mercury or above. Blood pressure can be lowered by following the **DASH diet**—a dietary pattern moderate in sodium; high in potassium, magnesium, calcium, and fibre; and low in fat, saturated fat, and cholesterol.

The effect of diet on blood pressure • Figure 8.12

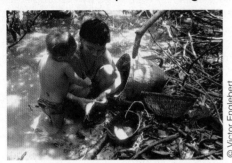

© Victor Englebert

- The Canadian diet is abundant in sodium and chloride from processed foods and table salt but generally low in potassium. A diet that is high in fresh fruits and vegetables will easily meet the body's potassium needs. Recommendations for health suggest that we increase our intake of potassium and consume less sodium.

4 Major Minerals and Bone Health 267

- Bone is a living tissue that is constantly changing. In young adulthood, **bone remodelling** favours an increase in bone density and the achievement of **peak bone mass**.

- **Age-related bone loss** occurs in adults when more bone is broken down than is made. Bone loss is accelerated in women after **menopause** and leads to **postmenopausal bone loss**. **Osteoporosis** occurs when bone mass is so low that it increases the risk of bone fractures.

- Most of the calcium in the body is found in bone, but calcium is also needed for such essential functions as nerve transmission, muscle contraction, blood clotting, and blood pressure regulation. Good sources of calcium in the Canadian diet include dairy products, fish consumed with bones, and leafy green vegetables. Low blood calcium causes the release of **parathyroid hormone (PTH)**, which affects the

amount of calcium excretion at the kidney, calcium absorption from the diet, and the release of calcium from bone through **bone resorption**. When blood calcium is high, **calcitonin** blocks calcium release from bone.

- Phosphorus is widely distributed in foods. It plays an important structural role in bones and teeth. Phosphorus helps prevent changes in acidity and is an essential component of phospholipids, ATP, DNA, and RNA.

- Magnesium is important for bone health and blood pressure regulation, and it is needed as a cofactor and to stabilize ATP. The best dietary sources are whole grains and green vegetables.

- Sulphur is found in protein and is part of the structure of certain vitamins and of glutathione, which protects cells from oxidative damage.

Bone mass and osteoporosis • Figure 8.16

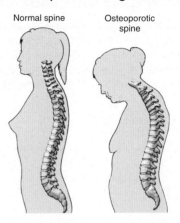

Normal spine   Osteoporotic spine

5 Trace Minerals 276

- Iron functions as part of **hemoglobin, myoglobin**, and proteins in energy metabolism. The amount of iron absorbed depends on the form of iron and other dietary components. **Heme iron**, found in meats, is more absorbable than nonheme iron, which is the only form found in plant foods. **Iron deficiency anemia** causes fatigue and decreased work capacity. The amount of iron transported from the intestinal cells to body cells depends on the amount needed. **Iron overload** can occur if too much iron is absorbed, and is typically due to the genetic condition **hemochromatosis**. If iron levels are too high, the heart and liver can be damaged, and diabetes and cancer are more likely. A single large dose of iron is toxic and can be fatal.

- Copper functions in proteins that affect iron and lipid metabolism, synthesis of connective tissue, antioxidant capacity, and iron transport. High levels of zinc can cause a copper deficiency. A copper deficiency can result in anemia and bone abnormalities. Seafood, nuts, seeds, and whole-grain breads and cereals are good sources of copper.

- Zinc is needed for the activity of many enzymes, and zinc-containing proteins are needed for gene expression. Good sources of zinc include red meats, eggs, dairy products, and whole grains. The amount of zinc in the body is regulated primarily by the amount absorbed and lost through the small intestine. Zinc deficiency depresses immunity. Too much zinc depresses immune function and contributes to copper and iron deficiency.

- Selenium is part of the antioxidant enzyme **glutathione peroxidase** and is needed for the synthesis of **thyroid hormones**. Dietary sources include seafood, eggs, organ meats, and plant foods grown in selenium-rich soils. Selenium deficiency causes muscle discomfort and weakness and is associated with **Keshan disease**. Low selenium intake has been linked to increased cancer risk.

- Iodine is an essential component of thyroid hormones, which regulate metabolism in the body. **Thyroid stimulating hormone** acts on the thyroid gland to promote the synthesis of thyroid hormones when levels drop in the blood. The best sources of iodine are seafood, foods grown near the sea, and **iodized salt**. When iodine is deficient, the **thyroid gland** enlarges, forming a **goiter**. Iodine deficiency also affects growth and development and is associated with **cretinism** in young children. The use of iodized salt

has reduced the incidence of iodine deficiency worldwide. However, the consumption of **goitrogens**, found in cabbage and cassava, increases the risk of iodine deficiency.

- Chromium is needed for normal insulin action and glucose utilization. Dietary sources of chromium include liver, brewer's yeast, nuts, and whole grains.

- Fluoride is necessary for the maintenance of bones and teeth and the prevention of **dental caries**. Dietary sources of fluoride include fluoridated drinking water, toothpaste, tea, and marine fish consumed with bones. Too much fluoride causes **fluorosis** in children.

Iron deficiency • Figure 8.25

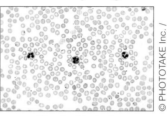
Normal red blood cells

© PHOTOTAKE Inc. / Alamy

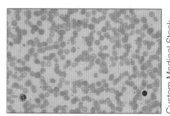
Iron deficiency anemia

Custom Medical Stock Photo

Key Terms

- **age-related bone loss** 269
- **aldosterone** 262
- **antidiuretic hormone (ADH)** 253
- **blood pressure** 251
- **bone remodelling** 267
- **bone resorption** 271
- **calcitonin** 271
- **cofactors** 260
- **cretinism** 286
- **DASH (Dietary Approaches to Stop Hypertension) diet** 263
- **dehydration** 250
- **dental caries** 287
- **diuretic** 256
- **electrolytes** 260
- **fluorosis** 288

- **glutathione peroxidase** 283
- **goiter** 284
- **goitrogens** 286
- **heme iron** 277
- **hemochromatosis** 281
- **hemoglobin** 276
- **hypertension** 262
- **hyponatremia** 255
- **iodized salt** 286
- **ions** 258
- **iron deficiency anemia** 278
- **iron overload** 281
- **Keshan disease** 283
- **major minerals** 257
- **menopause** 269
- **minerals** 257

- **myoglobin** 276
- **osteoporosis** 269
- **parathyroid hormone (PTH)** 270
- **peak bone mass** 269
- **postmenopausal bone loss** 269
- **prehypertension** 263
- **sodium chloride** 261
- **solutes** 251
- **solvent** 253
- **thirst** 251
- **thyroid gland** 284
- **thyroid hormones** 284
- **thyroid-stimulating hormone** 284
- **trace minerals** 257
- **water intoxication** 255

Critical and Creative Thinking Questions

1. Why might a thirsty sailor who drank seawater die of dehydration?

2 Sahr works at a desk. The only exercise she gets is when she takes care of her nieces and nephews one weekend a month. Her typical diet includes a breakfast of cereal, tomato juice, and coffee. She has a snack of doughnuts and coffee at work, and for lunch she joins her co-workers for a fast-food cheeseburger, fries, and a milkshake. When she gets home, she snacks on a pop and peanuts or chips. Dinner is usually a TV dinner and a

glass of milk. A recent physical exam indicated that her blood pressure is elevated. What dietary and lifestyle changes would you recommend to help Sahr lower her blood pressure?

3. Use food labels to identify three processed foods you commonly eat that contain more than 10% of the Daily Value for sodium per serving. What less-processed choices can you substitute for these foods? If you typically consumed one serving of each of these processed foods per day, by how much would the substitutions lower your sodium intake?

4. Many people in Canada must limit milk consumption due to lactose intolerance. What foods can they include in their diets to help meet their calcium needs?

5. The following table shows the incidence of hip fractures in different groups within a population of older adults. Use your knowledge of bone physiology to explain the differences observed.

Population group	Annual incidence of hip fracture per 1,000 people
Caucasian women	30
Caucasian men	13
Black women	11
Black men	7

6. A researcher asked his new technician to prepare a diet for his laboratory animals. The technician is interrupted several times while mixing the diet and is unfamiliar with the scale he is using to weigh the diet ingredients. After the diet is fed to the animals for several months, they begin to show signs of anemia. An error in diet preparation is suspected. Use the diet ingredients listed below to suggest which trace mineral deficiencies or excesses could cause anemia. What vitamin deficiencies can cause anemia?

Diet Ingredients

Starch, sucrose, casein (protein), corn oil, mixed plant fibres, vitamin A, vitamin D, vitamin E, vitamin K, B vitamin mix, calcium, sodium, potassium, magnesium, chloride, zinc, iron, iodine, selenium, copper, manganese, chromium, molybdenum.

7. Lin has just been diagnosed with anemia that is believed to be due to a deficiency in her diet. The total amount of hemoglobin in her blood is low, as is her hematocrit (the percentage of her blood that is made up or red blood cells). What other information will help determine which nutrient deficiency is the cause?

8. Evaluate your risk of developing osteoporosis based on your age, ethnicity, gender, diet, and lifestyle.

What is happening in this picture?

This photo shows astronaut Pete Conrad riding a stationary bike during his 28-day stay aboard Skylab in 1973. Weight-bearing exercise and adequate nutrient intake are important for the maintenance of bone.

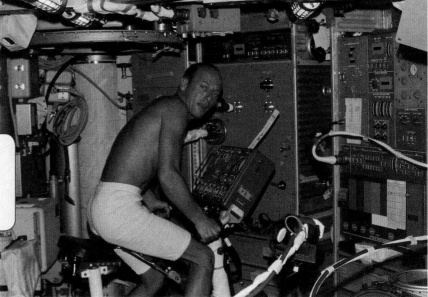

NASA/National Geographic Stock

Think Critically

1. Why is scheduled exercise even more important for bone health in space than it is on Earth?
2. What nutrients other than calcium might be of particular concern for bone health in an astronaut? Why?

Self-Test

(Check your answers in Appendix J.)

1. In a sedentary individual, most water is lost via _____.
   a. evaporation from the skin and lungs
   b. sweat
   c. saliva
   d. urine
   e. feces

2. _____ will increase water needs.
   a. A high-salt diet
   b. A high-protein diet
   c. A high-fibre diet
   d. A very low-calorie diet
   e. All of the above

3. If the concentration of solutes in your blood increases (i.e., the blood is more concentrated), which one of the following is most likely to occur?
   a. You will lose more water in the urine.
   b. Antidiuretic hormone will be released.
   c. You will begin to sweat.
   d. Your body temperature will go up.
   e. You will feel hungry.

4. The risk of high blood pressure is increased by _____.
   a. obesity
   d. sedentary lifestyle
   b. family history
   e. all of the above
   c. high-salt diet

5. Which one of the following is occurring at the point labelled with the arrow?

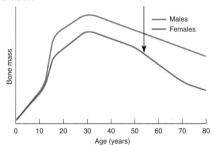

a. Bone formation is occurring more rapidly than bone breakdown.
b. Peak bone mass has been reached.
c. Bone breakdown exceeds bone formation due to normal aging.
d. Bone loss is accelerated after menopause.

6. Which of the following statements about iron is false?
   a. When iron levels are high, more iron is eliminated from the body in the urine.
   b. Heme iron is better absorbed than non-heme iron.
   c. Iron is a part of the oxygen-carrying protein hemoglobin.
   d. Iron is a part of the oxygen-storage protein myoglobin.
   e. Red meat is a good source of heme iron.

7. Hemochromatosis is treated with iron supplements.
   a. True
   b. False

8. Which of the following does not occur when blood calcium levels drop too low?
   a. More calcium is excreted in the urine.
   b. Bone is broken down, releasing calcium into the blood.
   c. Vitamin D is activated by the kidney.
   d. Parathyroid hormone is released.
   e. Intestinal absorption of calcium increases.

9. Which of the following is a function of iodine?
   a. It is an antioxidant.
   b. It is needed for insulin action.
   c. It is a component of the thyroid hormones.
   d. It is a component of superoxide dismutase.
   e. It is needed to cross-link collagen.

10. Women of childbearing age need more iron than men of the same age because they _____.
    a. are more active
    b. are growing
    c. lose more iron in the digestive tract
    d. have more muscle mass
    e. lose iron through menstruation

11. Which of the following statements about zinc is false?
    a. The amount that moves from the intestinal cells into the blood is regulated.
    b. Phytates present in grain products enhance zinc absorption.
    c. Zinc is involved in regulating protein synthesis.
    d. Zinc is part of the protein that allows vitamin A to affect gene expression.
    e. Zinc is absorbed better from meat than from plant foods.

12. Which of the following statements about selenium is false?
    a. It is part of the antioxidant enzyme glutathione peroxidase.
    b. It reduces some of the need for vitamin E.
    c. The amount in grain depends on the selenium content of the soil where it is grown.
    d. Low intakes are linked to a type of heart disease called Keshan disease.
    e. It is needed for the mineralization of bones and teeth.

13. The woman shown here has a deficiency of which of the following minerals?
    a. calcium
    b. iodine
    c. iron
    d. chromium
    e. magnesium

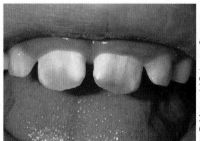

© Mike Goldwater / Alamy

14. Chromium increases the effectiveness of _____.
    a. insulin
    d. antidiuretic hormone
    b. thyroid hormone
    e. parathyroid hormone
    c. thyroid-stimulating hormone

15. Which of the following is most likely to have caused the condition shown here?
    a. living in a community that does not have fluoridated water
    b. taking calcium supplements
    c. swallowing toothpaste
    d. absorbing too much iron

Dr. P. Marazzi / Science Source

THE PLANNER ✓

Review your Chapter Planner on the chapter opener and check off your completed work.

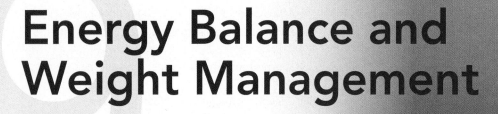

Energy Balance and Weight Management

A person's weight is not a reflection of his or her worth as a human being. Unfortunately, the opposite belief is often expressed in the media and in our culture. It is implied that we need to achieve a certain level of thinness or muscularity to be considered attractive. This inferred societal ideal is in sharp contrast to how our environment affects our food consumption and physical activity behaviours. Managing our weight has become a paradox: we are expected to be thin, but we live in an environment that promotes the patterns of overeating and physical inactivity associated with obesity.

Everywhere you look, you can see multiple influences to eat more and move less. Stores are lined with nutrient-poor, high-calorie foods. An increase in the use of electronic devices and motorized transport has decreased physical activity levels. Historically, people worked in labour-intensive jobs and cooked their own meals at home. Now, sedentary office jobs are the norm, and we consistently turn to calorically dense convenience foods to support our busy lifestyles.

The increase in the weight of Canadians over the past four decades has led to an increase in the cases of heart disease, type-2 diabetes, some cancers, depression, and decreased quality of life. If our higher weights are associated with so many health concerns, why are Canadians heavier than ever? Many people argue that we just need to "eat better" and "exercise more," but the answer is not that simple! Complex arrays of biological, psychological, and environmental factors increase a person's likelihood to be overweight.

All is not lost however! It is possible to control weight and lower our risk of disease by changing ourselves, our minds, and our relationships with food and physical activity. We also need to become aware of our external environment and evaluate how we can effectively change it to minimize the risk of obesity in the population.

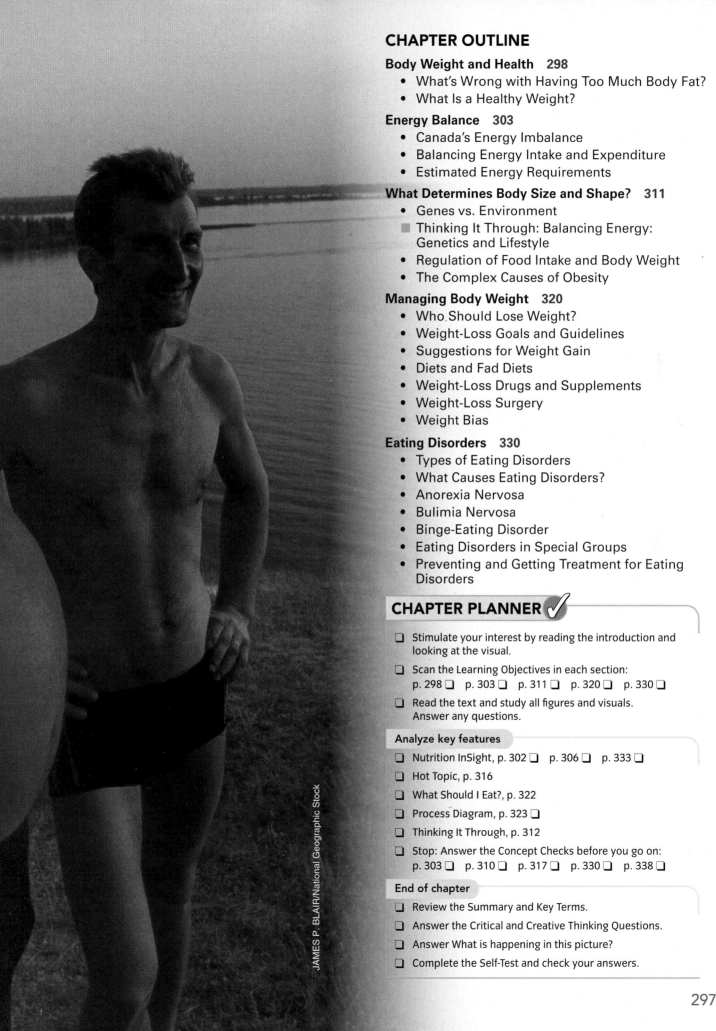

CHAPTER OUTLINE

CHAPTER PLANNER ✓

☐ Stimulate your interest by reading the introduction and looking at the visual.

☐ Scan the Learning Objectives in each section:
p. 298 ☐   p. 303 ☐   p. 311 ☐   p. 320 ☐   p. 330 ☐

☐ Read the text and study all figures and visuals. Answer any questions.

Analyze key features

☐ Nutrition InSight, p. 302 ☐   p. 306 ☐   p. 333 ☐

☐ Hot Topic, p. 316

☐ What Should I Eat?, p. 322

☐ Process Diagram, p. 323 ☐

☐ Thinking It Through, p. 312

☐ Stop: Answer the Concept Checks before you go on:
p. 303 ☐   p. 310 ☐   p. 317 ☐   p. 330 ☐   p. 338 ☐

End of chapter

☐ Review the Summary and Key Terms.

☐ Answer the Critical and Creative Thinking Questions.

☐ Answer What is happening in this picture?

☐ Complete the Self-Test and check your answers.

JAMES P. BLAIR/National Geographic Stock

Body Weight and Health

LEARNING OBJECTIVES

1. **Discuss** the obesity epidemic in Canada.

2. **Name** six chronic disorders that are more common in obese individuals than in lean individuals.

3. **Calculate** your BMI and determine whether it indicates increased health risks.

4. **Distinguish** visceral from subcutaneous body fat.

Many Canadians struggle with their weight, and more and more of us are in weight categories that increase our risk of disease. Since the decline of tobacco use in the past few decades, obesity has gained speed as one of the most significant lifestyle-related predictors of early mortality. It is estimated that about 60 percent of Canadian adults are **overweight** or **obese**.[1] Between the late 1970s and 2004, rates of obesity almost doubled from 14 percent of the Canadian adult population to 23 percent.[1] This increase does not affect all Canadians equally. The largest increases have been observed in Saskatchewan, Newfoundland and Labrador, and New Brunswick[1] (**Figure 9.1**). In Canada, men are still more likely than women to be obese, but female obesity rates have shown a significant increase over time. Low-income women are more likely to be obese than high-income women, but, surprisingly, the opposite trend is observed in Canadian males.[2] Also, ethnicity and immigrant status are also associated with different obesity rates. Aboriginal people have the highest obesity rates in Canada, followed by Latin Canadians and Caucasian Canadians.[3] Canadians whose ethnic background is East Asian, Southeast Asian, or South Asian have the lowest rates.

Compared with Canadians who have lived here for some time, recent immigrants to Canada have lower weights for their height and better health outcomes overall, a trend that has been coined "the healthy immigrant effect." This effect seems to disappear over time, as immigrants' weights rise once they have become integrated into Canada's **obesogenic environment**.[5]

Obesity is also a growing concern worldwide. The world is becoming heavier, with the average person's weight

> **overweight** Being too heavy for one's height, usually due to an excess of body fat. Overweight is defined as having a body mass index (ratio of weight to height squared) of 25 to 29.9 kg/m².
>
> **obese** Having excess body fat. Obesity is defined as having a body mass index (ratio of weight to height squared) of 30 kg/m² or greater.
>
> **obesogenic environment** A setting that promotes excessive energy intake and low levels of physical activity, resulting in an increase in obesity rates.

Distribution of obesity in Canada • Figure 9.1

Obesity rates vary across Canada. Higher rates of obesity are evidenced in certain Maritime provinces and Saskatchewan. Also, rural areas have higher proportions of obese individuals compared with more densely populated urban centres.[4]

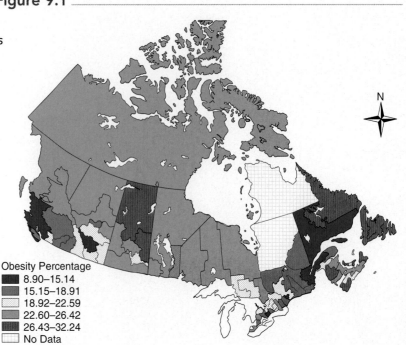

Obesity Percentage
- 8.90–15.14
- 15.15–18.91
- 18.92–22.59
- 22.60–26.42
- 26.43–32.24
- No Data

Ask Yourself

Why are the rates of obesity higher in rural areas of Canada than in urban centres?

Chronic Diseases in Canada, Volume 30, no. 1, December 2009, Socio-demographic and geographic analysis of overweight and obesity in Canadian adults using the Canadian Community Health Survey (2005) http://www.phac-aspc.gc.ca/publicat/cdic-mcbc/30-1/ar_01-eng.php Public Health Agency of Canada, 2005. Reproduced with the permission of the Minister of Public Works and Government Services Canada, 2012

Health consequences of excess body fat • Figure 9.2

Obesity-related health complications, such as those highlighted here, have reached epidemic proportions in Canada and around the world.

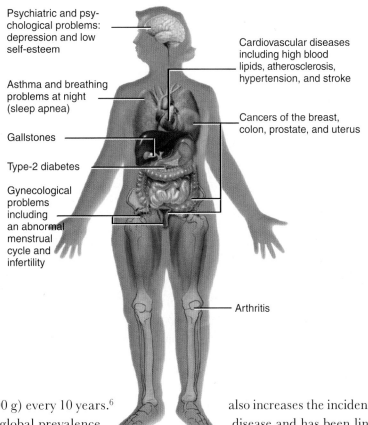

Psychiatric and psychological problems: depression and low self-esteem

Asthma and breathing problems at night (sleep apnea)

Gallstones

Type-2 diabetes

Gynecological problems including an abnormal menstrual cycle and infertility

Cardiovascular diseases including high blood lipids, atherosclerosis, hypertension, and stroke

Cancers of the breast, colon, prostate, and uterus

Arthritis

rising just over one pound (500 g) every 10 years.[6] Between 1980 and 2008, the global prevalence of obesity doubled from 6 percent to 12 percent. (Half of this increase occurred in the period between 2000 and 2008 alone.) During these three decades, overweight rates also increased from 25 percent of the population to 34 percent.[7] The increase in obesity rates is such an important trend that the word *globesity* has been coined to reflect the escalation of global obesity and overweight. Around the world, approximately 1.5 billion adults are overweight, and 500 million of them are obese.[6] The World Health Organization projects that by 2015, approximately 2.3 billion adults will be overweight and more than 700 million will be obese.[8] Once considered a problem only in high-income countries, overweight and obesity are now on the rise in low and middle-income countries, particularly in urban settings.

What's Wrong with Having Too Much Body Fat?

Having too much body fat increases a person's risk of developing a host of chronic health problems, including high blood pressure, heart disease, high blood cholesterol, type-2 diabetes, gallbladder disease, arthritis, sleep disorders, respiratory problems, menstrual irregularities, and cancers of the breast, uterus, prostate, and colon (**Figure 9.2**). Obesity

also increases the incidence and severity of infectious disease and has been linked to poor wound healing and surgical complications. The more excess body fat you have, the greater your health risks. The longer you carry excess fat, the greater the risks; individuals who gain excess weight at a young age and remain overweight throughout life face the greatest health risks.

Being overweight also has psychological and social consequences. Negative stereotypes about overweight and obese individuals may decrease their likelihood of feeling accepted or comfortable in social settings. Also, overweight and obese individuals of any age are more likely to experience depression, negative self-image, and feelings of inadequacy.[9] The physical health consequences of excess body fat may not manifest themselves as disease for years, but the psychological and social problems are experienced every day.

Because a higher weight status increases health problems, it also increases health care costs. Estimates suggest that, in direct costs alone, overweight and obesity cost the Canadian government approximately $6 billion a year, which represents 4.1 percent of our national health care expenditures.[10] Since our health care system already faces concerns about budgetary sustainability, it is now more important than ever to focus on preventative efforts to reduce disease risk.

How healthy is your BMI? • Figure 9.3[11]

Underweight is also associated with increased risk of early death, but not all thin people are at risk.[12] People who are naturally lean have a lower incidence of certain chronic diseases and do not face increased health risks due to their low body weight. However, low body fat due to starvation, eating disorders, or a disease process can decrease energy reserves and reduce the ability of the immune system to fight disease.

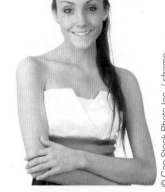

© Can Stock Photo Inc. / sframe

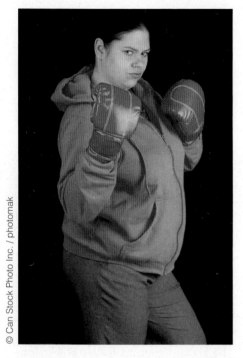

© Can Stock Photo Inc. / photomak

Classification of Obesity (World Health Organization Cut-Offs)

BMI (kg/m²)	Classification	Risk of associated health concerns
<18.5	Underweight	Low (but increased risk of other clinical problems)
18.5–24.9	Normal weight	Average
≥25	Overweight	
25–29.9	Pre-obese	Increased
30–34.9	Obese class 1	Moderate
35–39.9	Obese class 2	Severe
≥40	Obese class 3	Very severe

World Health Organization. WHO Global Database on Body Mass Index (BMI), 2011. Available online at http://apps.who.int/bmi/index.jsp?introPage=intro_3.html. Accessed March 15, 2011.

A high BMI may be caused by either too much body fat or a large amount of muscle. Therefore, for muscular athletes, BMI does not provide an accurate estimate of health risk. Both of the individuals pictured below have a BMI of 33, but only the man on the right has excess body fat. The high body weight of the man on the left is due to his large muscle mass. His body fat and, hence, his disease risk, is low. ▼

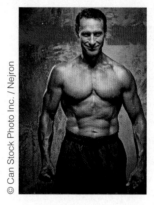

© Can Stock Photo Inc. / Nejron

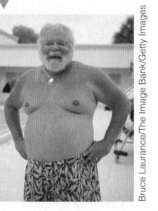

Bruce Laurance/The Image Bank/Getty Images

▲ BMI is a useful tool to help people assess how healthy their weight is, but it cannot provide a full picture of overall health status or of an individual's risk of disease. For example, a person who is overweight according to BMI but consumes a healthy diet and exercises regularly may be more fit and at a lower health risk than a person with a BMI in the healthy range who is sedentary and eats a poor diet.

What Is a Healthy Weight?

healthy weight
The weight that minimizes health risks and promotes overall health.

lean body mass
Body mass attributed to non-fat body components such as bone, muscle, and internal organs; also called *fat-free mass*.

Medically speaking, a **healthy weight** is a weight that minimizes health risks. Although a healthy weight is often associated with physical appearance, a person who follows sound nutritional and physical activity practices can be considered healthy at a wide range of weights. Your body weight is the sum of the weight of your fat and your **lean body mass**. Some body fat is essential for health, but too much increases your risk for numerous chronic health problems. How much weight and fat is too much depends on your genetics, age, gender, lifestyle, and the location of your fat.

Body mass index (BMI) The most common tool for assessing the healthfulness of body weight is the **body mass index (BMI)**, which is determined by dividing body weight (in kilograms) by height (in metres) squared. A healthy BMI for adults is between 18.5 and 24.9 kg/m² (**Figure 9.3**). People with a BMI in this range have the lowest health risks.

body mass index (BMI) A measure of body weight relative to height that is used to compare body size with a standard.

You can calculate your BMI according to either of these equations:

$$BMI = \text{Weight in kilograms}/(\text{Height in metres})^2$$

or

$$BMI = [\text{Weight in pounds}/(\text{Height in inches})^2] \times 703$$

Body composition **Body composition**, which refers to the relative proportions of fat and lean tissue that make up the body, affects the risks associated with excess body weight. Having more than the recommended percentage of body fat increases health risks, whereas having more lean body mass does not. In general, women store more body fat than men do, so the level of body fat that is considered healthy for women is higher than the level that is considered healthy for men. A healthy level of body fat for a young adult female is between 21 and 32 percent of total weight; for young adult males, it is between 8 and 19 percent.[13] With aging, lean body mass decreases and body fat increases, even if body weight remains the same. Some of this change may be prevented through exercise.

Body fat percentage is a better measure of obesity than BMI because it indicates how much of a person's weight is composed of fat. Many have accordingly argued that we should use another standard for assessing the risk posed by a person's size. The problem is that methods of determining body composition (**Figure 9.4**) require specialized

Techniques for measuring body composition • Figure 9.4

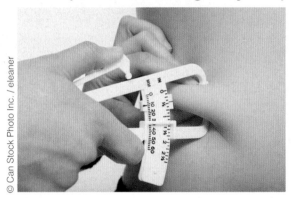

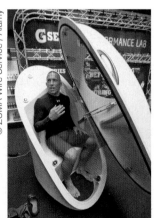

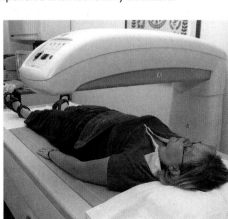

Underwater weighing. Underwater weighing relies on the fact that lean tissue is denser than fat tissue. The difference between a person's weight on land and his or her weight underwater is used to calculate body density; the higher a person's body density, the less fat he or she has. Underwater weighing is accurate but can't be used for small children or for ill or frail adults.

Skinfold thickness. Skinfold thickness uses calipers to measure the thickness of the fat layer under the skin at several locations. This technique assumes that the amount of fat under the skin is representative of total body fat. It is fast, easy, and inexpensive but can be inaccurate if not performed by a trained professional.

Air displacement. The BOD POD measures the amount of air displaced by the body in a closed chamber and uses this measurement along with body weight to determine body density, which is related to body fat mass. This method is accurate and easy for the subject but expensive and not readily available.

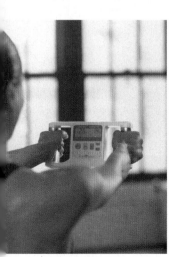

Bioelectric impedance. Bioelectric impedance analysis measures an electric current travelling through the body. It is based on the fact that current moves easily through lean tissue, which has a high water content, but is slowed by fat, which resists current flow. Bioelectric impedance devices are often used in gyms to assess the body fat percentage of gym-club members. These measurements are fast, easy, and painless but can be inaccurate if the amount of body water is higher or lower than typical. For example, the percentage of body fat obtained using bioelectric impedance will be artificially high in someone who has been sweating heavily.

© PHOTOTAKE Inc. / Alamy

Dual energy X-ray absorptiometry (DXA). DXA distinguishes among various body tissues by measuring differences in levels of X-ray absorption. A single investigation can accurately determine total body mass, bone mineral mass, and body fat percentage, but the apparatus is expensive and not readily available.

Keith/Custom Medical Stock Photo Custom Medical Stock Photo/Newscom

a. People who carry their excess fat around and above the waist have more visceral fat. Those who carry their extra fat below the waist, in the hips and thighs, have more subcutaneous fat. In the popular literature, these body types have been dubbed "apples" and "pears," respectively.

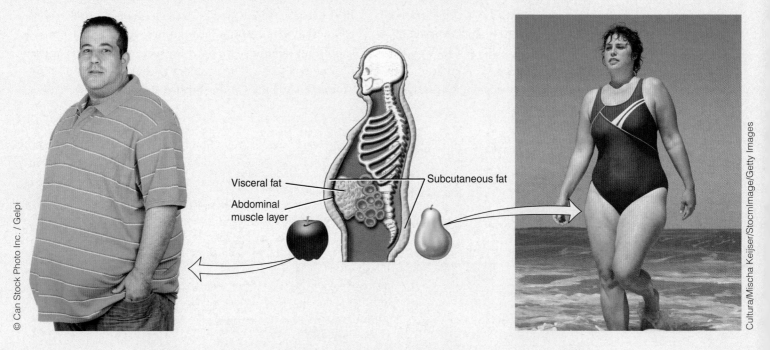

Visceral fat

Abdominal muscle layer

Subcutaneous fat

© Can Stock Photo Inc. / Gelpi

Cultura/Mischa Keijser/StocmImage/Getty Images

b. Waist circumference is indicative of the amount of visceral fat, the type of fat that is associated with increased health risk. Waist measurements and BMI are used to estimate the health risk associated with excess body fat. These waist circumference "cutoffs" are not useful in patients with a BMI of 35 kg/m² or greater.

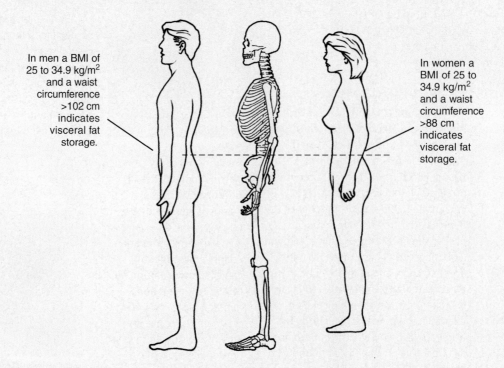

In men a BMI of 25 to 34.9 kg/m² and a waist circumference >102 cm indicates visceral fat storage.

In women a BMI of 25 to 34.9 kg/m² and a waist circumference >88 cm indicates visceral fat storage.

equipment, training, or both, and are more expensive, more time-consuming, and more involved than using an equation such as BMI, which requires only two easily determined inputs. BMI is therefore useful for population-level assessment of weight status, especially since most of the world has adopted it as a health measure.

Individuals should consider not only their BMI number but what that BMI comprises. When a person is muscular or has a larger frame, he or she may have a BMI that indicates being overweight or obese, despite having less body fat than someone with less muscle mass and a smaller bone size and a BMI that indicates a healthy weight.

Location of body fat BMI neither differentiates between fatty and lean tissue, nor indicates *where* an individual carries his or her weight. Excess **subcutaneous fat**, which is adipose tissue located under the skin, does not increase health risk as much as does excess **visceral fat**, which is adipose tissue located around the organs in the abdomen. Generally, fat in the hips and lower body is subcutaneous, whereas fat in the abdominal region is primarily visceral. Visceral fat is more metabolically active than subcutaneous fat, releasing dozens of biologically active substances that can contribute to disease.[14] An increase in visceral fat is associated with a higher incidence of heart disease, high blood cholesterol, high blood pressure, stroke, diabetes, and breast cancer.

> **waist circumference** A measurement of the tendency for visceral fat deposition. A waist circumference higher than 102 cm for men and 88 cm for women is associated with a greater risk of disease.

Waist circumference can be an effective tool for determining whether weight is deposited in a subcutaneous or visceral pattern (**Figure 9.5b**). It can be determined by placing a measuring tape around the waist at the top of the hip bone. A woman with a waist circumference of more than 88 cm and a man with a waist circumference of more than 102 cm are more likely to have a visceral fat deposition pattern associated with increased health risk. This measure is often used both independently and in addition to BMI as a more predictive measure of not only overall disease risk but of cardiovascular disease risk specifically. The cut-off points are meant for the general population. Members of ethnic groups and individuals who have smaller body frames may have a visceral fat pattern associated with increased health risk, even if they are below these cut-off points.

Whether your extra fat is deposited in a subcutaneous or visceral pattern is primarily determined by your genes.[15] For this reason, you cannot specifically target a certain area, such as the abdominals, for weight loss. Visceral fat storage is more common in men than in women, but after menopause, women's amount of visceral fat increases. Age and environment also influence where fat is stored.[16] Visceral fat storage increases with age. Stress, tobacco use, and alcohol consumption predispose people to visceral fat deposition, whereas weight loss and exercise reduce the amount of visceral fat.

CONCEPT CHECK STOP

1. **How** has the incidence of overweight and obesity changed in Canada over the past few decades?

2. **What** are the health consequences of excess body fat?

3. **How** is BMI flawed in measuring the health status of an individual?

4. **Where** is visceral fat located?

Energy Balance
LEARNING OBJECTIVES

1. **Identify** lifestyle factors that have led to weight gain among Canadians.
2. **Explain** the principle of energy balance.
3. **Describe** the components of energy expenditure.
4. **Calculate** your EER at various levels of activity.

Countless environmental factors in Canada promote an excess intake of calories and a reduced level of activity. These factors have affected the **energy balance** of Canadians; as a result, we are gaining fat and weight. According to the principle of energy balance, if you

> **energy balance** The amount of energy consumed in the diet compared with the amount of energy expended by the body over a given period.

consume the same amount of energy—or calories—as you burn, your body weight will remain the same. If you consume more energy than you expend, you will gain weight; and if you expend more energy than you consume, you will lose weight. This picture of energy balance is far too simple because our biology plays a significant role in whether we will put on weight and the rate at which we will gain weight. Some people can consume excess calories, never exercise, and not gain weight. Conversely, others have a biology that promotes weight gain, and excess calories are quickly converted into body fat. Although the principle of energy balance is not an exact science, it provides valuable insight into what drives whether an individual will gain or lose weight.

Canada's Energy Imbalance

Over the past 40 years, changes in environmental and social factors have affected what we eat, how much we eat, and how physically active we are. Food is plentiful and continuously available, and little physical activity is required in our daily lives. Simply put, more Canadians are overweight than ever before because we are eating more and burning fewer calories than we used to.

Eating more When deciding on what or how much to eat, the healthy choice is rarely the easy one. If you look around a typical Canadian city or town, you will see many examples of our living in an obesogenic environment. Grocery stores are lined with highly processed foods that are high

> **appetite** The *psychological* drive to consume food that is independent of hunger.
>
> **hunger** The *physiological* drive to consume food that is triggered by internal signals.

in calories and fat. Everywhere you go, you are exposed to fast-food restaurants, coffee shops, vending machines, and food advertisements. Moreover, unhealthy, high-calorie foods are often less expensive than healthier choices, and many stores offer discounts for buying foods in bulk amounts. Because **appetite** is triggered by external cues, such as the sight or smell of food, it is usually appetite, and not **hunger**, that urges us to stop for an ice cream cone on a summer afternoon or gives in to the smell of freshly baked cinnamon buns while strolling through the mall, even after we have eaten a large dinner.

In addition to having more enticing choices available to us, we consume more calories today because portion sizes have increased (**Figure 9.6**).[17] The more food that is put in front of us, the more we eat.[18] We

Portion distortion • Figure 9.6

a. Portion sizes have dramatically increased over the years and are continuing to increase. The burgers and French fries served in fast-food restaurants today are two to five times larger than they were when fast food first appeared about 40 years ago. Soft-drink serving sizes have also escalated. A large fast-food soft drink today typically contains three-quarters of a litre, providing over 300 kcal entirely from sugar. Also, 500-mL and 710-mL bottles have replaced 340-mL cans in many vending machines, further promoting overconsumption.

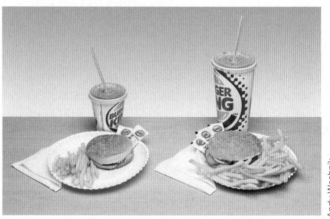

Andy Washnik

40 years ago   Today

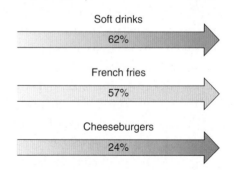

Soft drinks
62%

French fries
57%

Cheeseburgers
24%

Percent increase in portion size

b. In 2012, Tim Hortons decided to rename its beverage sizes and add another extra-large size. Now, when you order a medium French Vanilla Cappuccino, you receive a larger 414-mL size, weighing in at 420 kcal, rather than the former, smaller 295-mL size offering 300 kcal.

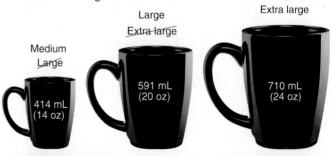

Extra small
Small
237 mL (8 oz)

Small
Medium
296 mL (10 oz)

Medium
Large
414 mL (14 oz)

Large
Extra large
591 mL (20 oz)

New Extra large
710 mL (24 oz)

Ask Yourself

Will the change in the naming of Tim Hortons sizes affect your intake?

tend to eat in units, such as one cookie, one sandwich, or one bag of chips, regardless of the size of the unit. When we are presented with larger units, we eat more.

Social changes over the past few decades have also contributed to the increase in the number of calories Canadians consume. Busy schedules and an increase in the number of both single-parent households and households with two working parents mean that many families are often too rushed to cook meals at home. As a result, prepackaged, convenience, and fast-food meals have become mainstays. These foods are typically higher in energy and fat than foods prepared at home.

Moving less Along with Canada's rising energy intake, there has been a decline in the amount of energy Canadians expend, both at work and at play. It is estimated that only 15 percent of Canadians are getting the recommended amounts of physical activity.[19] Fewer Canadian adults today work in jobs that require physical labour. People drive to work rather than walk or bike, take elevators instead of stairs, use dryers rather than hang clothes outside, and cut the lawn with riding mowers rather than using push mowers. Even farm life has become less physically demanding because of the increased use of machinery to maximize output. All these simple changes reduce the amount of energy we expend daily. Canadians are also less active during their leisure time because busy schedules, commuting, and long days at work leave little time or desire for active recreation. At the end of a long and busy day, many people sit in front of television sets, video games, and computers.

Inactivity is an issue not just for overweight or obese individuals but for all Canadians. Although overweight and obese Canadians are typically less active than Canadians with a healthy weight, both groups spend a similar amount of time in pursuits requiring a moderate to vigorous level of activity.[19] Also, overweight or obese individuals carry more weight when they are active, so they burn more calories. If the total daily caloric burn of normal weight individuals were compared with the caloric burn of obese and overweight individuals, the two groups would be even more similar. This similarity suggests that although inactivity contributes to the obesity epidemic, something else, namely a high caloric intake, is likely the main behaviour-related cause of higher weights. It is quite frankly very easy to out-eat exercise, but nearly impossible to out-exercise overeating. This by no means suggests that physical activity isn't important for a healthy weight or a healthy life. Rather, it suggests that physical inactivity isn't the main lifestyle-related driving force behind the obesity epidemic; it is more likely that the cause is excessive energy intake.

Balancing Energy Intake and Expenditure

The energy needed to fuel your body comes from the food you eat and the energy stored in your body. You use this energy to stay alive, process your food, move, and grow.

Energy intake The amount of energy you consume depends on what and how much you eat and drink. The carbohydrate, fat, protein, and alcohol consumed in food and drink all contribute energy: 4, 9, 4, and 7 kcal per gram, respectively (**Figure 9.7a**). Although vitamins, minerals, and water are essential nutrients, they do not provide energy. You can determine your calorie intake by reading food labels and by looking up caloric values in a food composition table or database (**Figure 9.7b, c**).

Energy expenditure The total amount of energy used by the body each day is called **total energy expenditure**. It includes the energy needed to maintain basic body functions and to fuel physical activity and process food. For children who are growing and for pregnant women, total energy expenditure includes the energy used to form new tissues. In lactating women, it includes the energy used to produce milk. A small amount of energy is also used to maintain body temperature in a cold environment.

For most people, about 60 to 75 percent of total energy expenditure is used for **basal metabolism**. Basal metabolism includes all the essential metabolic reactions and life-sustaining functions needed to keep our bodies functioning, such as breathing, circulating blood, regulating body temperature, synthesizing tissues, removing waste products, and sending nerve signals. The rate at which energy is used for these basic functions is the **basal metabolic rate (BMR)**.

basal metabolism The energy expended to maintain an awake, resting body that is not digesting food or being physically active.

basal metabolic rate (BMR) The rate of energy expenditure under resting conditions. It is measured after 12 hours without food or exercise.

What you weigh is determined by the balance between how much energy you take in and how much energy you expend.

a. The number of kilocalories in a food depends on how much carbohydrate, fat, and protein it contains. This taco contains 9 g of protein, 16 g of carbohydrate, and 13 g of fat. Its energy content is

(9 g × 4 kcal/g protein)
+ (16 g × 4 kcal/g carbohydrate)
+ (13 g × 9 kcal/g fat)
= 217 kcal.

Two tacos would then be 434 kcal, approximately 1/6 of a man's daily caloric needs and 1/5 of a woman's daily caloric needs.

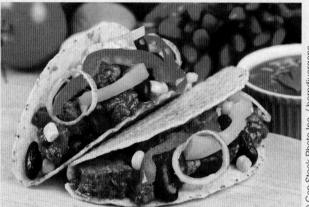

© Can Stock Photo Inc. / berndjuergens

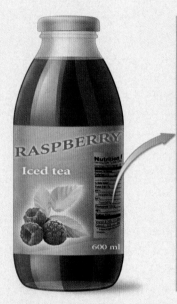

Nutrition Facts
Valeur nutritive
Per 250 ml / par 250 ml

Amount Teneur	% Daily Value % valeur quotidienne
Calories / Calories 100	
Fat / Lipides 0.5 g	1 %
Saturated / saturés 0 g + Trans / trans 0 g	0 %
Cholesterol / Cholestérol 0 mg	
Sodium / Sodium 0 mg	0 %
Carbohydrate/ Glucides 26 g	9 %
Sugars / Sucres 25 g	
Protein/ Protéines 3 g	
Vitamin A / Vitamine A	2 %
Vitamin C / Vitamine C	10 %
Calcium / Calcium	0 %
Iron / Fer	2 %

b. The Nutrition Facts panel shows the kilocalories, per serving. To understand how many kilocalories your portion contains, check the serving size and compare it with the net quantity declaration on the label. Often the portions of foods and beverages that people consume are larger than the servings listed on the label. As a result, we often consume more calories than we think we are consuming.

Ask Yourself

If you drank this entire bottle of iced tea, how many kilocalories would you have consumed?

c. Some people have no idea how many kilocalories are in some of their favourite fast foods. Typically, the more cream, fat, and sugar a product has, the more kilocalories it has. A better understanding of the caloric content of food will increase individuals' ability to more effectively control their energy intake.

Food Item	Energy (kcal)
McDonald's French Fries Large	500
McDonald's Big Mac	540
Wendy's Baconator Double	940
Burger King Whopper	670
Burger King Onion Rings (medium)	320
Subway 15-cm Meatball Marinara	570
Dairy Queen Turtle Pecan Cluster Blizzard Large	1460
Starbucks Double Choclatey Chip Frappuccino blended beverage (475 ml)	500
Tim Hortons Chocolate-Glazed Timbit	70
Tim Hortons Chocolate Macadamia Nut Cookie	240

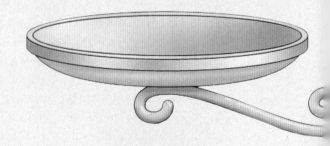

Energy in

d. The hood in the photo below collects expired air. Because aerobic metabolism uses oxygen and produces carbon dioxide, measures of these gases in expired air can be used to estimate energy expenditure. To estimate the energy expended for basal metabolism, measures are taken in the morning, in a warm room, before rising, and at least 12 hours after food intake or activity. For convenience, measurements are often made after only five to six hours without food or exercise. This measurement, called the **resting metabolic rate (RMR)**, yields values that are about 10 to 20 percent higher than BMR values.[28]

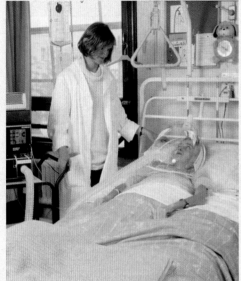

St. Bartholomew's Hospital/Science/Custom Medical Stock Photo

Factors that affect basal metabolism	Effect
Higher lean body mass	↑
Greater height and weight	↑
Male gender	↑
Pregnancy	↑
Lactation	↑
Growth	↑
Low-calorie diet	↓
Starvation	↓
Fever	↑
Low thyroid hormone levels	↓
Stimulant drugs such as caffeine and tobacco	↑
Exercise	↑

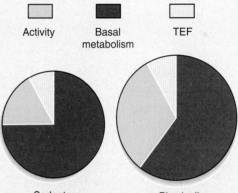

Activity   Basal metabolism   TEF

e. Sedentary people must plan their intake carefully so it does not exceed their energy expenditure. More active people burn more calories through activity so they can eat more and still maintain their weight. Very active people, such as professional athletes, can actually burn more calories through activity than they do for basal metabolism.

Sedentary person (1,800 kcal/day)

Physically active person (2,200 kcal/day)

© Can Stock Photo Inc. / anitapatterson

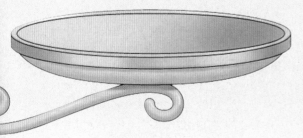

Energy out

f. The amount of energy used to process the food we eat varies depending on the size and composition of the meal. A bigger meal produces a greater thermic effect of food (TEF). A high-fat meal yields a lower TEF than a meal high in carbohydrate or protein because dietary fat can be used and stored more efficiently.[29]

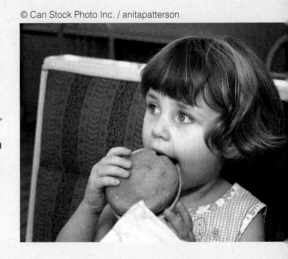

The energy expended for basal metabolism does *not* include the energy needed for physical activity or for the digestion and absorption of food (**Figure 9.7d**).

BMR is primarily determined by genetics and is the main reason why two individuals may have identical patterns of food consumption and physical activity, but differ in their tendencies for weight gain. BMR increases as body weight increases and as muscle mass increases (Figure 9.7d). BMR is generally higher in men than in women because men have a greater amount of lean body mass. BMR decreases with age, partly because of the decrease in lean body mass that occurs as we get older. BMR is also lower when calorie intake is consistently less than the body's needs.[20] When individuals lose weight, their BMR drops, meaning they will need to permanently lower their daily caloric intake to maintain their new weight.

Physical activity is the second major component of total energy expenditure. In most people, physical activity accounts for a smaller proportion of total energy expenditure than basal metabolism does, about 15 to 30 percent of energy requirements (**Figure 9.7e**). The energy we expend in physical activity includes both planned exercise and daily activities such as walking to work, typing, performing yard work, work-related activities, and

> **non-exercise activity thermo-genesis (NEAT)** The energy expended for everything we do other than sleeping, eating, or sports-like exercise.

even fidgeting. This **non-exercise activity thermogenesis (NEAT)** includes the energy expended for everything that is not sleeping, eating, or sports-like exercise. It accounts for the majority of the energy expended for activity and varies enormously, depending on an individual's environment, occupation, and daily movements.

An endless number of activities can contribute to your physical activity needs for the day. To be physically active, it is not necessary to belong to a gym or to go for a run. Moderate to vigorous intensity activities that promote healthy hearts, bones, and weights can be achieved by walking the dog briskly, gardening, taking the stairs over the elevator, or hiking through one of Canada's many beautiful landscapes.

The amount of energy used for an activity depends on the length of time it is performed, how strenuous the activity is, and the size of the person. More strenuous activities, such as jogging, use more energy than do less strenuous activities, such as walking. If you walk for an hour, you will probably burn as many calories as you would by jogging for 30 minutes (Appendix G).

We also use energy to digest food and to absorb, metabolize, and store the nutrients from food. The energy used for these processes is called either the **thermic effect of food (TEF)** or **diet-induced thermogenesis**. This energy expenditure causes body temperature to rise slightly for several hours after a person has eaten. The energy required for

> **thermic effect of food (TEF)** or **diet-induced thermogenesis** The energy required for the digestion of food and absorption, metabolism, and storage of nutrients.

TEF is estimated to be about 10 percent of energy intake but can vary, depending on the amounts and types of nutrients consumed (**Figure 9.7f**).

The basics of weight gain and weight loss

According to the principle of energy balance, if you consume more energy than you expend, the excess energy is stored for later use (**Figure 9.8**). A small amount of energy is stored as glycogen in liver and muscle, but most is stored as fat in **adipocytes**, which make up adipose tissue. Adipocytes

> **adipocytes** Cells that store fat.

contain large fat droplets (see Figure 5.10b). The cells increase in size and number as they accumulate more fat, and they shrink as fat is removed, but *do not decrease in number*. If, over the long term, intake exceeds need, the adipocytes will enlarge and divide, and the amount of body fat will increase, causing weight gain. A person with a larger initial number of adipocytes has a greater capacity to store fat. Most adipocytes are formed during infancy and adolescence, but excessive weight gain can cause the formation of new adipocytes at any time of life. The human body theoretically has a limitless ability to make fat cells.

Stored energy is retrieved and used when energy intake is reduced. To maintain a steady supply of blood glucose, liver glycogen breaks down (see Figure 9.8). Glucose is also supplied by the breakdown of small amounts of body protein, primarily muscle protein, to yield amino acids. These amino acids can then be used to make glucose or produce ATP. Energy for tissues that don't require glucose is provided by the breakdown of stored fat. Nutrients consumed in the next meal replenish these stores, but as the result of prolonged energy restriction, fat and protein are lost, and body weight is reduced. An energy deficit of about 3,500 kcal will result in the loss of approximately 500 g (1 lb.) of adipose tissue.

Storing and retrieving energy • Figure 9.8

If energy balance is your goal, you want to ensure that the total amount of calories consumed from all sources does not exceed the total amount of calories expended as a result of three factors: BMR, the thermic effect of food, and physical activity. Excess energy consumed as dietary fat is easily stored as body fat. Excess energy consumed as dietary carbohydrate is stored as glycogen or converted into fat. Excess energy consumed as dietary protein is converted into body fat. If your goal is weight loss, you need to watch your total caloric intake from *all* sources. When you eat less than you need to fuel BMR and physical activity, you retrieve energy from these stores. Liver glycogen and a small amount of body protein break down to supply glucose, and triglycerides in adipose tissue break down to supply fatty acids for energy.

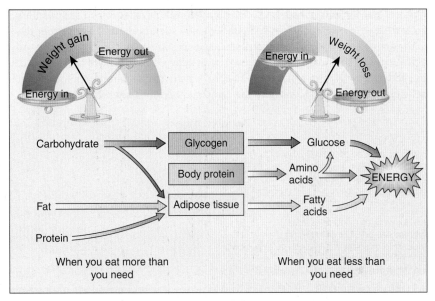

Estimated Energy Requirements

The current recommendation for energy intake in Canada is the *estimated energy requirement* (*EER*; see Chapter 2), the number of kilocalories needed for a healthy individual to maintain his or her weight.[28] EER is calculated using equations that take into account gender, age, height, weight, activity level, and life stage, all of which affect calorie needs.

To calculate your EER, first determine your physical activity level.[30] Do this by keeping a daily log of your activities and recording the amount of time spent on each activity. Use **Figure 9.9** to help translate the amount of time you spend engaged in moderate-intensity or vigorous activity into an activity level (sedentary, low active, active, or high active). Each activity level corresponds to a numerical physical activity (PA) value that can be used to calculate your EER. For example, if you spend about an hour a day walking (a moderate-intensity activity) or about 45 minutes jogging (a vigorous activity), you are in the active category and should use the active PA value corresponding to your age and gender to calculate your EER.

Activity level has a significant effect on calorie needs. For example, a 22-year-old man who is 183 cm (6 feet) tall and weighs 85 kg (185 lb.) needs about 2,770 kcal per day if he is at a sedentary activity level but almost 600 more kcal if he is at an active level.

Once you have determined your physical activity level, calculate your EER by entering your age, weight, height, and PA value (see Figure 9.9) into the appropriate EER prediction equation. You will need to know your height in metres and your weight in kilograms to do so. **Table 9.1** provides equations for normal-weight adults age 19 and older. Equations for other groups are in Appendix A.

EER prediction equations for adults ≥19 years   Table 9.1

Gender	EER prediction equation*
Men	EER = 662 − (9.53 × Age in yrs) + PA [(15.91 × Weight in kg) + (539.6 × Height in m)]
Women	EER = 354 − (6.91 × Age in yrs) + PA [(9.36 × Weight in kg) + (726 × Height in m)]

For example, if you are an active 19-year-old male who weighs 72.7 kg (160 lb.) and is 1.75 m (5' 9") tall, then the equation is applied as follows:
EER = 662 − (9.53 × 19 yrs) + 1.25([15.91 × 72.7 kg] + [539.6 × 1.75 m]) = 3,107 kcal/day

*These equations are appropriate for determining EER in normal-weight individuals. Equations that predict the amount of energy needed for weight maintenance in overweight and obese individuals are also available (see Appendix A).

What are your physical activity level and PA value? • Figure 9.9

Physical activity level, which is used to calculate EER, is categorized as sedentary, low active, active, or very active. A sedentary person spends about 2.5 hours per day engaged in the activities of daily living, such as housework, homework, and yard work. Adding activity moves the person into the low-active, active, or very-active category. Activity can be moderate or vigorous or a combination of the two; compared to moderate-intensity activity, vigorous activity will burn the same number of calories in less time.

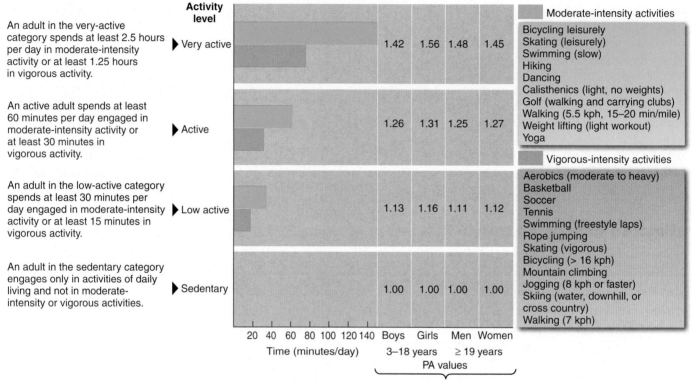

An adult in the very-active category spends at least 2.5 hours per day in moderate-intensity activity or at least 1.25 hours in vigorous activity.

An active adult spends at least 60 minutes per day engaged in moderate-intensity activity or at least 30 minutes in vigorous activity.

An adult in the low-active category spends at least 30 minutes per day engaged in moderate-intensity activity or at least 15 minutes in vigorous activity.

An adult in the sedentary category engages only in activities of daily living and not in moderate-intensity or vigorous activities.

Activity level

▶ Very active   1.42   1.56   1.48   1.45

▶ Active   1.26   1.31   1.25   1.27

▶ Low active   1.13   1.16   1.11   1.12

▶ Sedentary   1.00   1.00   1.00   1.00

20 40 60 80 100 120 140   Boys   Girls   Men   Women
Time (minutes/day)   3–18 years   ≥ 19 years
PA values

Each physical activity level is assigned a numerical physical activity (PA) value that can then be used in the EER calculation.

Moderate-intensity activities
Bicycling leisurely
Skating (leisurely)
Swimming (slow)
Hiking
Dancing
Calisthenics (light, no weights)
Golf (walking and carrying clubs)
Walking (5.5 kph, 15–20 min/mile)
Weight lifting (light workout)
Yoga

Vigorous-intensity activities
Aerobics (moderate to heavy)
Basketball
Soccer
Tennis
Swimming (freestyle laps)
Rope jumping
Skating (vigorous)
Bicycling (> 16 kph)
Mountain climbing
Jogging (8 kph or faster)
Skiing (water, downhill, or cross country)
Walking (7 kph)

Ask Yourself

What are your activity level and corresponding PA value?

CONCEPT CHECK   **STOP**

1. **Which** is more likely the lifestyle-related factor driving the obesity epidemic: high caloric intake or physical inactivity?

2. **Where** in the body is most energy stored when intake exceeds expenditure?

3. **Which** component of energy expenditure is the easiest to modify?

4. **What** is your EER?

What Determines Body Size and Shape?

LEARNING OBJECTIVES

1. **Discuss** genetic and environmental factors that affect body weight.

2. **List** four physiological signals that determine whether you feel hungry or full.

3. **Describe** how hormones regulate body fat levels.

4. **Discuss** factors that cause some people to gain weight more easily than others.

You are probably shaped like your mother or father. This is because the information that determines body size and shape is contained in the genes you inherit from your parents (**Figure 9.10**). Some of us inherit long, lean bodies, and others inherit huskier builds and the tendency to gain weight. Genes involved in regulating body weight have been called **obesity genes** because variations in these genes determine the likelihood of becoming obese. Scientists have identified more than 200 genes that are associated with body weight regulation; an estimated 20 or 30 of these genes may contribute to obesity in humans.[30] These genes are responsible for the production of proteins that affect your appetite and therefore how much food you eat, how much energy you expend, and the way your body stores fat. But genes are not the only factor; regardless of your genetic background, the lifestyle choices you make play an important role in determining what you weigh.

Genes vs. Environment

The genes you inherit have a significant influence on your body weight. If one or both of your parents is obese, your risk of becoming obese is increased by a factor of two or three, and the risk increases with the magnitude of the obesity. By studying identical twins, who have the same genetic makeup, researchers have been able to determine that about 75 percent of the variation in BMI can be attributed to genes.[31, 32] The remaining 25 percent is determined by the environment where you live and the lifestyle choices you make (see the *Thinking It Through* feature).

Genes determine body shape • Figure 9.10

The genes we inherit from our parents are important determinants of our body size and shape. The boy on the left inherited his father's long, lean body, whereas the boy on the right has his father's huskier build and will likely have a tendency to be overweight throughout his life.

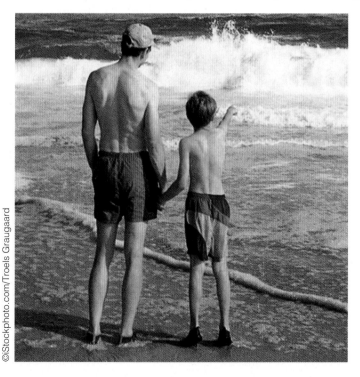

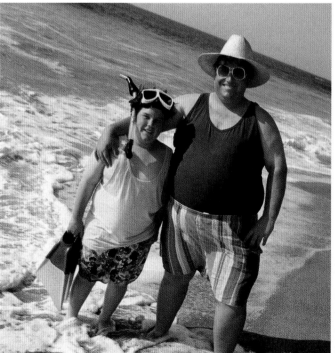

THINKING IT THROUGH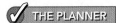

Balancing Energy: Genetics and Lifestyle

Lucia was a chubby baby. In her teens, she continued to be slightly overweight. Because her parents are both obese, no one was surprised by Lucia's size. During her first year of university, she gained 5 kg (10 lb) and became resigned to the inevitability that she would be obese like her parents. Then she noticed that the choices many of her thinner friends made—both in the foods they ate and how they spent their free time—differed from the choices she made. She decided to make some changes.

Lucia, now 23 years old, is 163 cm (5′4″) tall and weighs 70 kg (155 lb).

What is her BMI? Is it in the healthy range? What does BMI not tell us?

▼

Your answer: _____

_____

By recording and analyzing her food intake for three days, Lucia determines that she consumes about 2,450 kcal every day. By keeping an activity log, she estimates that a typical day includes 30 minutes of walking rapidly around campus—a moderate-intensity activity.

What is her EER?

(Tip: Make sure you use height in metres and weight in kilograms)

▼

Your answer: _____

_____

How does Lucia's EER compare with her intake? Is she in energy balance?

▼

Your answer: _____

_____

Lucia decides to start playing tennis four days a week again and to cut down on her portions at meals. Meal A, shown below, was once her typical lunch, and Meal B is her new lunch.

How can Meal B have fewer calories even though it looks like more food?

▼

Your answer: _____

_____

Why might Meal B satisfy hunger just as well as or better than Meal A?

▼

Your answer: _____

_____

If Lucia adds an additional 30 minutes of moderate-intensity exercise five days a week, by how much will her EER increase?

▼

Your answer: _____

_____

Do you think Lucia is destined to be overweight? Explain your answer.

▼

Your answer: _____

_____

(Check your answers in Appendix I.)

Meal A

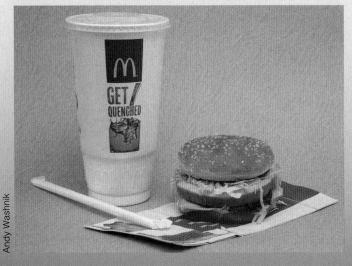

Andy Washnik

Meal B

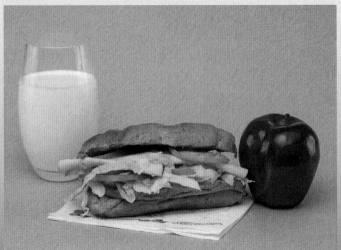

Andy Washnik

When individuals who are genetically susceptible to weight gain find themselves in an environment where food is appealing and plentiful and physical activity is easily avoided (like many Canadian towns or cities), obesity is a likely outcome. It is, however, not the only possible outcome. If you inherit genes that predispose you to being overweight but carefully monitor your diet and exercise regularly, you can maintain a healthy weight. Individuals with no genetic tendency toward obesity can also become overweight if they consume a high-calorie diet and get little exercise. The interplay between genetics and lifestyle is illustrated by the higher incidence of obesity in Pima Indians living in Arizona than in a genetically similar group of Pima Indians living in Mexico (**Figure 9.11**).[33]

Regulation of Food Intake and Body Weight

To regulate weight and body fat at a constant level, the body must be able to respond both to short-term changes in food intake and to long-term changes in the amount of stored body fat. Signals related to food intake affect hunger, **satiety**, and **satiation** (**Figure 9.12**) over a short period—from meal to meal—whereas signals from adipose tissue trigger the brain to adjust both food intake and energy expenditure for long-term weight regulation.

Regulating how much we eat at each meal

How do you know how much to eat for breakfast or when it is time to eat lunch? The physical sensations of hunger or satiation that determine how much you eat at each meal are triggered by signals from the gastrointestinal tract, levels of nutrients and hormones circulating in the blood, and messages from the brain.[36] Some signals are sent before you eat to tell you that you are hungry, some signals are sent while food is in

satiety After a meal has been consumed, the feeling of fullness that determines the length of time before the desire to eat returns.

satiation While eating, the feeling of fullness and satisfaction that eliminates the desire to continue eating.

Genes vs. environment • Figure 9.11

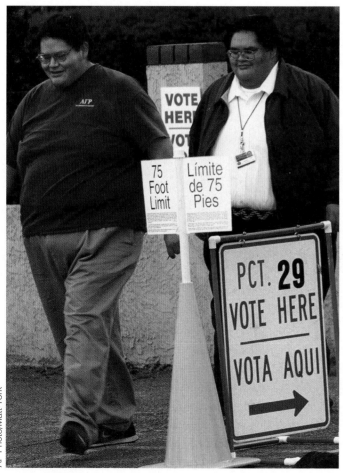

AP Photo/Matt York

a. Genetic analysis of the Pima Indian population living in Arizona identified the genes that may be responsible for this group's tendency to store excess body fat.[34] When this genetic susceptibility is combined with a lifestyle that includes high-calorie foods and demands little physical activity, the outcome is the strikingly high incidence of obesity seen in this population.

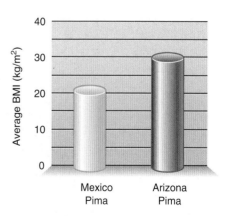

b. The Pima Indians of Mexico share the same genetic susceptibility to obesity as the Arizona Pimas but are farmers who work in the fields and consume the food they grow.[35] Although the Mexican group has higher rates of obesity than would be predicted from their diet and exercise patterns, which suggests they possess genes that favour fat storage, they are significantly less obese than the Arizona Pimas.[33]

a.

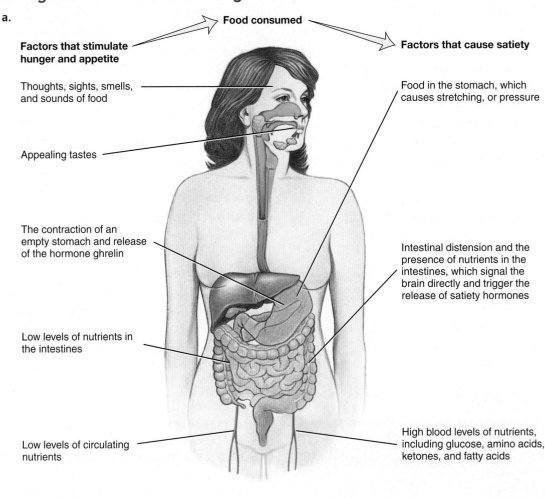

Food consumed

Factors that stimulate hunger and appetite

Factors that cause satiety

Thoughts, sights, smells, and sounds of food

Food in the stomach, which causes stretching, or pressure

Appealing tastes

The contraction of an empty stomach and release of the hormone ghrelin

Intestinal distension and the presence of nutrients in the intestines, which signal the brain directly and trigger the release of satiety hormones

Low levels of nutrients in the intestines

Low levels of circulating nutrients

High blood levels of nutrients, including glucose, amino acids, ketones, and fatty acids

b. Hunger is the physiological drive to consume food that promotes food consumption. Satiation is the feeling of fullness experienced while eating that makes an individual stop eating. Satiety is the feeling of fullness experienced after a meal has been consumed that influences how long it takes before that person is hungry again.

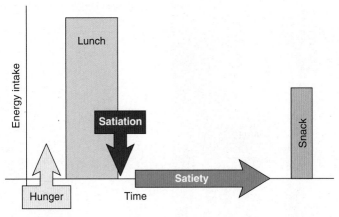

the gastrointestinal tract, and others occur when nutrients are circulating in the bloodstream (Figure 9.12).

The hormone **neuropeptide Y** promotes feeding behaviours and an increased storage of energy as adipose tissue. It is implicated in the development of obesity. Regardless of when you ate breakfast and how much you ate, the hormone **ghrelin** may cause you to feel hungry around lunchtime by stimulating the release of neuropeptide Y.

Ghrelin, which is produced by the stomach, is believed to stimulate the desire to eat at usual mealtimes. Blood levels of ghrelin rise an hour or two before a meal and drop very low after a meal. Ghrelin levels also rise when we don't get enough sleep, thereby promoting an increased appetite during the day and a potentially larger caloric consumption.[37] Another hormone, peptide YY, causes a reduction in appetite. It is released from the gastrointestinal tract after a meal, and the amount released is proportional to the number of kilocalories consumed.[38]

Psychological factors can also affect how much you consume. Some people eat excessively for comfort and to relieve stress, independent of internal cues. Others lose their appetite when they experience these emotions. Psychological distress can alter the mechanisms that regulate food intake. Also, a growing body of evidence suggests that some people may have a physical and psychological addiction to food, which promotes larger food intake patterns (see *Hot Topics*). If psychology is driving poor food-related behaviour, these factors need to be acknowledged and addressed before positive change can be made.

Regulating how much we weigh over the long term
If we consistently consume more calories than we require, our overconsumption can cause an increase in body weight and fatness. To return fatness to the former healthy level, the body must be able to monitor how much fat is present. Some of this information comes from hormones.

Leptin is a good example of a hormone that can affect body weight. Leptin is produced by the adipocytes. The amount of leptin produced is proportional to the size of the adipocytes, and the effect of leptin on energy intake and expenditure depends on the amount of leptin released. When a person loses weight, fat is lost from adipocytes, and less leptin is released, causing an increase in food intake and a decrease in energy expenditure, promoting future weight regain. When a person gains weight, the adipocytes accumulate fat, and more leptin is released, triggering events that decrease food intake and increase energy expenditure (**Figure 9.13**).

Leptin and body fat • Figure 9.13

a. Mouse studies have helped us to better understand how leptin is used in chronic energy balance. As shown in the diagram, the effect of leptin depends on how much of it is present. When the mouse loses weight, fat is lost from adipocytes, and less leptin is released. The result is an increase in food intake and a decrease in energy expenditure, promoting future weight regain. When the mouse gains weight, the adipocytes accumulate fat, and more leptin is released, triggering events that decrease food intake and increase energy expenditure.

Mice that inherit a defective leptin gene may produce no leptin. For these mice, even when the adipocytes enlarge, the leptin levels do not increase. The lack of leptin continues to signal the mouse to eat more and expend less energy. ▼

ORNL

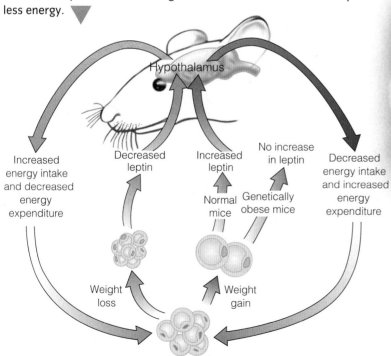

Adipocytes at specific size

b. The mouse on the left inherited a defective leptin gene, so it produces no leptin. For these mice, even when the adipocytes enlarge, the leptin levels do not increase. The lack of leptin continues to signal the mouse to eat more and expend less energy. The mouse on the right also inherited a defective leptin gene, but treatment with leptin injection returned its weight to normal.

Think Critically

What might happen to a mouse with a defect that causes overproduction of leptin?

HOT TOPIC

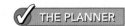

Can individuals be addicted to food?

For some people, appropriately regulating their food consumption is a relatively simple task: they eat when they are hungry and they rarely overconsume. For others, food consumption is a central focus of their daily thoughts and they regularly experience an overwhelming compulsion to overconsume, even in the absence of hunger.

A growing body of evidence suggests that food-seeking behaviour may be similar to drug-seeking behaviour. Some even argue that food addiction (or dependency) should be listed in the American Psychiatric Association's *Diagnostic and Statistical Manual of Mental Disorders* (DSM).

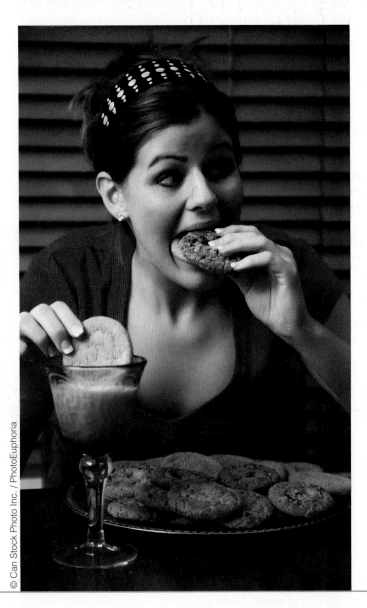

© Can Stock Photo Inc. / PhotoEuphoria

Those who propose that food addiction is a legitimate disorder argue that food, specifically highly palatable, processed food, can have a similar effect on the reward systems in the brain that are also implicated in drug abuse. For example, sugar can stimulate the brain's dopamine reward system, the same system that is implicated in the observed effects of cocaine and amphetamine use.[41] Brain imaging scans have shown that both obese individuals and drug addicts have a lower number of receptors for dopamine, which increases their craving for substances (i.e., certain foods) that, in turn, increase dopamine.[41]

In addition to the neurological support for the idea of food addiction, many argue that food seeking has similar behavioural signs and symptoms as drug seeking. According to the *DSM-IV-TR*, an individual is diagnosed with a substance dependency when a sufficient amount of the following criteria are met:

Diagnostic Criteria for Substance Dependence

- Tolerance: more of the drug is needed to achieve the desired effect
- Withdrawal: physical symptoms are evidenced when an individual stops using the substance
- The individual continues to use the drug despite the negative physical and psychological consequences they experience
- The individual takes more of the substance and abuses it for a longer period of time than intended
- The individual has a persistent desire to reduce their use
- The individual spends a great deal of time thinking about the substance or trying to acquire it
- The individual reduces the importance of other activities in favour of the substance

Ask Yourself

Which of these criteria may be found in a compulsive overeater?

Whether or not people with a strong food-seeking behaviour are actually addicted to food remains a controversial topic. For instance, it is debatable whether such concepts as withdrawal and tolerance can appropriately be applied to food consumption. This area of research is still relatively new, and more studies are required before we can fully understand the potential ability of foods to drive addictive behaviour.

Unfortunately, leptin regulation, like other regulatory mechanisms, is much better at preventing weight loss than at preventing weight gain. Obese individuals generally have high levels of leptin, but these levels are not effective at reducing caloric intake and increasing energy expenditure, a condition known as leptin resistance.[39]

Despite regulatory mechanisms that act to keep our weight stable, changes in physiological, psychological, and environmental factors can cause the level at which body weight is maintained to change, usually increasing it over time. This effect supports the hypothesis that the mechanisms that defend against weight loss are stronger than those that prevent weight gain.[40]

The Complex Causes of Obesity

Most people attribute the obesity epidemic in Canada to individual lifestyle behaviours: namely, we eat too much and exercise too little. If only it were that simple! For one, we have just learned that genes play a significant role in influencing weight status. Also, a diverse group of environmental, physiological, social, and psychological factors promote the increase in weight status evidenced in Canada and most parts of the world. The Foresight obesity map (**Figure 9.14a**) is a conceptual model that illustrates the complex array of factors that interact to promote obesity. It attributes the worldwide rise in obesity to seven main causal domains: physiology, food consumption, food production, individual physical activity, environmental physical activity, individual psychology, and social psychology.

CONCEPT CHECK **STOP**

1. **What** is the role of genes in regulating body weight?

2. **Why** do we feel hungry at about the same times every day?

3. **What** happens to our leptin levels when we lose weight?

4. **What** main factors drive the obesity epidemic?

The complex, interrelated causes of obesity • Figure 9.14

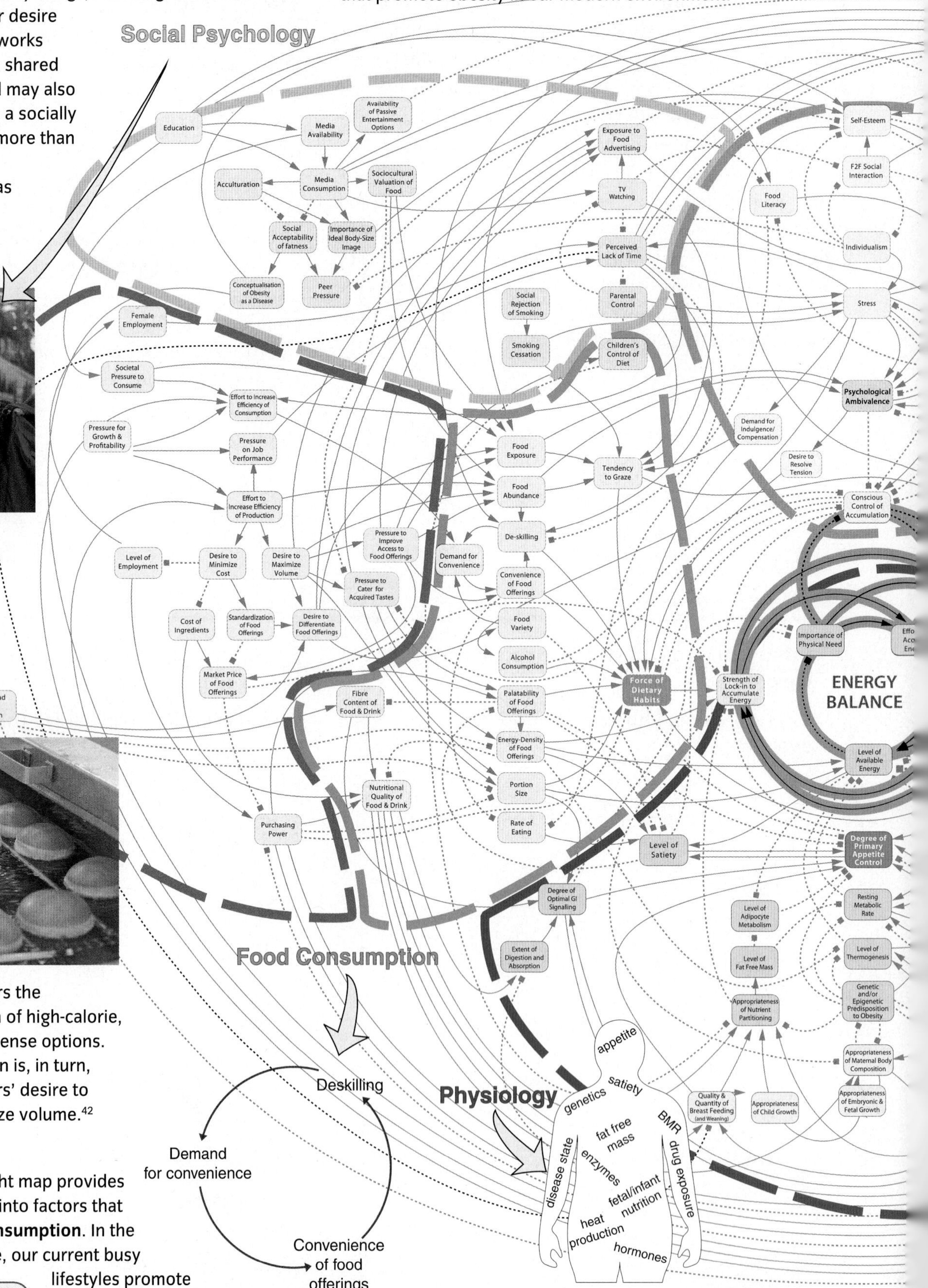

b. Social psychology refers to many things, including the influence of media and advertisements on our desire to consume more. Our social networks can influence our weight through shared activities and eating patterns and may also influence what we consider to be a socially acceptable weight. In a study of more than 12,000 participants, it was found that having a close friend who was obese increased an individual's risk for obesity by approximately 50 percent![43]

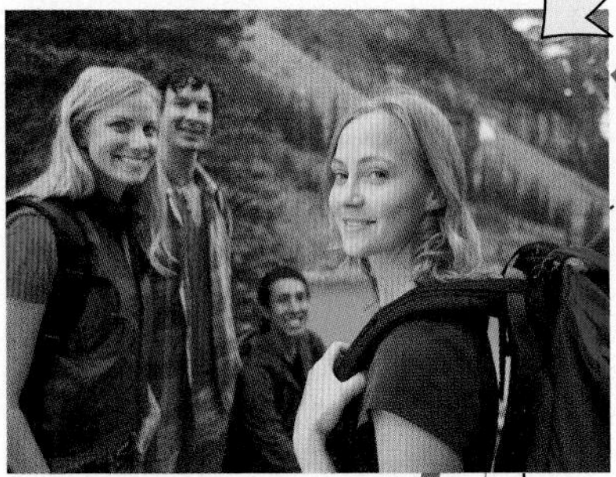

© Can Stock Photo Inc. / Leaf

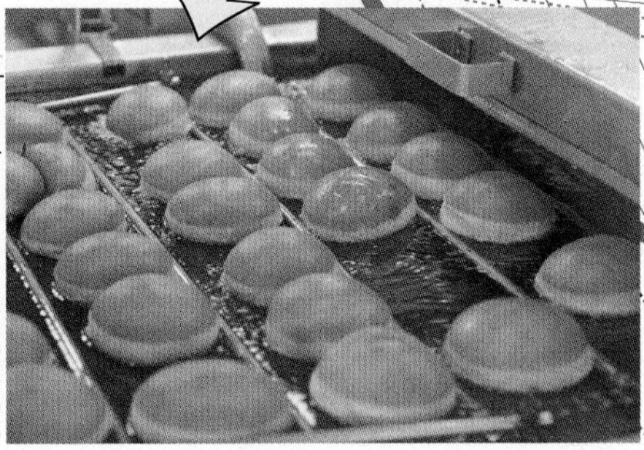

a. This Foresight obesity web[42] illustrates the complex array of factors that promote obesity in our modern environment.

Food Production

© Can Stock Photo Inc. / lindaparton

h. Food production favours the production and distribution of high-calorie, high-fat, and low-nutrient-dense options. This type of food production is, in turn, influenced by manufacturers' desire to minimize costs and maximize volume.[42]

g. The Foresight map provides further insight into factors that affect **food consumption**. In the above example, our current busy lifestyles promote an increased demand for convenience foods, which is met by food producers. Our access to all these convenience foods reduces our need to learn how to cook. Since we don't have these skills, we continue to demand convenience foods, and the cycle continues.

Deskilling → Convenience of food offerings → Demand for convenience → (cycle)

Ask Yourself

How can we break the cycle of convenience foods?

f. A complex array of **physiological factors** influence our appetite, our metabolic rate, and our tendency to either gain or lose weight. These factors vary greatly across the population and are often related to genetics. The environment of the womb can also have an effect on an offspring's predisposition for obesity.

Labels in the web: Social Psychology, Education, Media Availability, Availability of Passive Entertainment Options, Acculturation, Media Consumption, Sociocultural Valuation of Food, Social Acceptability of fatness, Importance of Ideal Body-Size Image, Conceptualisation of Obesity as a Disease, Peer Pressure, Female Employment, Societal Pressure to Consume, Pressure for Growth & Profitability, Effort to Increase Efficiency of Consumption, Pressure on Job Performance, Level of Employment, Desire to Minimize Cost, Desire to Maximize Volume, Effort to Increase Efficiency of Production, Pressure to Improve Access to Food Offerings, Pressure to Cater for Acquired Tastes, Demand for Convenience, Cost of Ingredients, Standardization of Food Offerings, Desire to Differentiate Food Offerings, Market Price of Food Offerings, Demand for Health, Fibre Content of Food & Drink, Nutritional Quality of Food & Drink, Purchasing Power, Food Production, Food Consumption, Convenience of Food Offerings, Food Variety, Alcohol Consumption, Palatability of Food Offerings, Energy-Density of Food Offerings, Portion Size, Rate of Eating, Food Exposure, Food Abundance, De-skilling, Tendency to Graze, Exposure to Food Advertising, TV Watching, Perceived Lack of Time, Parental Control, Children's Control of Diet, Social Rejection of Smoking, Smoking Cessation, Self-Esteem, F2F Social Interaction, Food Literacy, Individualism, Stress, Psychological Ambivalence, Demand for Indulgence/Compensation, Desire to Resolve Tension, Conscious Control of Accumulation, Force of Dietary Habits, Strength of Lock-in to Accumulate Energy, ENERGY BALANCE, Importance of Physical Need, Level of Available Energy, Level of Satiety, Degree of Optimal GI Signaling, Extent of Digestion and Absorption, Degree of Primary Appetite Control, Resting Metabolic Rate, Level of Thermogenesis, Level of Adipocyte Metabolism, Level of Fat Free Mass, Appropriateness of Nutrient Partitioning, Genetic and/or Epigenetic Predisposition to Obesity, Appropriateness of Maternal Body Composition, Quality & Quantity of Breast Feeding (and Weaning), Appropriateness of Child Growth, Appropriateness of Embryonic & Fetal Growth, Physiology, appetite, satiety, genetics, fat free mass, disease state, enzymes, heat production, hormones, fetal/infant nutrition, drug exposure, BMR

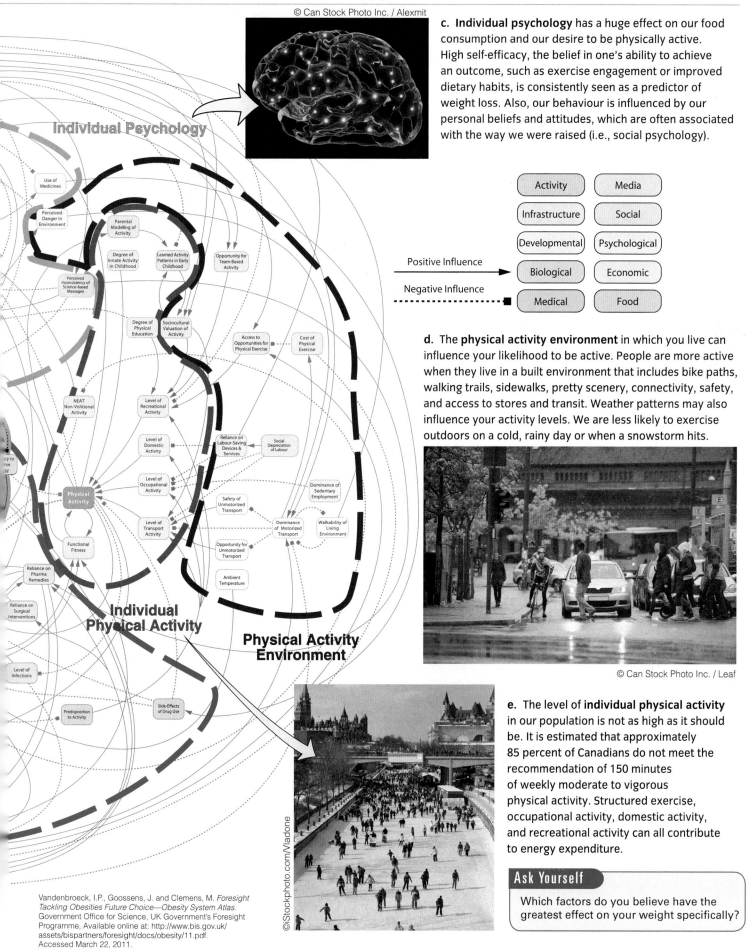

© Can Stock Photo Inc. / Alexmit

Individual Psychology

Individual Physical Activity

Physical Activity Environment

c. Individual psychology has a huge effect on our food consumption and our desire to be physically active. High self-efficacy, the belief in one's ability to achieve an outcome, such as exercise engagement or improved dietary habits, is consistently seen as a predictor of weight loss. Also, our behaviour is influenced by our personal beliefs and attitudes, which are often associated with the way we were raised (i.e., social psychology).

Activity	Media
Infrastructure	Social
Developmental	Psychological
Biological	Economic
Medical	Food

Positive Influence →

Negative Influence ∙∙∙∙∙∙∙∙∙∙∙∙∙∙∙■

d. The **physical activity environment** in which you live can influence your likelihood to be active. People are more active when they live in a built environment that includes bike paths, walking trails, sidewalks, pretty scenery, connectivity, safety, and access to stores and transit. Weather patterns may also influence your activity levels. We are less likely to exercise outdoors on a cold, rainy day or when a snowstorm hits.

© Can Stock Photo Inc. / Leaf

e. The level of **individual physical activity** in our population is not as high as it should be. It is estimated that approximately 85 percent of Canadians do not meet the recommendation of 150 minutes of weekly moderate to vigorous physical activity. Structured exercise, occupational activity, domestic activity, and recreational activity can all contribute to energy expenditure.

©iStockphoto.com/Vladone

Ask Yourself

Which factors do you believe have the greatest effect on your weight specifically?

Vandenbroeck, I.P., Goossens, J. and Clemens, M. *Foresight Tackling Obesities Future Choice—Obesity System Atlas.* Government Office for Science, UK Government's Foresight Programme, Available online at: http://www.bis.gov.uk/ assets/bispartners/foresight/docs/obesity/11.pdf. Accessed March 22, 2011.

What Determines Body Size and Shape? 319

Managing Body Weight

LEARNING OBJECTIVES

1. **Evaluate** an individual's weight and medical history to determine whether weight loss is recommended.

2. **Discuss** the recommendations for the rate and amount of weight loss.

3. **Distinguish** between a good weight management program and a fad diet.

4. **Explain** how medications and surgery can affect weight.

Managing your body weight to keep it in the healthy range requires a proper balance between energy intake and energy expenditure. For some people, weight management may mean avoiding weight gain as they age by making healthy food choices, controlling portion size, and maintaining an active lifestyle. For others, it may mean making major lifestyle changes to first reduce their weight to the healthy range and then to keep it there. Although weight loss may seem like a cumbersome process to some, positive behaviour change is much more likely when individuals are ready to change, when they reduce their individual barriers, customize their plan to their current lifestyle, and focus on their individual strengths.

Who Should Lose Weight?

These days, just about everybody wants to lose a bit of weight, but not everyone needs to lose weight to be healthy. The risks associated with carrying excess weight are related to the proportion of fatty vs. lean tissue, the degree of the excess, the location of the excess fat, and the presence of other diseases or risk factors that often accompany excess body fat. A person with a healthy BMI may still require weight loss if his or her body fat percentage is above the recommended levels. Also, an individual with an overweight or obese BMI may not need to lose excess weight for health if his or her weight is mostly due to large muscles or bones and if the individual engages in a healthy dietary pattern and ample physical activity. Rather than focusing on losing weight, it is more important to focus on promoting the healthy behaviours that promote a healthy body composition.

Weight-Loss Goals and Guidelines

Before you engage in a specific weight-loss regimen, an important first question to ask yourself is, "Why do I want to lose weight?" Is it to reduce your risk of disease and promote health, or is it to achieve a certain perceived ideal of beauty? A person can be healthy at a wide range of weights. Your focus should be to encourage behaviours that promote health, not to become skinny.

Five hundred grams (1 lb.) of adipose tissue provide about 3,500 kcal. Theoretically, then, to lose 500 g (1 lb.) of fat requires decreasing food intake and/or increasing energy expenditure by this amount. According to this theory of energy balance, to lose 500 g (1 lb.) in a week, you will need to have a negative caloric balance of approximately 500 kcal per day. The story is not that simple, however, because some people require a larger negative balance to achieve weight loss.

People who are at a weight that increases their risk of disease can significantly reduce their risk by losing as little as 5 to 15 percent of body weight.[45] Losing weight slowly, at a rate of 250 g to 1 kg (1/2 to 2 lb.) per week, helps to ensure that most of what is lost is fat and not lean tissue. The more severe energy restrictions that are needed for rapid weight loss lead to greater losses of water and protein and can cause a significant drop in BMR, making it more difficult to keep the weight off and may potentially lead to repeated cycles of weight loss and gain (**Figure 9.15**).

Decreasing energy intake A diet restricted in calories and balanced in nutrients promotes overall health and is associated with the achievement and maintenance of a healthy weight. People who successfully lose weight and keep it off tend to restrict certain high-calorie foods, decrease the amount of calories they consume, and sometimes count calories.[46] They are also more likely to resist overindulging on the weekends and holidays, and they typically exhibit a similar eating pattern every week and throughout the year. Furthermore, successful weight-loss maintainers regularly eat breakfast and have fewer periods when they lose control over their energy intake.

Portion control, hunger control, and a realistic understanding of the caloric values of food can also help with caloric restriction. Even a small reduction in portion size at each meal can have a large overall effect. Controlling hunger may also be accomplished by eating foods that promote

Yo-yo dieting • Figure 9.15

Repeated cycles of weight loss and gain, referred to as *weight cycling*, or *yo-yo dieting*, decrease the likelihood of success in future attempts at weight loss.[44]

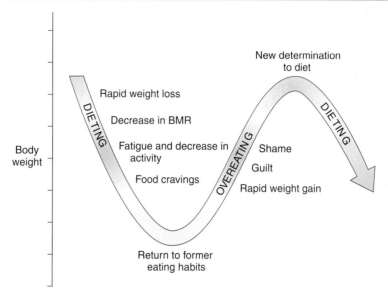

Body weight

DIETING

Rapid weight loss

Decrease in BMR

Fatigue and decrease in activity

Food cravings

Return to former eating habits

OVEREATING

New determination to diet

DIETING

Shame

Guilt

Rapid weight gain

satiation and satiety, such as fibre-rich foods and foods that are high in protein, healthy fats, and a mixture of nutrients.

Because individual psychology can strongly affect eating patterns, a good question to ask yourself is, "Why am I eating? Is it hunger, boredom, or is it to feed an emotion?" Sometimes the reasons people overeat are because of larger psychological issues that they are not addressing; those issues may first need to be identified and dealt with before making a change to eating patterns. For example, if depression is driving binge-eating behaviours, the depression may need to be treated before a reduction in binge eating is observed.

If long-term success is desired, an individual must make realistic and positive changes that can *permanently* fit into his or her life. If a plan is unsustainable, then success will be short term. Individuals who diet short term, stop exercising, and revert to their previous unhealthy behaviours, will tend to regain any weight that was lost.[46]

Clearly, Canadians as a whole, both those who are overweight and those who aren't, overconsume calories. Also clear is that each of us has a completely different set of factors that influence our behaviours, be it biological, social, or psychological. As much as the causes of overeating vary, so do the solutions. What works for one individual will not necessarily work for another. **Motivational interviewing** is one technique that may help individuals to successfully identify the motivators of change and the proper tool set required to implement those changes (see Appendix E).

Increasing physical activity Physical activity is associated with a reduced risk of cardiovascular disease, a reduced risk of some cancers, and a reduced risk of all-cause mortality, and is recommended for *all* individuals regardless of their weight. Furthermore, exercise increases energy expenditure and therefore makes weight loss easier. A study of thousands of weight-loss maintainers found that people who were successful at sustaining weight loss typically engage in approximately one hour of moderate to vigorous intensity activity per day.[46] Only 10 percent of those who had lost weight and kept it off did so through diet alone.

If food intake remains the same, adding enough exercise to expend an extra 200 kcal five days a week may result in the loss of 500 g (1 lb.) in about three-and-a-half weeks, but results may vary among individuals. Because exercise promotes muscle development and muscle is metabolically active tissue, increased muscle mass increases energy expenditure. In addition, physical activity improves overall fitness, body image, body tone, and relieves boredom and stress. It's pretty much one of the best things you can include in your life!

A significant psychological predictor of weight loss is exercise self-efficacy[47]: an individual's belief in his or her ability to exercise. Our exercise intrinsic motivation, or our internal motivation to exercise, is another psychological predictor of success.[47] Examples of intrinsic exercise motivators include the belief that exercise is fun, awareness that exercise reduces the risk of disease, and a desire for improved fitness and quality of life.

Different activities burn varying amounts of kilocalories, but many activities can be successful for the achievement of a healthy body and weight (see Appendix G). An effective physical activity plan includes regular moderate to vigorous physical activity and exercises that strengthen muscles and bone. You don't need to "go to the gym" to promote a healthy weight (but if you enjoy the gym, go for it!). The best types of physical activity are those activities that you enjoy and that you can and will engage in throughout your life. Approximately 80 percent of successful weight-loss maintainers reported that their primary form of physical activity is walking.[46] The benefits of exercise are discussed more fully in Chapter 10.

Psychological modification A significant number of people who lose weight do so by modifying their behaviour in the short term and, once the weight is lost, they revert to their old habits, leading to weight regain. To adopt the behaviours that lead to the long-term achievement of a healthy weight, an individual must change some of the unhealthy thought processes that influenced the original negative behaviour. This change is facilitated by having proper goals and attitudes about wanting to lose weight (i.e., to promote health and to reduce disease risk) and by having the right social support and **self-efficacy**. To successfully promote change, behaviour change goals should be specific, realistic, and attainable.

> **self-efficacy** An individual's belief in his or her ability to achieve a certain outcome.

The importance of making permanent behaviour changes is a central theme to this chapter. However, before you change your behaviour, you may first need to change your mind and the way you think. Some people believe they are unable to exercise, they are destined to be overweight, or they are unable to decrease their caloric intake. These thought processes and many others may limit a person's ability to change. Maladaptive thoughts can influence our feelings, which can then influence our behaviours.

One method of improving the thinking patterns associated with making significant changes to a person's behaviour is **cognitive behavioural therapy (CBT)**. In this form of psychotherapy, patients are encouraged to examine their current thought patterns and how they promote negative feelings and behaviours (**Figure 9.16**).

WHAT SHOULD I EAT?
Weight Management

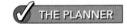
✔ THE PLANNER

Watch your calories!
- Check labels to see whether your portion matches the serving size on the label.
- Have one scoop of ice cream instead of two.
- Don't eat mindlessly! Think about how tasty food is while you are eating it, and don't eat it too quickly.
- Don't supersize—choose a small drink and a small order of fries.
- Pour chips or crackers into a one-serving bowl rather than eating right from the bag or box.
- Stick with water. Try not to drink your calories, especially if they come from beverages with a high-calorie and fat content.
- Take your lunch instead of eating out.
- Have a conversation over family dinner, and take your time to eat slowly and enjoy the company.
- When you eat out, share an entrée with a friend, or take some home for lunch the next day.

Balance intake with exercise
- Go for a bike ride.
- Look up one of the many (free) Disc Golf courses online, and play a round or two with some friends on a Sunday afternoon.

- Take a walk during your lunch break or after dinner.
- Play tennis; you don't need to be good to get plenty of exercise.
- Get off the bus one stop early.
- Be active! Take the stairs, walk, and bike whenever you can, and spend less time sitting in general.

Change your brain
- Use constant reinforcing self-talk to motivate your positive behaviours.
- Remind yourself why eating better and exercising more is important to you.
- Identify your strengths that will help you succeed.
- Surround yourself with people who also eat well and enjoy exercise. Being in the company of similar people can help to nurture positive behaviours so they become simply something you do.
- Focus on the benefits, not the challenges, of change.
- Know that you can change. We *all* have the *physical* ability to change our behaviours, but we are often held back by our *mental* insecurities. You are physically able to change, and that is a fact.

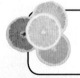
Use iProfile to calculate the number of kilocalories you consume as between-meal snacks.

ABCs of behaviour modification • Figure 9.16

Behaviour modification is based on the theory that behaviours involve three factors: antecedents or cues that lead to a behaviour, the behaviour itself, and the consequences of the behaviour. These factors are referred to as the ABCs of behaviour modification. The steps shown here can be used to identify and change undesirable behaviours.

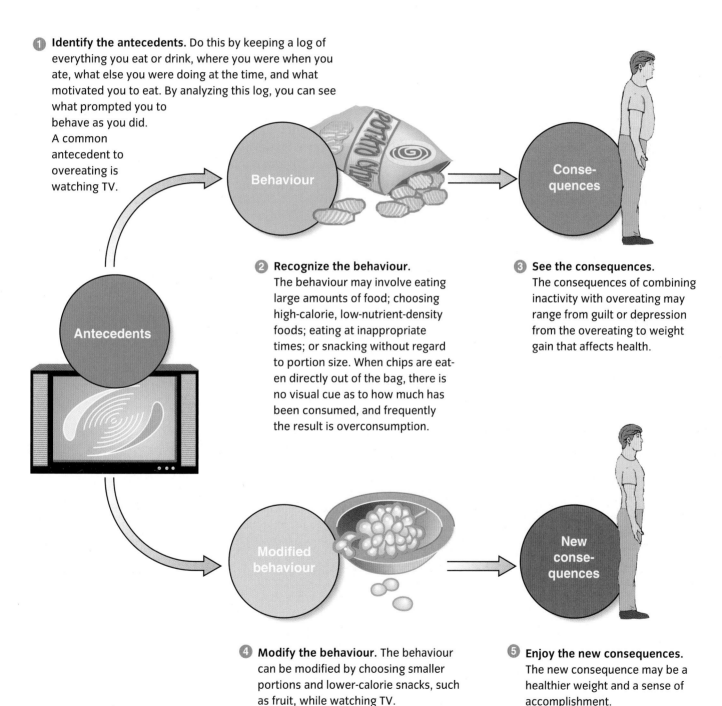

1 **Identify the antecedents.** Do this by keeping a log of everything you eat or drink, where you were when you ate, what else you were doing at the time, and what motivated you to eat. By analyzing this log, you can see what prompted you to behave as you did. A common antecedent to overeating is watching TV.

Behaviour

Conse-quences

Antecedents

2 **Recognize the behaviour.** The behaviour may involve eating large amounts of food; choosing high-calorie, low-nutrient-density foods; eating at inappropriate times; or snacking without regard to portion size. When chips are eaten directly out of the bag, there is no visual cue as to how much has been consumed, and frequently the result is overconsumption.

3 **See the consequences.** The consequences of combining inactivity with overeating may range from guilt or depression from the overeating to weight gain that affects health.

Modified behaviour

New conse-quences

4 **Modify the behaviour.** The behaviour can be modified by choosing smaller portions and lower-calorie snacks, such as fruit, while watching TV.

5 **Enjoy the new consequences.** The new consequence may be a healthier weight and a sense of accomplishment.

Patients are then provided with new ways of thinking (e.g., "I actually *am* capable of doing this," "Eating healthy foods can actually be enjoyable," "My weight does not determine my value as an individual") that can help them to promote change. They are also taught to recognize situations that provoke negative thoughts and behaviours, and develop new positive strategies for managing those situations without turning to food.

Not everyone can afford psychotherapy or has access to it. For such people, motivational interviewing may also promote positive psychological modification.

Suggestions for Weight Gain

As difficult as weight loss is for some people, weight gain can be equally elusive for people who are underweight. The first step toward weight gain is a medical evaluation to rule out medical reasons for low body weight. This step is particularly important when weight loss occurs unexpectedly. If the low body weight is due to low energy intake or high energy expenditure, the typical suggestion is to gradually increase consumption of energy-dense foods. Energy intake can be increased by eating meals more frequently;

by adding healthy, high-calorie between-meal snacks, such as nuts, peanut butter, or milkshakes; and by replacing low-calorie drinks, such as water and diet beverages, with 100 percent fruit juices and milk. Conversely, increasing caloric intake by consuming high-fat, high-sodium, low-fibre meals is not recommended. Although these practices may help an individual to gain weight, they may also increase their risk for chronic diseases such as heart disease, cancer, and type-2 diabetes.

Any weight-gain program should include strength-training exercises to encourage a gain in muscle rather than a gain in fat. This approach requires extra calories to fuel the activity needed to build muscles. These recommendations apply to individuals who are naturally thin and have trouble gaining weight on the recommended energy intake. However, this dietary approach may not promote weight gain for those who limit their intake because of an eating disorder.

Diets and Fad Diets

Want to lose 5 kg (10 lb.) in just five days? What dieter wouldn't? People who are desperate to lose weight fall prey

Distinguishing between healthy diets and fad diets Table 9.2	
A healthy diet . . .	**A fad diet . . .**
Promotes a healthy dietary pattern that meets nutrient needs, includes a variety of foods, suits food preferences, and can be maintained throughout life.	Limits food selections to a few food groups or promotes rituals such as eating only specific food combinations. As a result, it may be limited in certain nutrients and in variety.
Promotes a reasonable weight loss of 250 g to 1 kg (½ to 2 lb.) per week and does not restrict kilocalories to less than 1,200 per day.	Promotes rapid weight loss of much more than 1 kg (2 lb.) per week.
Promotes or includes physical activity.	Advertises weight loss without the need to exercise.
Is flexible enough to be followed when eating out and includes foods that are easily obtained.	May require a rigid menu or avoidance of certain foods or may include "magic" foods that promise to burn fat or speed up metabolism.
Does not require costly supplements.	May require the purchase of special foods, weight-loss patches, expensive supplements, creams, or other products.
Promotes a change in behaviour. Teaches new eating habits. Provides social support.	Does not recommend changes in activity and eating habits, recommends an eating pattern that is difficult to follow for life, or provides no support other than a book that must be purchased.
Is based on sound scientific principles and may include monitoring by qualified health professionals.	Makes outlandish and unscientific claims, does not support claims that it is clinically tested or scientifically proven, claims that it is new and improved or is based on some new scientific discovery, or relies on testimonials from celebrities or connects the diet to trendy places such as Beverly Hills.

to all sorts of diets that promise quick fixes. They willingly eat a single food for days at a time, select foods on the basis of special fat-burning qualities, and consume odd combinations at specific times of the day. Most diets, no matter how outlandish, will promote weight loss because they reduce energy intake. Even diets that focus on modifying fat or carbohydrate intake or promise to allow unlimited amounts of certain foods work because total intake is reduced. The true test of the effectiveness of a weight-loss plan is whether it promotes weight loss that can be maintained over the long term.

Effective weight-management programs encourage healthy behaviour changes that promote a healthy weight. When selecting a program, look for one that is based on sound nutrition and exercise principles; suits your individual preferences in terms of food choices, time, and costs; and promotes long-term lifestyle changes. Quick fixes and fad diets are tempting, but if the program's approach cannot be followed for a lifetime, it is unlikely to promote successful weight management (**Table 9.2**). Believe it or not, the multibillion-dollar weight-loss industry has virtually no regulation, and eager consumers who seek quick weight loss fixes may be easily misled.

The various commercial diet plans include exchange list programs, plans that reduce the carbohydrates or fat content of a diet, herbal remedies, medically supervised programs, and plans that sell liquid or pre-portioned meals (**Figure 9.17**). All these methods can cause weight

Common dieting methods • Figure 9.17

a. Some diet plans regulate calories by recommending certain numbers of servings from specific food lists. Foods that are in the same exchange list, such as rice, bread, and potatoes, are similar in their energy and macronutrient content, so they can be exchanged for one another. These plans include a variety of foods and are likely to meet nutrient needs. They teach meal-planning skills that are easy to apply away from home and can be used over the long term. ▼

 = 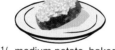 =

$^1/_3$ cup rice	1 slice bread	$^1/_2$ medium potato, baked
80 kilocalories 15 g carbohydrate 3 g protein 0–1 g fat	80 kilocalories 15 g carbohydrate 3 g protein 0–1 g fat	80 kilocalories 15 g carbohydrate 3 g protein 0–1 g fat

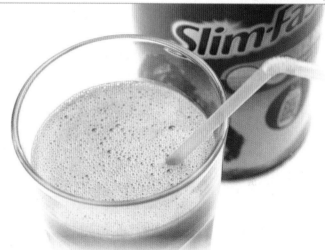

c. Because fat is high in calories, consuming a low-fat diet typically reduces calorie intake. Low-fat diets can include large quantities of fresh fruits and vegetables, which are low in fat and calories and high in nutrients and phytochemicals. But, just because a food is low in fat does not mean it can be consumed in unlimited amounts. In the 1990s, low-fat cookies, crackers, and cakes flooded the market. These foods were low in fat but not necessarily low in energy. When eaten in excess, they may contribute to weight gain ▼

▲ **b.** Pre-portioned meals or liquid formulas make it easier to eat less, but they are not practical when travelling or eating out, and they do not teach the food-selection skills needed to make a long-term lifestyle change. Programs that rely exclusively on liquid formulas are not recommended without medical supervision.

d. Where are the rice and potatoes? Low-carbohydrate diets limit bread and grains, fruits, some vegetables, and milk while allowing unlimited quantities of meats and fats. Weight loss occurs on these diets because people eat less. This may be due to metabolic changes that suppress appetite, but intake is also reduced because of the monotony of the food choices.[51] ▼

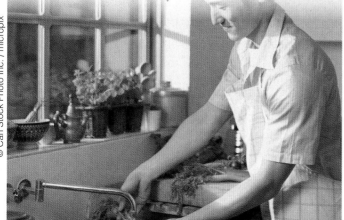

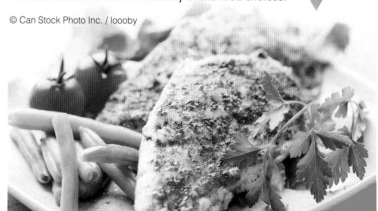

loss in the short term by limiting, in one way or another, the number of kilocalories consumed. However, none of these methods has ever been scientifically proven to promote long-term weight loss in the majority of its clients. Also, some may have negative side effects to the body or may simply cost an unsustainable amount of money.

Exchange lists give clients an idea of the caloric density of foods without specifically counting calories, although the idea is similar. Diets that severely restrict a specific nutrient, such as carbohydrates, often do not meet the basic needs of the body, may cause symptoms of deficiency, and can rarely be maintained in the long term. Other diets that provide herbal supplements cost customers thousands of dollars and require the purchase of supplements that are based on poor science. Dieters typically show short-term weight-loss success, but these results are rarely maintained in the long term, and most people regain the weight after completion of the program.

Even commercial programs that are medically supervised have shown little efficacy over the long term and can cost consumers more than $600 a month. Lastly, eating pre-portioned or liquid meals doesn't teach people how to reduce their caloric intake in real-life settings. Also, the cost of pre-portioned food can be upwards of $500 per month, and these foods are often full of preservatives and an unhealthy balance of nutrients. Many of the above diets are strict and unrealistic for incorporating into one's life for the long term. These diets may lead dieters into negative cycles of yo-yo dieting. The true test of whether a diet will be effective long term is whether the reduced caloric intake is nutritionally sound and can be maintained once the program is completed.

Weight-Loss Drugs and Supplements

Specific drugs are sometimes prescribed to promote weight loss in obese individuals. These drugs work by either blocking fat absorption or altering neural circuits. Fat blockers such as orlistat (brand name Xenical) promote modest weight loss in obese individuals by decreasing fat and, therefore, also decreasing calorie absorption. However, if the overweight individual doesn't learn to also avoid fatty foods, the result can be abdominal cramping, flatulence, and an inability to control fecal secretions. Also, because the absorption of the fat-soluble vitamins A, D, E, and K require fat, orlistat promotes a decrease in the dietary intake of these vitamins.

Phentermine (trade name Adipex) has been shown to reduce weight when used periodically. This drug has a slightly elevated potential for drug abuse and is prescribed for use only for one year at maximum. Sibutramine, which is marketed under the brand names Meridia and Reductil, was initially marketed as an antidepressant. Although it was later found to be ineffective for depression, it promotes weight loss by increasing satiety. In October 2010, sibutramine was voluntarily withdrawn from Canadian pharmacies after a randomized control trial showed that patients with a history of heart disease slightly increased their risk of a heart attack or stroke after sibutramine treatment.[52] Both sibutramine and phentermine are amphetamine derivatives that suppress appetite and, like all amphetamines, increase heart rate. An increase in heart rate puts more strain on the heart muscle and is associated with hypertension, a leading risk factor for heart attacks and strokes. Health Canada will continue to monitor all weight-loss drugs to ensure they meet the requirements of the Food and Drugs Act and do not increase risk of disease.

Like prescription drugs, over-the-counter weight-loss medications are regulated by Health Canada under the Food and Drugs Act. They must adhere to strict guidelines regarding the dose per pill and the effectiveness of the ingredients. Health Canada has approved only a limited number of substances for sale as non-prescription weight-loss medications. One such substance is a non-prescription version of orlistat, which became available in 2007 under the brand name Alli. Alli blocks fat absorption by disabling the fat-digesting enzyme lipase. Risks associated with its use are similar to the risks of taking orlistat. As with prescription medications, any weight loss that occurs with over-the-counter weight-loss medications is often regained when the product is no longer consumed.

In addition to weight-loss drugs, hundreds of dietary supplements claim to promote weight loss. As with other dietary supplements, weight-loss supplements are *not* strictly regulated by Health Canada, so their safety and effectiveness may not have been carefully tested. Weight-loss supplements often include herbal sources of compounds that are contained in prescription medications, some of which are powerful drugs with dangerous side effects. Do not assume that a product is safe simply because it is labelled "herbal" or "all natural."

Weight-loss supplements that contain soluble fibre promise to reduce the amount you eat by filling up your stomach. Although they are safe, little evidence supports the claim that they promote weight loss.[55] Hydroxycitric acid, conjugated linoleic acid, and chromium picolinate are weight-loss supplements that promise to enhance fat loss by altering metabolism to prevent the synthesis and deposition of fat. None of these supplements has been shown to effectively promote weight loss in humans.[56–58] Supplements that boost energy expenditure, often called "fat burners," can be effective but have serious and potentially life-threatening side effects. One of the most popular and controversial herbal fat burners is ephedra, a stimulant that increases blood pressure and heart rate and constricts blood vessels. Due to safety concerns, it was banned by Health Canada in 2001 (**Figure 9.18**). After the ban was instituted, supplement manufacturers substituted other herbal products, such as bitter orange, which contains similar stimulants and therefore may have similar side effects.[59] Fat burners also typically contain guarana, an herbal source of caffeine. Green tea extract is another popular supplement used to boost metabolism and aid weight loss. It appears to be safe if used in appropriate amounts, but studies have not shown it to enhance weight loss.[60, 61]

Some dietary supplements result in weight loss through water loss—either because these supplements are diuretics or because they cause diarrhea. These supplements decrease body weight primarily through *water* loss but do not cause a decrease in body *fat*. Herbal laxatives found in weight loss teas and in supplements include senna, aloe, buckthorn, rhubarb root, cascara, and castor oil. Overuse of these substances can have serious side effects, including nausea, diarrhea, vomiting, stomach cramps, chronic constipation, fainting, and severe electrolyte imbalances, which can lead to cardiac arrhythmia and death.[62]

The dangers of fat burners • Figure 9.18

In 2003, Baltimore Orioles pitcher Steve Bechler died of complications from heatstroke following a spring training workout. It was concluded that ephedra played a significant role in his death. Ephedra use is associated with serious side effects such as hypertension, arrhythmia, heart attack, stroke, and seizure.[53] Shortly after this episode, the U.S. Food and Drug Administration banned the sale of products containing ephedra,[54] which had already been banned for sale in Canada in 2001. The Canadian ban occurred following such adverse effects as heart attack, stroke, and sudden death, which were observed in more than 60 people. Ephedra is still banned for sale in Canada, except at a limited dosage in certain nasal decongestants. Although ephedra abuse still occurs, it has decreased substantially since the ban. A further decrease may be observed by further educating the public about the severe cardiovascular threats of ephedra and possibly by imposing a complete ban on it.

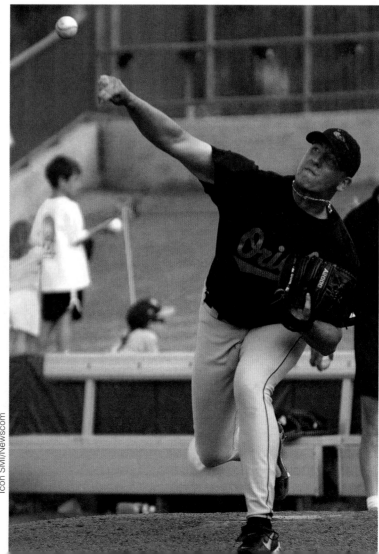

Mark Goldman/Icon SMI 749/Mark Goldman/Icon SMI/Newscom

Weight-Loss Surgery

Many surgical procedures decrease body weight by altering the gastrointestinal tract to reduce food intake and absorption. These surgical approaches are recommended only in cases when individuals are at great risk of dying from the complications of obesity. Included in this group are individuals who fit the definition of Class 3 obesity (BMI $\geq$ 40 kg/m²) and those with a BMI between 35 and 40 kg/m² who have other life-threatening conditions that could be remedied by weight loss. At present, the most popular surgical approaches to treating obesity are **gastric bypass** and **adjustable gastric banding** (**Figure 9.19**), collectively known as bariatric surgeries.

Bariatric surgery is more effective than

gastric bypass A surgical procedure that reduces the size of the stomach and bypasses a portion of the small intestine.

adjustable gastric banding A surgical procedure in which an adjustable band is placed around the upper portion of the stomach to limit the volume that the stomach can hold and the rate of stomach emptying.

Gastric bypass and banding • Figure 9.19

a. Gastric bypass involves bypassing part of the stomach and small intestine by connecting the intestine to the upper portion of the stomach. Food intake is reduced because the stomach is smaller, which promotes satiation, and absorption is reduced because the small intestine is shortened. Gastric bypass entails short-term surgical risks and a long-term risk of nutrient deficiencies because the shorter digestive path can reduce micronutrient absorption. ▼

b. Gastric banding involves surgically placing an adjustable band around the upper part of the stomach, creating a small pouch. The narrow opening between the stomach pouch and the rest of the stomach slows the rate at which food leaves the pouch. Weight loss is promoted because the amount of food that can be consumed at one time is reduced, thereby slowing digestion. Gastric banding entails less surgical risk than other types of weight-loss surgery and is more easily reversible. ▼

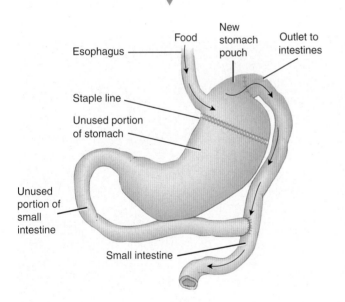

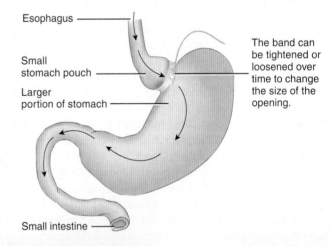

c. Significant weight loss is usually achieved 18 to 24 months after weight-loss surgery. NBC's *Today Show* weather anchor, Al Roker, lost 45 kg (100 lb.) after undergoing gastric bypass surgery. Some weight gain is common after two to five years. Even after surgery, the types and amounts of food consumed must be limited to maintain the lower weight.

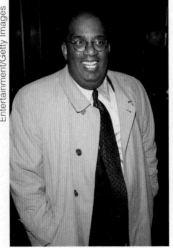

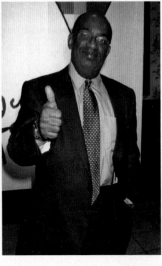

Nick Elgar/Staff/Getty Images Entertainment/Getty Images

© Gregory Pace/Corbis

most conventional treatments for obesity, such as prescribing exercise and diet modification to patients. Weight loss is greater in patients who have undergone bariatric surgery, and this surgery can be effective at minimizing or controlling type-2 diabetes, hypertension, and high blood cholesterol, and can improve overall quality of life and reduce medication costs associated with obesity comorbidities.[63, 64] Bariatric surgery is, however, not without its limitations. First, patients must reduce their weight before they can undergo the surgery. Also, complications associated with the surgery occur in one in five patients and may require follow-up surgery.[65] In the case of gastric bypass surgery, these complications may include ulcers, blockage of the stomach opening, leakage of the connection between the stomach and the intestines, pneumonia, and blood clots.[66]

In those patients who do not experience complications from the surgery, other concerns must be considered. Nutrient absorption may be affected, and the individual may require daily supplementation. Also, if food intake is not limited, the outcome may be chronic diarrhea, gas, foul-smelling stools, and changes in bowel habits.[66]

Gastric bypass surgery is covered by the Canadian health care system, but it is not available in every province, and is not insured in the territories.[67] Gastric banding is insured only in Alberta and New Brunswick, but private facilities exist for those willing to pay out of pocket. Canada has approximately 30 bariatric surgery centres, 12 of which are private. The cost of gastric banding at a private facility ranges from $13,000 to $18,000, and has a relatively low wait list of one month, compared with the three- to five-year wait for publicly funded gastric bypass surgery.[67]

Although bariatric surgery is a cost-effective treatment of obesity,[68] it is not without risks and should not be considered a simple solution to the obesity epidemic. This surgery is recommended only in extreme cases of obesity.

Another popular surgical procedure for reducing body fat is **liposuction**. This procedure involves inserting a large hollow needle under the skin into a fat deposit and literally vacuuming out the fat. Liposuction is considered a cosmetic procedure and does not significantly reduce overall body weight. Also, if the former behaviours that promoted the original weight gain are not altered, the individual may easily regain the weight after surgery.

Weight Bias

Internationally, Canada has a reputation for being an inclusive country that is accepting of a diverse group of people. We are world leaders in positive attitudes about people who have different ethnicities and different sexual orientations. Although many Canadians have negative attitudes toward discrimination based on ethnicity or sexual orientation, **weight bias** is still prevalent and has shown a marked increase in the past few decades.[69] Harmful stereotypes against obese individuals include beliefs that they are lazy, lack self-control, are stupid, are unsuccessful, and have no willpower. You may think that making fun of overweight people is funny or acceptable, but the truth of the matter is that such attitudes simply are not funny or acceptable, and they are making things worse.

> **weight bias** Negative attitudes toward overweight or obese individuals that affect social interactions.

Weight bias can affect how overweight individuals are treated at work, at school, and at home.[69] According to overweight subjects, family members are the people most likely to show weight bias, followed by doctors.[69] For instance, parents of obese children are less likely to help their child buy a car or pay for school;[70] health care professionals often have negative attitudes toward obese people, including beliefs that they are undisciplined, lazy, lack willpower, and are non-compliant in treatment.[69] This bias may account for an obese individual's unwillingness to be treated by or to seek advice from a medical professional and may possibly exacerbate the obese person's condition.[69] Obese adults may also face disadvantages in getting a job, in the amount they earn, and in promotions. Weight bias can be overt and in the form of name-calling, teasing, or bullying but it can also be subtle and may take the form of judging looks.

Also, the media often portray obese individuals in a negative light. An analysis of media portrayals of obese individuals showed that they were often pictured headless, from the side or rear angle, with less clothing, or with clothing that doesn't fit, and rarely engaging in healthy behaviours[71] (**Figure 9.20**). Although some believe that bias against overweight individuals may motivate them to change their behaviour, the opposite has actually been found. Potential consequences of weight bias on the individual include binge eating, higher caloric intake, less program compliance, and weight gain.[69]

Everyone needs to recognize that obesity is a disease caused by a complex array of factors, from the biological to the psychological and environmental, and that some people are at a higher risk than others. A healthy-weight individual may have exactly the same or worse eating and physical activity behaviours than an obese individual, but does not suffer the same stigmas. Weight bias is not justified and is as unacceptable as racial bias, and should not be tolerated.

Media portrayals of overweight individuals typically show them in unflattering lights, contributing to weight bias.

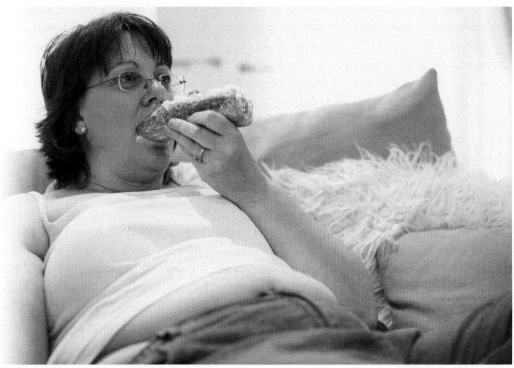

© Can Stock Photo Inc. / monkeybusiness

CONCEPT CHECK STOP

1. **Why** is weight loss not recommended for everyone with a BMI above the healthy range?

2. **How** much weight loss per week is recommended?

3. **What** are some characteristics of a good weight-loss program?

4. **How** does gastric bypass cause weight loss?

Eating Disorders

LEARNING OBJECTIVES

1. **Distinguish** among anorexia, bulimia, and binge-eating disorder.

2. **Describe** demographic and psychological factors associated with an increased risk of developing an eating disorder.

3. **Discuss** how body ideal and the media affect the incidence of eating disorders.

4. **Explain** what is meant by the binge/purge cycle.

hat and how much people eat varies, depending on social occasions, emotions, time limitations, hunger, and the availability of food. People generally eat when they are hungry, choose foods that they enjoy, and stop eating when they are satisfied. Abnormal or disordered eating occurs when a person is overly concerned with food, eating, body size, and body shape. When the emotional aspects of food and eating and the associated

eating disorder A psychological illness characterized by specific abnormal eating behaviours, often intended to control weight.

psychological causes overpower the role of food as nourishment, an **eating disorder** may develop. Eating disorders affect physical and nutritional health and psychosocial functioning. If untreated, eating disorders can be fatal.

Types of Eating Disorders

Mental health guidelines define three categories of eating disorders: **anorexia nervosa**, **bulimia nervosa**, and **eating disorders not otherwise specified (EDNOS)**, which includes **binge-eating disorder** and other abnormal eating behaviours that don't qualify as anorexia or bulimia (**Table 9.3**).

anorexia nervosa An eating disorder typically characterized by self-starvation, a distorted body image, and abnormally low body weight.

What Causes Eating Disorders?

We do not completely understand what causes eating disorders, but we do know that genetic, psychological, and socio-cultural factors contribute to their development (**Figure 9.21**). Eating disorders can be triggered by traumatic events, such as sexual abuse, or by day-to-day occurrences, such as teasing or judgemental comments by a friend or a coach. Eating disorders occur in people of all ages, races, and socio-economic backgrounds, but some groups are at greater risk than others. For example, women are more likely than men to develop eating disorders. Canadian eating disorder rates are estimated to be similar to those seen in the United States where approximately 3 percent of girls and women are affected.[72] Professional dancers, models, and others who are concerned about maintaining a low body weight are more likely to develop eating disorders.[72] Eating

bulimia nervosa An eating disorder characterized by the consumption of a large amount of food at one time (binge eating) followed by purging behaviours such as self-induced vomiting to prevent weight gain.

binge-eating disorder An eating disorder characterized by recurrent episodes of binge eating in the absence of compensatory behaviour such as purging or overexercising.

Distinguishing among eating disorders Table 9.3

Characteristic	Eating disorder: Anorexia nervosa	Bulimia nervosa	Binge-eating disorder
Prevalence	1% females, 0.3% males	1.5% females, 0.5% males	3.5% females, 2% males
Body weight	Below normal (<85% of recommended)	Usually normal	Above normal
Binge eating	Possibly	Yes, at least twice a week for three months	Yes, at least twice a week for six months
Purging, excessive exercising, or use of laxatives	Possibly	Yes, at least twice a week for three months	No
Restricts food intake	Yes	Yes	Yes
Body image	Dissatisfaction with body and distorted image of body size	Dissatisfaction with body and distorted image of body size	Dissatisfaction with body and distorted image of body size
Fear of being fat	Yes	Yes	Possibly
Self-esteem	Low	Low	Low
Menstrual abnormalities	Absence of at least three consecutive periods	No	No
Typical age of onset	Preadolescence/adolescence	Adolescence/young adults	Adults of all ages

Factors contributing to eating disorders • Figure 9.21

Eating disorders are caused by a combination of genetic, psychological, and socio-cultural factors. Although these disorders are not necessarily passed from parent to child, the genes that a person inherits contribute to personality traits and other psychological and biological characteristics that can predispose a person to developing an eating disorder. When placed in the right socio-cultural environment, an individual who carries such genes will be more likely than others to develop an eating disorder.

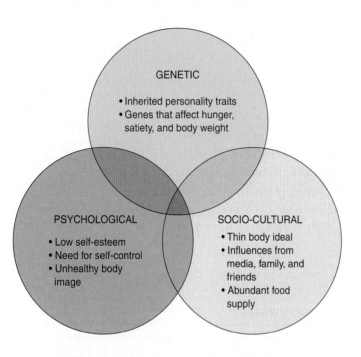

GENETIC
- Inherited personality traits
- Genes that affect hunger, satiety, and body weight

PSYCHOLOGICAL
- Low self-esteem
- Need for self-control
- Unhealthy body image

SOCIO-CULTURAL
- Thin body ideal
- Influences from media, family, and friends
- Abundant food supply

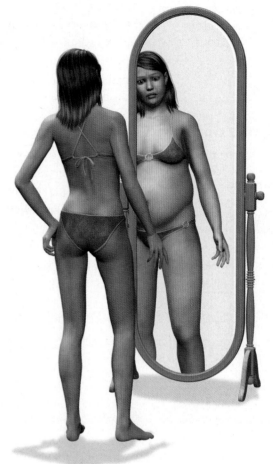

disorders commonly begin in adolescence, when physical, psychological, and social development occurs rapidly.

Psychological issues People with eating disorders often have low self-esteem. *Self-esteem* refers to the judgements people make and maintain about themselves—a general attitude of approval or disapproval as to one's self-worth and capability. A poor **body image**

> **body image** The way a person perceives and imagines his or her body.

contributes to low self-esteem. Eating disorders are characterized not only by dissatisfaction with one's body but also by a distorted body image (**Figure 9.21**). Someone with a distorted body image is unable to accurately judge the size of his or her own body. Thus, even if a young woman achieves a body weight comparable to or lower than that of a fashion model, she may continue to see herself as fat and may strive to lose more weight.

People with eating disorders are often perfectionists who set very high standards for themselves and strive to

be in control of their bodies and their lives. Despite their many achievements, they may feel inadequate, defective, and worthless. They may use their relationship with food to gain control over their lives and to boost their self-esteem. They believe that controlling their food intake and weight demonstrates their ability to control other aspects of their lives and solves other problems. Even if they feel insecure, helpless, or dissatisfied in other aspects of their lives, they can successfully control their food intake, weight, and body size.

Socio-cultural issues What is considered as an "ideal" body differs across cultures and has changed throughout history (**Figure 9.22**). Cultural ideals about body size are linked to body image and the incidence of eating disorders.[73] Eating disorders occur in societies where food is abundant and the body ideal is to be thin. They do not occur in societies where food is scarce and people worry about where their next meal is coming from.

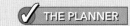
a. A fuller figure is still desirable in many cultures. Young women in these cultures, such as the Zulu of South Africa, may struggle to gain weight to achieve what is viewed as the ideal female body. As television images of very thin Western women become more accessible, the Zulu cultural view of plumpness as desirable may change.[75]

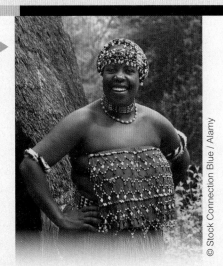

© Stock Connection Blue / Alamy

b. Thinness has not always been the beauty standard in North America. This timeline shows how the female body ideal has changed over the years. As female models, actresses, and other cultural icons have become thinner over the past several decades, the incidence of eating disorders has increased.

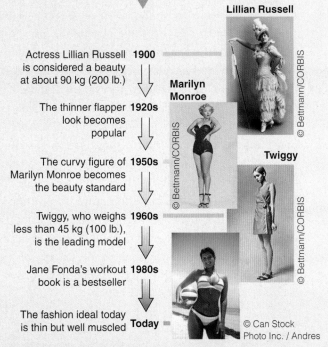

Lillian Russell

Actress Lillian Russell **1900** is considered a beauty at about 90 kg (200 lb.)

Marilyn Monroe

The thinner flapper **1920s** look becomes popular

The curvy figure of **1950s** Marilyn Monroe becomes the beauty standard

Twiggy

Twiggy, who weighs **1960s** less than 45 kg (100 lb.), is the leading model

Jane Fonda's workout **1980s** book is a bestseller

The fashion ideal today **Today** is thin but well muscled

© Bettmann/CORBIS

© Bettmann/CORBIS

© Bettmann/CORBIS

© Can Stock Photo Inc. / Andres

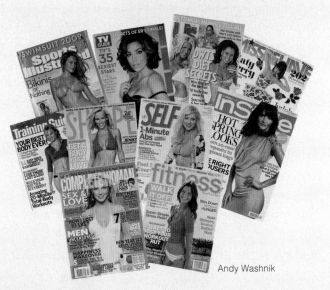

Andy Washnik

c. The fashion models whom women may emulate have unhealthy BMIs and are unrealistic models of perfection. Forty years ago, the average weight of a model was 8 percent lower than that of an average woman; today, the difference is more than 25 percent.[76]

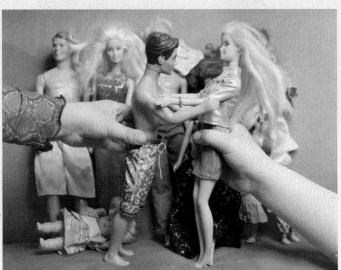

© Johner Images / Alamy

d. The toys that children play with set a cultural standard for body ideal. Girls playing with Barbie dolls want to be like Barbie when they grow up, and boys playing with Superman, Batman, or GI Joe action figures want to be like Superman, Batman, or GI Joe. Children's wanting to be like these toys includes wanting to look like them. Unfortunately, Barbie's measurements would be virtually unachievable if she were life-sized. The same is true of the big chest, muscular arms and legs, and flat stomach with "six-pack" abs seen on male action figures.

North American culture today is a culture of thinness. Messages about what society views as a perfect body—the ideal that we should strive for—are constantly delivered by television, the Internet, movies, magazines, advertisements, and even toys. Tall, lean fashion models adorn billboards and magazine covers. Thinness is associated with beauty, success, intelligence, and vitality. A young woman can feel overwhelmed when facing a future in which she must be independent, land a prestigious job, maintain a successful love relationship, bear and nurture children, manage a household, and keep up with fashion trends. Unable to master all these roles, she may look for some aspect of her life that she can control. Food intake and body weight are natural choices because thinness is associated with success. Messages about how we should look are difficult to ignore and can create pressure to achieve this ideal body. But it is a standard that is very difficult to meet—and contributes to disturbances in body image and eating behaviour.

Although men currently represent a small percentage of people with eating disorders, their numbers are increasing.[74] This trend is likely due to increasing pressure to achieve an ideal male body. Advertisements directed at men are showing more and more exposed skin, with a focus on well-defined abdominal and chest muscles.

Anorexia Nervosa

Anorexia means lack of appetite, but in the case of the eating disorder anorexia nervosa, it is the desire to be thin that leads to decreased food intake. Anorexia nervosa is characterized by severe weight loss, **amenorrhea**, constipation, and restlessness. The average age of onset is 17 years. People with anorexia nervosa have a 5 percent death rate in the first two years, and the death rate can reach 20 percent in untreated individuals.[72]

amenorrhea
Delayed onset of menstruation or the absence of three or more consecutive menstrual cycles.

The psychological component of anorexia nervosa revolves around an overwhelming fear of gaining weight, even in individuals who are already underweight. Anorexia is also characterized by disturbances in body image or perception of body size that prevent those with this disorder from seeing themselves as underweight even when they are dangerously thin. No matter how much weight they lose, they do not gain self-respect, inner assurance, or the happiness they seek. Therefore, they continue to restrict their intake and use additional behaviours to lose weight.

The most obvious behaviours associated with anorexia are those that contribute to the maintenance of a body weight that is 15 percent or more below normal. These behaviours include restriction of food intake, binge-eating and purging episodes, and, in some patients, strange eating rituals. A person with anorexia may also exercise excessively and feel guilty if they cannot exercise (**Figure 9.23**). They may link exercise and eating, so a certain amount of exercise earns them the right to eat, and if they eat too much, they must pay the price by adding more exercise.

The first obvious physical manifestation of anorexia is weight loss. As weight loss becomes severe, symptoms

A day in the life of an anorexic • Figure 9.23

For individuals with anorexia, food and eating become an obsession. In addition to restricting the total amount of food they consume, they develop personal diet rituals, limiting certain foods and eating them in specific ways. Although they do not consume very much food, they are preoccupied with food and spend an enormous amount of time thinking about it, talking about it, and preparing meals for others. Instead of eating, they may move food around the plate and cut it into tiny pieces.

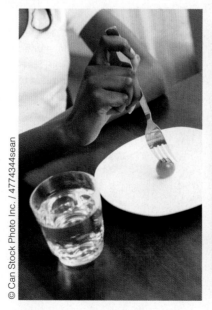

© Can Stock Photo Inc. / 4774344sean

Personal Journal
For breakfast today I had a cup of tea. For lunch I ate some lettuce and a slice of tomato, but no dressing. I cooked dinner for my family. I love to cook, but it is hard not to taste. I tried a new chicken recipe and served it with rice and asparagus. I even made a chocolate cake for dessert but I didn't even lick the bowl from the frosting. When it came time to eat, I only took a little. I told my mom I nibbled while cooking. I pushed the food around on my plate so no one would notice that I only ate a few bites. I was good today — I kept my food intake under control. The scale says I have lost 20 pounds but I still look fat.

of starvation begin to appear. Starvation affects mental function, causing the person to become apathetic, dull, exhausted, and depressed. Fat stores are depleted. Other symptoms that appear include muscle wasting, inflammation and swelling of the lips, flaking and peeling of skin, growth of fine hair (called lanugo) on the body, and dry, thin, brittle hair on the head. In females, estrogen levels drop, and menstruation becomes irregular or stops. In males, testosterone levels decrease. In the final stages of starvation, the person experiences abnormalities in electrolyte and fluid balance and cardiac irregularities. Suppression of the immune function leads to infection, which further increases nutritional needs.

The goal of treatment for anorexia nervosa is to help resolve the psychological and behavioural problems underlying the disorder while providing for physical and nutritional rehabilitation. Treatment requires an interdisciplinary team of nutritional, psychological, and medical specialists and typically requires years of therapy. The goal of nutrition intervention is to promote weight gain by increasing energy intake and expanding dietary choices.[77] In severe cases, people who have anorexia are hospitalized, and their food intake and exercise behaviours are controlled. Some people with anorexia make full recoveries, but about half have poor long-term outcomes—remaining irrationally concerned about weight gain and never achieving a normal body weight. Some patients with anorexia also transition to bulimia nervosa.[77] Anorexia is associated with both early mortality from malnutrition and suicide.

It has the highest mortality risk of any type of psychiatric illness, including depression and schizophrenia.[78]

Bulimia Nervosa

The term *bulimia nervosa* was coined in 1979 by a British psychiatrist who suggested that bulimia consists of powerful urges to overeat in combination with a morbid fear of becoming fat and avoidance of the fattening effects of food by inducing vomiting, abusing purgatives, or both.[79]

Like anorexia, bulimia is characterized by an intense fear of becoming fat and a negative body image, accompanied by a distorted perception of body size. Because self-esteem is highly tied to impressions of body shape and weight, people with bulimia may blame all their problems on their appearance, believing that if they can achieve their ideal weight, all their problems will disappear. They may engage in continuous dieting, which leads to a preoccupation with food.

Bulimia typically begins with food restriction motivated by the desire to be thin or by guilt concerning a previous episode of binging. Overwhelming hunger may finally cause the dieting to be interrupted by a period of overeating. Eventually, a pattern develops that consists of semi-starvation interrupted by periods of gorging. During a binge-eating episode, a person with bulimia experiences a sense of lack of control. Binges usually last less than two hours, occur in secrecy, and involve rapid food intake. Eating stops when the food runs out, or when pain, fatigue, or an interruption intervenes (**Figure 9.24**).

A day in the life of a bulimic • Figure 9.24

The amount of food consumed during a binge varies but can be in the range of 1,000 to 4,000 kcal in a single sitting, while a normal young woman may consume only about 2,000 kcal in an entire day. Self-induced vomiting is the most common purging behaviour. At first, a physical manoeuvre such as sticking a finger down the throat is needed to induce vomiting, but patients eventually learn to vomit at will. Binging and purging are followed by intense feelings of guilt and shame.

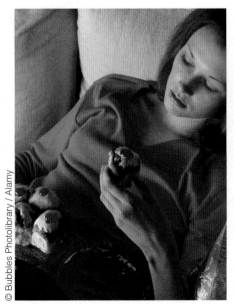

© Bubbles Photolibrary / Alamy

Personal Journal
Today started well. I stuck to my diet through breakfast, lunch, and dinner, but by 8 PM I was feeling depressed and bored. I thought food would make me feel better. Before I knew it I was at the convenience store buying two cartons of ice cream, a large bag of chips, a package of cookies, a half dozen chocolate bars, and a litre of milk. I told the clerk I was having a party. But it was a party of one. Alone in my dorm room, I started eating the chips, then polished off the cookies and chocolate bars, washing them down with milk and finishing with the ice cream. Luckily no one was around so I was able to vomit without anyone hearing. I feel weak and guilty but also relieved that I got rid of all those calories. Tomorrow, I will start a new diet.

After binge episodes, people who have bulimia use various behaviours to eliminate the extra calories and prevent weight gain. Some use behaviours such as fasting or excessive exercise, but most use purging behaviours, such as vomiting or taking laxatives, diuretics, or other medications. Self-induced vomiting does eliminate some of the food before the nutrients have been absorbed, but only a fraction of the ingested kilocalories are eliminated. Considering that a person who has bulimia may take in thousands of kilocalories in a single sitting, it is not a surprise that they are not overly thin. Laxatives and diuretics are sometimes also used, but they do not cause significant fat loss. Nutrient absorption is almost complete before food enters the colon, where laxatives have their effect. The weight loss associated with laxative abuse is due to dehydration. Diuretics also cause water loss, but via the kidney rather than the gastrointestinal (GI) tract.

It is the purging portion of the binge/purge cycle that is most hazardous to health. Vomiting brings stomach acid into the mouth. Frequent vomiting affects the gastrointestinal tract by causing tooth decay, sores in the mouth and on the lips, swelling of the jaw and salivary glands, irritation of the throat and esophagus, and changes in stomach capacity and the rate of stomach emptying.[72] It also causes broken blood vessels in the face due to the force of vomiting, electrolyte imbalance, dehydration, muscle weakness, and menstrual irregularities. Laxative and diuretic abuse can also cause dehydration and electrolyte imbalance.

The overall goal of therapy for people with bulimia nervosa is to reduce or eliminate bingeing and purging behaviour by separating the patients' eating behaviours from their emotions and their perceptions of success and to promote eating in response to hunger and satiety. People with bulimia must resolve their psychological issues related to body image and their sense of lack of control over eating. Nutritional therapy must address physiological imbalances caused by purging episodes and provide education on nutrient needs and how to meet them. Treatment has been found to speed recovery, especially when it is provided soon after symptoms begin, but for some women this disorder may remain a chronic problem throughout life.[80]

Binge-Eating Disorder

Binge-eating disorder is the most common eating disorder. Whereas anorexia and bulimia are uncommon in men, they account for about 40 percent of binge-eating disorder cases. This disorder is most common in overweight individuals (**Figure 9.25**). Individuals with binge-eating disorder engage in recurrent episodes of binge eating but do not regularly engage in compensatory behaviours such as vomiting or excessive exercise.

The major complications of binge-eating disorder are the health problems associated with obesity, which include diabetes, high blood pressure, high cholesterol levels, gallbladder disease, heart disease, and certain types of cancer.

A day in the life of a binge eater • Figure 9.25

People with binge-eating disorder often seek help for their weight rather than for their disordered eating pattern. An estimated 10 to 15 percent of people enrolled in commercial weight-loss programs suffer from this disorder.[81]

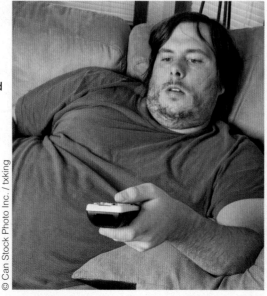

Personal Journal
I got on the scale today. What a mistake! My weight is up to 120 kg. I hate myself for being so fat. Just seeing that I gained more weight made me feel ashamed – all I wanted to do was bury my feelings in a box of cookies and a carton of ice cream. Why do I always think the food will help? Once I started eating I couldn't stop. When I finally did I felt even more disgusted, depressed, and guilty. I am always on a diet but it is never long before I lose control and pig out. I know my eating and my weight are not healthy but I just can't seem to stop.

© Can Stock Photo Inc. / txking

Treatment of binge-eating disorder often requires counselling due to the underlying psychological issues that drive this disorder. These issues must first be identified and dealt with before binge-eating behaviour is reduced. Counselling can also help improve body image and self-acceptance and address potential socio-environmental triggers.

Eating Disorders in Special Groups

Although anorexia and bulimia are most common in women in their teens and 20s, eating disorders occur in both genders and all age groups. Both male and female athletes are at high risk for eating disorders, with an incidence rate of 10 to 20 percent.[72, 82] Eating disorders also occur during pregnancy and are becoming more frequent among younger children due to social values about food and body weight. They also occur in individuals with diabetes.[83] A number of less common eating disorders appear in special groups within the general population (**Table 9.4**).

Preventing and Getting Treatment for Eating Disorders

Because eating disorders are often triggered by weight-related criticism, eliminating this type of behaviour can have a major impact on prevention. Another important target for reducing the incidence of eating disorders is

Other eating disorders	Table 9.4	
Eating disorder	**Who is affected**	**Characteristics and consequences**
Anorexia athletica	Athletes in weight-dependent sports such as dance, figure skating, gymnastics, track and field, cycling, wrestling, and horse racing	Engaging in compulsive exercise to lose weight or maintain a very low body weight. Can lead to more serious eating disorders and serious health problems, including kidney failure, heart attack, and death.
Female athlete triad	Female athletes in weight-dependent sports	A triad of disordered eating, amenorrhea, and osteoporosis. The energy restriction, along with high levels of exercise, causes amenorrhea. Low estrogen levels then interfere with calcium balance, eventually causing reductions in bone mass and an increased risk of bone fractures (discussed further in Chapter 10).
Night-eating syndrome	Obese adults and those experiencing stress	A disorder that involves consuming most of the day's calories late in the day or at night. People with this disorder—which contributes to weight gain—are tense, anxious, upset, or guilty while eating. A similar disorder, in which a person may eat while asleep and have no memory of the events, is called nocturnal sleep-related eating disorder (NS-RED) and is considered a sleep disorder, not an eating disorder.
Pica	Pregnant women, children, people with psychiatric disturbances and developmental disabilities, people whose family or ethnic customs include eating certain non-food substances, people who are hungry and try to ease hunger and cravings with non-food substances	Craving and eating non-food items such as dirt, clay, paint chips, plaster, chalk, laundry starch, coffee grounds, and ashes. Depending on the items consumed, pica can cause perforated intestines and contribute to mineral deficiencies or intestinal infections.
Insulin misuse (diabulimia)	People with type-1 diabetes	Type-1 diabetes is a disease that forces patients to focus on food portions and body weight. This may cause some to become preoccupied with their weight and to control it by withholding insulin. Without insulin, glucose cannot enter cells to provide fuel, blood levels rise, and weight drops. Uncontrolled blood sugar can lead to blindness, kidney disease, heart disease, nerve damage, and amputations.

the media. Altering the unrealistically thin body ideal presented by the media would likely decrease the incidence of eating disorders. Even with such an intervention, however, eating disorders are unlikely to go away entirely. Education through schools and communities about the symptoms and complications of eating disorders can help people identify friends and family members who are at risk and persuade those with early symptoms to seek help.

The first step in preventing individuals from developing eating disorders is to recognize those who are at risk. Early intervention can help prevent these individuals from developing serious eating disorders. People who are predisposed to developing an eating disorder often have excessive concerns about body weight, have friends who are preoccupied with weight, are teased about their weight by peers, and have family problems.

Once an eating disorder has developed, the person usually does not get better on his or her own. The actions of family members and friends can help people who have eating disorders to get help before their health is impaired. But it is not always easy to persuade a friend or relative with an eating disorder to seek help. People with eating disorders are good at hiding their behaviours and denying the problem, and they often do not want help. When confronted, one person might be relieved that you are concerned and willing to help, whereas another might be angry and defensive. When approaching someone about an eating disorder, make it clear that you are not forcing the person to do anything she or he doesn't want to do. Continued encouragement can help some people agree to seek professional help.

CONCEPT CHECK

1. **Which** eating disorder is characterized by extreme weight loss? Which is characterized by excess weight?

2. **What** is the main difference between bulimia and binge-eating disorder?

3. **What** is meant by body image?

4. **How** does a food binge differ from "normal" overeating?

Summary

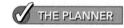

1 Body Weight and Health   298

- More Canadians today are **overweight** and **obese** than ever before. Excess body fat increases the risk of chronic diseases such as type-2 diabetes, heart disease, high blood pressure, and certain types of cancer.

- **Body mass index (BMI)** can be used to evaluate the health risks of a particular body weight and height. Measures of **body composition** can be used to determine the proportion of a person's weight that is due to fat. Excess **visceral fat** is a greater health risk than excess **subcutaneous fat**.

Techniques for measuring body composition • Figure 9.4

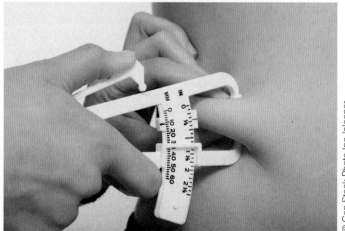

2 Energy Balance 303

- Canadians are getting larger because they are consuming more calories due to poor food choices and larger portion sizes and because they are moving less due to modern lifestyles in which computers, cars, and other conveniences reduce the amount of energy expended in work and play.

- The principle of **energy balance** states that if energy intake equals energy expenditure, body weight will remain constant. Energy is provided to the body by the carbohydrate, fat, and protein in the food we eat. This energy is used to maintain **basal metabolic rate (BMR)**, to support activity, and for the **thermic effect of food (TEF)**. When excess energy is consumed, it is stored, primarily as fat in **adipocytes**, causing weight gain. When energy in the diet does not meet needs, energy stores in the body are used, and weight is lost.

- The energy needs of healthy people can be predicted by calculating their estimated energy requirements (EER). EER depends on gender, age, life stage, height, weight, and level of physical activity.

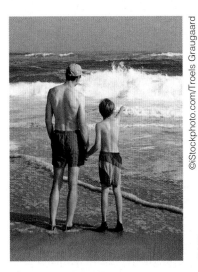

Genes determine body shape • Figure 9.10

- Inheriting an efficient metabolism or expending less energy through **non-exercise activity thermogenesis (NEAT)** may contribute to obesity.

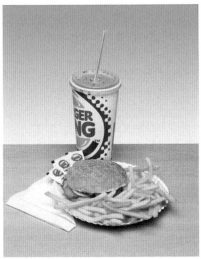

Portion distortion • Figure 9.6

Andy Washnik

3 What Determines Body Size and Shape? 311

- The genes people inherit affect their body size and shape. Body weight is also affected by environmental factors and personal choices concerning the amount and type of food consumed and the amount and intensity of exercise performed.

- **Hunger** and **satiety** from meal to meal are regulated by signals from the gastrointestinal tract, hormones, and levels of circulating nutrients. Signals from fat cells, such as the release of **leptin**, regulate long-term energy intake and expenditure.

4 Managing Body Weight 320

- Weight loss is recommended for those with a BMI above the healthy range who have excess body fat or a large waist circumference or who have health conditions associated with obesity. A loss of 5 to 15 percent of body weight significantly improves health outcomes.

- Weight management involves adjusting energy intake and expenditure to lose or maintain weight and **behaviour modification** to keep weight in a healthy range over the long term. To lose 500 g (1 lb.) of adipose tissue, energy expenditure must be increased or intake decreased by approximately 3,500 kcal. Slow, steady weight loss of 250 g to 1 kg (½ to 2 lb.) weekly is more likely to be maintained than rapid weight loss.

- If **underweight** is not due to a medical condition, weight gain can be accomplished by increasing energy intake and resistance training to increase muscle mass.

- A good weight-loss program promotes physical activity and a wide variety of nutrient-dense food choices, does not require the purchase and consumption of special foods or combinations of foods, and can be followed for life.

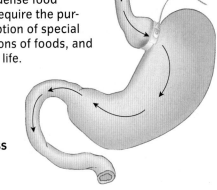

Gastric bypass and banding • Figure 9.19

• Drug therapy and surgery are recommended only for those whose health is seriously compromised by their body weight. Currently, the most popular surgical approaches to treating obesity are **gastric bypass** and **adjustable gastric banding**.

5 Eating Disorders   330

• **Eating disorders** are psychological disorders that involve dissatisfaction with body weight. **Anorexia nervosa** involves self-starvation, resulting in an abnormally low body weight. **Bulimia nervosa** is characterized by repeated cycles of **binge eating** followed by **purging** and other behaviours to prevent weight gain. **Binge-eating disorder** is characterized by bingeing without purging. People with this disorder are typically overweight.

• Eating disorders are caused by a combination of genetic, psychological, and socio-cultural factors. The lean body

A day in the life of an anorexic • Figure 9.23

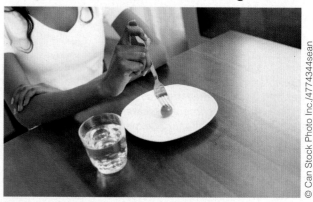

© Can Stock Photo Inc./4774344sean

ideal in North America is believed to contribute to disturbances in **body image** that lead to eating disorders. Treatment involves medical, psychological, and nutritional intervention to stabilize health, change attitudes about body size, and improve eating habits while supplying an adequate diet.

Key Terms

- adipocytes 308
- adjustable gastric banding 328
- amenorrhea 334
- anorexia nervosa 331
- appetite 304
- basal metabolic rate (BMR) 305
- basal metabolism 305
- binge-eating disorder 331
- body composition 301
- body image 332
- body mass index (BMI) 300
- bulimia nervosa 331

- cognitive behavioural therapy (CBT) 322
- eating disorder 331
- eating disorders not otherwise specified (EDNOS) 331
- energy balance 303
- food consumption 318
- food production 318
- gastric bypass 328
- ghrelin 314
- healthy weight 300
- hunger 304
- individual physical activity 319
- individual psychology 319

- lean body mass 300
- leptin 315
- liposuction 329
- motivational interviewing (MI) 321
- neuropeptide Y 314
- non-exercise activity thermogenesis (NEAT) 308
- obese 298
- obesity genes 311
- obesogenic environment 298
- overweight 298
- physical activity environment 319
- physiological factors 318

- resting metabolic rate (RMR) 307
- satiation 313
- satiety 313
- self-efficacy 322
- social psychology 318
- subcutaneous fat 303
- thermic effect of food (TEF) or diet-induced thermogenesis 308
- total energy expenditure 305
- underweight 300
- visceral fat 303
- waist circumference 303
- weight bias 329

Critical and Creative Thinking Questions

1. If a race of humans evolved on an island where food was always abundant, how might this environment affect the frequency of different types of genes that affect the regulation of body weight?

2. Using your knowledge of food intake regulation, explain why drinking a large glass of water will make you feel less hungry for a short time but not for more than an hour or so.

3. Suppose you have been invited to offer advice to your municipal planning committee. What recommendations would you make to help promote physical activity? What recommendations would you make for your local secondary school to encourage physical activity and healthy eating?

4. Design a weight-loss plan for someone who is 40 years old and 20 kg (40 lb.) overweight.

5. A late-night TV advertisement promotes a diet pill that will cause a weight loss of 5 kg (10 lb.) in the first week. Assuming that you did not change your physical activity, how many kilocalories would you need to eliminate from your diet *each day* to lose 5 kg (10 lb.) of adipose tissue in a week? Based on your calculation, do you think it is possible to lose 5 kg (10 lb.) of fat in one week? Why or why not?

6. Alissa is 22 years old and has a BMI in the healthy range. Discuss the steps she can take to prevent weight gain as she ages.

7. Discuss how bulimia might affect each side of the energy balance equation.

What is happening in this picture?

Sumo wrestlers train for many hours each day and eat huge quantities of food. The result is a high BMI and a large waist but surprisingly little visceral fat.

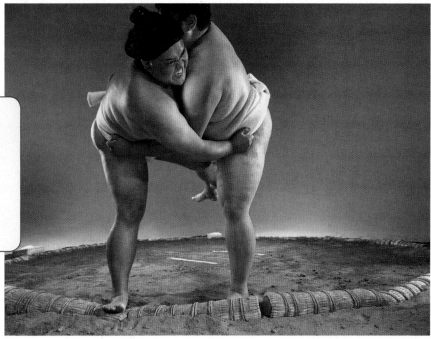

© Corbis RF Best/Alamy

Think Critically

1. Why do these individuals have a low level of visceral fat?
2. Do you think they are at risk for diabetes and heart disease?
3. What type of fat is hanging over the belts of these wrestlers?
4. What may happen if these wrestlers retire and stop exercising but keep eating large amounts of food?

Self-Test

(Check your answers in Appendix J.)

1. Which statement about basal metabolic rate (BMR) is false?

  a. In an average person, it is the largest component of energy expenditure.

  b. It includes the energy needed for kidney function and heartbeat.

  c. It includes the energy needed for exercise.

  d. It is measured in a warm room before rising, after 12 hours without food or exercise.

  e. It is the energy expended to keep an awake, resting body alive.

2. Excess body fat increases the risk of _____.

  a. diabetes

  b. high blood cholesterol

  c. certain cancers

  d. high blood pressure

  e. all of the above

3. To calculate a person's BMI, you need to know the person's _____.

  a. height and weight

  b. age and activity level

  c. lean body mass and waist circumference

  d. gender and weight

  e. gender and body composition

4. Which of the following has not contributed to the rising incidence of overweight and obesity in Canada?

    a. Canadians use less energy in the activities of their daily lives than they used to.

    b. Portion sizes of our food have increased.

    c. We have ready access to food 24 hours a day.

    d. Our genetics have changed significantly.

    e. The number of people who work at jobs requiring strenuous physical labour has decreased.

5. The method of determining body composition shown here relies on what principle to determine the amount of body fat?

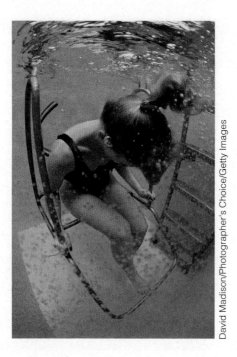

David Madison/Photographer's Choice/Getty Images

    a. Fat is less dense than water.

    b. Fat does not conduct electricity.

    c. The amount of subcutaneous fat is representative of total body fat.

    d. The extent to which X-rays penetrate fat is different from the extent to which they penetrate other tissues.

6. Which statement about EER is false?

    a. It is the amount of energy needed to maintain body weight.

    b. It is the amount of energy you expend daily.

    c. It increases if you lose weight.

    d. It decreases in adults as they get older.

    e. It increases if you exercise more.

7. Which statement about leptin is false?

    a. Someone with a defective leptin gene will most likely be obese.

    b. More leptin is released as adipocytes enlarge.

    c. Low leptin levels stimulate food intake and reduce energy expenditure.

    d. Most human obesity is due to abnormalities in the leptin gene.

    e. Leptin is better at defending against weight loss than against weight gain.

8. Long-term healthy weight loss is based on all of the following principles except _____.

    a. increasing physical activity

    b. adopting lifelong changes in eating habits

    c. eating specific combinations of foods that increase the number of calories burned

    d. keeping portion sizes moderate

    e. making nutrient-dense choices

9. Which statement about the type of body fat labelled by the letter A is false?

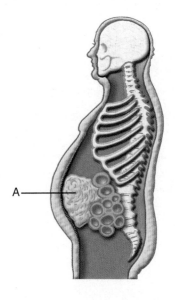

    a. This type of fat storage increases the risk of heart disease, diabetes, and high blood pressure.

    b. This type of fat storage can be reduced by eating grapefruit.

    c. This type of fat storage increases after menopause.

    d. This type of fat storage is more common in men than women.

    e. This type of fat storage can be reduced through exercise.

10. This chart most likely shows the distribution of energy expenditure in which of the following people?

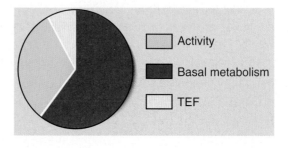

Activity

Basal metabolism

TEF

a. a cyclist who trains for six hours a day

b. an office worker who gets no exercise other than gardening

c. a young adult who works out for 90 minutes a day

d. an elderly man who is bedridden

11. True or false: It is possible for someone who is 20 kg (50 lb.) overweight to be in energy balance.

a. True

b. False

12. True or false: Everyone with a BMI in the overweight or obese range is at risk for weight-related health problems.

a. True

b. False

13. Which of the following is not a characteristic of anorexia nervosa?

a. a fear of gaining weight

b. a normal body weight

c. a preoccupation with food

d. an abnormal menstrual cycle

e. a distorted body image

14. Which group is least likely to develop anorexia nervosa?

a. ballet dancers

b. fashion models

c. female gymnasts

d. actresses

e. middle-aged men

15. What is the most common eating disorder in Canada?

a. pica

b. binge eating disorder

c. anorexia nervosa

d. bulimia nervosa

e. selective eating disorder

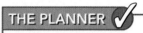
THE PLANNER ✓

Review your Chapter Planner on the chapter opener and check off your completed work.

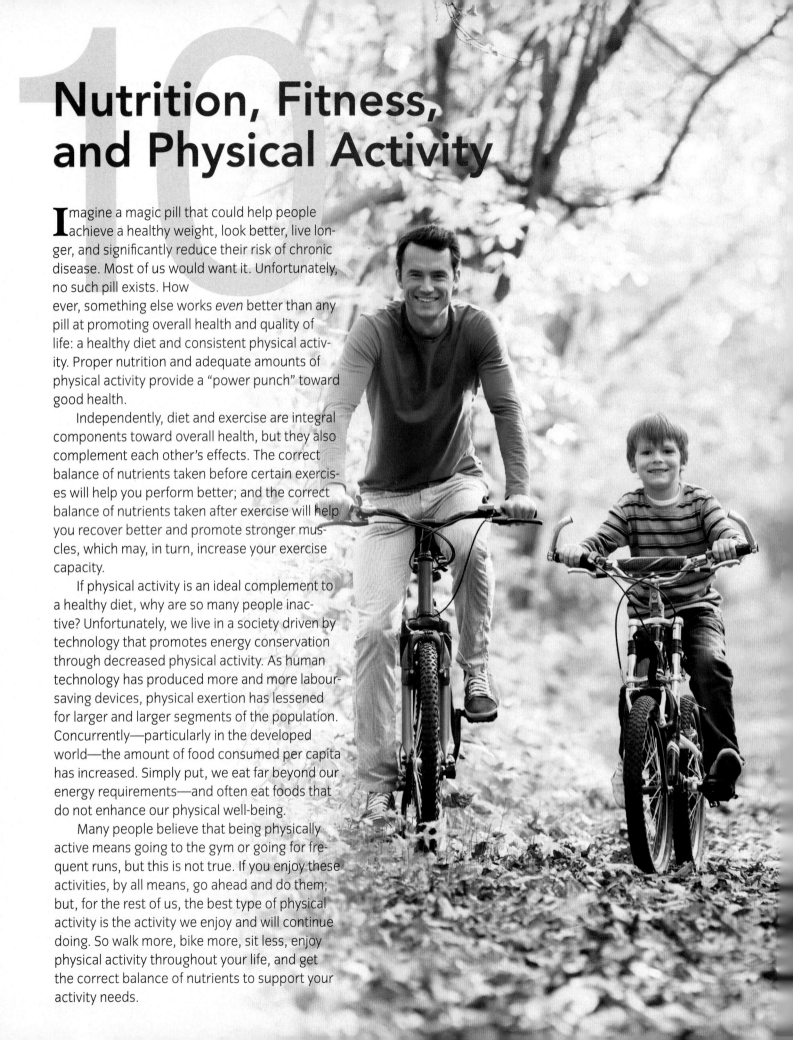

Nutrition, Fitness, and Physical Activity

Imagine a magic pill that could help people achieve a healthy weight, look better, live longer, and significantly reduce their risk of chronic disease. Most of us would want it. Unfortunately, no such pill exists. However, something else works *even* better than any pill at promoting overall health and quality of life: a healthy diet and consistent physical activity. Proper nutrition and adequate amounts of physical activity provide a "power punch" toward good health.

Independently, diet and exercise are integral components toward overall health, but they also complement each other's effects. The correct balance of nutrients taken before certain exercises will help you perform better; and the correct balance of nutrients taken after exercise will help you recover better and promote stronger muscles, which may, in turn, increase your exercise capacity.

If physical activity is an ideal complement to a healthy diet, why are so many people inactive? Unfortunately, we live in a society driven by technology that promotes energy conservation through decreased physical activity. As human technology has produced more and more labour-saving devices, physical exertion has lessened for larger and larger segments of the population. Concurrently—particularly in the developed world—the amount of food consumed per capita has increased. Simply put, we eat far beyond our energy requirements—and often eat foods that do not enhance our physical well-being.

Many people believe that being physically active means going to the gym or going for frequent runs, but this is not true. If you enjoy these activities, by all means, go ahead and do them; but, for the rest of us, the best type of physical activity is the activity we enjoy and will continue doing. So walk more, bike more, sit less, enjoy physical activity throughout your life, and get the correct balance of nutrients to support your activity needs.

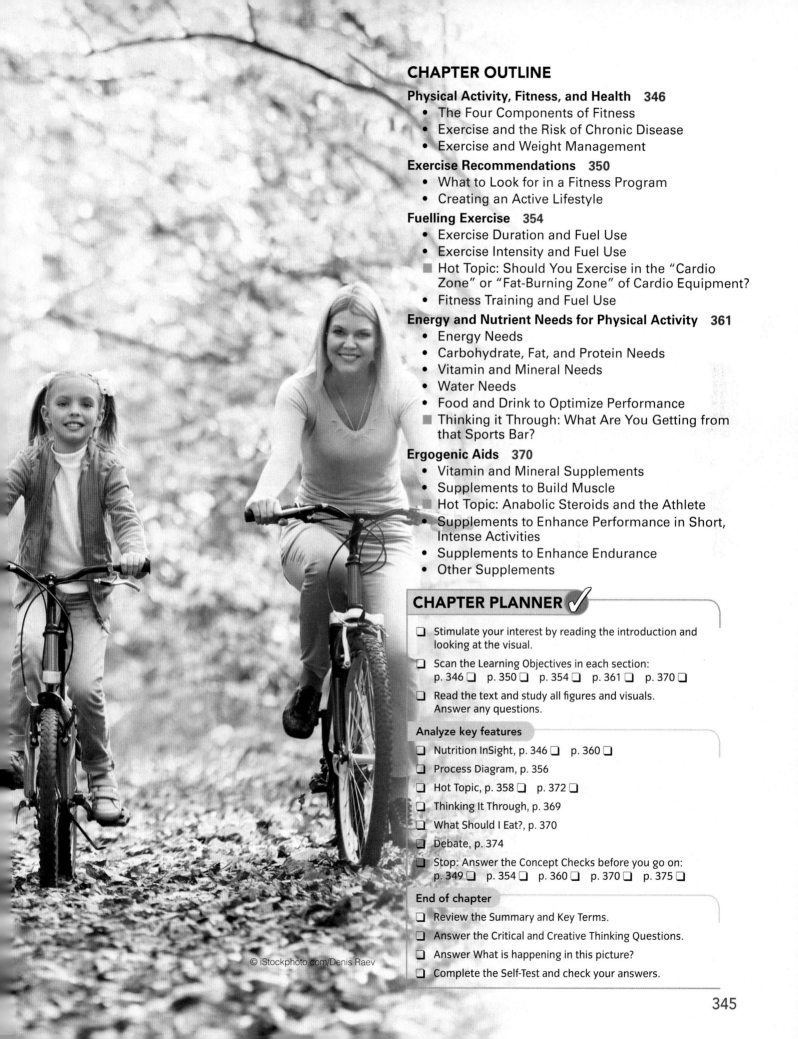

CHAPTER OUTLINE

CHAPTER PLANNER ✓

© iStockphoto.com/Denis Raev

345

Physical Activity, Fitness, and Health

LEARNING OBJECTIVES

1. **Describe** the characteristics of a fit individual.
2. **Explain** what is meant by the overload principle.
3. **Evaluate** the impact of exercise on health.
4. **Discuss** the role of exercise in weight management.

Exercise improves your **fitness** and overall health. This is true whether your fitness goal is to be able to walk around the block easily or to

> **fitness** A set of attributes related to the ability to perform routine physical activities without undue fatigue.

perform optimally in athletic competitions. This is also true regardless of weight. People of *all* sizes can benefit physically, mentally, and socially from regular physical activity. Exercise, along with a healthy diet, is important in maintaining health and reducing the risk of chronic diseases such as cardiovascular disease, type-2 diabetes, and obesity.

Many people are afraid of starting an exercise program because they are inexperienced or don't feel able enough. The great thing about exercise is the more you do it, the more your body adapts and grows to make it and future challenges easier and easier. When you exercise, changes occur in your body: You breathe harder, your

---

Nutrition InSight   The components of fitness • Figure 10.1

a. Cardiorespiratory endurance: The cardiovascular and respiratory systems are strengthened by **aerobic exercise**, such as jogging, bicycling, and swimming. Aerobic exercises maximize oxygen usage and elevate your breathing and heart rate. They are intense enough to train your heart and lungs, but are moderate enough

> **cardiorespiratory endurance** The efficiency with which the body delivers to cells the oxygen and nutrients needed for muscular activity and transports waste products from cells.
>
> **aerobic capacity** The maximum amount of oxygen that can be consumed by the tissues during exercise. Also called maximal oxygen consumption, or VO_2 max.

to be sustained for a prolonged period of time. In addition to increasing the amount of oxygen-rich blood that is pumped to your muscles, regular aerobic exercise increases your muscles' ability to use oxygen to produce adenosine triphosphate (ATP). Your body's maximum ability to generate ATP using aerobic metabolism is called your **aerobic capacity**, or VO_2 max. Aerobic capacity is a function of the ability of the cardiorespiratory system to deliver oxygen to the cells and the ability of the cells to use oxygen to produce ATP. The greater your aerobic capacity, the more intense activity you can perform before lack of oxygen affects your performance.

© Can Stock Photo Inc. / Wollwerth

b. Muscular strength and endurance: Greater **muscle strength** enhances the ability to perform tasks such as pushing or lifting. In daily life, this type of strength is needed to lift a 4-L jug of milk off the top shelf of the refrigerator with one hand, carry a full garbage can out to the curb, or move a couch into your new apartment. Greater **muscle endurance** enhances your ability to continue repetitive muscle

> **muscle strength** The amount of force that can be produced by a single contraction of a muscle.
>
> **muscle endurance** The ability of a muscle group to continue muscle movement at a sub-maximal intensity over time.
>
> **strength training exercise** or **resistance training exercise** Activities that are specifically designed to increase muscle strength, endurance, and size.

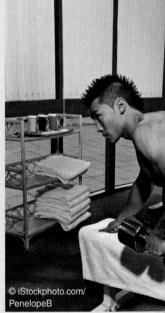

© iStockphoto.com/ PenelopeB

activity, such as shovelling snow or raking leaves. Muscle strength and endurance are increased by repeatedly using muscles in activities that require moving against a resisting force. This type of exercise is called either **strength-training exercise** or **resistance-training exercise** and includes such activities as weightlifting and calisthenics.

heart beats faster, and your muscles stretch and strain. If you exercise regularly, you adapt to the exercise you perform and, as a result, you can continue for a few minutes longer, lift a heavier weight, or stretch a millimetre farther. This response is known as the **overload principle**. To see improvements, you need to push yourself beyond what you are already capable of doing. For example, if you struggle to run a given distance three times a week, in a few weeks, you will be able to run farther and it will feel easier; if you lift heavy books for a few days, by the next week, you will have more muscle and will be able to lift more books more easily. These adaptations improve your overall fitness.

> **overload principle**
> The concept that the body adapts to the stresses placed on it.

The Four Components of Fitness

A person's fitness is defined by his or her cardiorespiratory endurance, strength, flexibility, and body composition (**Figure 10.1**). A fit person can continue an activity for a longer period than an unfit person can before fatigue forces a stop to the activity, but fitness is more than just stamina. Being fit also reduces the risk of chronic disease and makes weight management easier.

Exercise and the Risk of Chronic Disease

Regular exercise and a healthy diet not only make everyday tasks easier but can also prevent or delay the onset of chronic conditions such as cardiovascular disease, hypertension, type 2 diabetes, colon cancer, breast

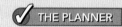
THE PLANNER

c. Flexibility determines your range of motion—how far you can bend and stretch muscles and ligaments. Being flexible makes everyday tasks easier and can improve athletic performance. Too-tight muscles, tendons, and ligaments restrict motion at the joints, decreasing stride or stroke length and increasing the amount of energy needed to move the joints. Regularly moving limbs, the neck, and the torso through their full range of motion helps increase and maintain flexibility. Flexibility also helps maintain a wide range of motion throughout life and into older age, can improve performance in certain activities, and may reduce your risk of injuries such as pulled muscles and strained tendons. ▼

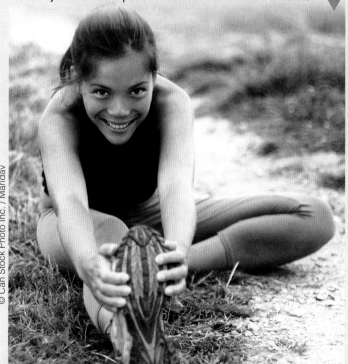

© Can Stock Photo Inc. / Maridav

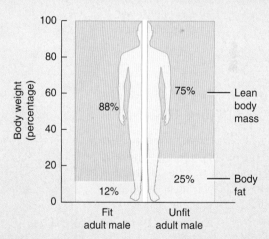

▲ **d. Body composition** Individuals who are physically fit have a greater proportion of muscle and a smaller proportion of fat than do unfit individuals of the same weight. Body composition also takes into account bone mass. A person with higher amounts of bone and muscle mass than fat mass are at decreased risk of disease. Body composition is therefore a better measure of overall health status than weight or body mass index. The amount of body fat a person has is affected by gender and age. In general, women have more stored body fat than men. For young adult women, the desirable amount of body fat is 21 to 32% of total weight; in adult men, the desirable amount is 8 to 19%.[1]

cancer, and bone and joint disorders (**Figure 10.2**).[2] The health benefits of exercise are so great that they can even overcome some of the health risks of carrying excess body fat. Exercise reduces overall mortality, regardless of whether the person is lean, normal weight, or obese.[2] So, even if you don't lose much weight, you'll still receive important benefits from continuing to exercise.

In addition to decreasing the risk of disease, exercise improves mood and self-esteem and increases vitality and overall well-being.[3] Exercise has also been shown to reduce depression and anxiety and to improve the quality of life.[4] The mechanisms involved are not clear, but one hypothesis suggests that exercise produces positive changes in certain neurotransmitters, the chemical messengers in the brain that are altered in individuals with mental illness. Another hypothesis relates to the production of **endorphins**. Exercise stimulates the release of these chemicals, which some believe are natural mood enhancers that play a role in triggering what athletes describe as an exercise high. The endorphins

endorphins Compounds that cause a natural euphoria and reduce the perception of pain under certain stressful conditions.

that lead to this state of exercise euphoria may also aid relaxation, pain tolerance, and appetite control. Evidence on the exercise–endorphin association isn't conclusive, however, and a high level of exercise may be needed to produce an endorphin response. The mental benefits of exercise may also relate to the feeling of accomplishment and increased ability that comes with exercise. If exercise takes place in a social setting, such as a group fitness class, the social interaction may also produce benefits to mental health.

Exercise and Weight Management

Exercise makes weight management easier because it increases both energy needs and lean body mass. During exercise, energy expenditure can rise well above the resting rate, and some of this increase persists for many hours after activity slows.[5] Over time, regular exercise increases lean body mass. Even at rest, lean tissue uses more energy than fat tissue; therefore, the increase in lean body mass increases metabolic rate. A significant impact on total energy expenditure

Health benefits of physical activity • Figure 10.2

Exercise improves strength and endurance, reduces the risk of chronic disease, aids weight management, reduces sleeplessness, improves self-image, and helps relieve stress, anxiety, and depression.

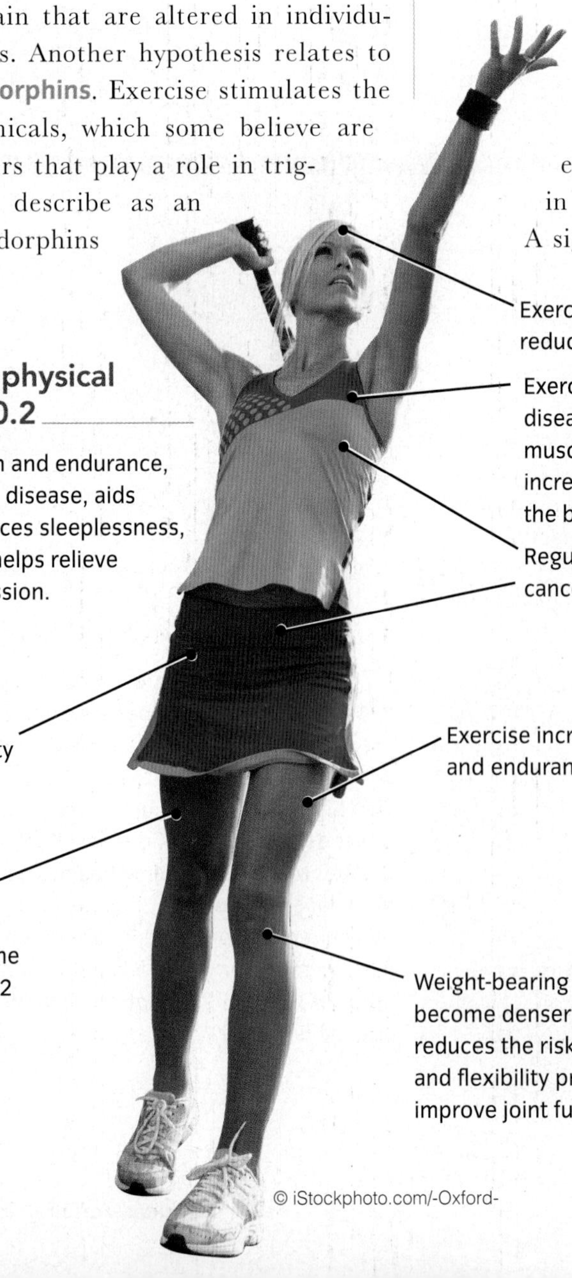

Exercise improves flexibility and balance.

Exercise increases the sensitivity of tissues to insulin and decreases the risk of developing type 2 diabetes.

Exercise improves mental health and reduces the risk of mental illness.

Exercise reduces the risk of cardiovascular disease because it strengthens the heart muscle, lowers blood pressure, and increases HDL (good) cholesterol levels in the blood.

Regular exercise reduces the risk of colon cancer and breast cancer.

Exercise increases muscle mass, strength, and endurance.

Weight-bearing exercise stimulates bones to become denser and stronger and therefore reduces the risk of osteoporosis. The strength and flexibility promoted by exercise can help improve joint function.

© iStockphoto.com/-Oxford-

Exercise increases energy expenditure • Figure 10.3

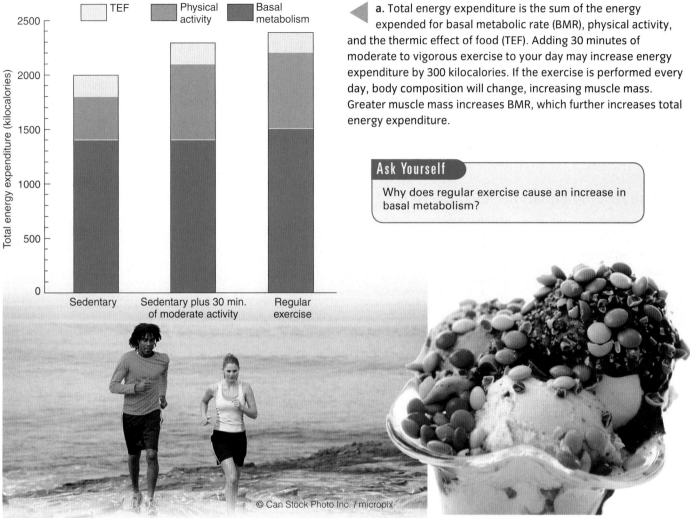

a. Total energy expenditure is the sum of the energy expended for basal metabolic rate (BMR), physical activity, and the thermic effect of food (TEF). Adding 30 minutes of moderate to vigorous exercise to your day may increase energy expenditure by 300 kilocalories. If the exercise is performed every day, body composition will change, increasing muscle mass. Greater muscle mass increases BMR, which further increases total energy expenditure.

Ask Yourself

Why does regular exercise cause an increase in basal metabolism?

© Can Stock Photo Inc. / micropix

© Can Stock Photo Inc. / yekophotostudio

b. Although exercise increases energy expenditure, moderate caloric intake is also required to achieve and maintain a healthy weight. The average person burns approximately 300 kilocalories in 30 minutes of running at a moderate-to-high intensity. It takes less time for that same person to easily consume a large ice cream dessert, like the one featured above, which may weigh in at more than 1,500 kilocalories five times the energy just expended in the 30-minute run!

results from the combination of increased energy output during exercise, the rise in energy expenditure that persists for a period after exercise, and the increase in metabolic needs over the long term (**Figure 10.3a**). The more energy you expend, the more food you can consume to maintain the same healthy weight. While exercise does increase the daily caloric intake required to maintain weight, it doesn't provide an unlimited licence to consume calories (**Figure 10.3b**). As discussed in Chapter 9, exercise is an essential component of any weight-reduction program: It increases energy needs, promotes loss of body

fat, and slows the loss of lean tissue that occurs with energy restriction.

CONCEPT CHECK

1. **What** distinguishes a fit person from an unfit person?

2. **How** does exercise affect heart health?

3. **How** does exercise help with weight management?

Exercise Recommendations

LEARNING OBJECTIVES

1. **Describe** the amounts and types of exercise recommended to improve health.
2. **Plan** a fitness program that can be integrated into your daily routine.
3. **Explain** overtraining syndrome.

Most Canadians do not exercise regularly. Only about 15% of Canadians get the recommended amount of physical activity each week.[6] To reduce the risk of chronic disease, public health guidelines advise at least 150 minutes of moderate to vigorous physical activity weekly, accumulated in intervals of at least 10 minutes at a time[7] (**Figure 10.4**).

Exercise recommendations • Figure 10.4

a. Everyday activities and aerobic exercise provide the base for an active lifestyle. They also decrease the risk of disease and improve overall quality of life.

Canadian Physical Activity Guidelines

FOR ADULTS - 18 – 64 YEARS

Guidelines

 To achieve health benefits, adults aged 18-64 years should accumulate at least 150 minutes of moderate- to vigorous-intensity aerobic physical activity per week, in bouts of 10 minutes or more.

 It is also beneficial to add muscle and bone strengthening activities using major muscle groups, at least 2 days per week.

 More physical activity provides greater health benefits.

Let's Talk Intensity!

Moderate-intensity physical activities will cause adults to sweat a little and to breathe harder. Activities like:

- Brisk walking
- Bike riding

Vigorous-intensity physical activities will cause adults to sweat and be 'out of breath'. Activities like:

- Jogging
- Cross-country skiing

Being active for at least **150 minutes** per week can help reduce the risk of:

- Premature death
- Heart disease
- Stroke
- High blood pressure
- Certain types of cancer
- Type 2 diabetes
- Osteoporosis
- Overweight and obesity

And can lead to improved:

- Fitness
- Strength
- Mental health (morale and self–esteem)

Pick a time. Pick a place. Make a plan and move more!

- ☑ Join a weekday community running or walking group.
- ☑ Go for a brisk walk around the block after dinner.
- ☑ Take a dance class after work.
- ☑ Bike or walk to work every day.
- ☑ Rake the lawn, and then offer to do the same for a neighbour.
- ☑ Train for and participate in a run or walk for charity!
- ☑ Take up a favourite sport again or try a new sport.
- ☑ Be active with the family on the weekend!

Now is the time. Walk, run, or wheel, and embrace life.

 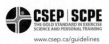

This recommendation is equivalent to 30 minutes of moderate exercise, such as jogging, spinning, or hiking, on most days.

Greater health benefits can be obtained by exercising more vigorously or for a longer duration. To promote maintenance of a healthy body weight, more exercise is often required. It is also recommended that Canadians include at least two days of physical activity that trains the bones and muscles each week.[7]

If you can't find the time or motivation to exercise for one hour a day, do not give up. Even a small amount of exercise is better than none.

b. Considered separately from physical inactivity, sedentary behaviours comprise a disease risk factor that increases your risk for future health concerns. Canada is one of the only countries in the world to recommend that children minimize the time spent in sedentary behaviours. A major recommendation of the sedentary guide is that children should not spend more than two hours at a time in sedentary pursuits, such as watching TV or playing video games.

Canadian Sedentary Behaviour Guidelines

FOR CHILDREN - 5 – 11 YEARS

Guidelines

For health benefits, children aged 5–11 years should minimize the time they spend being sedentary each day. This may be achieved by

 Limiting recreational screen time to no more than 2 hours per day; lower levels are associated with additional health benefits.

 Limiting sedentary (motorized) transport, extended sitting and time spent indoors throughout the day.

The lowdown on the slowdown: what counts as being sedentary?

Sedentary behaviour is time when children are doing very little physical movement. Some examples are:

- Sitting for long periods
- Using motorized transportation (such as a bus or a car)
- Watching television
- Playing passive video games
- Playing on the computer

Spending less time being sedentary can help children:

- Maintain a healthy body weight
- Do better in school
- Improve their self-confidence
- Have more fun with their friends
- Improve their fitness
- Have more time to learn new skills

Cutting down on sitting down. Help children swap sedentary time with active time!

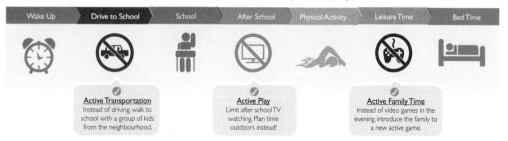

Active Transportation
Instead of driving, walk to school with a group of kids from the neighbourhood.

Active Play
Limit after school TV watching. Plan time outdoors instead!

Active Family Time
Instead of video games in the evening, introduce the family to a new active game.

There is no time like right now for children to get up and get moving!

 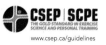

www.csep.ca/guidelines

What to Look for in a Fitness Program

A complete fitness program includes aerobic exercise for cardiovascular conditioning, stretching exercises for flexibility, and resistance exercises to increase muscle strength and endurance and to maintain or increase muscle mass.[7, 8] The program should be integrated into an active lifestyle that includes a variety of everyday activities, enjoyable recreational activities, and a minimum amount of time spent in sedentary activities (Figure 10.4).

Moderate or vigorous aerobic exercise should be performed most days of the week. An activity is aerobic if it raises your heart rate to 60 to 85% of your **maximum heart rate**; when you exercise at an intensity in this range, you are said to be in your **aerobic zone (Figure 10.5)**. For a sedentary individual who is begin-

maximum heart rate The maximum number of beats per minute that the heart can attain.

ning an exercise program, mild exercise such as walking can raise the heart rate into the aerobic zone. As fitness improves, more intense activity is needed to raise the heart rate to this level.

Aerobic activities of different intensities can be combined to meet recommendations and achieve health benefits. The total amount of energy expended in physical activity depends on the intensity, duration, and frequency of the activity. Vigorous physical activity, such jogging, raises heart rate to the high end of the aerobic zone (70 to 85%), leads to more improved fitness, and burns more calories per unit of time than moderate intensity activity, such as walking, which raises heart rate only to the low end of the zone (60 to 69%).

Individuals should structure their fitness program based on their needs, goals, and abilities. For example, some people might prefer a short, intense workout, such as

Calculating your aerobic zone • Figure 10.5

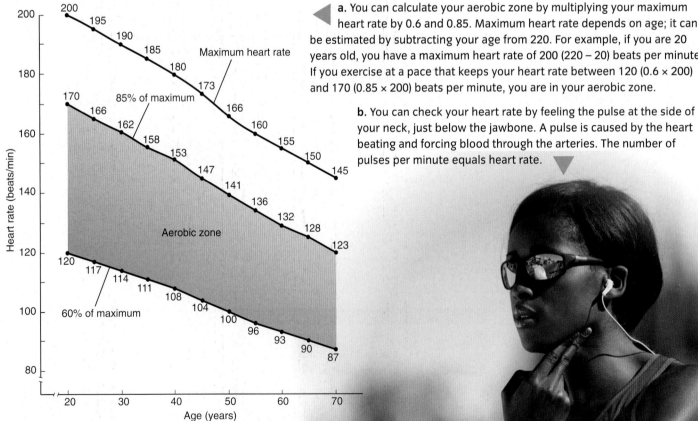

a. You can calculate your aerobic zone by multiplying your maximum heart rate by 0.6 and 0.85. Maximum heart rate depends on age; it can be estimated by subtracting your age from 220. For example, if you are 20 years old, you have a maximum heart rate of 200 (220 − 20) beats per minute. If you exercise at a pace that keeps your heart rate between 120 (0.6 × 200) and 170 (0.85 × 200) beats per minute, you are in your aerobic zone.

b. You can check your heart rate by feeling the pulse at the side of your neck, just below the jawbone. A pulse is caused by the heart beating and forcing blood through the arteries. The number of pulses per minute equals heart rate.

© iStockphoto.com/Andrew Rich

Interpreting Data

What is the aerobic zone for someone who is 30? What happens to the range when this person turns 40?

30 minutes of running, while others would prefer to work out for a longer time, at a lower intensity, such as a one-hour walk. Some may choose to complete all their exercise during one session, while others may spread their exercise throughout the day, in shorter bouts. For reducing the risk of chronic disease, three short bouts of 10-minute duration can be as effective as a continuous bout of 30 minutes.[8] The physical activity recommendations can be met through a combination of intensities, such as a brisk 30-minute walk three days a week, jogging for 20 minutes on two separate days a week, and increasing non-motorized transportation throughout the week.

Strength training can be performed less often than aerobic exercise. Strength training is needed about two days a week, depending on the goals of the individual. If an individual wants to gain larger muscle mass for increased athletic ability or overall fitness, an extra day or two may be required. Intense strength training, however, should not be done on consecutive days, especially training that works on the same muscle group. The rest between sessions gives the muscles time to respond to the stress by growing stronger. Muscles that aren't allowed to recover are more susceptible to injury and will not grow as effectively. How a person trains determines how their muscles will improve. For example, when training with weights, increasing the amount of weight lifted increases muscle strength, whereas increasing the number of repetitions improves muscle endurance. Also, flexibility exercises should be incorporated into a healthy lifestyle that includes aerobic and resistance training. Flexibility exercises can be performed two to seven days each week. Time spent stretching does not count toward meeting aerobic or strength training guidelines.

Creating an Active Lifestyle

Incorporating exercise into your day-to-day life may require a change in lifestyle, which is not always easy. Many people avoid exercise because they do not enjoy it, they do not want to join an expensive health club, they have little motivation to exercise alone, or they find exercise inconvenient and uncomfortable. Important steps in starting and maintaining an exercise program include finding an exercise you enjoy, setting aside a time that is realistic and convenient, making an exercise schedule, and finding a place that is appropriate and safe (**Table 10.1**). Find effective ways to increase your everyday activity level, such as riding your bike to class or work rather than driving, taking a walk during your lunch break, and throwing the Frisbee around or playing catch with your friends or family.

Suggestions for starting and maintaining an exercise program   Table 10.1
Start slowly. Set specific, attainable goals. Once you have met them, add more.
• Walk around the block after dinner. • Get off the bus or subway one stop early. • Use half of your lunch break to exercise. • Do a few biceps curls each time you take the milk out of the refrigerator.
Make your exercise fun and convenient.
• Opt for activities you enjoy—golfing and dancing may be more fun for you than using a treadmill in the basement. • Find a partner to exercise with and schedule regular exercise dates. • Choose times that fit your schedule.
Stay motivated.
• Vary your routine—swim one day and mountain bike the next. • Challenge your strength or endurance once or twice a week and do moderate workouts on other days. • Track your progress by recording your activity. • Reward your success with a new book, movie, or workout clothes, not food.
Keep your exercise safe.
• Warm up before you start. • Cool down when you are done. • Don't overdo it—alternate hard days with easy days, and take a day off when you need it. • Listen to your body and stop before an injury occurs.

The goal is to gradually make lifestyle changes that increase physical activity. Key to a consistently active life is choosing enjoyable activities that you'll want to keep doing.

Before beginning an exercise program, check with your physician to be sure that your plans are appropriate for you, considering your medical history (**Figure 10.6**).

Exercise is for everyone • Figure 10.6

Almost anyone of any age can exercise, no matter where they live, how old they are, or their physical limitations.

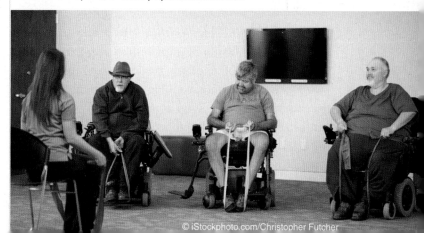

© iStockphoto.com/Christopher Futcher

If you choose to exercise outdoors rather than in a gym, reduce or curtail exercise in hot, humid weather to avoid heat-related illness. In cold weather, wear clothing that allows for evaporation of sweat while providing protection from the cold. Start each exercise session with a warm-up, such as walking or easy jogging, which will increase blood flow and nutrient delivery to the muscles. End with a cool-down period, such as walking or stretching, to prevent muscle cramps and reduce heart rate.

Don't overdo it. If you don't rest enough between exercise sessions, fitness and performance will not improve. During rest, the body replenishes energy stores, repairs damaged tissues, and builds and strengthens muscles. In athletes, excessive training without sufficient rest to allow for recovery can lead to **overtraining syndrome**. The most common symptom of this condition is fatigue that limits workouts and is felt even at rest. Some athletes experience decreased appetite, weight loss, muscle soreness,

> **overtraining syndrome** A collection of emotional, behavioural, and physical symptoms that occurs when the amount and intensity of exercise exceeds an athlete's capacity to recover.

increased frequency of viral illnesses, and increased incidence of injuries. Athletes who overtrain may become moody, easily irritated, or depressed. They may also experience altered sleep patterns or lose their competitive desire and enthusiasm. Overtrained athletes may be incapable of improving their fitness further and may even show setbacks in their abilities. Overtraining syndrome typically occurs only in serious athletes who are training extensively, but rest is essential for anyone who is working to increase fitness.

CONCEPT CHECK

1. **How** much aerobic exercise is recommended to reduce the risk of chronic disease?
2. **What** is your aerobic zone? Who is at risk for overtraining syndrome?

Fuelling Exercise

LEARNING OBJECTIVES

1. **Compare** the fuels used to generate ATP by anaerobic and aerobic metabolism.
2. **Discuss** the effect of exercise duration and intensity on the type of fuel used.
3. **Describe** the physiological changes that occur in response to exercise.

One of the factors that affect fuel use and the ability to sustain activity is whether the nature of exercise is aerobic or anaerobic. Long-distance running is an example of an aerobic activity because it is conducted at a constant, rhythmic pace over a sustained period of time. The nature of this activity allows the body to effectively coordinate oxygen delivery to the tissues with oxygen needs, making

it an aerobic (i.e., *with oxygen*) activity. In the presence of oxygen, cells can use oxygen and energy-yielding nutrients such as glucose, fatty acids, and amino acids to produce ATP, the energy currency of the cell.

Exercises such as weightlifting and sprinting are typically done at high intensities and for short periods of time. Your body therefore cannot effectively learn how to coordinate oxygen needs and delivery. Therefore, the majority of ATP needs to be produced anaerobically (i.e., *without oxygen*). Anaerobic metabolism is limited because only glucose can be used to fuel activity. Also, when activity is sustained at high intensities for too long a duration, lactic acid builds up, leading to an intense burning sensation in the exercising muscles. The buildup of lactic acid can also lead to an increase in the acidity of the blood, which promotes the urge to vomit. Luckily, the buildup of lactic acid is reversible. When oxygen becomes available

Anaerobic vs. aerobic metabolism • Figure 10.7

In the absence of oxygen, ATP can be produced only by anaerobic metabolism. **Anaerobic metabolism** can produce ATP very rapidly but must use glucose as a fuel. Anaerobic metabolism produces **lactic acid**, which can be used as a fuel for **aerobic metabolism**. When oxygen is present, the majority of ATP is produced by aerobic metabolism. Aerobic metabolism can use any fuel: carbohydrate, fat, or protein. It is slower but more efficient at generating ATP than anaerobic metabolism.

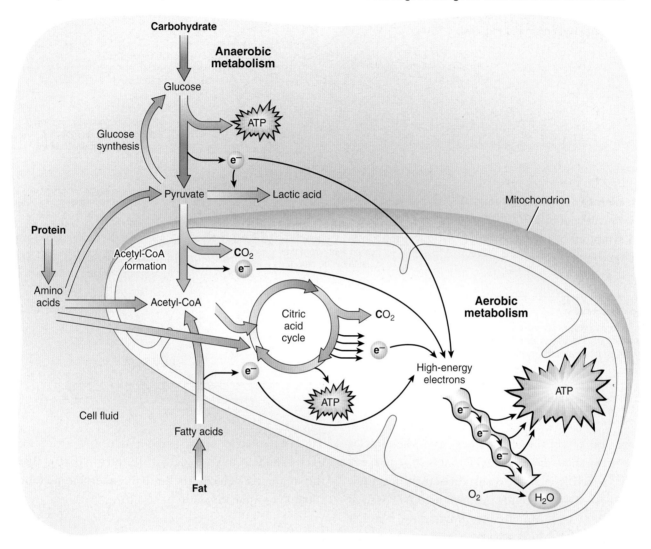

again, such as when exercise intensity is decreased, aerobic metabolism is favoured and the excess lactic acid is removed (**Figure 10.7**).

The amount of ATP produced depends on whether anaerobic or aerobic metabolism takes place, which, in turn, depends on the availability of oxygen. Oxygen is inhaled by the lungs and delivered to the muscle by the blood (**Figure 10.8**). When you are at rest, your muscles do not need much energy, and your heart and lungs are able to deliver enough oxygen to meet your energy needs using aerobic metabolism. When you exercise, your muscles need more energy. To increase the amount of energy provided by aerobic metabolism, you must increase the amount of oxygen delivered to the muscles, which your body accomplishes by increasing both heart rate and breathing rate. The ability of the circulatory and respiratory systems to deliver oxygen to tissues is affected by how long an activity is performed, the intensity of the activity, and the physical conditioning of the exerciser.

Exercise Duration and Fuel Use

When you take the first steps of your morning jog, your muscles increase their activity, but your heart and lungs have not yet had time to step up their delivery of oxygen

Increasing oxygen delivery • Figure 10.8

When you exercise, your muscles demand more oxygen. Your body responds by breathing faster and deeper to take in more oxygen and by increasing heart rate to deliver more oxygen to your muscles.

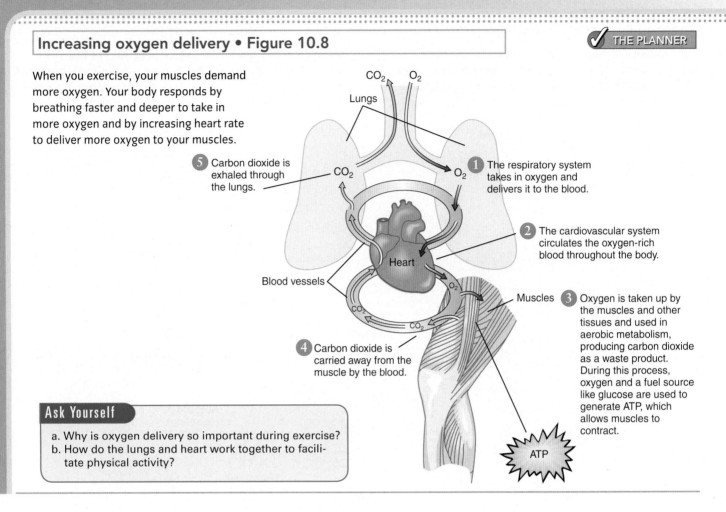

5 Carbon dioxide is exhaled through the lungs.

1 The respiratory system takes in oxygen and delivers it to the blood.

2 The cardiovascular system circulates the oxygen-rich blood throughout the body.

3 Oxygen is taken up by the muscles and other tissues and used in aerobic metabolism, producing carbon dioxide as a waste product. During this process, oxygen and a fuel source like glucose are used to generate ATP, which allows muscles to contract.

4 Carbon dioxide is carried away from the muscle by the blood.

Ask Yourself

a. Why is oxygen delivery so important during exercise?
b. How do the lungs and heart work together to facilitate physical activity?

---

to the muscles. To get the energy they need, the muscles must rely on the small amount of ATP that is stored in resting muscle, which is enough to sustain activity for a few seconds. As the stored ATP is used up, enzymes break down another high-energy compound, **creatine phosphate**, which converts ADP (adenosine diphosphate) to ATP, allowing your activity to continue. But, like the amount of ATP, the amount of creatine phosphate stored in the muscle at any time is small and soon runs out (**Figure 10.9**).

> **creatine phosphate** A compound stored in muscle that can be broken down quickly to make ATP.

Short-term energy: Anaerobic metabolism After about 15 seconds of exercise, the ATP and creatine phosphate in your muscles are used up, but your heart rate and breathing have not increased enough to deliver more oxygen to the muscles. At this point, to gain more energy, your muscles must produce the additional ATP without oxygen—that is, anaerobically (see Figure 10.7).

This anaerobic metabolism can produce ATP very rapidly but is fuelled only by glucose (**Figure 10.10**). Because the amount of glucose is limited, anaerobic metabolism cannot continue indefinitely.

Long-term energy: Aerobic metabolism When you have been exercising for two to three minutes, your breathing and heart rate have increased to supply more oxygen to your muscles, which allows aerobic metabolism to predominate. Aerobic metabolism produces ATP at a slower rate than anaerobic metabolism, but aerobic metabolism is much more efficient, producing about 18 times more ATP for each molecule of glucose! As a result, glucose is used more slowly than in anaerobic metabolism. In addition, aerobic metabolism can use fatty acids, and amino acids from protein, to generate ATP (Figure 10.10).

In a typical adult, about 90% of stored energy is found in adipose tissue; this store provides an ample supply of fatty acids. When you continue to exercise at a low to moder-

Changes in the source of ATP over time • Figure 10.9

The main source of the ATP that fuels muscle contraction changes over the first few minutes of exercise.

Instant energy
During the first few seconds of exercise, the muscles get energy from stored ATP. Then, for the next 10 seconds or so, creatine phosphate stored in the muscles is broken down to form more ATP.

Short-term energy
Anaerobic metabolism of glucose, obtained either from the blood or from muscle glycogen, becomes the predominant source of ATP when creatine phosphate stores have been depleted. Thirty seconds into the activity, anaerobic pathways are operating at full capacity.

Long-term energy
After about two to three minutes, oxygen delivery to the muscles has increased enough to support aerobic metabolism, which uses fatty acids and glucose to produce ATP.

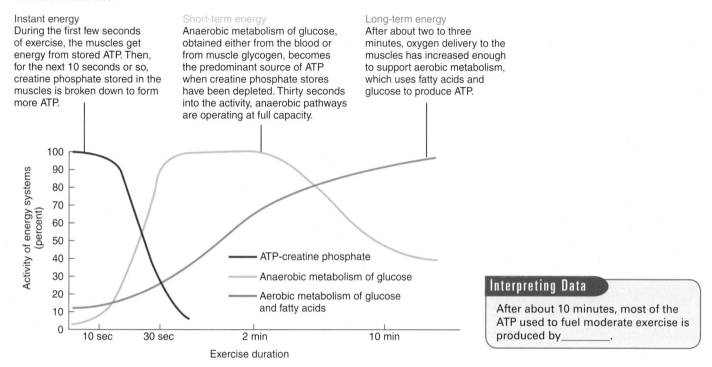

— ATP-creatine phosphate
Anaerobic metabolism of glucose
Aerobic metabolism of glucose and fatty acids

Interpreting Data
After about 10 minutes, most of the ATP used to fuel moderate exercise is produced by_____.

Fuels for anaerobic and aerobic metabolism • Figure 10.10

The glucose available to fuel muscle contraction comes from muscle glycogen breakdown or blood glucose. Blood glucose levels are maintained by the breakdown of liver glycogen, glucose synthesis by the liver, and carbohydrate consumed during exercise. Some of the fatty acids used as fuel come from triglycerides stored in the muscle, but most come from adipose tissue. The amino acids available to the body come from the digestion of dietary proteins and from the breakdown of body proteins.

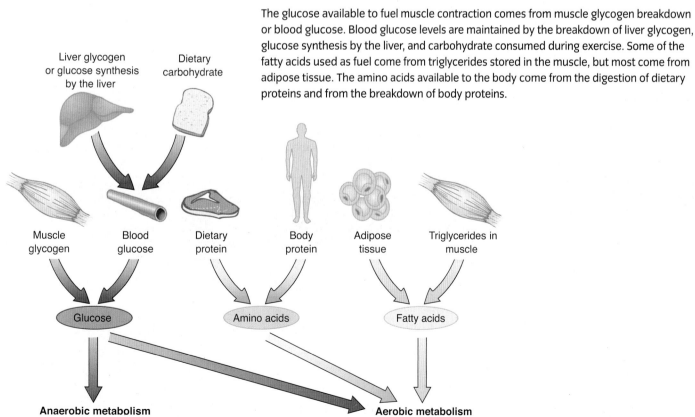

ate intensity, aerobic metabolism predominates, and fatty acids become the primary fuel source for your exercising muscles (**Figure 10.11**). When you pick up the pace, the relative amount of ATP generated by anaerobic versus aerobic metabolism and the fuels you burn will change.

Protein as a fuel for exercise Although protein is not considered a major energy source for the body, even at rest, small amounts of amino acids are used for energy. The amount increases if your diet does not provide enough total energy to meet your needs, if you consume more protein than you need, or if you are involved in endurance exercise (see Chapter 6).

When the nitrogen-containing amino group is removed from an amino acid through the process of deamination, the remaining carbon compound can be broken down to produce ATP by aerobic metabolism or, in some cases, used to make glucose (see Figure 10.7). Exercise

that continues for many hours increases the use of amino acids both as an energy source and as a raw material for glucose synthesis. Strength training does not increase the use of protein for energy, but it does increase the demand for amino acids for muscle building and repair.

Exercise Intensity and Fuel Use

The energy contributions from anaerobic and aerobic metabolism combine to ensure that your muscles get enough ATP to meet the demands placed on them. The relative contribution of each type of metabolism depends on the intensity of your activity. With low-intensity activity, sufficient ATP can be produced by aerobic metabolism so that both glucose and fatty acids can be used by the muscles. With intense exercise, more ATP is needed, but the oxygen delivered to the muscles and used by the muscles becomes limited, so the muscles must gain the additional

HOT TOPIC

THE PLANNER

Should you exercise in the "cardio zone" or "fat-burning zone" of cardio equipment?

Have you ever jumped onto a treadmill and chosen the workout that puts you in the "fat-burning zone" rather than the "cardio zone" because you wanted to lose weight? The fat-burning zone is a lower-intensity aerobic workout that keeps your heart rate between about 60 and 69% of maximum. The cardio zone is a higher-intensity aerobic workout that keeps heart rate between about 70 and 85% of maximum.

However, do you really burn more fat during a slow 30-minute jog in the fat-burning zone than during a vigorous 30-minute run in the cardio zone? While you do burn a higher *percentage* of calories from fat during a lower-intensity aerobic workout, you burn a lower amount of *total* calories.

When you pick up the pace and exercise in what the treadmill considers the cardio zone, you continue to burn fat. The graph shows that 50% of the calories burned come from fat during the lower-intensity workout (that is, in the fat-burning zone) and only 40% come from fat during the higher-intensity workout. Looking at the actual numbers of calories burned, however, shows that at the higher intensity, you burn just as much fat (about 150 Calories/hour) but a much greater number of calories overall.

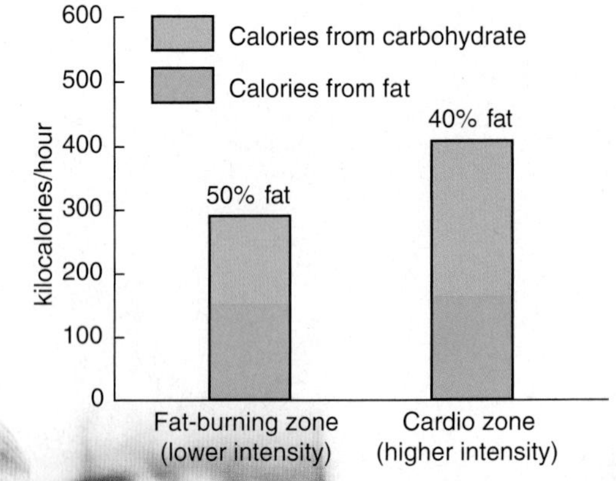

Calories from carbohydrate
Calories from fat

50% fat
40% fat

kilocalories/hour

600
500
400
300
200
100
0

Fat-burning zone (lower intensity)   Cardio zone (higher intensity)

Ask Yourself

Which workout will help you lose the most weight: 30 minutes in the cardio zone or 30 minutes in the fat-burning zone?

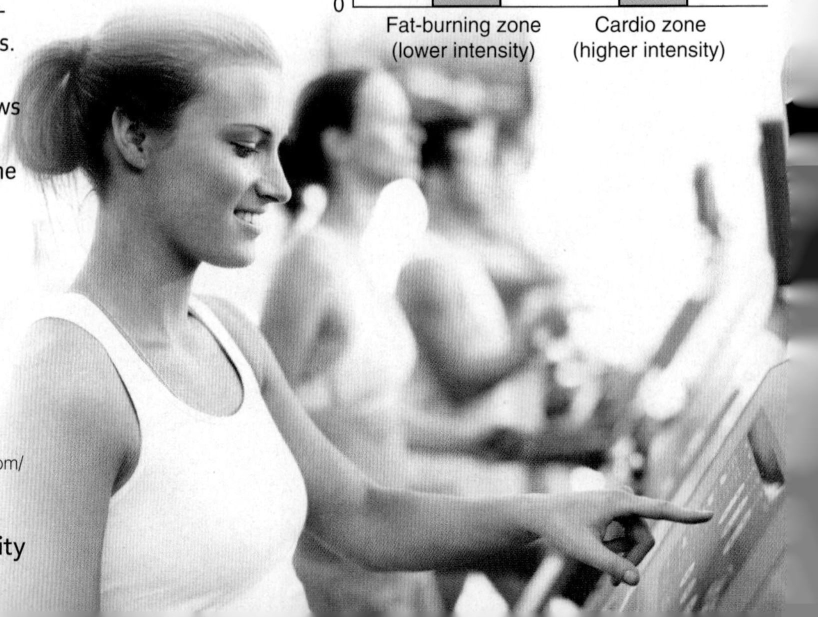

© iStockphoto.com/ Abel Mitja Varela

The effect of exercise intensity on fuel use • Figure 10.11

Exercise intensity determines the contributions of carbohydrate, fat, and protein—fuels for ATP production. At rest and during low- to moderate-intensity exercise, aerobic metabolism predominates, so fatty acids are an important fuel source. As exercise intensity increases, the proportion of energy supplied by anaerobic metabolism increases, so glucose becomes the predominant fuel. Keep in mind, however, that during exercise, the total amount of energy expended is greater than the amount expended at rest.

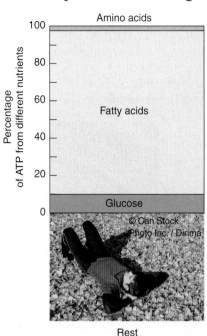
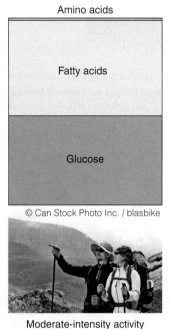
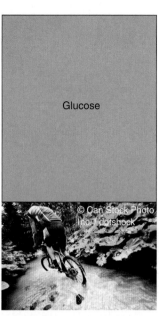

Rest   Moderate-intensity activity   High-intensity activity

ATP they need by using glucose for anaerobic metabolism (Figure 10.11).

Lower-intensity exercise relies on aerobic metabolism, which is more efficient than anaerobic metabolism and uses both glucose and fatty acids for energy. The body's fat reserves are almost unlimited, so if fat is the fuel, exercise can theoretically continue for a very long time. For example, it is estimated that a 60-kg (130-lb) woman has enough energy stored as body fat to run 1,600 km (1,000 miles).[9] However, even aerobic activity uses some glucose, which means that if exercise continues long enough, glycogen stores are eventually depleted, causing **fatigue**.

fatigue The inability to continue an activity at an optimal level.

Fatigue occurs much more quickly with high-intensity exercise than with lower-intensity exercise because more intense exercise relies more on anaerobic metabolism, which uses only glucose for fuel. Glycogen stores thus are rapidly depleted (**Figure 10.12**). Anaerobic metabolism also produces lactic acid. With low-intensity exercise, the small amounts of lactic acid produced are carried away from the muscles and used by other tissues as an energy source or converted back into glucose by the liver. During high-intensity exercise, the amount of lactic acid produced exceeds the amount that can be used by other tissues, leading to the lactic acid building up in the muscle and subsequently in the blood. Until recently, it was assumed that

Fatigue: "Hitting the wall" • Figure 10.12

Glycogen depletion is a concern for athletes because of the limited amount of stored glycogen available to produce glucose during exercise. When athletes run out of glycogen, they experience a feeling of overwhelming fatigue that is sometimes referred to as "hitting the wall," or "bonking."

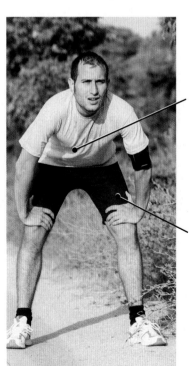

Between 60 and 120 grams of glycogen are stored in the liver; glycogen stores are highest just after a meal. Liver glycogen is used to maintain blood glucose between meals and during the night. Eating a high-carbohydrate breakfast will replenish the liver glycogen you used while you slept.

There are about 200 to 500 g of glycogen in the muscles of a 70-kg (154-lb) person. The glycogen in a muscle is used to fuel that muscle's activity.

© iStockphoto.com/William Perugini

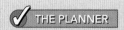
Aerobic training causes physiological changes in the cardiovascular system that increase the delivery of oxygen to cells. It also causes changes in the muscle cells that increase glycogen storage and the ability to use oxygen to generate ATP.

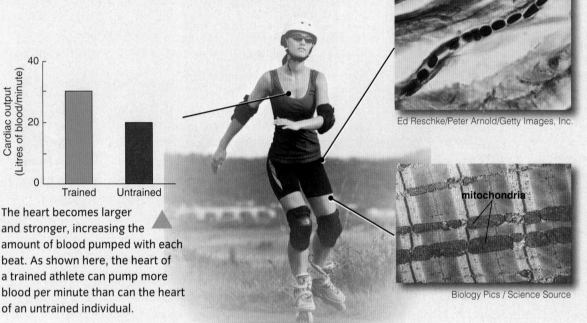

The heart becomes larger and stronger, increasing the amount of blood pumped with each beat. As shown here, the heart of a trained athlete can pump more blood per minute than can the heart of an untrained individual.

Ed Reschke/Peter Arnold/Getty Images, Inc.

The total blood volume and number of red blood cells expands, increasing the amount of hemoglobin, so that more oxygen can be transported. The number of capillary blood vessels in the muscles increases so that blood is delivered to muscles more efficiently.

Biology Pics / Science Source

mitochondria

The muscle increases its ability to store glycogen, and the number and size of muscle-cell mitochondria also increase. Because aerobic metabolism occurs in the mitochondria, the greater size and number of mitochondria increases the cell's capacity to burn fatty acids that produce AT

© iStockphoto.com/val_th

lactic acid buildup was the cause of muscle fatigue, but we now know that although lactic acid buildup is associated with fatigue, it does not cause it.[10] Fatigue most likely has many causes, including glycogen depletion, changes in the muscle cells, and changes in the concentrations of molecules and ions involved in muscle metabolism.

Fitness Training and Fuel Use

When you exercise regularly to improve your fitness, the training causes physiological changes in your body. The changes caused by repeated bouts of aerobic exercise increase the amount of oxygen that can be delivered to the muscles and the ability of the muscles to use oxygen to generate ATP by aerobic metabolism (**Figure 10.13**). This increased aerobic capacity allows fatty acids to be used for fuel, thereby sparing the glycogen and delaying

the onset of fatigue. Training aerobically also increases the amount of glycogen stored in the muscles. Because trained athletes store more glycogen and use it more slowly, they can sustain aerobic exercise for longer periods and at higher intensities than can untrained individuals.

CONCEPT CHECK

1. **What** fuels are used in anaerobic metabolism? In aerobic metabolism?

2. **What** type of metabolism does a marathon runner rely on?

3. **Why** is a trained athlete able to perform at a higher intensity for a longer time than an untrained person?

Energy and Nutrient Needs for Physical Activity

LEARNING OBJECTIVES

1. **Compare** the energy and nutrient needs of athletes and non-athletes.
2. **Explain** why athletes are at risk for iron deficiency.
3. **Discuss** the recommendations for food and drink during extended exercise.
4. **Plan** pre- and post-competition meals for a marathon runner.

Good nutrition is essential to performance, whether you are a marathon runner or a mall walker. Your diet must provide enough energy to fuel activity, enough protein to maintain muscle mass, sufficient micronutrients to permit utilization of the energy-yielding nutrients, and enough water to transport nutrients and cool your body. The major difference between the nutritional needs of a serious athlete and those of a casual exerciser is the amount of energy and water required.

Energy Needs

The amount of energy expended for any activity depends on the weight of the exerciser and the intensity, duration, and frequency of the activity (**Figure 10.14**). Whereas

Factors affecting energy expenditure
• Figure 10.14

This graph illustrates the impact of running pace and body weight on energy expenditure per hour. The longer an individual continues to run, the greater the amount of energy expended. Body weight affects energy needs because moving a heavier body requires more energy than moving a lighter body. Therefore, if the pace is the same, a 77-kg (170-lb) woman requires more energy to run for an hour than does a 57-kg (125-lb) woman.

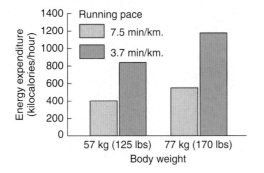

casual exercise may burn only 100 additional kilocalories a day, the training required for an endurance athlete, such as a marathon runner, may increase energy expenditure by 2,000 to 3,000 kilocalories per day. Some athletes require 6,000 kilocalories a day to maintain their body weight. In general, the more intense the activity, the more energy it requires; and the more time spent exercising, the more energy is expended (see Appendix G). For example, walking for 60 minutes involves less work than running for 60 minutes and therefore requires less energy.

Gaining or losing weight Body weight and composition can affect exercise performance. In sports such as football and weightlifting, a large amount of muscle is advantageous, and athletes may try to build muscle and increase body weight. Healthy weight gain can be achieved through a combination of increased energy intake from nutritious sources, adequate protein intake, and strength-training exercises, which promote an increase in lean tissue rather than fat.

In activities such as ballet, gymnastics, and certain running events, small, light bodies offer an advantage, so people involved in these activities may restrict their energy intake in an effort to maintain a low body weight. While a slightly leaner physique may be beneficial in these activities, dieting to maintain an unrealistically low weight may threaten health and performance. Athletes who need to lose weight should do so in advance of their most active season to prevent the calorie restriction from affecting their performance. The general guidelines for healthy weight loss should be followed: Reduce energy intake by 200 to 500 kilocalories per day, increase activity, and change the behaviours and thinking patterns that led to weight gain (see Chapter 9).

Unhealthy weight-loss practices Successful athletes are vulnerable to eating disorders because their motivation and self-discipline make them more susceptible to the pressure to lose weight in an effort to optimize their performance (see Chapter 9).[11] In athletes who develop anorexia nervosa, their restricted food intake can affect growth and maturation and impair their exercise performance. In athletes who develop bulimia, purging can lead to dehydration and electrolyte imbalance, which affect performance and put overall health at risk. In addition to restricting food intake or purging to keep body weight low, athletes are more likely than

Female athlete triad • Figure 10.15

Women with female athlete triad syndrome typically have low body fat; an increased risk of multiple or recurrent stress fractures; and irregular menstruation, a condition known as amenorrhea. Neither adequate dietary calcium nor the increase in bone mass caused by weight-bearing exercise can compensate for the bone loss caused by low estrogen levels. Treatment involves increasing energy intake and reducing activity so that menstrual cycles resume.[12]

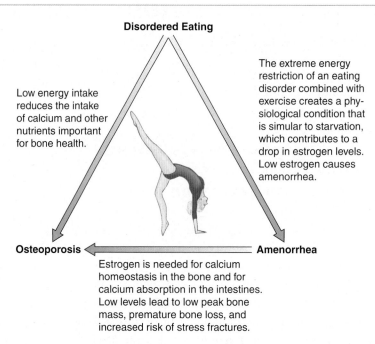

Disordered Eating

Low energy intake reduces the intake of calcium and other nutrients important for bone health.

The extreme energy restriction of an eating disorder combined with exercise creates a physiological condition that is simular to starvation, which contributes to a drop in estrogen levels. Low estrogen causes amenorrhea.

Osteoporosis ← **Amenorrhea**

Estrogen is needed for calcium homeostasis in the bone and for calcium absorption in the intestines. Low levels lead to low peak bone mass, premature bone loss, and increased risk of stress fractures.

non-athletes to engage in compulsive exercise behaviours in their efforts to increase energy expenditure.

In female athletes, the pressure to reduce body weight and fat in an effort to improve performance, achieve an ideal body image, and meet goals set by coaches, trainers, or parents may lead to a combination of symptoms referred to as the **female athlete triad**. This syndrome includes disordered eating patterns, amenorrhea, and disturbances in bone formation and breakdown that can lead to osteoporosis (**Figure 10.15**).

Athletes involved in sports that have weight classes, such as wrestling and boxing, are at high risk for unhealthy weight-loss practices because they are under pressure to lose weight before a competition so that they can compete in a lower weight class. Competing at the high end of a weight class is thought to offer an advantage over smaller opponents. To lose weight rapidly, these athletes may use sporadic diets that severely restrict energy intake or dehydrate themselves through such practices as vigorous exercise, fluid restriction, wearing of vapour-impermeable suits, or use of hot environments such as saunas and steam rooms to increase sweat loss. They may also resort to even more extreme measures, such as vomiting and the use of diuretics and laxatives. These practices can be dangerous and even fatal (**Figure 10.16**). They may impair performance and can adversely affect heart and kidney function, temperature regulation, and electrolyte balance.

Making weight • Figure 10.16

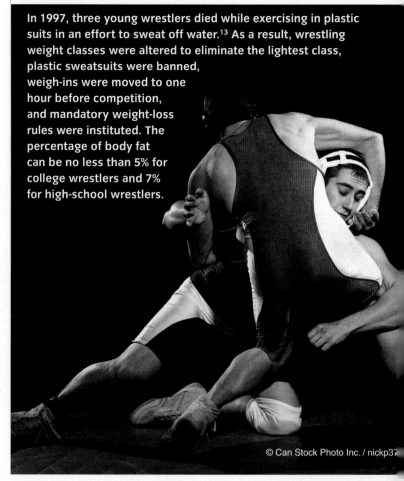

In 1997, three young wrestlers died while exercising in plastic suits in an effort to sweat off water.[13] As a result, wrestling weight classes were altered to eliminate the lightest class, plastic sweatsuits were banned, weigh-ins were moved to one hour before competition, and mandatory weight-loss rules were instituted. The percentage of body fat can be no less than 5% for college wrestlers and 7% for high-school wrestlers.

© Can Stock Photo Inc. / nickp37

Carbohydrate, Fat, and Protein Needs

In an athlete's diet, the source of energy consumed can be as important as the amount of energy consumed. To maximize glycogen stores and optimize performance, a diet that provides approximately 6 to 10 g of carbohydrate per kilogram of body weight per day (kg/day) is recommended for physically active individuals (**Figure 10.17**).[14] The recommended amount of fat is the same as the amount recommended for the general population—between 20 and 35% of energy.[14] To allow for enough consumption of carbohydrate, some athletes may need fat intakes at the lower end of this range. Diets that are very low in fat (less than 20% of calories) do not benefit performance. Protein is not a significant energy source, accounting for only about 5% of energy expended, but dietary protein is needed to maintain and repair lean tissues, including muscle. A diet in which 15 to 20% of calories come from protein will meet the needs of most athletes.

As discussed in Chapter 6, competitive athletes who participate in endurance or strength sports may require extra protein. In endurance events, such as marathons, protein is used for energy and to maintain blood glucose. Athletes participating in these events may benefit from 1.2 to 1.4 g of protein/kg/day. Athletes who participate in strength events require amino acids to synthesize new muscle proteins and may benefit from 1.2 to 1.7 g/kg/day.[14] While this amount is greater than the recommended daily allowance (RDA) of 0.8 g/kg/day, it is not greater than the amount of protein habitually consumed by athletes.[15]

Vitamin and Mineral Needs

An adequate intake of vitamins and minerals is essential for optimal performance. These micronutrients are needed for energy production, oxygen delivery, protection against oxidative damage, and repair and maintenance of body structures.

Exercise increases the amounts of many vitamins and minerals used both in metabolism during exercise and in repairing tissues after exercise. In addition, exercise may increase losses of some micronutrients. Nevertheless, most athletes can meet these needs by consuming the amounts of vitamins and minerals recommended for the general population. Because athletes must eat more food to satisfy their higher energy needs, they consume extra vitamins and minerals with these foods, particularly if they choose nutrient-dense foods. Athletes who restrict their intake in an effort to maintain a low body weight may be at risk for vitamin and mineral deficiencies.

Antioxidants and oxidative damage Exercise increases the amount of oxygen used by muscle and the rate of energy-producing metabolic reactions.[16] This increased oxygen use leads to a higher production of free radicals, which can lead to oxidative damage and contribute to muscle fatigue.[17] To protect the body from oxidative damage, muscle cells contain antioxidant defences, some of which may interact with dietary antioxidants such as vitamin C, vitamin E, beta carotene, and selenium. Despite the importance of antioxidants for health, there is little evidence that supplementation with antioxidants improves human athletic performance.[18]

Proportions of energy-yielding nutrients in an athlete's diet • Figure 10.17

The proportions of carbohydrate, fat, and protein recommended for the diets of physically active individuals are within the ranges recommended to the general public: about 45 to 65% of total energy from carbohydrate, 20 to 35% of energy from fat, and 10 to 35% of energy from protein.

Dietary fat is essential for health even though body fat stores contain enough energy to fuel even the longest endurance events. Most dietary fat should be from sources high in heart-healthy mono- and polyunsaturated fats.

An 85-kg (187-lb) man consuming 3,000 kilocalories, of which 15 to 20% is from protein, would be consuming 1.6 g of protein/kilogram body weight, enough to meet even the higher protein needs of a strength or an endurance athlete. This protein can come from either plant or animal sources.

The majority of calories should come from carbohydrate. Most of the carbohydrate should be from nutrient-dense choices such as whole grains, fruits, vegetables, and dairy products.

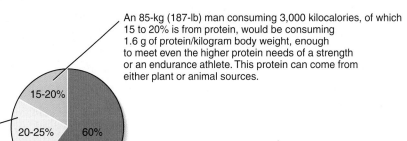

15-20%
20-25%
60%

Protein
Carbohydrate
Fat

Sports anemia • Figure 10.18

Training causes blood volume to expand to increase oxygen delivery, but the synthesis of red blood cells lags behind the increase in blood volume. The result is a decrease in the percentage of blood volume that is red blood cells. However, the total number of red blood cells stays the same or increases slightly, so the transport of oxygen is not impaired. As training progresses, the number of red blood cells increases to catch up with the increase in total blood volume.

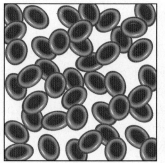
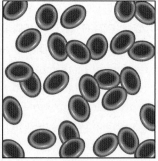

Normal   Sports anemia

Iron and anemia The body requires iron to form hemoglobin, myoglobin, and other iron-containing proteins that are essential for the production of energy by aerobic metabolism. Exercise increases the need for many of these proteins and may thereby increase iron needs. For example, exercise stimulates the production of red blood cells, so more iron is needed for hemoglobin synthesis. Some athletes may also face increased iron requirements because prolonged training can lead to increased iron loss through feces, urine, and sweat.[14]

Another cause of iron loss is the breaking of red blood cells due to the contraction of large muscles or the physical impact on the body in activities such as running. This type of red blood cell breakage is referred to as *foot-strike hemolysis*. It rarely causes anemia because most of the iron from these cells is recycled, and the breaking of red blood cells stimulates the production of new red blood cells.

Reduced iron stores are not uncommon in athletes.[19] Female athletes are at particular risk; their needs are higher than those of male athletes because they need to replace the iron lost in menstrual blood.[20] In athletes of both sexes, inadequate iron intake often contributes to low iron stores. Iron intake may be low in athletes who are attempting to keep their body weight down and in those who do not eat meat, which is an excellent source of readily absorbable heme iron. If iron deficiency progresses to anemia, the body's ability both to transport oxygen and to provide energy by aerobic metabolism is reduced, impairing both exercise performance and overall health.

Iron-deficiency anemia (see Chapter 8) should not be confused with **sports anemia**, which is an adaptation to training that does not seem to impair the delivery of oxygen to tissues (**Figure 10.18**). Although a specific iron RDA has not been set for athletes, the dietary reference intakes (DRIs) acknowledge that the requirement may be 30 to 70% higher for athletes than for the general population.[21]

Water Needs

Exercise increases water needs because of the increased water loss through sweat and from evaporation through the respiratory system. During exercise, most people drink only enough to satisfy their thirst, but this amount typically is not enough to replace the water lost. Therefore, many people end their exercise session in a state of dehydration and must restore fluid balance during the remainder of the day. Any weight loss between the beginning and end of an exercise session is almost entirely water loss. In other words, if you lost a kilogram during your session, you lost a kilogram of water (not fat), which will need to be replaced.

The risk of dehydration is greater in hot environments than in cold environments. However, dehydration may also occur when exercising in the cold because cold air tends to be dry, leading to greater evaporative losses from the lungs. In addition, insulated clothing worn in cold weather may increase sweat loss, and fluid intake may be reduced because a chilled athlete may be reluctant to drink a cold beverage. Also, female athletes who train in cold weather sometimes limit their fluid intake to avoid the inconvenience of having to remove clothing to urinate.[14]

Even when fluids are consumed at regular intervals throughout exercise, it may not be possible to drink enough to compensate for water losses. During exercise, water is needed to cool the body, to transport both oxygen and nutrients to the muscles, and to remove waste products from the muscles. Not consuming enough water to replace the water lost can be hazardous to the performance and health of even the most casual exerciser (**Figure 10.19**).

Dehydration and heat-related illnesses Dehydration occurs when water loss is great enough for blood volume and pressure to decrease, thereby reducing the ability of the circulatory system to deliver oxygen and nutrients to exercising muscles (see Chapter 8).

Dehydration and performance • Figure 10.19

As the severity of dehydration increases, exercise performance declines. Even mild dehydration—a water loss of 1 to 2% of body weight—can impair exercise performance. A 3% reduction in body weight decreases blood volume and thus can significantly reduce the amount of blood pumped with each heartbeat. This effect, in turn, reduces the circulatory system's ability to deliver oxygen and nutrients to cells and remove waste products.

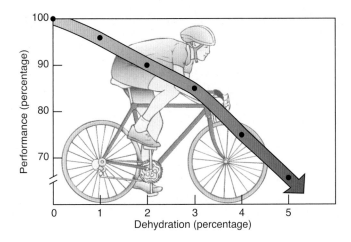

core body temperature rises above 40°C, causing the brain's temperature-regulation centre to fail. When heat stroke occurs, the individual does not sweat even though body temperature is rising. Heat stroke is characterized by elevated body temperature; hot, dry skin; extreme confusion; and unconsciousness. It requires immediate medical attention.

Exercising in hot, humid weather increases the risk of heat-related illnesses. As environmental temperature rises, the body has more difficulty dissipating heat; and as humidity rises, the body decreases its ability to cool itself through evaporation.

For example, southern Ontario typically has the highest average relative humidity in all of Canada. In the summer months, the relative humidity is typically around 75%, and the temperature often rises above 30°C. At these levels of heat and humidity, the dangers associated with heat-related illnesses are more likely, and extra caution should be taken to stay cool and hydrated.

---

heat-related illnesses Health conditions, including heat cramps, heat exhaustion, and heat stroke, which can occur due to an unfavourable combination of exercise, hydration status, and climatic conditions.

A decrease in blood volume also reduces blood flow to the skin and the amount of sweat produced, thus limiting the body's ability to cool itself. As a result, core body temperature can increase, escalating the risk of various **heat-related illnesses**.

Heat cramps are involuntary muscle spasms that occur during or after intense exercise, usually in the muscles involved in the exercise. These cramps are a form of heat-related illness caused by an imbalance of electrolytes in the muscle cell membranes. They can occur when water and salt are lost during extended exercise.

Heat exhaustion occurs when water loss causes blood volume to decrease so much that it is not possible both to cool the body and to deliver oxygen to active muscles. It is a form of heat-related illness characterized by a rapid but weak pulse, low blood pressure, disorientation, profuse sweating, and fainting. A person who is experiencing symptoms of heat exhaustion should stop exercising and move to a cooler environment.

Heat exhaustion can progress to **heat stroke**, the most serious form of heat-related illness. It occurs when

Hyponatremia Sweating helps us stay cool. But if the water and sodium lost in sweat are not replaced in the right proportions, the result may be low blood sodium, or hyponatremia (see Chapter 8). For most activities, sweat losses can be replaced with plain water, and lost electrolytes can be replaced during the meals following exercise. However, during endurance events, such as marathons, when sweating continues for many hours, both water and sodium need to be replenished. If an athlete replaces the lost fluid with plain water, the sodium that remains in the blood is diluted, causing hyponatremia. As sodium concentrations in the blood decrease, fluid moves into body tissues by osmosis, causing swelling. Fluid accumulation in the lungs interferes with gas exchange, and fluid accumulation in the brain can cause disorientation, seizure, coma, and death (**Figure 10.20**).

The risk of hyponatremia can be reduced by consuming a sodium-containing sports drink during long-distance events, increasing sodium intake several days prior to a competition, and avoiding Tylenol (acetaminophen), Aspirin (acetylsalicylic acid), Advil (ibuprofen), and other non-steroidal anti-inflammatory drugs, which may contribute to the development of hyponatremia by interfering with kidney function. The early symptoms of hyponatremia may be similar to those of dehydration: nausea, muscle cramps, disorientation, slurred speech, and confusion. A proper diagnosis is important because drinking water alone will worsen the problem. Mild symptoms of hyponatremia

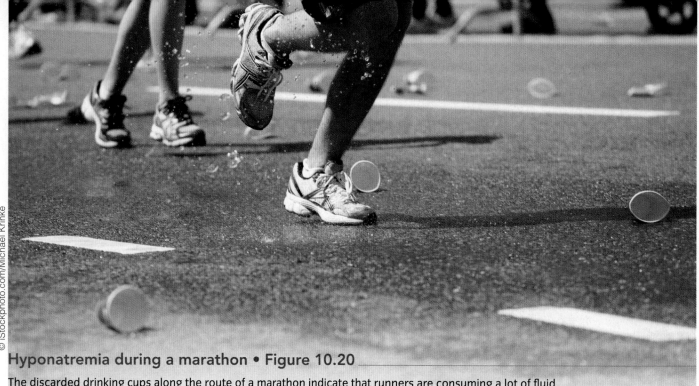

Hyponatremia during a marathon • Figure 10.20

The discarded drinking cups along the route of a marathon indicate that runners are consuming a lot of fluid. But if the runners drink too much plain water, they impair their health by changing the body's proportion of water and sodium. In 2002, a 28-year-old woman died after the Boston Marathon as a result of hyponatremia. A study done that year found that 13% of runners in the Boston Marathon had hyponatremia.[22]

can be treated by eating salty foods or drinking a sodium-containing beverage, such as a sports drink. More severe symptoms require medical attention.

Fluid recommendations for exercise Anyone who is exercising should consume extra fluids. Because thirst is not a reliable short-term indicator of the body's water needs, regular fluid breaks should be scheduled. Typically, however, exercising individuals ingest only about one-third to two-thirds of the amount of fluids that they lose in sweat.[23] To ensure hydration, adequate amounts of fluid should be consumed before, during, and after exercise.

Exercisers should drink generous amounts of fluid in the 24 hours before an exercise session and about 500 mL of fluid four hours before exercise. During exercise, whether casual or competitive, exercisers should try to drink enough fluid to prevent weight loss.[14] Drinking 175 to 350 mL of fluid every 15 to 20 minutes for the duration of the exercise should maintain adequate hydration. To restore lost water after exercise, each kilogram of weight lost should be replaced with 225 to 340 mL of fluid.[14]

The best type of beverage to consume during exercise depends on the duration of the exercise. For exercise lasting an hour or less, water is the only fluid needed, particularly if one of your exercise goals is weight management. A typical 500-mL sports drink provides about 100 to 150 kilocalories, so it will replace about half of the calories expended during your 30-minute ride on the stationary bicycle.

When exercise lasts more than 60 minutes, athletes are recommended to consume sports drinks or other beverages containing a small amount of carbohydrate (about 10 to 20 g of carbohydrate per 250 mL) and electrolytes (around 150 mg of sodium per 250 mL).[14] The carbohydrate is a source of glucose for the muscles and thus delays fatigue. Commercial sports drinks contain rapidly absorbed sources of carbohydrate, such as glucose, sucrose, or glucose polymers (chains of glucose molecules). The right proportion of carbohydrate to water is important. If the concentration of carbohydrate is too low, it will not help performance; if it is too high, it will delay stomach emptying. Water and carbohydrate trapped in the stomach do not benefit the athlete and may cause stomach cramps. Because fruit juices and soft drinks contain twice as much sugar as sports drinks, they are not recommended unless they are diluted with an equal volume of water. The sodium in sports drinks stimulates thirst, helps prevent hyponatremia, and enhances intestinal absorption of water and glucose. Flavoured beverages may also tempt athletes to drink more, helping to ensure adequate hydration.

Food and Drink to Optimize Performance

For most of us, a trip to the gym requires no special nutritional planning, but for competitive athletes, when and what they eat before, during, and after competition are as

Dietary carbohydrate and endurance • Figure 10.21

The amount of carbohydrate consumed in the diet affects the level of muscle glycogen and hence an athlete's endurance. This graph shows endurance capacity during cycling exercise after three days of three different diets: a low-carbohydrate diet (less than 5% carbohydrate), a normal diet (about 55% of energy from carbohydrate), and a high-carbohydrate diet (82% of energy from carbohydrate).[24]

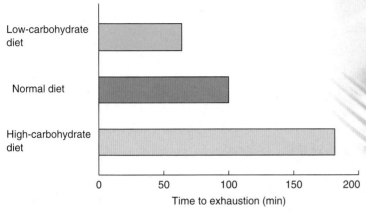

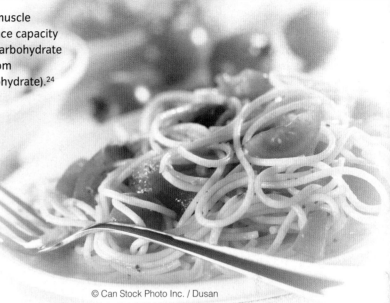

© Can Stock Photo Inc. / Dusan

important as a balanced overall diet. The type and amount of food eaten at these times may add or take away the extra seconds that can mean victory or defeat.

Maximizing glycogen stores

Glycogen stores are a source of glucose, and larger glycogen stores allow exercise to continue for longer periods. Glycogen stores and hence endurance are increased by increasing carbohydrate intake (**Figure 10.21**).

Serious endurance athletes who want to substantially increase their muscle glycogen stores before a competition may choose to follow a dietary regimen referred to as **glycogen supercompensation** or **carbohydrate (carbo-) loading**. This regimen involves resting for one to three days before competition while consuming a very high carbohydrate diet.[25,26] The diet should provide 10 to 12 g of carbohydrate/kg/day. For a 68-kg (150-lb) person, this amount is equivalent to about 700 g of carbohydrate per day. Having a stack of pancakes with syrup and a glass of juice for breakfast provides more than 200 g of carbohydrate. Many commercial high-carbohydrate beverages (50 to 60 g of carbohydrate in 250 mL) are available to help athletes consume the amount of carbohydrate recommended to maximize glycogen stores. (These beverages should not be confused with sports drinks that are designed to be consumed during competition, which contain only about 10 to 20 g of carbohydrate in 250 mL.) Trained athletes who follow a carbohydrate-loading regimen can double their muscle glycogen content.[26]

> **glycogen super-compensation** or **carbohydrate loading** A regimen designed to promote athletic endurance by increasing muscle glycogen stores beyond their usual capacity.

Although glycogen supercompensation is beneficial to endurance athletes, it provides no benefit, and even has some disadvantages, for those exercising for less than 90 minutes. For every gram of glycogen in the muscle, about 3 g of water are also deposited. This water will cause weight gain and may cause some muscle stiffness. As glycogen is used, the water is released, which can be an advantage when exercising in hot weather; but the extra weight is a disadvantage for individuals competing in short-duration events. Also, the idea of "carbo-loading" may lead an individual to over-consume calories to an extent that cannot be expended through activity, thereby promoting fat gain.

What to eat before exercise

Meals eaten before exercise should maximize glycogen stores and provide adequate hydration, while minimizing digestion, hunger, and gastric distress. A pre-exercise meal should provide enough fluid to maintain hydration and should be high in carbohydrate (60 to 70% of calories). The carbohydrate will help maintain blood glucose and maximize glycogen stores. Muscle glycogen is depleted by activity, but liver glycogen is used to supply blood glucose and is depleted even during rest if no food is ingested.

This high-carbohydrate pre-exercise meal should contain about 300 kilocalories and be moderate in protein (10 to 20%), low in fat (10 to 25%), and low in fibre to

The precompetition meal • Figure 10.22

When we don't eat, our overnight liver glycogen stores are reduced, so eating is particularly important first thing on the morning of a competition. A high-carbohydrate meal, such as cereal, milk, and juice, two to four hours before competition will replenish liver glycogen stores. The effect of different foods should be tested during training, not during competition. A competitor should not try anything new on event day, as it may not be digested well. In addition to providing nutritional clout, your regular pre-training meal that includes "lucky" foods may provide an added psychological advantage.

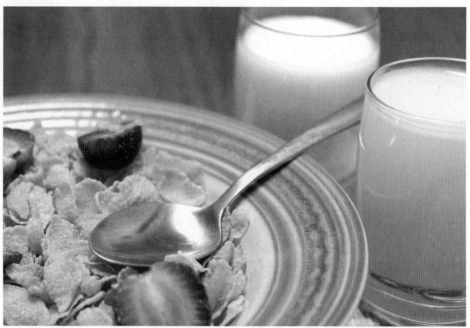

© iStockphoto.com/Jim Jurica

minimize gastrointestinal distress and bloating during competition (**Figure 10.22**). If exercise is being performed to promote a healthy weight, a smaller meal may be preferable. Athletes should avoid spicy foods, which can cause heartburn, and large amounts of simple sugars, which can cause diarrhea, unless they are accustomed to eating these foods. No matter what food is chosen for a pre-exercise meal, it shouldn't be eaten too soon before exercise, as digestion may cause cramps during the activity. A good rule of thumb is to eat at least an hour before exercise.

What to eat during exercise Most people don't need to eat while they exercise. But if the activity is intense and lasts longer than an hour, carbohydrate should be consumed during exercise to maintain glucose supplies. Carbohydrate consumption is particularly important for athletes who exercise in the morning, when liver glycogen levels are low.

Carbohydrate intake should begin shortly after exercise begins, and regular amounts should be consumed every 15 to 20 minutes during exercise. The carbohydrate should provide a combination of glucose and fructose. (Fructose alone is not as effective as the combination and may cause diarrhea.) This carbohydrate can be obtained from a sports drink, but consuming a solid-food snack or a carbohydrate gel with water is also appropriate. About 30 to 60 g of carbohydrate (the amount in a banana or an energy bar) each hour is recommended (see *Thinking it Through*).[14]

Snacks and sports drinks also provide sodium. Although the amounts of sodium lost in sweat during exercise lasting less than three to four hours are usually not enough to affect health or performance, a snack or beverage containing sodium is recommended for exercise lasting more than an hour to stimulate thirst, reduce the risk of hyponatremia, and improve glucose and water absorption.

What to eat after exercise When you stop exercising, your body shifts from the task of breaking down glycogen, triglycerides, and muscle proteins for fuel to the job of restoring muscle and liver glycogen, depositing lipids, and synthesizing muscle proteins. Meals eaten after exercise should replenish lost fluid, electrolytes, and glycogen and provide protein for building and repairing muscle tissue.

After exercise, the first priority for all exercisers is to replace fluid losses. For serious athletes competing on consecutive days, glycogen replacement is also a priority. To maximize glycogen replacement, a high-carbohydrate meal or drink should be consumed within 30 minutes after the competition and again every two hours for about six hours.[14] Ideally, the meals or drinks should provide about 1.0 to 1.5 g of easily absorbed carbohydrate per kilogram of body weight, which is about 50 to 100 g of carbohydrate for a 70-kg (154-lb) person—the equivalent of 500 mL of pasta or 500 mL of chocolate milk.[27] Consuming foods

THINKING IT THROUGH

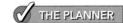

What Are You Getting from that Sports Bar?

Brad enjoys long-distance cycling. On weekends, he often goes on a 65- or 80-km ride, which takes him three to four hours. Despite the sports drink in his bike bottle, after about two hours, he gets hungry and fatigued, so he is looking for a snack that's easy to carry. He finds that some sports bars are high in protein and low in carbohydrate, some are high in carbohydrate and low in fat, and some have a more balanced ratio of carbohydrate, protein, and fat.

What type of bar will give Brad the energy he needs to continue his ride? Why?

▼

Carbohydrate is the fuel that is depleted during prolonged exercise. So if Brad wants to have the energy to keep pedalling, he should choose a high-carbohydrate bar. These are often called *energy bars* or *endurance bars*. They contain the carbohydrate needed to prevent hunger and maintain blood glucose during a sporting event. Brad should use the Nutrition Facts panel to select a bar that provides about 45 g of carbohydrate and no more than about 8 g of fat and 16 g of protein. Bars that are higher in fat or protein or lower in carbohydrate will not give him the blood glucose boost he needs to continue riding.

What are the advantages and disadvantages of sports bars?

▼

Your answer: _____

_____

With flavours such as chocolate coconut, tropical crisp, and sesame raisin crunch, many sports bars don't sound very different from chocolate bars. For about half the cost, Brad can buy a chocolate bar to put in his bike bag.

Based on the labels shown here, how do sports bars differ from chocolate bars?

▼

Your answer: _____

_____

Suggest a snack for Brad that is nutritionally comparable to a sports bar but less expensive.

▼

Your answer: _____

_____

(Check your answers in Appendix I.)

Nutrition Facts
Valeur nutritive
Per 1 bar(65 g) / par 1 barre (65 g)

Amount Teneur	% Daily Value % valeur quotidienne
Calories / Calories 230	
Fat / Lipides 2 g	3 %
Saturated / saturés 0.5 g + Trans / trans 0 g	3 %
Cholesterol / Cholestérol 0 mg	0 %
Sodium / Sodium 90 mg	4 %
Carbohydrate / Glucides 45 g	15 %
Fibre / Fibres 3 g	12 %
Sugars / Sucres 14 g	
Protein / Protéines 10 g	
Vitamin A / Vitamine A	0 %
Vitamin C / Vitamine C	100 %
Calcium / Calcium	30 %
Iron / Fer	35 %
Vitamin D / Vitamine D	0 %
Vitamin E / Vitamine E	100 %
Thiamin / Thiamine	100 %
Riboflavin / Riboflavine	100 %
Niacin / Niacine	100 %
Vitamin B$_6$ / Vitamin B$_6$	100 %
Folate / Folate	100 %
Vitamin B$_{12}$ / Vitamin B$_{12}$	100 %
Biotin / Biotine	100 %
Pantothenate / Pantothénate	100 %
Phosphorus / Phosphore	35 %
Magnesium / Magnésium	35 %
Zinc / Zinc	35 %
Copper / Cuivre	35 %
Chromium / Chrome	20 %

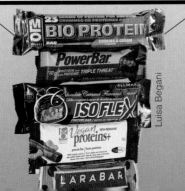

Luisa Begani

Nutrition Facts
Valeur nutritive
Per 1 bar (57 g) / par 1 barre (57 g)

Amount Teneur	% Daily Value % valeur quotidienne
Calories / Calories 271	
Fat / Lipides 14 g	21 %
Saturated / saturés 5 g + Trans / trans 0 g	26 %
Cholesterol / Cholestérol 5 mg	2 %
Sodium / Sodium 140 mg	6 %
Carbohydrate / Glucides 35 g	12 %
Fibre / Fibres 1 g	5 %
Sugars / Sucres 30 g	
Protein / Protéines 4 g	
Vitamin A / Vitamine A	2 %
Vitamin C / Vitamine C	0 %
Calcium / Calcium	5 %
Iron / Fer	2 %

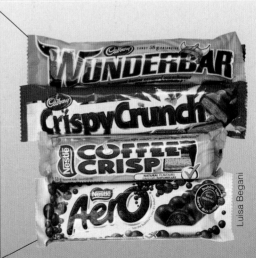

Luisa Begani

369

WHAT SHOULD I EAT?
Before, During, and After Exercise

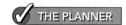 ✓ **THE PLANNER**

Before you exercise
- Fill a water bottle four hours before exercise and finish it before you start.
- Plan to eat whole-grain pasta but pass on the cream sauce.
- Eat a bowl of cereal with low-fat milk.

During your short workouts (≤60 min)
- Fill your water bottle with water.
- Take a swallow of water every 15 minutes.

During your long workouts (>60 min)
- Fill your water bottle with a sports drink.
- Take a sip of fluid at every sign or intersection to make sure you consume at least 175 mL of fluid every 15 min.

- Carry an apple and a bagel to snack on.
- Bring a sports bar that's high in carbohydrates.

When you are finished
- Restore fluid losses after exercise—215 to 325 mL for each kilogram of weight lost.
- Refuel with a sandwich or a plate of pasta and a glass of chocolate milk.

Use iProfile to plan a pre-competition meal that provides at least 50 g of carbohydrate

---

such as these that contain both carbohydrate and protein enhances glycogen synthesis even more than consuming carbohydrate alone.[28] The protein in post-exercise meals also provides the amino acids needed for muscle protein synthesis and repair (see *What Should I Eat?*).

The glycogen-restoring regimen just described can replenish muscle and liver glycogen within 24 hours of an athletic event and is critical for optimizing performance on the following day. Athletes who aren't competing again the next day can replenish their glycogen stores more slowly by consuming high-carbohydrate foods for the next day or so. About 600 g of carbohydrate, or about 8 to 10 g per kilogram of body weight, is recommended for the 24 hours after exercise.[14]

Most of us are not competitive athletes, so we don't need a special glycogen replacement strategy to ensure that our glycogen stores are replenished before our next visit to the gym. If your routine includes 30 to 60 minutes at the gym, a typical diet that provides about 55% of calories from carbohydrate will replace the glycogen used so that you will be ready for a workout again the next day.

CONCEPT CHECK

 STOP

1. **Why** might a low-carbohydrate diet be a poor choice for an endurance athlete?

2. **Why** are female athletes at particular risk for iron deficiency?

3. **How** much of what fluid should you drink during a two-hour bike ride?

4. **What** should an athlete eat as a pre-competition meal and why?

Ergogenic Aids
LEARNING OBJECTIVES

1. **Assess** the health risks associated with anabolic steroids.
2. **Explain** why creatine supplements affect sprint performance.
3. **Describe** one way in which a supplement might improve endurance.

*C*itius, altius, fortius—faster, higher, stronger—is the motto of the Olympic Games. For as long as there have been sporting events, athletes have yearned to gain a competitive edge. Everything from bee pollen and high-dose vitamins to ancient herbs and hormones has been used as an **ergogenic aid**.

> **ergogenic aid**
> A substance, appliance, or procedure that improves athletic performance.

The impact of diet and supplements on performance • Figure 10.23

This rainbow illustrates the relative impact of various nutrition strategies on exercise performance. Along with talent and hard work, the most significant benefit is achieved by eating a healthy overall diet. Foods and beverages that supply energy and ensure hydration during physical activity can provide additional benefits, whereas most ergogenic supplements provide little or no performance boost.

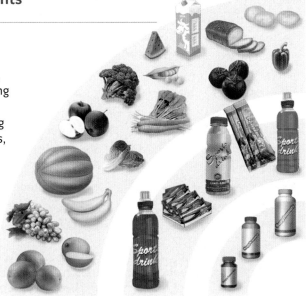

An overall healthy diet makes up the largest part of the rainbow

Sports foods and beverages used to refuel and rehydrate

A few specific supplements are beneficial in some cases

Athletes are willing to go to great lengths to improve their performance and are therefore susceptible to the lures of ergogenic supplements. Many of the vitamins, minerals, and other substances in these supplements help to provide energy for exercise or promote recovery from exercise. A few are beneficial for certain types of activities, but many carry more risks than benefits (**Figure 10.23**). When considering whether to use an ergogenic supplement, or any other type of supplement, wise consumers weigh the health risks against the potential benefits (see Figure 7.35).

Vitamin and Mineral Supplements

Many of the promises made to athletes about the benefits of vitamin and mineral supplements are extrapolated from the biochemical functions of these micronutrients. For example, B vitamin supplements are promoted to enhance ATP production because of their roles in muscle energy metabolism. Vitamin B6, vitamin B12, and folic acid are promoted for aerobic exercise because they help to transport oxygen to exercising muscle. These vitamins are needed for energy metabolism, and a deficiency of one or more will interfere with ATP production and impair athletic performance. That being said, providing more than the recommended amount does not deliver more oxygen to the muscle, cause more ATP to be produced, or enhance athletic performance.

Supplements of vitamin E, vitamin C, and selenium are promoted to athletes because of their antioxidant functions. As discussed earlier, exercise increases oxidative processes and therefore increases the production of free radicals, which cause cellular damage and have been associated with fatigue. However, antioxidant supplements have not been found to improve performance.[18]

Supplements of chromium (chromium picolinate) and vanadium (vanadyl sulfate) are marketed to increase lean body mass and decrease body fat. Chromium is needed for insulin action, and insulin promotes protein synthesis. However, studies have not consistently demonstrated that supplemental chromium has any effect on muscle strength, body composition, or other aspects of health (see Chapter 8).[29] Vanadium is also believed to assist the action of insulin, but there is no evidence that supplemental vanadium increases lean body mass.[30]

Supplements to Build Muscle

Protein supplements are often marketed to athletes with the promise of enhancing muscle growth or improving performance. Adequate protein is necessary for muscle growth, but consuming extra protein, either as food or supplements, does not increase muscle growth or strength. Muscles enlarge in response to exercise stress. The protein provided by expensive supplements will not meet an athlete's needs any better than the protein found in a balanced diet. If an athlete's diet provides enough energy, it usually provides enough protein without a supplement.

Growth hormone is appealing to athletes because it increases muscle protein synthesis and because its name inherently suggests increased muscle mass. Despite these physiological and psychological effects, however, growth hormone has not been shown to have ergogenic benefits.[31] Prolonged use of growth hormone can cause heart dysfunction, high blood pressure, and excessive growth of some body parts, such as hands, feet, and facial features. Growth hormone is on the World Anti-Doping Agency's list of banned substances.

Supplements of the amino acids ornithine, arginine, and lysine are marketed with the promise that they will stimulate the release of growth hormone and, in turn, enhance the growth of muscles. Large doses of these amino acids have been shown to stimulate the release of growth hormone. However, growth hormone levels in the blood of athletes taking these amino acids are no greater than levels typically resulting from exercise alone. Also, supplements of these amino acids have not been found to cause greater increases in muscle mass and strength than can be achieved through strength-training exercise alone.[32,33]

Anabolic steroids accelerate protein synthesis. When taken in conjunction with exercise and an adequate diet, anabolic steroids cause increases in muscle size and strength. However, anabolic steroids have extremely dangerous side effects (see *Hot Topic*), which has led to

> **anabolic steroids**
> Synthetic fat-soluble hormones that mimic testosterone and are used to increase muscle strength and mass.

HOT TOPIC

✓ THE PLANNER

Anabolic steroids and the athlete

Athletes looking at this photograph see the bulging muscles and enhanced performance that can be achieved with anabolic steroid use, but these are not the only effects of anabolic steroids. These drugs make the body believe that natural testosterone is being produced, and, therefore, as shown in the diagram, the body shuts down its own testosterone production. Natural testosterone stimulates and maintains the male sexual organs and promotes the development of bones and muscles and the growth of skin and hair. The synthetic testosterone in anabolic steroids has a greater effect on muscle, bone, skin, and hair than it does on sexual organs. Without natural testosterone, the sexual organs are not maintained, which leads to shrinkage of the testicles and a decrease in sperm production.[35]

In adolescents, the use of anabolic steroids causes cessation of bone growth and stunted height. Anabolic steroid use may also cause oily skin and acne, water retention in the tissues, yellowing of the eyes and skin, coronary artery disease, liver disease, and sometimes death. Users may experience psychological and behavioural side effects, such as violent outbursts and depression, possibly leading to suicide.[35]

When testosterone levels are low, the hypothalamus releases a hormone that stimulates the anterior pituitary to release a hormone that increases the production of testosterone by the testes. High levels of either natural or synthetic testosterone inhibit the release of the stimulatory hormone from the hypothalamus, shutting down the synthesis of natural testosterone.

Ask Yourself

Why does anabolic steroid use promote muscle development but cause the testes to shrink?

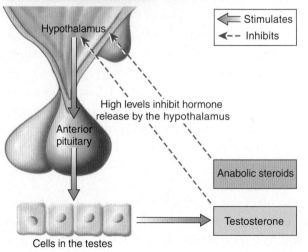
© iStockphoto.com/softservegirl

Despite the risks, in the United States, between 1 million and 3 million athletes have used anabolic steroids.[36] Anabolic steroids are controlled substances and are banned by the International Olympic Committee, the National Collegiate Athletic Association (NCAA), and most other sporting organizations.[37] In Canada, if someone is convicted of buying or selling these controlled substances, they may be sentenced to up to 18 months in jail.

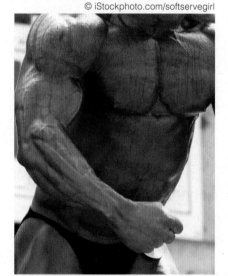

→ Stimulates
⟵-- Inhibits

Hypothalamus

High levels inhibit hormone release by the hypothalamus

Anterior pituitary

Anabolic steroids

Cells in the testes

Testosterone

their being regulated as controlled substances. **Steroid precursors**, which are compounds that can be converted into steroid hormones in the body, are also classified as controlled substances. The best known of these is androstenedione, often referred to as "andro." It was launched to public prominence when professional baseball player Mark McGwire announced his use of androstenedione during the 1998 major league baseball season, when he hit 70 home runs, breaking the league's single-season home-run record. Contrary to marketing claims, the use of andro or other steroid precursors has not been found to increase testosterone levels or produce any ergogenic effects, and they may cause some of the same side effects as anabolic steroids.[34]

Supplements to Enhance Performance in Short, Intense Activities

Numerous supplements are marketed to athletes who seek to improve their performance in activities that depend on quick bursts of intense activity. Supplements of β-hydroxy-β-methylbutyrate, known as HMB, claim to increase strength and muscle growth and improve muscle recovery; however, the outcome of research studies has been variable. Overall, studies have found a small increase in strength in previously untrained men, but the effects in trained weightlifters are trivial, as is the effect of HMB on body composition.[38]

Bicarbonate may provide some advantage for intense activities. Because bicarbonate acts as a buffer in the body,

some believe that supplementing it will neutralize acid, thereby delaying fatigue and enabling improved performance. Taking sodium bicarbonate (which is simply baking soda typically found in the kitchen cupboard) before exercise has been found to improve performance and delay exhaustion in sports that entail intense exercise lasting only one to seven minutes, such as sprint cycling, but it is of no benefit for lower-intensity aerobic exercise.[39] Just because baking soda is an ingredient in your cookies does not mean that it is risk-free. Many people experience abdominal cramps and diarrhea after taking sodium bicarbonate, and other possible side effects have not been carefully researched.

One of the most popular ergogenic supplements is **creatine**. This nitrogen-containing compound is found primarily in muscle, where it is used to make creatine phosphate (**Figure 10.24**). Higher levels of creatine and creatine phosphate provide more quick energy for short-term maximal exercise. Creatine supplementation has been shown to improve performance in high-intensity exercise lasting 30 seconds or less. It is therefore beneficial for exercise that requires explosive bursts of energy, such as sprinting and weightlifting, but not for long-term endurance activities, such as marathons.[40]

Athletes also take creatine supplements to increase muscle mass and strength. Some of the increase in lean body mass is believed to be due to water retention related to creatine uptake in the muscle. In addition, an increase in muscle mass and strength may occur in response to the greater amount and intensity of training that may be

Creatine boosts creatine phosphate • Figure 10.24

Creatine can be synthesized in the liver and kidneys and is also provided by meat and milk consumed in the diet. The more creatine consumed, the greater the amount of creatine stored in the muscles. Increasing creatine intake through supplement use has been shown to increase levels of muscle creatine and creatine phosphate, which is made from creatine.[40] During short bursts of intense activity, the creatine phosphate can be converted back into creatine, transforming ADP to ATP for muscle contraction.

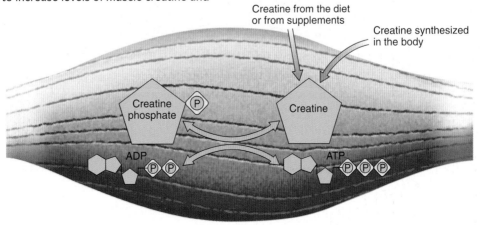

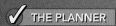
The Issue: Energy drinks are sold alongside sports drinks, and manufacturers of these beverages often sponsor athletes and athletic events. Should they be used as ergogenic aids? Is drinking them a safe way to improve your game?

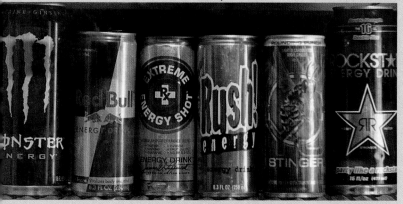

© Tony Cenicola/The New York Times/ReduxStock

Energy drinks have been available for purchase in Canada only since 2004, but the popularity of such drinks as Red Bull, Monster, and Full Throttle has soared over the past decade. They promise to keep you alert to study, work, drive, party all night, and perhaps excel at your next athletic competition. The main ingredients in these drinks are sugar and caffeine. Glucose is an important fuel for exercise, and caffeine is known to enhance endurance, so these drinks may seem like an ideal ergogenic aid.

A traditional sports drink, like Gatorade, contains about 28 g of sugar in 500 mL; a typical energy drink provides twice this much (55 to 60 g). Since carbohydrate fuels activity, it may seem that the additional sugar would provide energy for prolonged exercise. But more is not always better during activity. The double load of sugar cannot be absorbed quickly, and unabsorbed sugar in the stomach can cause gastrointestinal distress and slow fluid absorption.

The caffeine content of energy drinks ranges from 50 to 500 mg per can or bottle. Caffeine is an effective ergogenic aid that enhances endurance when consumed before or during exercise.[46] But too much caffeine, referred to as caffeine intoxication, causes nervousness, anxiety, restlessness, insomnia, gastrointestinal upset, tremors, increased blood pressure, and rapid heartbeat. Numerous cases of caffeine-associated death, seizure, and cardiac arrest have occurred after consumption of energy drinks.[47–49] Even if the caffeine in an energy drink increases endurance, depending on when it is consumed, it can also affect timing and coordination and hurt overall performance. These effects are of particular concern because a recent *Consumer Reports* analysis found that approximately one-third of reviewed energy drinks contained caffeine levels significantly higher than were declared on their labels.[50] Caffeine is also a diuretic; at the levels contained in these drinks, it may contribute to dehydration, particularly in first-time users. Because of caffeine's potential for toxicity at high doses, Health Canada is currently considering limiting the amount of caffeine in these beverages to a maximum level of 180 mg per container, regardless of size.[51]

Energy drinks often contain other ingredients that promise to improve performance, such as B vitamins, taurine, guarana, and ginseng. B vitamins are needed to produce ATP, so they are marketed to enhance energy production from sugar. But unless you are deficient in these vitamins, drinking them in an energy drink will not enhance your ATP production. Taurine is an amino acid that may reduce the amount of muscle damage and improve exercise performance and capacity, but not all research supports these claims.[52] Guarana is an herbal ingredient that contains caffeine and small amounts of the stimulants theobromine and theophylline. The extra caffeine from guarana (which is not included in the caffeine content listed for these beverages) may contribute to caffeine toxicity. Ginseng is also claimed to have performance-enhancing effects, but these effects have not been demonstrated scientifically.[52] In general, the amounts of these ingredients are too small to have much effect, and the safety of consuming them in combination with caffeine prior to or during exercise has yet to be established.[52]

Ask Yourself

a. So should you down an energy drink before your next competition? They do provide a caffeine boost, but is it so much caffeine that you also risk dehydration, high blood pressure, and heart problems?

b. Energy drinks provide sugar to fuel activity, but will they upset your stomach? What about the herbal ingredients—do they offer a benefit you are looking for?

---

achieved: Increased muscle creatine permits greater training intensity, which leads to greater muscle hypertrophy.[41]

Long-term creatine supplementation appears to be safe at intakes of up to 5 g per day, but the safety of higher doses over the long term has not been established.[42] Ingestion of creatine before or during exercise is not recommended, and Health Canada has advised that consumers, especially those who are pregnant, consult a physician before using creatine.

Supplements to Enhance Endurance

Sprinters and weightlifters can benefit from increases in creatine phosphate levels, but endurance athletes are more concerned about running out of glycogen. Glycogen is spared when fat is used as an energy source, allowing exercise to continue for a longer time before glycogen is depleted and fatigue sets in. Supplements that increase the amount of fat or oxygen available to the muscle cell are used to increase endurance.

Carnitine supplements are marketed as fat burners—substances that increase the utilization of fat during exercise. Carnitine is needed to transport fatty acids into the mitochondria, where they are used to produce ATP by aerobic metabolism. However, enough carnitine is made in the body to ensure efficient use of fatty acids. Carnitine supplements have not been shown to increase endurance.[43]

Medium-chain triglycerides (MCT) are composed of fatty acids with medium-length carbon chains (8 to 10 carbons). These fatty acids can be absorbed directly into the blood without first being incorporated into chylomicrons. They are therefore absorbed quickly, causing blood fatty acids levels to rise and thereby increasing the availability of fat as a fuel for exercise. Nevertheless, research has not found that supplementation with MCT increases endurance, spares glycogen, or enhances performance.[44]

Caffeine is a stimulant found in coffee, tea, some soft drinks, and energy drinks (see *Debate: Energy Drinks and Performance*).[45] Consuming 3 to 6 mg of caffeine per kilogram of body weight, an amount equivalent to about half a litre of percolated coffee, up to an hour before exercising and then consuming smaller doses of caffeine during exercise (1 to 2 mg/kg) has been shown to improve endurance.[40] Caffeine enhances the release of fatty acids. When fatty acids are used as a fuel source, less glycogen is used, and the onset of fatigue is delayed. Athletes who are unaccustomed to caffeine respond better than those who consume it routinely. Caffeine also improves concentration and enhances alertness, but in some athletes, it may impair performance by causing gastrointestinal upset.

Caffeine may be effective, but consuming excess caffeine before a competition is illegal. The International Olympic Committee prohibits athletes from competing when caffeine levels in the urine are 12 μg/mL or greater. For urine caffeine to reach this level, an individual would need to drink six to eight cups of coffee in a two-hour period. Caffeine is also found in pill form; NoDoz contains about 100 mg of caffeine per tablet—about the same amount as in a cup of coffee.

Athletes have also used the hormone erythropoietin, known as EPO, to enhance endurance. Natural erythropoietin is produced by the kidneys and stimulates cells in the bone marrow to differentiate into red blood cells. EPO can enhance endurance by increasing the ability to transport oxygen to the muscles. It therefore increases aerobic capacity and spares glycogen. However, too much EPO can cause production of too many red blood cells, which can lead to excessive blood clotting, heart attacks, and strokes. EPO was banned in 1990, after it was linked to the deaths of more than a dozen cyclists.[53] However, cyclists and other athletes continue to use EPO illegally.

Recently, various sports—cycling in particular—have seen a crackdown on the use of performance-enhancing supplements. Also, it has been discovered that many of the competitors in previous Tour de France competitions used banned substances to enhance their performance, including the famous American athlete, Lance Armstrong. As we continue to learn more details about the extent of the doping controversy, one thing is for certain: the tolerance for cyclists who use these illegal substances is decreasing substantially, and much shame has been brought to these athletes and their sport because of the ongoing scandal.

Other Supplements

In addition to the supplements discussed thus far, hundreds of other products are marketed to athletes, although most have no effect on performance. For example, brewer's yeast is a source of B vitamins and some minerals but has not been found to have any ergogenic properties. Likewise, no evidence has been found to support claims that bee pollen or wheat germ oil enhance performance. Royal jelly, a substance that worker bees produce to help the queen bee grow larger and live longer, does not appear to enhance athletic capacity in humans. Supplements of DNA and RNA are marketed to aid in tissue regeneration. DNA and RNA are needed to synthesize proteins, but are not required in the diet, and DNA and RNA supplements do not help replace damaged cells.

Herbal products are also marketed to athletes. Most have not been studied extensively for their ergogenic effects, so the evidence of their benefits is only anecdotal. Because many herbs can harm both health and performance, athletes should consider the risks before using these products.

CONCEPT CHECK

1. **How** do anabolic hormones affect the production of testosterone?
2. **Why** are creatine supplements not helpful for endurance athletes?
3. **How** does EPO affect performance?

Summary

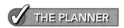

1 Physical Activity, Fitness, and Health 346

- Regular exercise improves **fitness**. An individual's level of fitness depends on his or her **cardiorespiratory endurance**, **muscle strength**, **muscle endurance**, flexibility, and body composition.

- Regular exercise can reduce the risk of chronic diseases such as obesity, heart disease, diabetes, and osteoporosis. It can also reduce overall mortality even in obese individuals.

- Exercise helps manage body weight by increasing energy expenditure and by increasing the proportion of body weight that is lean tissue.

The components of fitness • Figure 10.1

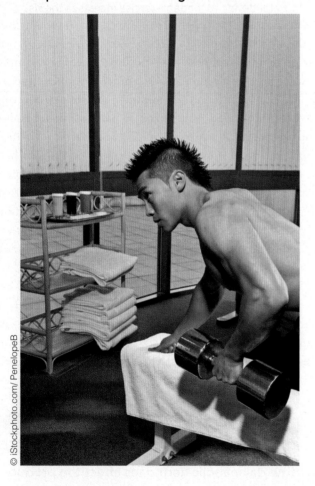

© iStockphoto.com/ PenelopeB

2 Exercise Recommendations 350

- Health Canada recommends 150 minutes of moderate to vigorous physical activity per week, accumulated in intervals of 10 minutes or more. A well-designed fitness program involves aerobic exercise, stretching, and strength-training exercises.

- An exercise program should include activities that are enjoyable, convenient, and safe. Rest is important to allow the body to recover and rebuild. In serious athletes, inadequate rest can lead to **overtraining syndrome**.

Calculating your aerobic zone • Figure 10.5

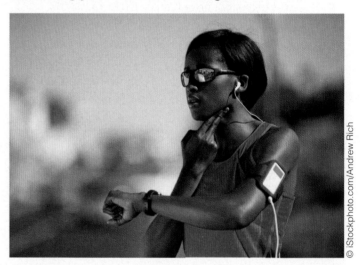

© iStockphoto.com/Andrew Rich

3 Fuelling Exercise 354

- During the first 10 to 15 seconds of exercise, ATP and **creatine phosphate** stored in the muscle provide energy to fuel activity. During the next two to three minutes, the amount of oxygen at the muscle remains limited, so ATP is generated by the **anaerobic metabolism** of glucose. After a few minutes, the delivery of oxygen at the muscle increases, and ATP can be generated by **aerobic metabolism**. Aerobic metabolism is more efficient than anaerobic metabolism and can utilize glucose, fatty acids, and amino acids as energy sources. The use of protein as an energy source increases when exercise continues for many hours.

- For short-term, high-intensity activity, ATP is generated primarily from the anaerobic metabolism of glucose from glycogen stores. Anaerobic metabolism uses glucose more rapidly and produces **lactic acid**. Both of these factors are associated with the onset of **fatigue**. For lower-intensity exercise of longer duration, aerobic metabolism predominates, and both glucose and fatty acids are important fuel sources.

- Fitness training causes changes in the cardiovascular system and muscles that improve oxygen delivery and utilization, allowing aerobic exercise to be sustained for longer periods at higher intensity.

Changes in the source of ATP over time • Figure 10.9

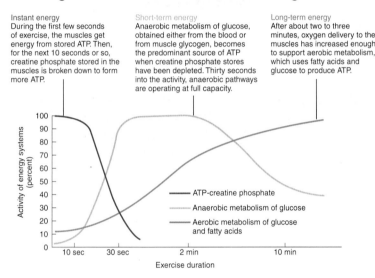

Instant energy
During the first few seconds of exercise, the muscles get energy from stored ATP. Then, for the next 10 seconds or so, creatine phosphate stored in the muscles is broken down to form more ATP.

Short-term energy
Anaerobic metabolism of glucose, obtained either from the blood or from muscle glycogen, becomes the predominant source of ATP when creatine phosphate stores have been depleted. Thirty seconds into the activity, anaerobic pathways are operating at full capacity.

Long-term energy
After about two to three minutes, oxygen delivery to the muscles has increased enough to support aerobic metabolism, which uses fatty acids and glucose to produce ATP.

- ATP-creatine phosphate
- Anaerobic metabolism of glucose
- Aerobic metabolism of glucose and fatty acids

4 Energy and Nutrient Needs for Physical Activity 361

- The diet of an active individual should provide sufficient energy to fuel activity. The pressure to compete and maintain a body weight that is optimal for their sport puts some athletes at risk for eating disorders. A combination of excessive exercise and energy restriction puts female athletes at risk for the **female athlete triad**.

- To maximize glycogen stores, optimize performance, and maintain and repair lean tissue, a diet providing about 60% of energy from carbohydrate, 20 to 25% of energy from fat, and about 15 to 20% of energy from protein is recommended.

- Sufficient vitamins and minerals are needed to generate ATP from macronutrients to maintain and repair tissues and to transport oxygen and wastes to and from the cells. Most athletes who consume a varied diet that meets their energy needs are also able to meet their vitamin and mineral needs. Those who restrict their food intake may be at risk for deficiencies. Fitness training increases the body's iron losses and leads to increased iron needs, which put many athletes, particularly female athletes, at risk for iron deficiency.

- Water is needed to ensure that the body can be cooled and that nutrients and oxygen can be delivered to body tissues. If water intake is inadequate, dehydration can lead to a decline in exercise performance and increase the risk of **heat-related illness**. Adequate fluid intake before exercise ensures that athletes begin their exercise well hydrated. Fluid intake during and after exercise must replace water lost in sweat and from evaporation through the lungs. Plain water is an appropriate fluid to consume for most exercise. Beverages containing carbohydrate and sodium are recommended for exercise lasting more than an hour. Drinking plain water during extended exercise increases the risk of hyponatremia.

- Competitive endurance athletes may benefit from **glycogen supercompensation (carbohydrate loading)**, which maximizes glycogen stores before an event. Meals eaten before competition should help ensure adequate hydration, provide moderate amounts of protein, be high enough in carbohydrate to maximize glycogen stores, be low in fat and fibre to speed gastric emptying, and satisfy the psychological needs of the athlete. During exercise, athletes need beverages and food to replace lost fluid and provide carbohydrate and sodium. Post-competition meals should replace lost fluids and electrolytes, provide carbohydrate to restore muscle and liver glycogen, and provide protein for muscle protein synthesis and repair.

Dietary carbohydrate and endurance • Figure 10.21

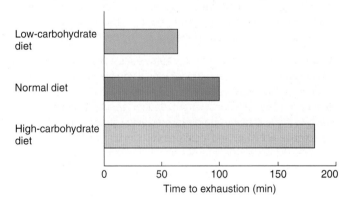

5 Ergogenic Aids   370

- Many types of **ergogenic aids** are marketed to improve athletic performance. Some are beneficial for certain types of activity, but many offer little or no benefit. Athletes should use an individual risk–benefit analysis to determine whether taking a supplement is appropriate.

- **Anabolic steroids** combined with resistance-training exercise increase muscle size and strength, but these supplements are illegal and have dangerous side effects.

- **Creatine** supplementation has been shown to improve performance in short-duration, high-intensity exercise. Caffeine use can improve performance in endurance activities, but high doses are illegal during athletic competitions.

Creatine boosts creatine phosphate • Figure 10.24

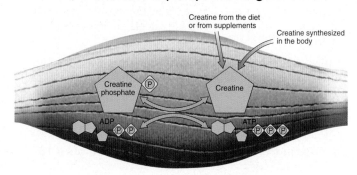

Key Terms

- aerobic capacity 346
- aerobic exercise 346
- aerobic metabolism 355
- aerobic zone 352
- anabolic steroids 372
- anaerobic metabolism 355
- cardiorespiratory endurance 346
- creatine 373

- creatine phosphate 356
- endorphins 348
- ergogenic aid 370
- fatigue 359
- female athlete triad 362
- fitness 346
- glycogen supercompensation or carbohydrate loading 367
- heat cramps 365

- heat exhaustion 365
- heat stroke 365
- heat-related illnesses 365
- lactic acid 355
- maximum heart rate 352
- muscle endurance 346
- muscle strength 346
- overload principle 347

- overtraining syndrome 354
- sports anemia 364
- steroid precursors 373
- strength-training exercise or resistance-training exercise 346

Critical and Creative Thinking

1. On the way to an out-of-town soccer match, Diego's team stops at a fast-food restaurant. It is only about an hour before game time. Most of the boys have burgers, fries, and a soft drink. How might this food affect their performance in the game? What do you recommend they do differently for the next match?

2. Evaluate your weekly physical activity. Does it meet the current exercise recommendations? Would you classify yourself as sedentary, low active, active, or very active? Do you include activities to enhance your strength, endurance, and flexibility? Can each of these activities be performed year-round? If not, suggest alternative activities and locations you can use during inclement weather. How can you improve on what you are currently doing?

3. Given that aerobic metabolism depends on the availability of oxygen, suggest an experiment to determine an athlete's aerobic capacity.

4. Use your knowledge of energy production and body energy stores to explain why during exercise cells rely more on glucose and fat for energy than on protein.

5. Two friends are running a marathon together. One participated in an intensive training program. The other was too busy and trained only a few hours a week. After about five minutes of running the marathon, they have settled into a slow, steady pace and are able to carry on a conversation. After an hour, the well-trained friend is feeling good and increases her pace. The untrained friend tries to keep up but is no longer able to talk, and after about 15 minutes is fatigued and needs to stop. Why does the untrained person tire faster?

6. David is beginning an exercise program. He plans to run before lunch and then play racquetball every night after dinner. When he begins his exercise program, he finds that he feels lethargic and hungry before his late-morning run. After running, he doesn't have much of an appetite, so he saves his lunch until mid-afternoon. He is still hungry enough to eat dinner at home with his family but finds that when he goes to play racquetball, he has stomach cramps and feels too full. His typical diet consists of the following:

     Breakfast: Orange juice, coffee

     Lunch: Ham and cheese sandwich, potato chips, soft drink, cookies

Dinner: Steak, baked potato with sour cream and butter, green beans in butter sauce, salad with Italian dressing, whole milk

How can David change his diet to better suit his exercise program? Do you think David will be able to stick with this exercise program? Why or why not? Suggest some changes to make David's exercise program more convenient and more balanced.

7. Use the Internet to do a risk–benefit analysis of an ergogenic aid. List the risks and benefits, then write a conclusion, stating why you would or would not take this substance.

What is happening in this picture?

During competitive events, cyclists often ride their bikes for six or more hours a day. This rider is collecting water bottles from his team's car. He will carry these ahead and deliver them to the other cyclists on his team.

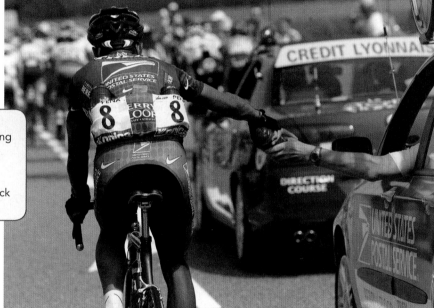

Think Critically

1. How much might someone need to drink during six hours of cycling?
2. What type of fluid do you think is in the water bottles? Why?
3. What type of food might the riders want to pick up from their team car?

Doug Pensinger/Staff/Getty Images Sport/Getty Images, Inc.

Self-Test

(Check your answers in Appendix J.)

1. Which bar indicates the proportion of energy obtained from glucose, fatty acids, and amino acids that is suitable to be used as fuel while studying for an exam?

  a. A   b. B   c. C

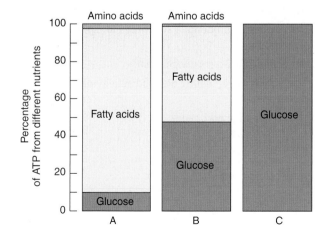

2. Which of the following statements about aerobic exercise is false?

  a. It increases heart rate.

  b. It requires oxygen in metabolism.

  c. It can use fat as a fuel.

  d. It is performed at an intensity low enough to carry on a conversation.

  e. It includes activities such as weightlifting and sprinting.

3. If an athlete loses a lot of water and salt in sweat but drinks only water, he is at risk for _____.

  a. hypertension

  b. hypodermic

  c. hyperactivity

  d. hyponatremia

  e. dehydration

4. Andreas is 30 years old. He would like to exercise at an intensity that ensures he is in his aerobic zone. Use the following graph to determine the heart rate range that is appropriate for Andreas.

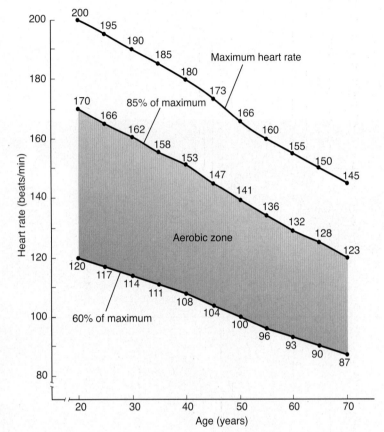

a. 114 to 162
b. 114 to 190
c. 120 to 170
d. 87 to 120
e. 123 to 170

5. The source of fuel in the first few seconds of exercise is
_____.
a. ATP and creatine phosphate
b. stored glycogen
c. glucose made by the liver
d. fatty acids
e. protein

6. Which statement is true of the energy system indicated by the arrow?

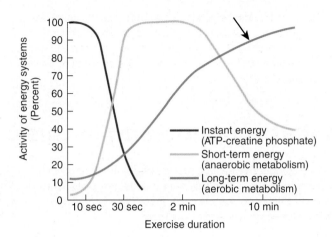

a. It provides energy for the first 10 to 15 seconds of activity.
b. It can use glucose, amino acids, and fatty acids to produce ATP.
c. It produces ATP rapidly but inefficiently.
d. It can use only glucose to generate ATP.

7. Which nutrient can be used to produce energy in the absence of oxygen?
a. protein
b. fatty acids
c. glucose
d. B vitamins
e. lactic acid

8. The female athlete triad consists of _____.
a. iron deficiency anemia, disordered eating, and excess menstrual blood loss
b. disordered eating, amenorrhea, and osteoporosis
c. dieting, excessive exercise, and folate deficiency
d. iron, calcium, and zinc deficiency

9. Which of the following statements about carbohydrate loading is false?
a. It provides a competitive advantage for sprinters and weightlifters.
b. It causes short-term weight gain.
c. It involves manipulating diet and activity patterns before an event.
d. It can enhance endurance.

10. Which of the following is a goal of pre-competition meals?

    a. maximizing fat stores

    b. increasing muscle mass

    c. keeping the stomach full

    d. maximizing glycogen

11. True or false: A fit person will have a higher percentage of lean tissue than an unfit person of the same body weight.

    a. True

    b. False

12. The best fluid to consume during a marathon is _____.

    a. plain water

    b. fruit juice

    c. a sports drink containing glucose and sodium

    d. a protein shake

13. Which best describes how creatine supplements might enhance performance?

    a. They increase the amount of creatine phosphate in the muscle.

    b. They increase the transport of fatty acids into the mitochondria.

    c. They increase delivery of oxygen to the muscle.

    d. They eliminate free radicals.

14. How much and how often should athletes drink during exercise?

    a. as much as they can

    b. enough to prevent weight loss

    c. 250 mL every hour

    d. nothing unless exercise lasts more than 60 minutes

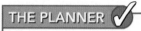

THE PLANNER ✓

Review your Chapter Planner on the chapter opener and check off your completed work.

Nutrition during Pregnancy and Infancy

Healthy nutritional practices are critical for optimal functioning throughout life, from conception to old age. To meet nutritional needs and promote overall health, a diet should be rich in natural foods, such as vegetables, fruits, and lean proteins, and moderate in fats and overall calories. This dietary pattern is also appropriate for pregnant women, but they also have other special considerations.

Nutrition in early life is critical to the future health of a child. For instance, overnutrition during pregnancy may result in a larger baby and may increase that baby's future risk for such chronic diseases as obesity and type-2 diabetes. On the other hand, inadequate nutrition during pregnancy produces an undernourished infant who may never catch up to its healthy peers.

Factors that can compromise fetal nutrition include low maternal weight gain, lack of prenatal visits, obesity, and major chronic illnesses in the mother. Nutrient deficiencies and excesses can also negatively affect a fetus. For example, insufficient iodine during pregnancy has been linked to brain damage in the baby; insufficient iron creates an increased risk of anemia; and excessive vitamin A causes an increased risk of birth defects of the head, face, heart, and brain. Eating a balanced and moderate diet can help prevent these defects.

The responsibility of the mother does not stop when the infant is born. The 40 weeks of a pregnancy produce a needy newborn who requires a lengthy period of care. Breast milk provides optimal nutrition for a growing infant, and a breastfeeding mother's diet continues to affect the nutrition of her child. In addition, the quality of infant nutrition can affect both growth in the early years and the potential for developing chronic diseases later in life.

Having a healthy pregnancy is one of the first and most important steps a mother can take to ensure her child leads a healthy and enjoyable life.

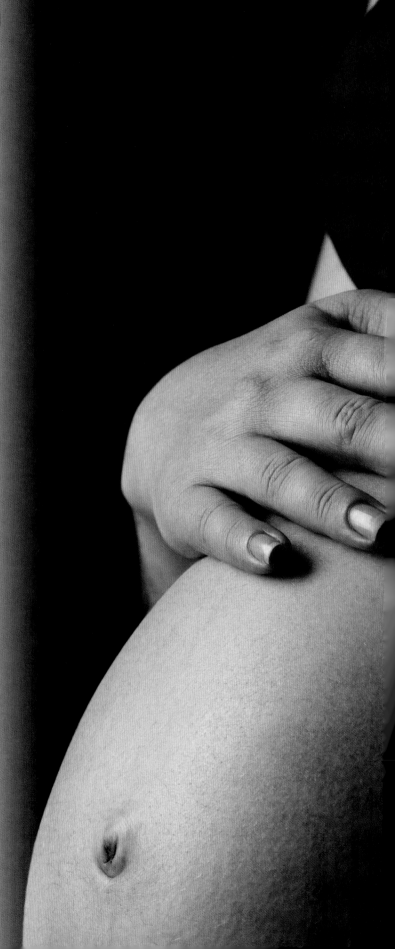

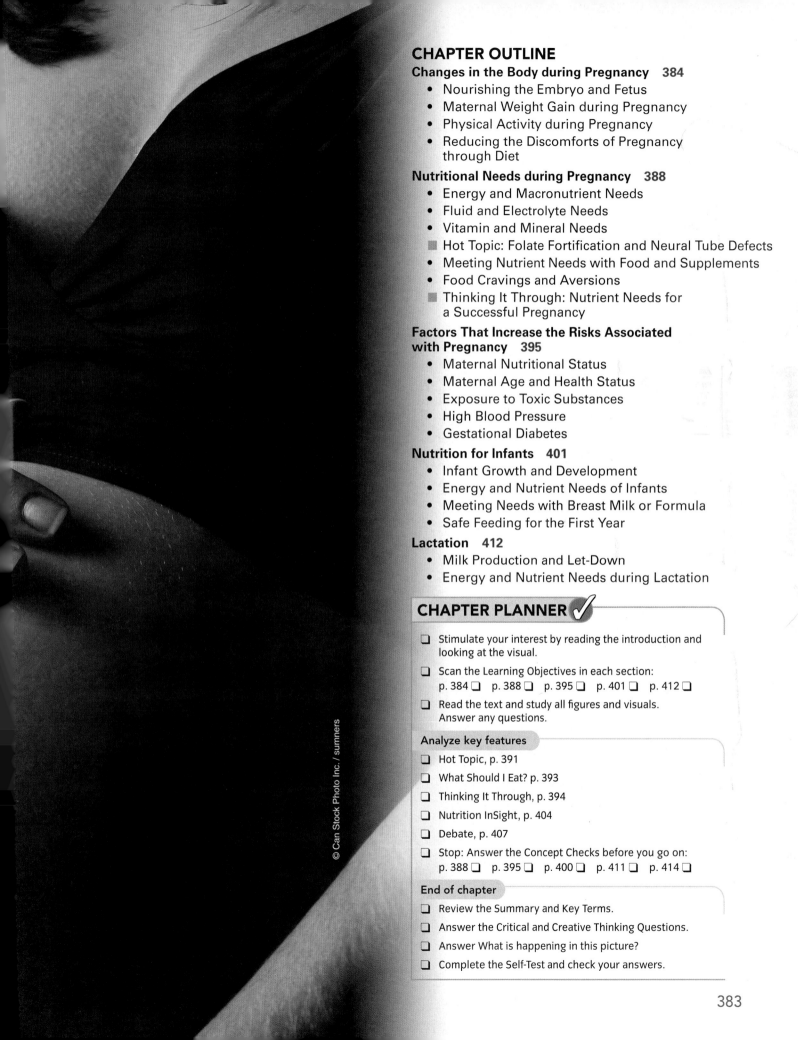

CHAPTER OUTLINE

CHAPTER PLANNER ✓

- ❑ Stimulate your interest by reading the introduction and looking at the visual.
- ❑ Scan the Learning Objectives in each section:
  p. 384 ❑   p. 388 ❑   p. 395 ❑   p. 401 ❑   p. 412 ❑
- ❑ Read the text and study all figures and visuals. Answer any questions.

Analyze key features

- ❑ Hot Topic, p. 391
- ❑ What Should I Eat? p. 393
- ❑ Thinking It Through, p. 394
- ❑ Nutrition InSight, p. 404
- ❑ Debate, p. 407
- ❑ Stop: Answer the Concept Checks before you go on:
  p. 388 ❑   p. 395 ❑   p. 400 ❑   p. 411 ❑   p. 414 ❑

End of chapter

- ❑ Review the Summary and Key Terms.
- ❑ Answer the Critical and Creative Thinking Questions.
- ❑ Answer What is happening in this picture?
- ❑ Complete the Self-Test and check your answers.

© Can Stock Photo Inc. / sumners

Changes in the Body during Pregnancy

LEARNING OBJECTIVES

1. **Describe** how the embryo and fetus are nourished.

2. **Discuss** why modest weight gain is important during pregnancy.

3. **Explain** why morning sickness, heartburn, and constipation are common during pregnancy.

W hether we end up with a height of 193 cm (6′4″) or 160 cm (5′3″), we all began as a single cell that resulted from the union of a sperm and an egg. Over the course of about 40 weeks, this cell grew and developed into a fully formed human baby. Prenatal growth and development are carefully orchestrated processes that require adequate supplies of all the essential nutrients to progress normally.

In the days after **fertilization**, the single cell divides rapidly to form a ball of cells. The cells then begin to differentiate and move to form body structures. During these early steps in development, this ball of cells obtains the nutrients it needs from the fluids around it.

> **fertilization** The union of a sperm and an egg.

About a week after fertilization, the developing embryo begins burrowing into the lining of the uterus, and by two weeks, **implantation** is complete and it is now an **embryo**.

Nourishing the Embryo and Fetus

The embryonic stage of development lasts until the eighth week after fertilization. During this time, the cells differentiate to form the multitude of specialized cell types that make up the human body. At the end of this stage, the embryo is about 3 cm long and has a beating heart. The fundamentals of all major external and internal body structures have been formed.

The early embryo receives its nourishment by breaking down the lining of the uterus, but this source is soon inadequate to meet its growing needs. After about five weeks, the **placenta** takes over the role of nourishing the embryo (**Figure 11.1**). The placenta also secretes hormones that are necessary to maintain pregnancy.

> **implantation** The process by which a developing embryo embeds itself in the uterine lining.
>
> **embryo** The developing human from two through eight weeks after fertilization.

> **placenta** An organ produced from maternal and embryonic tissues. It secretes hormones, transfers nutrients and oxygen from the mother's blood to the fetus, and removes metabolic wastes.

The placenta • Figure 11.1

The placenta is made up of branchlike projections that extend from the embryo into the uterine lining, placing maternal and fetal blood in close proximity. The placenta allows nutrients and oxygen to pass from maternal blood to fetal blood and waste products to be transferred from fetal blood to maternal blood. Fetal blood travels to and from the placenta via the umbilical cord.

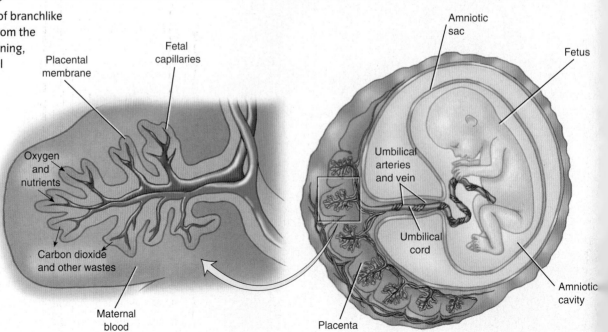

From the ninth week on, the developing offspring is a **fetus**. During the fetal period, structures formed during the embryonic period grow and mature. The placenta continues to nourish the fetus until birth. During this time, the length of the fetus increases from about 3 cm to around 50 cm. The fetal period usually ends after 40 weeks with the birth of an infant weighing 3 to 4 kg (6.5 to 8.8 lb.).[1]

> **fetus** A developing human from the ninth week after fertilization to birth.

Unfortunately, not all pregnancies go according to plan, and some infants are born too small or too early. Infants who are born on time but have failed to grow well in the uterus are said to be **small for gestational age**. Those born before 37 weeks of gestation are said to be **preterm**, or **premature**. Both of these situations can occur for a variety of reasons, including poor maternal nutrition. Whether born too soon or too small, **low-birth-weight** infants and **very-low-birth-weight** infants are at increased risk for illness and early death (**Figure 11.2**).[2]

> **low birth weight** A birth weight less than 2.5 kg (5.5 lb.).
>
> **very low birth weight** A birth weight less than 1.5 kg (3.3 lb.).

Low-birth-weight infants • Figure 11.2

Low-birth-weight and very-low-birth-weight infants require special care and a special diet so they can continue to grow and develop. Today, with advances in medical and nutritional care, infants born as early as 25 weeks of gestation and those weighing as little as 1 kg (2.2 lb.) can survive.

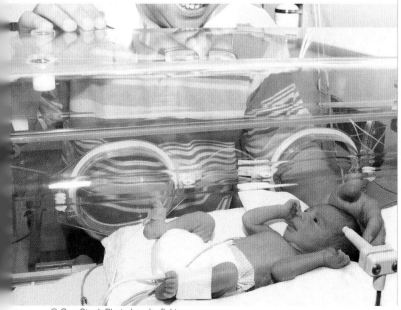

© Can Stock Photo Inc. / reflekta

Maternal Weight Gain during Pregnancy

During pregnancy, a woman's body undergoes many changes to support the growth and development of her child. Her blood volume increases by 50%. The placenta develops to allow nutrients to be delivered to the fetus and to produce hormones that orchestrate other changes in the mother's body. The amount of body fat increases to provide the energy needed late in pregnancy. The uterus enlarges, muscles and ligaments relax to accommodate the growing fetus and allow for childbirth, and the breasts develop in preparation for **lactation**. All these changes naturally result in weight gain (**Figure 11.3a**), but a woman's weight during pregnancy

> **lactation** Production and secretion of milk.

should not increase too excessively; otherwise, both she and her child may experience complications during and after pregnancy.

Some women take the saying "eating for two" a little too literally and believe a significant increase in caloric intake and weight is acceptable or perhaps even healthy. Although a pregnant woman will have an increased need for food, this food should be consumed moderately. After the third month of pregnancy, Health Canada recommends increasing daily food intake by *only* two or three food guide servings.[3] Eating beyond this level may lead to unhealthy weight gain, which leads to future complications not only for the mother but also for the child. A healthy, normal-weight woman should gain 11 to 16 kg (25 to 35 lb.) during pregnancy.[4] The rate of weight gain is as important as the amount gained. Little gain is expected in the first three months, or **trimester**—usually about 0.9 to 1.8 kg (2 to 4 lb.). In the second and third trimesters, the recommended maternal weight gain is about 0.5 kg (1 lb.) per week. All pregnant women should gain weight at a slow, steady rate, but the recommended weight gain for women who are underweight and women who are overweight or obese at conception is, respectively, higher and lower than for normal-weight women (**Figure 11.3b**).[1,4,5]

Being underweight by 10% or more at the onset of pregnancy or gaining too little weight during pregnancy will increase the risk of producing a low-birth-weight baby.[6] Excess weight, whether present before conception or gained during pregnancy, can also compromise pregnancy outcome. Excess weight increases the mother's risks for high blood pressure, diabetes, a difficult delivery, and the need for a **Caesarean section**; it also increases the risk of

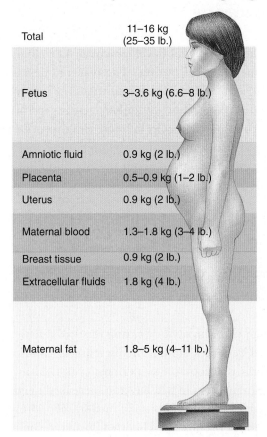

Total	11–16 kg (25–35 lb.)
Fetus	3–3.6 kg (6.6–8 lb.)
Amniotic fluid	0.9 kg (2 lb.)
Placenta	0.5–0.9 kg (1–2 lb.)
Uterus	0.9 kg (2 lb.)
Maternal blood	1.3–1.8 kg (3–4 lb.)
Breast tissue	0.9 kg (2 lb.)
Extracellular fluids	1.8 kg (4 lb.)
Maternal fat	1.8–5 kg (4–11 lb.)

b. Although a similar pattern of weight gain is recommended for women who, at the start of pregnancy, are normal weight, underweight, overweight, or obese, their recommendations for total weight gain differ.[1]

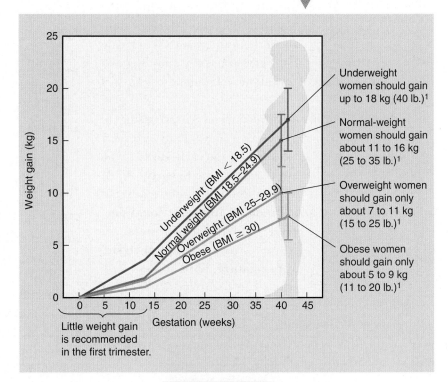

Underweight women should gain up to 18 kg (40 lb.)[1]

Normal-weight women should gain about 11 to 16 kg (25 to 35 lb.)[1]

Overweight women should gain only about 7 to 11 kg (15 to 25 lb.)[1]

Obese women should gain only about 5 to 9 kg (11 to 20 lb.)[1]

Little weight gain is recommended in the first trimester.

a. The weight of an infant at birth accounts for about 25% of total weight gain during pregnancy. The balance of weight gain is accounted for by the placenta, amniotic fluid, and changes in maternal tissues, including enlargement of the uterus and breasts, expansion of the volume of blood and other extracellular fluids, and increased fat stores.

Interpreting Data

How much weight should be gained during pregnancy by a woman with a BMI of 27?

---

large for gestational age
Weighing more than 4 kg (8.8 lb.) at birth.

having a **large-for-gestational-age** baby.[7] Excessive prenatal weight gain also increases the mother's long-term risk for obesity; and mounting evidence suggests it may also increase the risk that the baby will be overweight in childhood and later in life.[8-10] This effect—of a mother gaining too much weight during pregnancy, thereby increasing her offspring's risk for obesity—has been termed "the developmental origin of obesity."[10] However, dieting during pregnancy is not advised, even for obese women. If possible, excess weight should be lost before the pregnancy begins or, alternatively, after the child has been born and weaned.

Physical Activity during Pregnancy

In terms of overall health, physical activity goes hand in hand with proper nutrition; this guideline is typically also true during pregnancy. In the past, pregnant women were sometimes advised to avoid physical activity for fears that it could hurt the developing fetus. We now know that moderate physical activity can be beneficial to both the pregnant mother and her offspring. Physical activity during pregnancy can improve digestion, mood, and self-image; reduce stress; prevent excess weight gain, low back pain, and constipation; reduce the risk of diabetes and high blood pressure; and speed recovery from childbirth.[4] Guidelines have been developed to maximize the benefits of exercise during pregnancy and minimize the risks of injury to mother and fetus. In general, women who were physically active before becoming pregnant can continue a program of about 30 minutes of carefully chosen moderate exercise per day, making changes where appropriate.[4,11] Women who weren't active before pregnancy should slowly add low-intensity, low-impact activities, such as swimming, walking, and prenatal yoga.[11] These changes can help ensure a healthy pregnancy, lower the risk of weight gain, improve how the mother feels, and set the stage for the long-term adoption of an active lifestyle.[4] Because intense exercise can limit the delivery of oxygen and nutrients to the fetus, intense exercise should be limited.

Reducing the Discomforts of Pregnancy through Diet

The physiological changes that occur during pregnancy can cause uncomfortable side effects.

During the first trimester of pregnancy, many women experience nausea and vomiting, which is referred to as **morning sickness**, although symptoms can occur at any time during the day or night. Morning sickness is thought to be related to hormones that are released early in pregnancy. Unfortunately, the acidic nature of the vomit associated with the condition can lead to tooth decay in the mother. After an episode has occurred, women should therefore rinse their mouth with water or fluoride.[4] The symptoms of morning sickness may be alleviated by eating small, frequent snacks of dry, starchy foods, such as plain crackers or bread. In most women, the symptoms of morning sickness decrease significantly after the first trimester, but, for some women, the symptoms last for the entire pregnancy and, in severe cases, women may require intravenous nutrition.

The hormones produced during pregnancy to relax the uterine muscles also relax the muscles of the gastrointestinal tract. This relaxation, along with crowding of the organs by the growing baby, can cause heartburn and constipation (**Figure 11.4**). Heartburn can be reduced

Crowding of the gastrointestinal tract • Figure 11.4

During pregnancy, the uterus enlarges and pushes higher into the abdominal cavity, exerting pressure on the stomach and intestines.

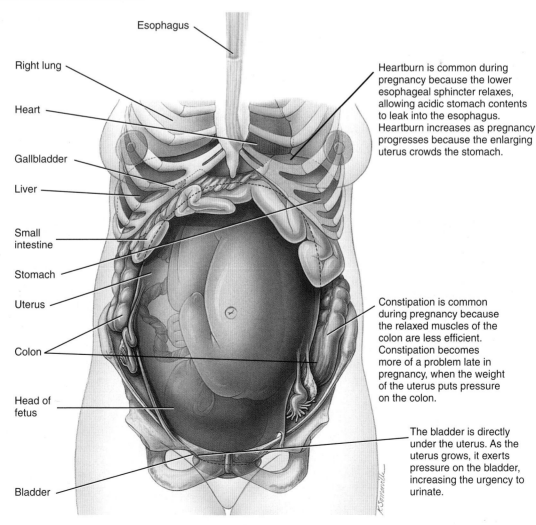

Esophagus

Right lung

Heart

Gallbladder

Liver

Small intestine

Stomach

Uterus

Colon

Head of fetus

Bladder

Heartburn is common during pregnancy because the lower esophageal sphincter relaxes, allowing acidic stomach contents to leak into the esophagus. Heartburn increases as pregnancy progresses because the enlarging uterus crowds the stomach.

Constipation is common during pregnancy because the relaxed muscles of the colon are less efficient. Constipation becomes more of a problem late in pregnancy, when the weight of the uterus puts pressure on the colon.

The bladder is directly under the uterus. As the uterus grows, it exerts pressure on the bladder, increasing the urgency to urinate.

by limiting high-fat foods, which leave the stomach slow-ly; avoiding foods containing substances that are known to cause heartburn, such as caffeine and chocolate; eating small, frequent meals; and remaining upright after eating. Constipation can be prevented by maintaining a moderate level of physical activity and consuming plenty of fluids and high-fibre foods. Hemorrhoids are common during pregnancy as a result of both constipation and changes in blood flow.

CONCEPT CHECK

1. **How** are nutrients and oxygen transferred from mother to fetus?

2. **How** does a mother's weight during pregnancy affect the birth weight of her child?

3. **Why** do heartburn and constipation tend to increase later in pregnancy?

Nutritional Needs during Pregnancy

LEARNING OBJECTIVES

1. **Compare** the energy and protein needs of pregnant and non-pregnant women.
2. **Explain** why pregnancy increases the need for many vitamins and minerals.
3. **Discuss** the use of dietary supplements during pregnancy.

During pregnancy, the mother's diet must provide all of her nutrients in addition to those nutrients needed for the baby's growth and development. Because the increase in nutrient needs is greater than the increase in caloric needs, a nutrient-dense diet is essential.

Energy and Macronutrient Needs

Although pregnant women are eating for two, they don't need to eat twice as much as they normally do. During the first trimester, energy needs are not increased from the recommended levels for non-pregnant women. During the second and third trimesters, an additional two to three food guide servings per day are recommended (**Figure 11.5**).[3]

During pregnancy, women should consume more protein, which is needed for the synthesis of new blood cells, formation of the placenta, enlargement of the uterus and breasts, and growth of the baby (**Figure 11.6**). An additional 25 g of

Energy and macronutrient recommendations • Figure 11.5

This graph illustrates the percentage increase above non-pregnant levels in the recommended daily intake of energy, protein, carbohydrate, fibre, essential fatty acids, and water for a 25-year-old pregnant woman in her third trimester.

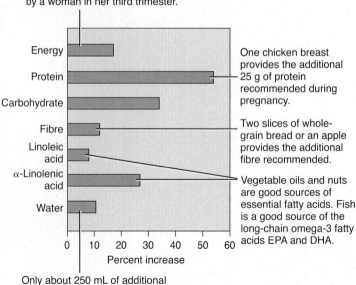

A snack of a sandwich, an apple, and a glass of milk will easily add the extra calories needed by a woman in her third trimester.

One chicken breast provides the additional 25 g of protein recommended during pregnancy.

Two slices of whole-grain bread or an apple provides the additional fibre recommended.

Vegetable oils and nuts are good sources of essential fatty acids. Fish is a good source of the long-chain omega-3 fatty acids EPA and DHA.

Only about 250 mL of additional water is needed per day.

Micronutrient needs during pregnancy • Figure 11.6

The graph illustrates the percentage increase in recommended micronutrient intakes for a 25-year-old woman during the third trimester of pregnancy.

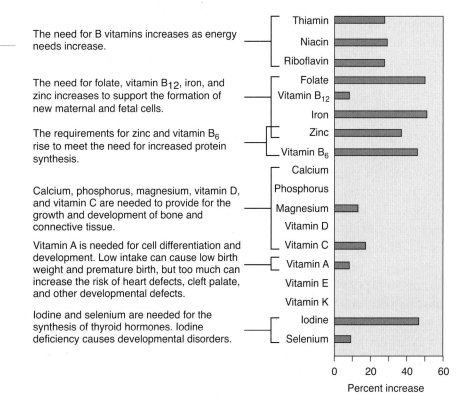

The need for B vitamins increases as energy needs increase.

The need for folate, vitamin B_{12}, iron, and zinc increases to support the formation of new maternal and fetal cells.

The requirements for zinc and vitamin B_6 rise to meet the need for increased protein synthesis.

Calcium, phosphorus, magnesium, vitamin D, and vitamin C are needed to provide for the growth and development of bone and connective tissue.

Vitamin A is needed for cell differentiation and development. Low intake can cause low birth weight and premature birth, but too much can increase the risk of heart defects, cleft palate, and other developmental defects.

Iodine and selenium are needed for the synthesis of thyroid hormones. Iodine deficiency causes developmental disorders.

protein above the recommended daily allowance (RDA) for non-pregnant women, or 1.1 g/kg/day, is recommended for the second and third trimesters of pregnancy.

To ensure sufficient glucose to fuel the fetal and maternal brains during pregnancy, the RDA for carbohydrate is increased by 45 g, to 175 g/day. If this carbohydrate comes from whole grains, fruits, and vegetables, it will also provide the additional 3 g of fibre per day, which is recommended during pregnancy.

Although women do not need to increase their total fat intake during pregnancy, additional amounts of the essential fatty acids linoleic and α-linolenic acid are recommended because these are incorporated into the placenta and fetal tissues. The long-chain polyunsaturated fatty acids docosahexaenoic acid (DHA) and arachidonic acid are important because they both support maternal health and are essential for the development of the eye and nervous system in the fetus.[12]

Despite increases in the recommended intakes of protein, carbohydrate, and specific fatty acids during pregnancy, the distribution of calories from protein, carbohydrate, and fat should remain about the same as the recommended distribution for the general population.

Fluid and Electrolyte Needs

During pregnancy, a woman will accumulate six to nine litres of water. Some of this water is intracellular, resulting from the growth of tissues, but most is due to increases in the volume of blood and the fluid between cells. The need for water increases from 2.7 L/day in non-pregnant women to 3 L/day during pregnancy.[13] Despite changes in the amount and distribution of body water during pregnancy, there is no evidence that pregnant women's requirements for potassium, sodium, and chloride differ from the requirements for non-pregnant women.

Vitamin and Mineral Needs

Many vitamins and minerals are needed for the growth of new tissues in both mother and child (see Figure 11.6). For many of these nutrients, the increased need is easily met through the extra food the mother consumes. For other nutrients, the increased need is met because their absorption is increased during pregnancy. For a few nutrients, including calcium, vitamin D, folate, vitamin B_{12}, iron, and zinc, there is a risk that the woman will not consume adequate amounts without supplementation.

Calcium and vitamin D During gestation, the fetus accumulates about 30 g of calcium, mostly during the last trimester, when the bones are growing rapidly and the teeth are forming. However, the adequate intake (AI) is not increased during pregnancy because calcium absorption doubles.[14] The AI for calcium can be met by consuming three to four servings of dairy products daily. Women who are lactose-intolerant can meet their calcium needs through yogurt, cheese, reduced-lactose milk, calcium-rich vegetables, calcium-fortified foods, and calcium supplements. Many pregnant women fail to consume adequate amounts of calcium, which increases their risk of developing preeclampsia.[15]

Adequate vitamin D is essential to ensure efficient calcium absorption. The RDA for vitamin D during pregnancy is 600 international units (IU) (15 μg/day), the same as for non-pregnant women.[14] Vitamin D deficiency is a particular risk for dark-skinned women living at latitudes greater than 40° north or south—which includes all of Canada.[16]

Folate and vitamin B$_{12}$ Folate is needed for the synthesis of DNA and hence for cell division. Adequate folate intake before conception and during early pregnancy is crucial because rapid cell division occurs in the first days and weeks of pregnancy.

Low folate levels increase the risk of abnormalities in the formation of the *neural tube*, which forms the baby's brain and spinal cord (see Chapter 7, Figure 7.15). Neural tube closure, a critical step in neural tube development, occurs between 21 and 28 days after conception, often before a woman knows she is pregnant. Accordingly, the Public Health Agency of Canada recommends all women capable of becoming pregnant consume a daily multivitamin that provides 400 μg of folic acid (the synthetic form of folate) in addition to consuming a varied diet that is rich in natural sources of folate, such as leafy greens, legumes, and orange juice.[4] This recommendation and the fortification of folate into many foods has significantly helped to decrease the incidence of neural tube defects in Canada over the past two decades (see *Hot Topic*).

Folate continues to be important even after the neural tube closes. Folate deficiency can cause megaloblastic (macrocytic) anemia in the mother and is associated with fetal growth retardation and premature and low-birth-weight infants.[19] During pregnancy, the RDA is 600 μg of dietary folate equivalents per day.[20]

Vitamin B$_{12}$ is essential for the regeneration of active forms of folate. A deficiency of vitamin B$_{12}$ can therefore result in megaloblastic (macrocytic) anemia. Based on the amount of vitamin B$_{12}$ transferred from mother to fetus during pregnancy and on the increased efficiency of vitamin B$_{12}$ absorption during pregnancy, the RDA for pregnancy is set at 2.6 μg/day.[20] This recommendation is easily met by consuming a diet containing even small amounts of animal products. Pregnant women who consume vegan diets must include vitamin B$_{12}$ supplements or foods fortified with vitamin B$_{12}$ to meet both their needs and those of the fetus.

Iron and zinc Iron needs are high during pregnancy because iron is required for the synthesis of hemoglobin and other iron-containing proteins in both maternal and fetal tissues. The RDA for pregnant women is 27 mg/day, 50% higher than the recommended amount for non-pregnant women.[21] Many women start pregnancy with diminished iron stores and quickly become iron-deficient, despite the increase of iron absorption during pregnancy and the decrease of iron losses because menstruation ceases. Because most of the transfer of iron from mother to fetus occurs during the last trimester, babies who are born prematurely may not have had time to accumulate sufficient iron.

A well-planned diet is needed to meet iron needs during pregnancy. Red meat is a good source of the more absorbable heme iron, and leafy green vegetables and fortified cereals are good sources of non-heme iron. Iron absorption can be enhanced by consuming citrus fruits, which are high in vitamin C; meat, which contains heme iron; or other foods that are good sources of non-heme iron. Iron supplements are typically recommended during the second and third trimesters, and iron is included in prenatal supplements.

Zinc is involved in the synthesis and function of DNA and RNA and the synthesis of proteins. It is therefore extremely important for growth and development. Zinc deficiency during pregnancy is associated with increased risks of fetal malformations, premature birth, and low birth weight.[22] Because zinc absorption is inhibited by high iron intake, iron supplements may compromise zinc status if the mother's diet is low in zinc. The RDA for zinc

HOT TOPIC

Folate fortification and neural tube defects

The pasta in this picture is made from a coarse flour called semolina, which has been fortified with niacin, thiamin, riboflavin, iron, and folic acid. In 1998, the Canadian and United States governments began requiring the addition of folic acid to pasta and other enriched grain products in an effort to increase the folic acid intake in women of childbearing age, with the goal of reducing the incidence of neural tube defects. Enriched grains were chosen for fortification because this target population regularly consumes pasta in sufficient amounts to make a difference. Because high folic acid intake can mask the symptoms of vitamin B_{12} deficiency, the amount added to enriched grains was kept low enough to avoid this problem in any segment of the population but high enough to reduce the risk of neural tube defects. This public health measure was a large success and has contributed to a reduction in the amount of neural tube defect by 50% in Canada and by 25% in the United States![17,18]

> **Ask Yourself**
>
> Why has the incidence of neural tube defects not been cut to zero?

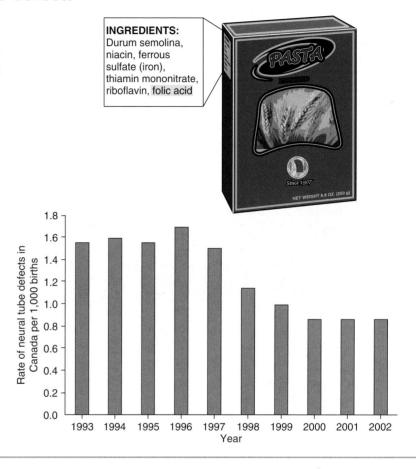

INGREDIENTS: Durum semolina, niacin, ferrous sulfate (iron), thiamin mononitrate, riboflavin, folic acid

---

is 13 mg/day for pregnant women age 18 and younger and 11 mg/day for pregnant women age 19 and older.[21] As is the case with iron, the zinc in red meat is more absorbable than zinc from other sources.

Meeting Nutrient Needs with Food and Supplements

The energy and nutrient needs of pregnancy can be met by following the recommendations of the Public Health Agency of Canada's *The Sensible Guide to a Healthy Pregnancy* (**Figure 11.7**).[4] The guide stresses the centrality of brightly coloured vegetables and fruits to a pregnant woman's diet, specifically recommending the consumption of at least one dark green and one orange vegetable per day. Unrefined grains, those listed as "whole grain" on an ingredients list, should also have a significant place in the diet. Consuming the milk and milk alternatives servings can be met by drinking 250 mL of milk and another milk alternative, such as yogurt, each day. The consumption of milk and alternatives will also help meet the woman's increased protein needs, as will consuming low-fat meat and meat alternatives. Fish can also be consumed, but should be chosen wisely to minimize exposure to mercury and bacteria.

For all of the above foods and food groups, varieties that are low in fat, sodium, and added sugar should be chosen to provide the fetus with the best nutritional environment. You will note that many of these recommendations are almost identical to those found in *Eating Well with Canada's Food Guide*. The main difference is evidenced in the number of servings recommended for pregnant

The Sensible Guide to a Healthy Pregnancy, produced by the Public Health Agency of Canada, is a useful resource for understanding the changes that take place in the female body during gestation. In the guide, you will find recommendations for proper dietary, physical activity, and emotional health practices during pregnancy.

Visit Health Canada's Web site to find out how to choose fish that are low in mercury so that you and your baby can take advantage of the benefits of eating fish while minimizing the risks from mercury.

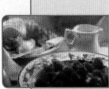
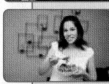
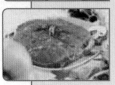

Next Steps

Aim for three meals a day with healthy snacks in between.

Check out Canada's Food Guide to see how many servings of each food group you need each day.

Take a multivitamin every day. Make sure it has 0.4 mg of folic acid and also contains iron. A health care provider can help you find the multivitamin that is right for you.

COMMON QUESTIONS ABOUT PRENATAL NUTRITION

How much weight should I gain while I'm pregnant?

It depends on how much you weighed before you got pregnant. The following recommendations are based on your Body Mass Index (BMI) before you became pregnant. BMI is a number based on a comparison of your weight to your height (BMI = weight (kg)/height (m)^2).

BMI	Recommended Weight Gain
Below 18.5	12.5 to 18 kg (28 to 40 pounds)
Between 18.5 and 24.9	11.5 to 16 kg (25 to 35 pounds)
Between 25.0 and 29.9	7 to 11.5 kg (15 to 25 pounds)
Over 30	5 to 9 kg (11 to 20 pounds)

If you are pregnant with more than one baby (twins, triplets) you will need to gain more weight. Your health care provider will be able to advise you.

women. The guide recommends increasing food intake by two or three food guide servings per day. In addition to eating a balanced diet, it is also recommended that a multivitamin with iron and 0.4 mg of folic acid be consumed daily. This prenatal supplement, however, must be taken along with, not in place of, a carefully planned diet (**Figure 11.8**) (see *Thinking It Through*).

Food Cravings and Aversions

Most women experience some food cravings and aversions during pregnancy. The foods most commonly craved are ice cream, sweets, candy, fruit, and fish (see *What Should I Eat?*). Common aversions include coffee, highly seasoned foods, and fried foods. It is not known why women experience these cravings and aversions. Some people suggest that hormonal or physiological changes during pregnancy—in particular, changes in taste and smell—may be the cause, but psychological and behavioural factors may also be involved.

Usually, the foods that pregnant women crave are not harmful and can be safely included in the diet to meet not only nutritional needs but also emotional needs and individual preferences. However, **pica** during pregnancy can lead to serious health consequences. Women with pica commonly consume such non-foods as clay, laundry starch, and ashes. Consuming large amounts of these substances can reduce their intake of nutrient-dense foods, inhibit nutrient absorption, increase the risk of consuming

pica An abnormal craving for and ingestion of non-food substances that have little or no nutritional value.

Prenatal supplements • Figure 11.8

Prenatal supplements typically do not provide enough calcium to meet the needs of a pregnant woman because, to do so, the tablet would need to be very large. These supplements also lack the protein needed for tissue synthesis; the complex carbohydrates needed for energy; the essential fatty acids for brain and nerve tissue development; fibre and fluid, which help prevent constipation; and the phytochemicals found in a healthy diet.

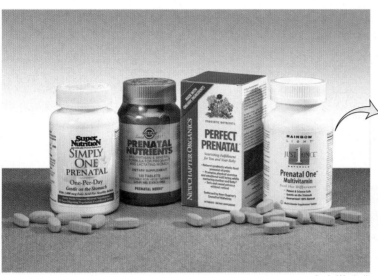

Andy Washnik

Supplement Facts

Per 1 Tablet

Amount	% Daily Value
Vitamin A (as beta carotene) 5000 IU	63%
Vitamin C (as ascorbic acid) 85 mg	100%
Vitamin D (as cholecalciferol) 400 IU	200%
Vitamin E (as d-alpha tocopheryl) acetate (Covitol™) 22 IU	67%
Vitamin K 90 mcg	100%
Thiamin 1.4 mg	100%
Riboflavin 1.6 mg	100%
Niacin (as niacinamide) 17 mg	100%
Vitamin B6 (as pyridoxine HCl) 2.6 mg	137%
Folic acid 1000 mcg	167%
Vitamin B12 (as cyanocobalamin) 2.6 mg	100%
Pantothenic Acid (as as d-calcium pantothenate) 6 mg	100%
Iron (as iron fumarate) 27 mg	100%
Iodine (kelp) 220 mcg	100%
Zinc (as monomethionine & gluconate) 11mg	100%
Selenium (as sodium selenate) 60 mcg	100%
Copper (as copper sulfate) 1000 mcg	100%
Calcium (as calcium carbonate) 200 mg	20%

* Daily Values based on RDAs for pregnant women ages 19-50
Other ingredients: stearic acid, vegetable stearate, silicon dioxide, croscarmellose sodium, microcrystalline cellulose, natural coating (contains hydroxypropyl methylcellulose, titanium dioxide, riboflavin, polyethylene glycol and polysorbate)

WHAT SHOULD I EAT?

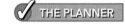 THE PLANNER

During Pregnancy

Make nutrient-dense choices
- Choose yogurt for a mid-morning snack.
- Add peanut butter to a banana to make a high-protein snack.
- Prepare a plate of pasta Florentine (with spinach)—it is both a natural and a fortified source of folate.

Drink plenty of fluids
- Drink a glass of milk to boost fluid and calcium intake.
- Keep a bottle of water at your desk or in your car.
- Relax with a cup of tea.

Indulge your cravings, within reason
- Savour some ice cream—it adds calcium and protein.
- Enjoy your cookies with a glass of low-fat milk.

 Use iProfile to plan a nutritious 300-Calorie snack for a pregnant woman.

THINKING IT THROUGH

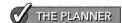

Nutrient Needs for a Successful Pregnancy

Erin is a sedentary 29-year-old at the end of her fourth month of pregnancy. She is 168 cm (5′6″) tall and weighed 64 kg (140 lb.) at the start of her pregnancy. She is concerned about gaining too much weight because her sister gained 23 kg (50 lb.) during her pregnancy and has had difficulty losing the excess weight since her baby was born. Erin would like to keep her weight gain below 9 kg (20 lb.).

Based on the graph below, how much weight would you recommend that Erin gain? Why would gaining only 9 kg (20 lb.) or as much as 23 kg (50 lb.) put the baby at risk?

▼

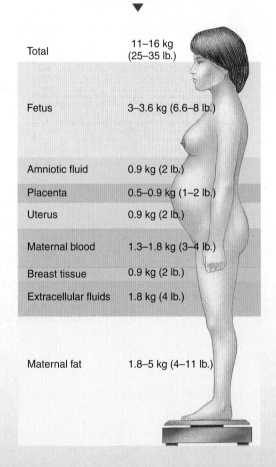

Total	11–16 kg (25–35 lb.)
Fetus	3–3.6 kg (6.6–8 lb.)
Amniotic fluid	0.9 kg (2 lb.)
Placenta	0.5–0.9 kg (1–2 lb.)
Uterus	0.9 kg (2 lb.)
Maternal blood	1.3–1.8 kg (3–4 lb.)
Breast tissue	0.9 kg (2 lb.)
Extracellular fluids	1.8 kg (4 lb.)
Maternal fat	1.8–5 kg (4–11 lb.)

Your answer: _____

_____

Erin's typical diet provides enough energy for a non-pregnant woman, but during her second and third trimesters, she needs to consume additional calories and nutrients. To decide what to add to her diet, Erin compares her typical intake to *Eating Well with Canada's Food Guide.* Her current diet includes four servings of grains, three servings of vegetables, two servings of fruit, 500 mL of milk, and 170 g of meat and beans.

How should the amounts of food from each food group be changed so that Erin meets her nutritional needs during the second trimester of her pregnancy?

▼

Your answer: _____

_____

Erin is taking a prenatal supplement but wonders whether her diet alone can meet her nutrient needs. She analyzes her diet and finds that she is meeting her needs for all nutrients except iron. Her current diet provides only 13.5 mg of iron—significantly less than the RDA of 27 mg for pregnant women.

Suggest some foods that Erin can include in her diet so she consumes an additional 13.5 mg of iron.

▼

Your answer: _____

_____

Is it reasonable for Erin to consume 27 mg of iron each day from her diet alone? Why or why not?

▼

Your answer: _____

_____

(Check your answers in Appendix I.)

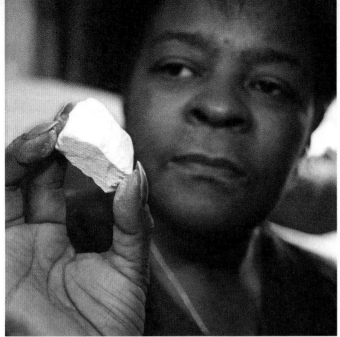

Pica • Figure 11.9

AP Photo/Michael DiBari, Jr.

This woman is eating a white clay called kaolin, which some women crave during pregnancy. Eating kaolin is also a traditional remedy for morning sickness. This example of pica may be related to cultural beliefs and traditions, but pica is also believed to be triggered by nutrient deficiencies, stress, and anxiety.

toxins, and cause intestinal obstructions. Complications of pica include iron-deficiency anemia, lead poisoning, and parasitic infestations.[23] Anemia and high blood pressure are more common in women with pica than among other pregnant women, but it is not clear whether pica is a result of these conditions or a cause. In newborns, anemia and low birth weight are often related to pica in the mother (**Figure 11.9**).

CONCEPT CHECK

1. **Why** is nutrient density so important during pregnancy?

2. **How** does calcium absorption change during pregnancy?

3. **What** nutrients are typically supplemented during pregnancy?

Factors That Increase the Risks Associated with Pregnancy

LEARNING OBJECTIVES

1. **Define** critical period in relation to fetal development.

2. **Discuss** how nutritional status can influence the outcome of pregnancy.

3. **Explain** how a pregnant woman's age and health status affect the risks associated with pregnancy.

4. **Describe** the effects of alcohol, mercury, and cocaine on the outcome of pregnancy.

5. **Assess** the risks associated with pregnancy-induced hypertension and gestational diabetes.

Approximately 375,000 children are born in Canada each year, and most of their mothers have healthy pregnancies.[24] Unfortunately, some babies are born with very low birth weight, and a small fraction of these babies may not make it through their first year of life. If complications during pregnancy are caught early, they can usually be managed, resulting in the delivery of a healthy baby.

Anything that interferes with embryonic or fetal development can cause a baby to be born too soon or too small or result in birth defects. The embryo and fetus are particularly vulnerable to damage because their cells are dividing rapidly, differentiating, and moving to form organs and other structures. Developmental errors can be caused by deficiencies or excesses in the maternal diet and by harmful substances that are present in the environment, consumed in the diet, or taken as medications or as recreational drugs. Any chemical, biological, or physical agent that causes a birth defect is called a **teratogen**. And because each organ system develops at a different time and rate, each has a **critical period** during which exposure to a teratogen is most likely to disrupt development and cause irreversible damage (**Figure 11.10**). Severe damage can result in miscarriage. Some women are at increased risk for complications during pregnancy because of their nutritional status, age, or pre-existing health problems. Others are at risk due to their exposure to harmful substances.

The critical periods of development differ for each body system. Because the majority of cell differentiation occurs during the embryonic period, during this time, exposure to teratogens can do the most damage, but vital body organs can still be affected during the fetal period. Of all babies born in Canada, 2 to 3% have a birth defect.[25]

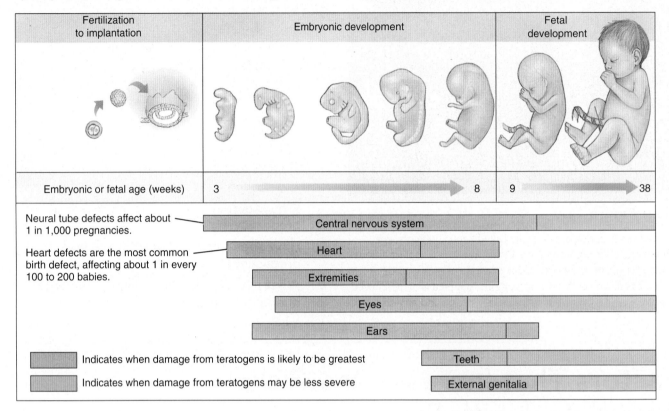

Neural tube defects affect about 1 in 1,000 pregnancies.

Heart defects are the most common birth defect, affecting about 1 in every 100 to 200 babies.

Fertilization to implantation | Embryonic development | Fetal development

Embryonic or fetal age (weeks): 3 → 8 | 9 → 38

Central nervous system
Heart
Extremities
Eyes
Ears
Teeth
External genitalia

Indicates when damage from teratogens is likely to be greatest

Indicates when damage from teratogens may be less severe

Maternal Nutritional Status

Before pregnancy, proper nutrition is important to enable conception and maximize the likelihood of a healthy pregnancy. Women with reduced body fat due to starvation diets, anorexia nervosa, or excessive exercise may have abnormal hormone levels. When hormone levels are too low, ovulation does not occur, and conception is not possible. Too much body fat can also reduce fertility by altering hormone levels. Deficiencies or excesses of specific nutrients can affect both fertility and the outcome of pregnancy.

During pregnancy, maternal malnutrition can cause fetal growth retardation, low birth weight, birth defects, premature birth, spontaneous abortion, or stillbirth. The effects of malnutrition vary, depending on when during the pregnancy it occurs.[26] As discussed earlier, inadequate folate intake in the first few weeks of pregnancy can affect neural tube development.[20] Too much vitamin A, particularly early in pregnancy, increases the risk of kidney problems and central nervous system abnormalities in the offspring.[21] To reduce the risk of excess vitamin A, supplements consumed during pregnancy should contain the vitamin A precursor, beta carotene, which is not damaging to the fetus.

Maternal malnutrition not only interferes with fetal growth and development but also causes changes that can affect the child's risk of developing chronic diseases later in life. Epidemiological studies suggest that, compared with normal-weight newborns, individuals who are small or disproportionately thin at birth and during infancy will, in adult life, have increased rates of heart disease, high blood pressure, stroke, high blood cholesterol, diabetes, obesity, and osteoporosis (**Figure 11.11**).[27] Maternal nutrition can also affect the future food preferences of an infant. Mothers who consume more varied diets can expose their offspring to a variety of flavours that the child may have an easier time accepting when they are later introduced. This concept of a "food bridge" also applies to the food a mother consumes while breastfeeding.

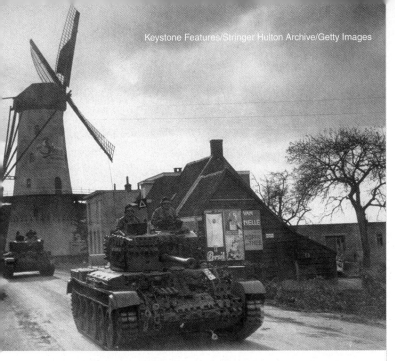

Effects of the Dutch famine • Figure 11.11

During World War II, an embargo on food transport to the Netherlands in the winter of 1944–45 caused the average food intake per person per day to drop below 1,000 kilocalories. As a result, pregnant women gave birth to smaller babies. In adulthood, the affected babies were more likely than others to have diabetes, heart disease, obesity, and other chronic diseases.[28]

Maternal Age and Health Status

Pregnancy places stresses on the body at any age, but these stresses have a greater impact on women in their teens and those age 35 or older. Because pregnant teens are still growing, their nutrient intake must meet their needs both for growth and for pregnancy. Pregnant teenagers are at increased risk of pregnancy-induced hypertension and are more likely to deliver preterm and low-birth-weight babies. Even teenagers who deliver normal-birth-weight infants may stop growing themselves.[29] To produce a healthy baby, a pregnant teenager needs early medical intervention and nutrition counselling (**Figure 11.12**). The rate of teenage pregnancy in Canada is fairly low compared with the rest of the world, and it continues to decline. The rate dropped 36.9% between 1996 and 2006 to 28 per 1,000 women.[30] This rate is less than half the rate of teenage pregnancies found in the United States and in England/Wales. In Canada, the rates from province to province can vary dramatically: for example, Saskatchewan has nearly twice the rate of teenage pregnancies as Newfoundland and Labrador.[30]

The nutritional requirements for older women during pregnancy are no different from those for women in their 20s, but pregnancy after age 35 carries additional risks. Older women are more likely to already have one or more medical conditions, such as cardiovascular disease, kidney disorders, obesity, or diabetes. These pre-existing conditions increase the risks associated with pregnancy. For example, a woman who has pre-existing high blood pressure is at increased risk for having a low-birth-weight baby, and a woman who has diabetes is more likely to have a baby who is large for gestational age. Older women are also more likely to develop gestational diabetes, pregnancy-induced hypertension, and other complications. They also have a higher incidence of low-birth-weight infants. In addition, their infants are more likely to have chromosomal abnormalities, especially Down syndrome. The frequency of twins and triplets is higher among older mothers, in part because of their greater

Nutrient needs of pregnant teens • Figure 11.12

Because the nutrient needs of pregnant teens differ from those of pregnant adults, the dietary reference intakes (DRIs) include a special set of nutrient recommendations for this age group. The percentage increase in micronutrient needs above non-pregnant levels is shown for 14- to 18-year-olds during their second and third trimesters of pregnancy.

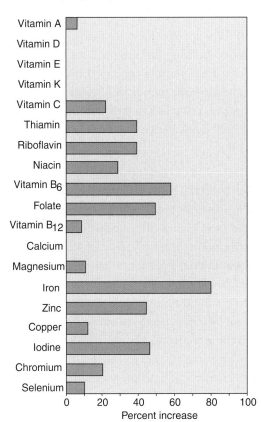

use of fertility treatments. Multiple pregnancies increase nutrient needs and the risk of pre-term delivery.

Women with a history of miscarriage or birth defects are also at increased risk. For example, a woman who has had past miscarriages is more likely to have another, and a woman who has had one child with a birth defect has an increased risk for defects in subsequent pregnancies. Another factor that increases risks is frequent pregnancies. An interval of less than 18 months between pregnancies increases the risk of delivering a small-for-gestational age infant. An interval of only three months increases the risk of a pre-term infant and the risk of neonatal death.[31] One reason for these increased risks is that the mother may not have replenished the nutrient stores depleted in her first pregnancy before becoming pregnant again.

Exposure to Toxic Substances

A pregnant woman's exposure to toxins in food, water, and the environment can affect the developing fetus. Even substances that seem innocuous can be dangerous. For example, herbal remedies, including herbal teas, should be avoided unless their consumption during pregnancy has been determined to be safe.[6]

Caffeine When consumed in excess, coffee and other caffeine-containing beverages have been associated with increased risks of miscarriage or low birth weight.[32] Health Canada recommends that women of child-bearing age consume less than 300 mg of caffeine per day, which is approximately equivalent to two 240-mL cups of coffee[4,33] (**Table 11.1**).

Mercury in fish Fish has both benefits and risks for pregnant women. It is a source of lean protein for tissue growth and of omega-3 fatty acids and iodine needed for brain development, but if it is contaminated with mercury, consumption during pregnancy can cause developmental delays and brain damage. Rather than avoid fish, pregnant women should be informed consumers. Exposure to mercury can be controlled by avoiding varieties of fish that are highest in mercury and limiting intake of fish that contain lower amounts mercury (**Table 11.2**). Raw fish such as oysters, clams, and sashimi should be avoided, as they have an increased risk of bacterial contamination.

Sources of caffeine	Table 11.1	
Food or medication	**Amount**	**Caffeine (mg)**
Coffee, regular brewed	240 mL	100–200
Coffee, decaffeinated	240 mL	3–12
Black tea, brewed	240 mL	40–120
Green tea, brewed	240 mL	8–30
Pepsi	591 mL	63
Mountain Dew	591 mL	91
Energy drink	250 mL	50–300
Hot chocolate	240 mL	7
Brownie	1	14
Chocolate bar	28 g	15
NoDoz	1 tablet	100
Excedrin	1 tablet	65
Empirin, Anacin	1 tablet	32

Food-borne illness The immune system is weakened during pregnancy, increasing susceptibility to and the severity of certain food-borne illnesses. *Listeria* infections are about 20 times more likely during pregnancy and are especially dangerous for pregnant women, often resulting in miscarriage, premature delivery, stillbirth, or infection of the fetus.[35] About one-quarter of babies born with *Listeria* infections do not survive. The bacteria are commonly found in unpasteurized milk, soft cheeses, and uncooked hot dogs and lunch meats (see Table 11.2).

Toxoplasmosis is an infection caused by a parasite. If a pregnant woman becomes infected, she can pass the infection to her unborn baby. Some infected babies develop vision and hearing loss, intellectual disability, and/or seizures. The toxoplasmosis parasite is found in cat feces, soil, and undercooked infected meat (see Table 11.2). Pregnant women should follow the safe food-handling recommendations discussed in Chapter 13.

Alcohol Alcohol consumption during pregnancy is one of the leading causes of preventable birth defects. Alcohol is a teratogen that is particularly damaging to the developing nervous system.[36] It also indirectly affects fetal growth and development because it is a toxin that reduces blood flow

Food safety during pregnancy[34] Table 11.2
Avoid eating swordfish, shark, king mackerel, or tilefish, which can be high in mercury.
Avoid drinking raw (unpasteurized) milk or consuming products made with unpasteurized milk, such as certain Mexican-style soft cheeses.
Avoid eating refrigerated smoked fish, cold deli salads, and refrigerated pâtés or meat spreads.
Avoid eating hot dogs unless they have been reheated to steaming hot.
Avoid eating raw or undercooked meat, poultry, fish, shellfish, or eggs.
Avoid eating unwashed fruits and vegetables, raw sprouts, or unpasteurized juice.
Avoid eating non-dried deli meats, such as bologna and turkey breast.
Ensure you are handling your food properly: cook food thoroughly, chill food in the refrigerator, separate animal products and plant products on different cutting surfaces, and wash all fruits and vegetables before eating them.

to the placenta, thereby decreasing the delivery of oxygen and nutrients to the fetus. Use of alcohol can also impair maternal nutritional status, further increasing the risks to the fetus.

Prenatal exposure to alcohol can cause a spectrum of disorders, depending on the amount, timing, and duration of the exposure. One of the most severe outcomes of alcohol use during pregnancy is delivery of a baby with **fetal alcohol syndrome (FAS)** (**Figure 11.13**). Not all babies who are exposed to alcohol while in the uterus have FAS, but many have some alcohol-related problems. **Alcohol-related neurodevelopment disorders (ARND)** are functional or mental impairments linked to prenatal alcohol exposure; **alcohol-related birth defects (ARBD)** are malformations in the skeleton or major organ systems. These conditions are less severe than FAS but occur about three times more often. Because alcohol consumption in each trimester has been associated with fetal abnormalities and NO level of alcohol consumption is known to be safe at any time, complete abstinence from alcohol is recommended during pregnancy.

In addition to avoiding alcohol, tobacco and certain drugs, such as cocaine and marijuana, should also be avoided during pregnancy. All of these drugs can cross the placenta and lead to profound negative effects on the offspring's development and future health.

fetal alcohol syndrome (FAS) A characteristic group of physical and mental abnormalities in an infant resulting from maternal alcohol consumption during pregnancy.

Dangers of alcohol use during pregnancy • Figure 11.13

This 3-year-old girl has the facial characteristics associated with fetal alcohol syndrome (FAS): a low nasal bridge, short nose, distinct eyelids, and thin upper lip. Newborns with FAS may be shaky and irritable, with poor muscle tone. Other problems associated with FAS include heart and urinary tract defects, impaired vision and hearing, and delayed language development. Below-average intellectual function is the most common and most serious effect.

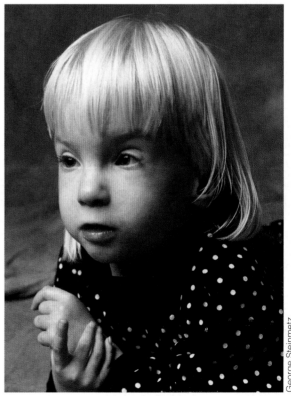

George Steinmetz

Factors That Increase the Risks Associated with Pregnancy 399

High Blood Pressure

About 5 to 10% of pregnant women experience high blood pressure during pregnancy. **Hypertensive disorders of pregnancy**, also known as **pregnancy-induced hypertension**, refer to a spectrum of conditions involving elevated blood pressure during pregnancy.[37] In the United States, high blood pressure accounts for more than 10% of pregnancy-related maternal deaths.[37] It is especially common in mothers under 18 and over 35 years of age, low-income mothers, and mothers with chronic hypertension or kidney disease.

About one-third of the hypertensive disorders of pregnancy are due to chronic hypertension that was present before the pregnancy, but the remainder are related to the pregnancy. The least problematic of these is **gestational hypertension**, an abnormal rise in blood pressure that occurs after the 20th week of pregnancy. Gestational hypertension may signal the potential for a more serious condition called **preeclampsia**. Preeclampsia is typically characterized by high blood pressure along with fluid retention and excretion of protein in the urine; it can result in a weight gain of several pounds within a few days. Some women, however, exhibit no symptoms or mistake them for common pregnancy symptoms. Preeclampsia is dangerous to the baby because it reduces blood flow to the placenta, and it is dangerous to the mother because it can progress to a more severe form of pregnancy-induced hypertension called **eclampsia**, in which life-threatening seizures occur. Women with preeclampsia require bed rest and careful medical monitoring. The condition usually resolves after delivery.

The causes of pregnancy-induced hypertension are not fully understood. At one time, low-sodium diets were prescribed to prevent preeclampsia, but studies have not found such diets to be beneficial in lowering blood pressure or preventing this condition.[13] Calcium may play a role in preventing pregnancy-induced hypertension; calcium supplements have been found to reduce the risk of high blood pressure and preeclampsia.[15]

> **peeclampsia**
> A condition characterized by elevated blood pressure, a rapid increase in body weight, protein in the urine, and edema. Also called *toxemia*.
>
> **eclampsia**
> Convulsions or seizures brought on by seriously high blood pressure during pregnancy (preeclampsia). Untreated, it can lead to coma or death.

Although calcium supplements are not routinely recommended for healthy pregnant women, additional dietary calcium may provide benefits for pregnant teens, individuals with inadequate calcium intake, and women who are known to be at risk of developing pregnancy-induced hypertension.[38]

Gestational Diabetes

Diabetes that develops in a pregnant woman is known as **gestational diabetes**. It is more common in obese women. Gestational diabetes usually resolves after the birth, but the mother has a 20 to 50% chance of developing diabetes in the next five to 10 years.[39] A woman with gestational diabetes requires treatment to normalize maternal blood glucose levels. Because glucose in the mother's blood passes freely across the placenta, when the mother's blood glucose levels are high, the growing fetus receives extra glucose and hence extra calories. The baby grows rapidly, placing it at risk for being large for gestational age and, consequently, at increased risk for difficult delivery and abnormal blood glucose levels at birth. Babies born to mothers with gestational diabetes are at increased risk of developing diabetes as adults.[40]

> **gestational diabetes** A condition characterized by high blood glucose levels that develop during pregnancy.

CONCEPT CHECK	STOP

1. **Why** does the effect of a given teratogen vary, depending on when a pregnant woman is exposed to it?

2. **How** does malnutrition during pregnancy affect the health of the child later in life?

3. **Why** do pregnant teenagers' requirements for some nutrients differ from the requirements for pregnant adult women?

4. **How** much alcohol can be safely consumed during pregnancy?

5. **How** does gestational diabetes in a mother affect the baby?

Nutrition for Infants

LEARNING OBJECTIVES

1. **Explain** how growth charts are used to monitor the nutritional well-being of infants.

2. **Discuss** the importance of choosing foods that are appropriate for a child's developmental stage.

3. **Compare** the benefits of breastfeeding and formula-feeding.

4. **List** three foods that should not be fed to infants and explain why.

After the umbilical cord is cut, a newborn must actively obtain nutrients rather than being passively fed through the placenta. The energy and nutrients an infant consumes must support his or her continuing growth and development, as well as his or her increasing activity level.

Infant Growth and Development

During **infancy**—the first year of life—growth is extremely rapid. Healthy infants follow standard patterns of growth—that is, whether a newborn weighs 3 kg (6.6 lb.) or 4 kg (8.8 lb.) at birth, the rate of growth should be approximately the same: rapid initially and slowing slightly as the infant approaches his or her first birthday. A rule of thumb is that an infant's birth weight should double by 4 months of age and triple by 1 year of age. In the first year of life, most infants increase their length by 50%. Growth is the best indicator of adequate nutrition in an infant.

Growth charts Growth charts can be used to compare an infant's growth with that of other infants of the same age (**Figure 11.14**).[41] The resulting ranking, or percentile, indicates where the infant's growth falls in relation to population standards. For example, if a newborn boy is at the 20th percentile for weight, 19% of newborn boys weigh less and 80% weigh more. Children usually remain at the same percentile as they grow. For instance, a child who is at the 50th percentile for height and the 25th percentile for weight generally remains close to these percentiles

throughout childhood. Small and premature infants often follow a pattern that is parallel to but below the growth curve for a period of time and then experience catch-up growth that takes them into the same range as children of the same age.

Slight variations in growth rate are normal, but a consistent pattern of not following the established growth curve or a sudden change in growth pattern is cause for concern and could indicate overnutrition or undernutrition. For example, a rapid increase in weight without an increase in height may indicate that the infant is being overfed. Because overweight children are more likely to be overweight as adults, this pattern of weight increase should be addressed early in life by establishing healthy eating behaviours and intake levels for a child to carry on throughout their life.

Growth that is slower than the predicted pattern indicates **failure to thrive**, a catch-all term for any type of growth failure in a young child. The cause may be a congenital condition, disease, poor nutrition, neglect, abuse, or psychosocial problems. The treatment is usually an individualized plan that includes adequate nutrition and careful monitoring by physicians, dietitians, and other health care professionals. Just as prenatal life has critical periods, infancy has critical periods when undernutrition can have permanent effects on growth and development. Malnutrition during infancy has a great impact on learning and behaviour because the first year of life is a critical period for brain development.

> **failure to thrive** Inability of a child's growth to keep up with normal growth curves.

Developmental milestones In addition to growing bigger, infants also develop physically, intellectually, and socially. Adequate nutrition is essential for achieving these developmental milestones, which, in turn, affect how the infant obtains nourishment. Although most of an infant's nutritional needs are met by breast milk or infant formula, solid and semi-solid foods can be gradually introduced into the diet starting at 4 to 6 months of life. By this time, the infant's feeding

Growth charts • Figure 11.14

This weight-for-age and length-for-age growth chart for boys and girls from birth to 24 months of age can be used to compare a child's weight and length at a particular age to standards for the general Canadian population. Growth charts for this age group are also available to monitor head circumference for age in boys and girls.

WHO GROWTH CHARTS FOR CANADA

GIRLS

BIRTH TO 24 MONTHS: GIRLS

Length-for-ageand Weight-for-agepercentiles

NAME: _____

DOB: _____ RECORD # _____

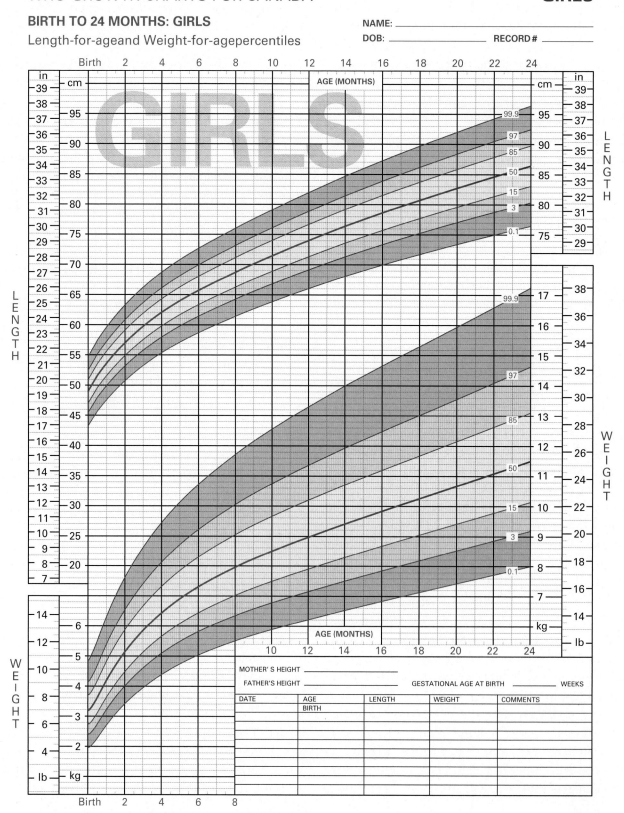

SOURCE: Based on the World Health Organization (WHO) Child Growth Standards (2006) and adapted for Canada by Dietitians of Canada, Canadian Paediatric Society, the College of Family Physicians of Canada and Community Health Nurses of Canada.

WHO GROWTH CHARTS FOR CANADA

BOYS

BIRTH TO 24 MONTHS: BOYS
Length-for-age and Weight-for-age percentiles

NAME: _____

DOB: _____ RECORD # _____

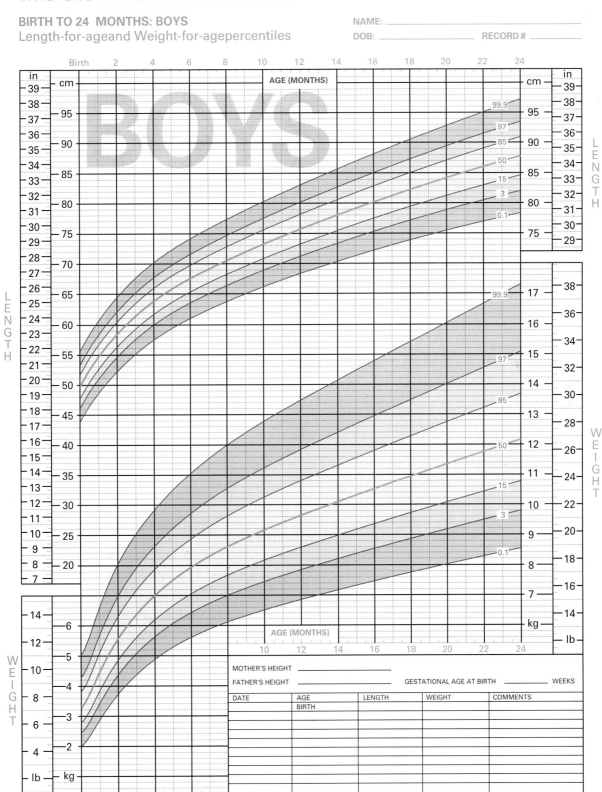

AGE (MONTHS)

LENGTH

WEIGHT

MOTHER'S HEIGHT _____

FATHER'S HEIGHT _____   GESTATIONAL AGE AT BIRTH _____ WEEKS

DATE	AGE	LENGTH	WEIGHT	COMMENTS
	BIRTH			

SOURCE: Based on the World Health Organization (WHO) Child Growth Standards (2006) and adapted for Canada by Dietitians of Canada, Canadian Paediatric Society, the College of Family Physicians of Canada and Community Health Nurses of Canada.

Nutrition InSight

Nourishing a developing infant • Figure 11.15

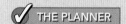

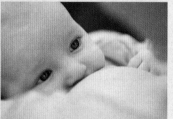 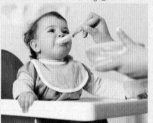 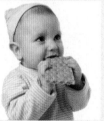 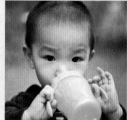

Age	Birth to 4 months	4 to 6 months	6 to 9 months	9 to 12 months
Developmental Milestones	The infant takes milk by means of a licking motion of the tongue called suckling, which strokes or milks the liquid from the nipple. Solid food placed in the mouth at an early age is usually pushed out as the tongue thrusts forward.	The tongue is held farther back in the mouth, allowing solid food to be accepted without being expelled. The infant can hold his or her head up and is able to sit, with or without support.	The infant can sit without support, chew, hold food, and easily move hand to mouth.	The infant can drink from a cup and feed him/herself.
Foods	Breast milk or iron-fortified infant formula.	Breast milk or formula, iron-fortified infant cereal. Rice cereal is usually the first solid food introduced because it is easily digested and less likely than other grains to cause allergies. After cereals, puréed vegetables and fruits can be introduced.	Breast milk or formula, iron-fortified infant cereal, puréed or strained vegetables, fruits, meats and beans, limited finger foods.	Breast milk or formula, iron-fortified infant cereal, chopped vegetables, soft fruits, meats and beans, fruit juice, nonchoking finger foods such as dry cereal, cooked pasta, and well-cooked vegetables.

abilities and gastrointestinal tract are mature enough to handle solid foods (**Figure 11.15**).

Energy and Nutrient Needs of Infants

The rapid growth and high metabolic rate of infants increase their need for energy, protein, and vitamins and minerals that are important for growth. Human milk and commercially produced formula are designed to meet infants' nutrient needs. Nevertheless, infants may still be at risk for deficiencies in iron, vitamin D, and vitamin K and for suboptimal levels of fluoride.

Energy and macronutrients Infants require more calories and protein per kilogram of body weight than do individuals at any other time of life (**Figure 11.16a**).[42] As infants grow older, their rate of growth slows, but they become more mobile, which increases the amount of energy they need for activity. Because infants change so much during the first year, energy recommendations are made for three age groups—0 to 3 months, 4 to 6 months, and 7 to 12 months—and nutrient recommendations are made for two age groups—0 to 6 months and 7 to 12 months.

The combination of high energy demands and a small stomach means that infants require an energy-dense diet. Healthy infants consume about 55% of their energy as fat during the first six months of life and 40% during the second six months. These percentages are far higher than the 20 to 35% of energy from fat recommended in the adult diet (**Figure 11.16b**). This energy-dense diet allows the small volume of food that fits in an infant's stomach to provide enough energy to meet the infant's needs.

Energy and macronutrient needs • Figure 11.16

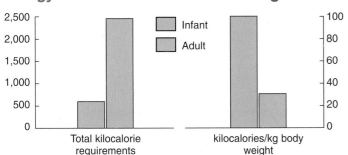

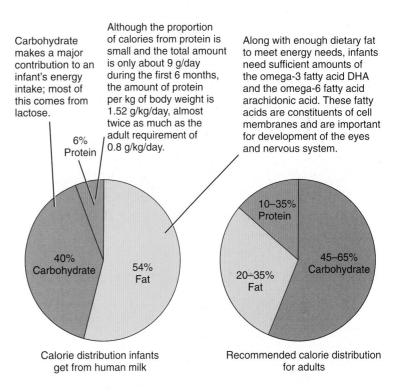

a. The total amount of energy required by an infant is less than the amount needed by an adult. When this amount is expressed as kilocalories per kilogram (kcal/kg) of body weight, however, infants require about three times more energy than an adult male.

Carbohydrate makes a major contribution to an infant's energy intake; most of this comes from lactose.

Although the proportion of calories from protein is small and the total amount is only about 9 g/day during the first 6 months, the amount of protein per kg of body weight is 1.52 g/kg/day, almost twice as much as the adult requirement of 0.8 g/kg/day.

Along with enough dietary fat to meet energy needs, infants need sufficient amounts of the omega-3 fatty acid DHA and the omega-6 fatty acid arachidonic acid. These fatty acids are constituents of cell membranes and are important for development of the eyes and nervous system.

b. Comparing the distribution of kilocalories from carbohydrate, fat, and protein in human milk with that recommended for an adult illustrates proportionally how much more fat infants need. As an infant grows and solid foods are introduced into the diet, the percentage of kilocalories from carbohydrate in the diet increases, and the percentage from fat decreases.

Calorie distribution infants get from human milk

Recommended calorie distribution for adults

Fluid needs

Infants have a higher proportion of body water than do adults, and they lose proportionately more water in urine and through evaporation. Urine losses are high because the kidneys are not fully developed and hence are unable to reabsorb as much water as adult kidneys. Water losses through evaporation are proportionately higher in infants than in adults because they have a larger surface area relative to body weight. As a result, they need to consume more water per unit of body weight than do adults. Nevertheless, healthy infants who are exclusively breastfed do not require additional water.[13] In older infants, some water is obtained from food and from beverages other than milk. When water losses are increased by diarrhea or vomiting, additional fluids may be needed.

Micronutrients at risk

Iron is the nutrient that is most commonly deficient in infants who are consuming adequate energy and protein. Iron deficiency usually is not a problem during the first six months of life because infants have iron stores at birth, and the iron in human milk, though not abundant, is very well absorbed. The AI for iron from birth to 6 months is 0.27 mg/day. After age 4 to 6 months, iron stores are depleted, but iron needs remain high. The RDA for infants 7 to 12 months old increases to 11 mg/day.[21] By this age, the diet of breastfed infants should contain other sources of iron. Formula-fed infants should be fed iron-fortified formula.

Breast milk is low in vitamin D. Therefore, it is recommended that breastfed infants and partially breastfed infants receive 400 IU (10 µg/day) of vitamin D beginning in the first few days of life and continuing until they are consuming about 1 L (4 cups) of vitamin D-fortified formula or milk daily.[14,43] Infant formulas contain at least 10 µg of vitamin D per litre of formula. Light-skinned infants can synthesize enough vitamin D if their faces are exposed to the sun for 15 minutes per day; a longer time is required for darker-skinned babies.

Infants are at risk for vitamin K deficiency because little vitamin K crosses the placenta and the infant's gut is sterile, so there are no bacteria to synthesize this vitamin. Because lack of vitamin K can cause bleeding, it is recommended that all newborns receive an intramuscular injection containing 0.5 to 1.0 mg of vitamin K within the six hours following birth, which provides enough of the vitamin to last until the intestines have been colonized with bacteria that synthesize it.[44]

Fluoride is important for tooth development, even before the teeth erupt. Breast milk is low in fluoride, and formula manufacturers use unfluoridated water to prepare liquid formula. Therefore, breastfed infants, infants who are fed premixed formula, and those who are fed formula mixed with low-fluoride water at home are often given fluoride supplements beginning at 6 months of age. In areas where drinking water is fluoridated, infants who are fed formula reconstituted with tap water should not be given fluoride supplements.

Meeting Needs with Breast Milk or Formula

Because of its health and nutritional benefits, breastfeeding is the recommended choice for the newborn of a healthy, well-nourished mother (see *Debate: DHA-Fortified Infant Formula*). Health professionals in Canada and the United States recommend exclusive breastfeeding for the first six months of life and breastfeeding with complementary foods for at least the first year and as long thereafter as mutually desired (**Figure 11.17**).[45,46] As infants begin consuming other foods, their demand for milk is reduced, and milk production decreases, but lactation can continue as long as suckling is maintained.

Whether infants are breastfed or formula-fed, they should be fed frequently, on demand. For breastfed infants, a feeding should last approximately 10 to 15 minutes at each breast. Bottle-fed newborns may consume less than 100 mL at each feeding; as the infant grows, the amount consumed will increase to 125 to 250 mL. A well-fed newborn, whether breastfed or bottle-fed, should urinate enough to soak six to eight diapers a day and gain about 0.15 to 0.23 kg (0.33 to 0.5 lb.) per week.

Breastfeeding vs. formula-feeding • Figure 11.17

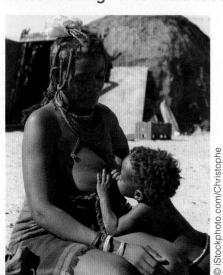

© Can Stock Photo Inc. / Feverpitched

a. After the first year, breastfeeding is not necessary to meet the infant's nutrient needs, but in developing nations, where other foods offered to young children are nutrient-poor, breastfeeding after the first year helps prevent malnutrition. The World Health Organization recommends breastfeeding for two years or more.[47] In both developed and developing nations, breastfeeding after the first year continues to provide nutrition, comfort, and an emotional bond between mother and child.

© iStockphoto.com/Christophe Cerisier

c. Infants should never be put to bed with a bottle because saliva flow decreases during sleep, and the formula remains in contact with the teeth for many hours. This causes **nursing bottle syndrome**, rapid and serious decay of the upper teeth. Usually the lower teeth are protected by the tongue.

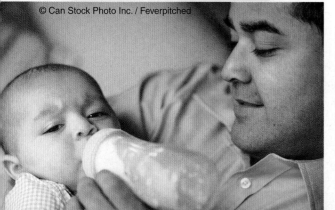

b. During bottle feeding, the infant's head should be higher than its stomach, and the bottle should be tilted so that there is no air in the nipple. Just as breastfed infants alternate breasts, bottle-fed infants should be held alternately on the left and right sides to promote equal development of the head and neck muscles.

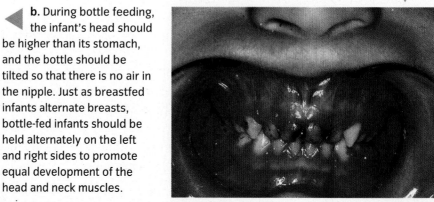

Custom Medical Stock Photo, Inc./K.L.Boyd DDS

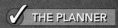
The Issue: The fatty acids docosahexaenoic acid (DHA) and arachidonic acid (ARA) are essential for development of the retina and brain. Some infant formulas in Canada are fortified with DHA and ARA, and advertisements suggest that they provide an advantage for infant development, but will these fortified formulas make babies smarter and improve their vision?

DHA and ARA are polyunsaturated fatty acids that can be made in the body from the essential α-linolenic acid (omega 3) and the essential linoleic acid (omega 6), respectively. Studies in animals indicate that DHA and ARA are found in high concentrations in the brain and retina and that they are needed for brain development and normal vision.[48] Accumulation of these fatty acids in the brain and retina occurs most rapidly between the third trimester of pregnancy and 24 months of age, so adequate amounts are crucial during this developmental period.

DHA and ARA are found in breast milk, so it seems logical that they should be added to infant formula. But, unlike most other nutrients, the amounts of DHA and ARA in breast milk are variable, depending on maternal diet, so it is unclear what constitutes optimal levels. The amounts of these fatty acids transferred to the fetus by the placenta during the third trimester may be enough to ensure adequate amounts for brain development.[48] Infants born at term are also capable of synthesizing DHA and ARA, so those fed unfortified formula may be able to meet their needs if they have enough α-linolenic acid and linoleic acid in their diet. But there is wide individual variation in the ability to convert α-linolenic acid to DHA, and, in some infants, conversion may be too low for optimal brain and visual development.[48] Infants born before term cannot synthesize enough of these fatty acids, so DHA and ARA must be included in formula for premature infants.

Will higher intakes of these fatty acids make children smarter? Numerous studies have explored the impact of postnatal intake of these fatty acids on intelligence and vision. Some have found that higher intakes of DHA increase blood levels of DHA in infants and are associated with improvements in cognitive development or vision compared to infants with lower intakes.[48-50] But not all studies agree. A study of 18-month-old babies found that feeding fortified formulas did not have a significant effect on mental or psychomotor development.[51] A review concluded that feeding infant formulas fortified with DHA and ARA has not been proven to result in benefits with regard to vision or cognition.[52]

Studies on the effects of fortified formulas are inconsistent for a variety of reasons. Differences may be due to variations in the DHA content of the formula, the duration of formula-feeding, and the methods used to assess visual acuity and cognitive development. Differences in children's intelligence may be due more to maternal or family characteristics, such as maternal IQ, than to the type of milk they are fed.[53]

In terms of brain and eye development, no one knows exactly how much DHA or ARA an infant needs. A direct link between the use of fortified formula and better vision or higher IQ compared with use of unfortified formula has yet to be established, but fortified formulas are generally recommended.[48,49] They may not make your baby smarter, but published literature has not demonstrated these formulas to be harmful for infants.[54] Breast milk is always better, so the biggest downside to fortified formulas is that advertising may make new mothers believe that formulas are as good as or better for their babies than breast milk.

Think Critically

Why is breast milk still better than these fortified formulas?

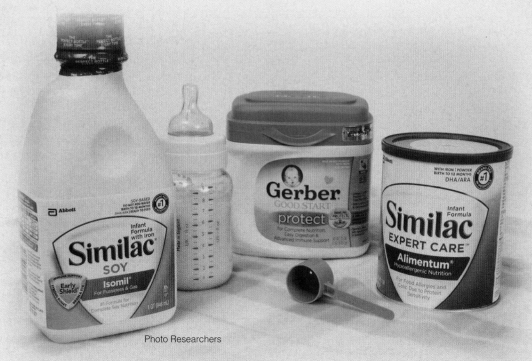

Photo Researchers

Nutrients in breast milk and formula Human milk is tailored to meet the needs of human infants. The composition of milk changes continuously to suit the needs of a growing infant. The first milk, called **colostrum**, which is produced by the breast for up to a week after delivery, has beneficial effects on the gastrointestinal tract, by acting as a laxative that helps the baby excrete the thick, mucous stool produced during life in the womb. Colostrum looks watery, but the nutrients it supplies meet the infant's needs until mature milk production begins. Mature breast milk contains an appropriate balance of nutrients in forms that are easily digested and absorbed. Infant formulas try to replicate human milk as closely as possible in an effort to match the growth, nutrient absorption, and other benefits associated with breastfeeding (**Table 11.3**).

colostrum The first milk, produced by the breast late in pregnancy and for up to a week after delivery. Compared with mature milk, it contains less fat and more water, protein, immune factors, minerals, and vitamins.

Health benefits of breastfeeding Despite infant formula having a nutritional profile similar to human milk, it can never exactly duplicate the composition of human milk. In breast milk, antibody proteins and immune-system cells pass from the mother to her child, providing

Nutritional composition of breast milk and infant formula Table 11.3

Nutrient	Amount in breast milk	Amount in formula	Comparisons
Protein (g/100 mL)	1.8	1.4	The relatively low protein content of human milk and formula protects the immature kidneys from a too-high load of nitrogen wastes. Alpha-lactalbumin, the predominant protein in human milk, forms a soft, easily digested curd in the infant's stomach. Most formula is made from cow's milk, modified to mimic the protein concentration and amino acid composition of human milk.
Fat (g/100 mL)	4	4.8	The fat in human milk is easily digested. Human milk is high in cholesterol and the essential fatty acids linoleic acid and α-linolenic acid, as well as their long-chain derivatives, arachidonic acid and DHA, which are essential for normal brain development, eyesight, and growth. The fat in formula is derived from vegetable oils and provides linoleic and α-linolenic acid. Some formulas are also supplemented with arachiconic acid and DHA.
Carbohydrate (g/100 mL)	7	7.3	Lactose, the primary carbohydrate in human milk and most formula, enhances calcium absorption. Because lactose is digested slowly, it stimulates the growth of beneficial acid-producing bacteria.
Sodium (mg/100 mL)	1.3	0.7	Because breast milk and formula are both low in sodium, the fluid needs of breastfed and formula-fed infants can be met without an excessive load on the kidneys.
Calcium (mg/100 mL)	22	53	The 2:1 ratio of calcium to phosphorus in breast milk and formula enhances calcium absorption.
Phosphorus (mg/100 mL)	14	38	
Iron (mg/100 mL)	0.03	0.1	Iron and zinc are present in limited amounts in breast milk but are readily absorbed. Most infant formulas are fortified with iron and zinc because the forms present are less absorbable than those in breast milk.
Zinc (mg/100 mL)	3.2	5.1	
Vitamin D (IU/100 mL)	4	41	Formulas are fortified with vitamin D, which is present at low levels in breast milk.

immune protection for the infant.[55] A number of enzymes and other proteins in breast milk prevent the growth of harmful microorganisms, and several of the carbohydrates in breast milk protect against viruses that cause diarrhea. One substance favours the growth of the beneficial bacterium *Lactobacillus bifidus* in the infant's colon; this bacterium inhibits the growth of disease-causing organisms. Growth factors and hormones present in human milk enhance digestion and promote maturation of the infant's gut and immune defences. In addition to the numerous health benefits that breastfeeding has for infants it has physical, emotional, and financial advantages for the mother (**Figure 11.18**).

When is formula-feeding better? Despite the benefits of breast milk, in some situations, formula-feeding may be the better option. Common illnesses such as colds and skin infections are not passed to the infant in breast milk, but tuberculosis, cytomegalovirus, and HIV infection are.[55,57] Some drugs can pass from the mother to the baby in breast milk, which means that women who take medications should ask their physician whether they can safely breastfeed. Because alcohol and drugs such as cocaine and marijuana can be passed to a baby in breast milk, alcoholic and drug-addicted mothers are counselled not to breastfeed. Nicotine from cigarette smoke is also rapidly transferred from maternal blood to milk, and heavy smoking may decrease the supply of milk.

Although alcoholic mothers are counselled not to breastfeed, occasional limited alcohol consumption while breastfeeding is probably not harmful if alcohol intake is timed to minimize the amount present in milk when the infant is fed. Alcohol is most concentrated an hour after consumption and is cleared from the milk at about the same rate at which it disappears from the bloodstream.

Feeding an infant with formula requires more preparation and washing than breastfeeding, but it can give the mother a break because other family members can share the responsibility. For preterm infants and infants with genetic abnormalities, formula may be the better option because special formulas are available to meet these infants' unique needs. If an infant is too small or weak to take a bottle, pumped breast milk or formula can be fed through a tube.

The benefits of breastfeeding • Figure 11.18

BENEFITS FOR INFANTS

- Provides optimum nutrition
- Enables strong bonding with mother
- Enhances immune protection
- Reduces allergies
- Decreases ear infections, respiratory illnesses, and asthma
- Reduces the likelihood of constipation, diarrhea, or chronic digestive diseases
- Reduces risk for sudden infant death syndrome (SIDS)
- Lowers risk for obesity, type-1 and -2 diabetes, heart disease, hypertension, high cholesterol, and childhood leukemia[56]
- Aids in the development of the facial muscles, speech development, and correct formation of the teeth
- Lessens the risk of overfeeding because the amount of milk consumed cannot be monitored visually

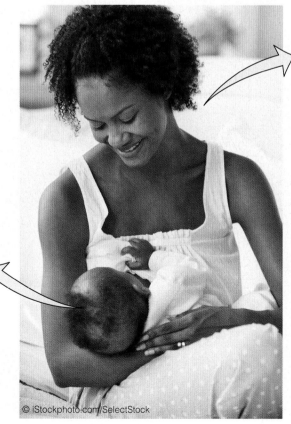

© iStockphoto.com/SelectStock

BENEFITS FOR MOTHERS

- Provides relaxing, emotionally enjoyable interaction; strengthens bonding with infant
- Reduces financial costs
- Requires less preparation and clean-up time; always available
- Causes uterine contractions that help the uterus return to its normal size more quickly after delivery
- Increases energy expenditure, which may speed return to prepregnancy weight
- Lowers risk of developing type-2 diabetes and breast and ovarian cancers[56]
- Improves bone density and decreases risk of fractures
- Inhibits ovulation, lengthening the time between pregnancies; however, breastfeeding cannot be relied on for birth control
- Decreases the risk of postpartum depression
- Enhances self-esteem in the maternal role

Safe Feeding for the First Year

Whether infants are breastfed or formula-fed, care must be taken to ensure that their needs are met and their food is safe. If proper measurements are not used when preparing formula, the infant may receive an excess or a deficiency of nutrients and an improper ratio of nutrients to fluid (**Figure 11.19a**). If the water and equipment used in preparing formula are not clean or if the prepared formula is left unrefrigerated, food-borne illness may result. Because sanitation is often lacking in developing nations, infections that lead to diarrhea and dehydration occur more frequently in formula-fed infants than in breastfed infants. Bacterial contamination is not a concern when a baby is breastfed, but care must be taken to avoid contamination when milk is pumped from the breast and stored for later feedings (**Figure 11.19b**).

Safe infant feeding • Figure 11.19

a. To avoid bacterial contamination, wash your hands before preparing formula. Clean bottles and bottle nipples by washing them in a dishwasher or placing them in boiling water for five minutes. Boil water for one to two minutes, then cool it before using the water to mix powdered formula or dilute concentrates. Cover and refrigerate opened cans of ready-to-feed and liquid concentrate formula and use the formula within the period indicated on the can. Prepare formula immediately before a feeding and discard any excess.

b. When breastfeeding isn't possible, milk can be pumped from the breast and fed from a bottle. To ensure the safety of pumped milk, wash hands, breast pumps, bottles, and bottle nipples. Breast milk that is not immediately fed to the baby can be kept refrigerated for 24 to 48 hours. Warming breast milk in a microwave is not recommended because microwaving destroys some of its immune properties and may result in dangerously hot milk. The best way to warm milk is by running warm water over the bottle.

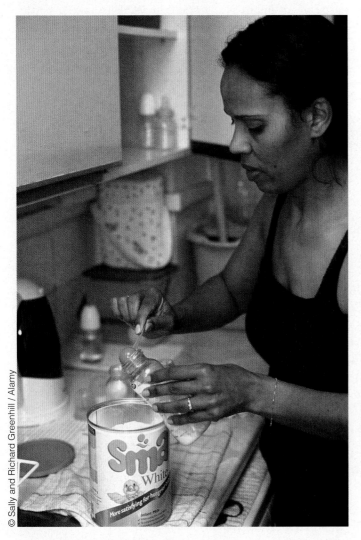

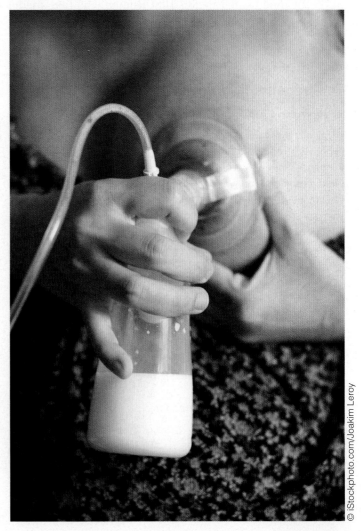

A concern unique to feeding breast milk is that substances in the maternal diet may pass into the milk and cause adverse reactions in the infant. For example, caffeine in the mother's diet can make the infant jittery and excitable, so a mother should avoid consuming large amounts of caffeine while breastfeeding. Most of these reactions seem to be unique to specific situations, so as long as a food does not affect the infant's health or response to feeding, it can be included in the mother's diet.

Food allergies Food allergies are common in infants because their digestive tracts are immature and therefore allow the absorption of incompletely digested proteins, which trigger a response from the immune system (see Chapters 3 and 6). Common allergies in infants include eggs, milk, peanuts, soy, tree nuts, and fish. Caregivers should watch for characteristic symptoms of a food allergy such as hives, swelling, vomiting, diarrhea, and/or difficulty breathing. After about 3 months of age, the risk of developing food allergies is reduced because incompletely digested proteins are less likely to be absorbed. Many children who develop food allergies before age 3 eventually outgrow them. Food allergies that appear after 3 years of age are more likely to continue throughout life.

Exclusive breastfeeding from age 4 to 6 months reduces an infant's risk of developing a food allergy.[58] If a formula-fed baby becomes allergic to the milk proteins used in the formula, soy formulas should be used. For infants who cannot tolerate soy protein, another option is a formula made from predigested proteins.

Introduction of solid foods Appropriate introduction of solid and semisolid foods can reduce the risk of an infant developing food allergies. The most commonly recommended first food is iron-fortified infant rice cereal mixed with formula or breast milk. This cereal is easily digested and rarely causes allergic reactions. After rice has been successfully added to the infant's diet, other grains can be introduced; wheat cereal is typically introduced last because it is the grain most likely to cause an allergic reaction. Each new food should be offered for a few days without the addition of any other new foods. Then, if an allergic reaction occurs, it is easier to determine which food caused the reaction. Foods that cause symptoms such as rashes, digestive upsets, or respiratory problems should be discontinued, and the symptoms should no longer be present before any other new foods are added.

Developmentally appropriate foods Foods that are offered to infants should be appropriate for their digestive and developmental abilities (see Figure 11.15). Cow's milk should never be fed to infants because it is too high in protein and too low in iron.[59] At 1 year of age, whole cow's milk can be offered; it can be used until 2 years of age, after which reduced-fat or low-fat milk can be used. As a child becomes familiar with more variety, food choices should be made from each of the food groups. To avoid choking, do not offer infants or toddlers foods that can easily lodge in the throat, such as carrots, grapes, and hot dogs.

Fruit juice can be fed from a cup when an infant is 9 to 10 months old, but excess quantities of apple and pear juice should be avoided because they contain sorbitol, a poorly absorbed sugar alcohol that can cause diarrhea. Added sugars should be offered in moderation to ensure a nutrient-dense diet. Unpasteurized honey should not be fed to children less than 1 year old because it may contain spores of *Clostridium botulinum*, the bacterium that causes botulism poisoning (discussed in Chapter 13). Older children and adults are not at risk from botulism spores because the environment in a mature gastrointestinal tract prevents the bacteria from growing.

CONCEPT CHECK

1. **What** does it mean if a child whose birth weight was in the 50th percentile is now in the 30th percentile for growth?
2. **When** can solid food be introduced into an infant's diet?
3. **Why** is breast milk the better choice for healthy mothers and babies?
4. **Why** is honey not recommended for infants?

Lactation

LEARNING OBJECTIVES

1. **Describe** the events that trigger milk production and let-down.

2. **Discuss** the energy and water needs of lactating women.

3. **Compare** the micronutrient needs of lactating women with those of non-pregnant, non-lactating women.

I f a woman chooses to breastfeed, she should be aware that her need for many nutrients is even greater during lactation than during pregnancy. The milk produced by a breast-feeding mother must meet all the nutrient needs of her baby, who is bigger and more active that he or she was in the womb. To meet these needs, a lactating woman must choose a varied, nutrient-dense diet.

Milk Production and Let-Down

Lactation involves both the synthesis of milk components—proteins, lactose, and lipids—and the movement of these components through the milk ducts to the nipple (**Figure 11.20**). Milk production and **let-down** are triggered by hormones that are released in response to an infant's suckling. The pituitary hormone **prolactin** stimulates milk production; the more the infant suckles, the more milk is produced. Let-down is caused by **oxytocin**, another pituitary hormone. Oxytocin release is also stimulated by suckling, but as nursing becomes more automatic, oxytocin release and let-down may occur in response to just the sight or sound of an infant. Oxytocin is also associated with social bonding, which may account for the emotional bond that forms between the mother and infant during breastfeeding. Let-down can be inhibited by nervous tension, fatigue, or embarrassment. Because let-down is essential for breastfeeding and makes suckling easier for the child, slow let-down can make feeding difficult.

> **let-down** The release of milk from the milk-producing glands and its movement through the ducts and storage sinuses.

Energy and Nutrient Needs during Lactation

Human milk contains about 70 kilocalories/100 millilitres (160 kilocalories/cup). During the first six months

Anatomy of milk production • Figure 11.20

Throughout pregnancy, hormones prepare the breasts for lactation by stimulating the enlargement and development of the milk ducts and milk-producing glands, called *alveoli* (*singular alveolus*). During lactation, milk travels from the alveoli through the ducts to the milk storage sinuses and then to the nipple.

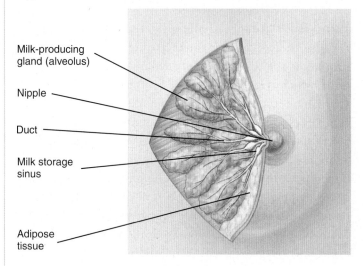

Milk-producing gland (alveolus)

Nipple

Duct

Milk storage sinus

Adipose tissue

of lactation, an average infant consumes 600 to 900 mL (about 2.5 to 4 cups)/day, so approximately 500 kilocalories are required from the mother each day. Much of this energy must come from the diet, but some can come from maternal fat stores. Because some of the energy for milk production comes from fat stores, the increase in recommended energy intake is lower during lactation than during pregnancy, even though total energy demands are greater (**Figure 11.21**). An additional 330 kilocalories/day above non-pregnant, non-lactating needs are recommended during the first six months of lactation, and an additional 400 kilocalories are recommended for the second six months. Beginning one month after birth, most lactating women lose 0.5 to 1 kg (1 to 2 lb.)/month for six months. Rapid weight loss is not recommended during lactation because it can decrease milk production.

To ensure adequate protein for milk production, the RDA for lactation is increased by 25 g/day. The recommended intakes of total carbohydrate, fibre, and the

Energy and macronutrient needs during lactation • Figure 11.21

This graph illustrates the percentage increase in energy and macronutrient recommendations for a 25-year-old woman during the third trimester of pregnancy and the first six months of lactation.

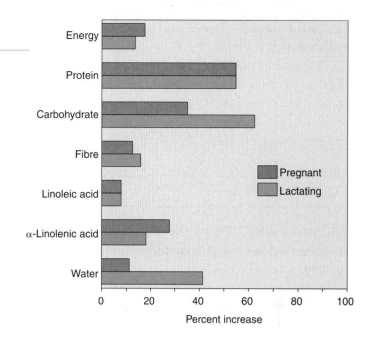

Micronutrient needs during lactation • Figure 11.22

This graph illustrates the percentage increase in vitamin and mineral recommendations for a 25-year-old woman during the third trimester of pregnancy and the first six months of lactation.

Folate needs are increased during lactation because this micronutrient is secreted in milk.

Because vitamin B_{12} may be deficient in the breast milk of vegan mothers, their infants should be given a vitamin B_{12} supplement.[20]

Increasing calcium intake during lactation does not prevent loss of calcium from maternal bones. Calcium supplements during lactation also do not affect the concentration of calcium in the milk or the minerals in the mother's bones.[6] The calcium lost from bones is restored after weaning.

Iron needs are not increased during lactation because little iron is lost in milk; moreover, iron losses are decreased in most lactating women because menstruation, which ceases during pregnancy, has not resumed. The RDA for lactation is 9 mg/day, half that of non pregnant, non-lactating women.[21]

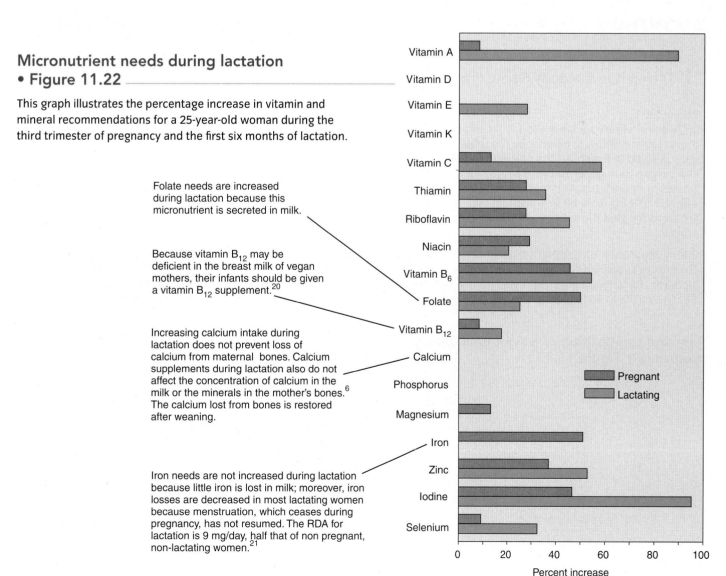

essential fatty acids linoleic and α-linolenic acid are also higher during lactation (see Figure 11.21).[42]

To avoid dehydration and ensure adequate milk production, lactating women need to consume about 1 L of additional water per day.[13] Consuming an extra glass of milk, juice, or water at each meal and when the infant nurses can help ensure adequate fluid intake. The recommended intakes for several vitamins and minerals are increased during lactation to meet the needs for synthesizing milk and to replace the nutrients secreted in the milk (**Figure 11.22**). Maternal intake of vitamins A, B_6, B_{12}, C, and D can affect the composition of milk. For other nutrients, including calcium and folate, levels in the milk are maintained at the expense of maternal stores.

CONCEPT CHECK STOP

1. **What** causes milk let-down?
2. **Where** does the energy for milk production come from?

3. **Why** is the recommended calcium intake for a new mother not increased while she is lactating?

Summary

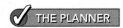 THE PLANNER

1 Changes in the Body during Pregnancy 384

- During the first eight weeks of development, all the organ systems necessary for life are formed in the **embryo**. Over the remaining weeks of pregnancy, the **fetus** grows, and organs develop and mature. The **placenta** transfers nutrients and oxygen from maternal blood to fetal blood and removes wastes from the fetus. At birth, a healthy baby weighs 3 to 4 kg (6.6 to 9 lb.). **Low-birth-weight** infants and infants who are **large for gestational age** are at increased risk of health problems.

- During pregnancy, the mother's body undergoes many changes to support the pregnancy and prepare for **lactation**. Recommended weight gain during pregnancy is 11 to 16 kg (25 to 35 lb.) for normal-weight women. Too little or too much weight gain can place both mother and baby at risk, but weight loss should never be attempted during pregnancy. Normal-weight, underweight, overweight, and obese mothers should all gain weight at a steady rate during pregnancy, but the total amount of weight gain recommended is different depending on prepregnancy weight.

- During healthy pregnancies, it can be beneficial and safe for the mother to participate in moderate-intensity exercise that does not increase the risk of abdominal trauma, falls, or joint stress.

- The hormones that direct changes in maternal physiology and fetal growth and development sometimes cause unwanted side effects, including **edema, morning sickness**, heartburn, constipation, and hemorrhoids.

Rate and composition of weight gain during pregnancy • Figure 11.3

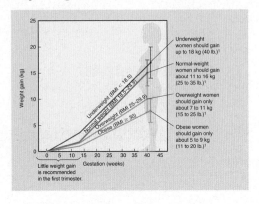

2 Nutritional Needs during Pregnancy 388

- During pregnancy, the requirements for energy, protein, carbohydrate, essential fatty acids, water, and many vitamins and minerals increase above non-pregnant levels.

- The AI for calcium is not increased because the increased need during pregnancy is met by an increase in absorption. Vitamin D deficiency is a concern, particularly for darker-skinned women. Adequate folic acid early in pregnancy reduces the risk of neural tube defects. Iron needs are high, and deficiency is common during pregnancy.

- *The Sensible Guide to a Healthy Pregnancy* can help pregnant women select foods to meet their nutritional needs. A prenatal supplement containing iron and folic acid and other vitamins and minerals is generally prescribed for all pregnant women.

- Food cravings are common during pregnancy. Most are harmless, but **pica** can reduce the intake of nutrient-dense foods, inhibit nutrient absorption, increase the risk of consuming toxins and infectious organisms, and cause intestinal obstructions.

Energy and macronutrient recommendations • Figure 11.5

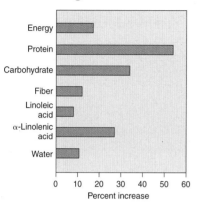

- **Hypertensive disorders of pregnancy** increase risk for the mother and baby. **Gestational hypertension** involves an increase in blood pressure during pregnancy. **Preeclampsia** is a more severe condition, characterized by edema, weight gain, and protein in the urine and can progress to life-threatening **eclampsia**. High blood glucose in the mother, called **gestational diabetes**, results in babies who are large for gestational age because extra glucose crosses the placenta from mother to baby.

Dangers of alcohol use during pregnancy • Figure 11.13

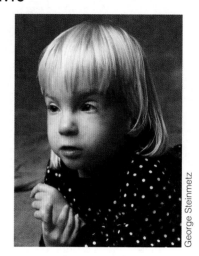

George Steinmetz

3 Factors That Increase the Risks Associated with Pregnancy 395

- The rapidly developing embryo and fetus are susceptible to damage from poor nutrition and physical, chemical, or other environmental **teratogens**. Malnutrition during pregnancy can cause fetal growth retardation, low infant birth weight, birth defects, premature birth, spontaneous abortion, and stillbirth.

- Pregnant teenagers are at increased risk because they are still growing themselves. Women over age 35 are at increased risk because they are more likely to have pre-existing health conditions and to develop gestational diabetes, pregnancy-induced hypertension, or other complications during pregnancy.

- Excessive caffeine intake can increase the risk of miscarriage. Following guidelines on fish consumption can minimize exposure to mercury, which can cause fetal brain damage. Pregnant women are particularly susceptible to food-borne illness and should follow safe food-handling recommendations. Alcohol consumption during pregnancy is a leading cause of brain damage and other birth defects. Exposure to cigarette smoke causes low birth weight and increases the risk of stillbirth, preterm delivery, and behavioural problems in the baby. The use of illegal drugs such as cocaine also increases the risk of low birth weight and birth defects.

4 Nutrition for Infants 401

- Growth is the best indicator of adequate nutrition in an infant. Healthy infants follow standard patterns of growth. Growth charts can be used to compare an infant's growth with the growth of other infants of the same age. Slow growth indicates **failure to thrive**, whereas excess weight gain may predispose a child to obesity. Adequate nutrition is essential for achieving developmental milestones and affect how an infant can obtain nourishment.

- Infants require more calories and protein per kilogram of body weight than at any other time of life. Fat and fluid needs are also proportionately higher than in adults. Infants are at risk for deficiencies of iron, vitamin D, and vitamin K, as well as low fluoride intake.

- Breast milk is the ideal food for infants. It meets nutrient needs; it is always available; it requires no special equipment, mixing, or sterilization; and it provides immune protection. Many infant formulas on the market are patterned after human milk and provide adequate nutrition to a baby. Formula is the better option when the mother is ill or is taking prescription or illicit drugs, or when the infant has special nutritional needs.

Nourishing a developing infant • Figure 11.15

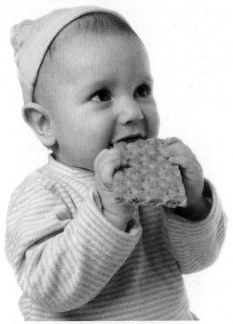

© Can Stock Photo Inc. / fanfo

- Introducing solid foods between 4 and 6 months of age adds iron and other nutrients to the diet. Newly introduced foods should be appropriate to the child's stage of development and offered one at a time to monitor for food allergies.

5 Lactation 412

- Milk production and **let-down** are triggered by hormones released in response to the suckling of an infant.

- Lactation requires energy and nutrients from the mother to produce adequate milk. The energy for milk production comes from the diet and maternal fat stores. Maternal needs for protein, fluid, and many vitamins and minerals are even greater during lactation than during pregnancy.

Anatomy of milk production • Figure 11.20

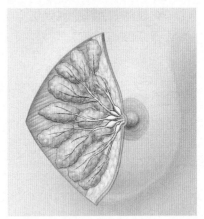

Key Terms

- alcohol-related birth defects (ARBD) 399
- alcohol-related neuro-development disorders (ARND) 399
- Caesarean section 385
- colostrum 408
- critical period 395
- eclampsia 400
- embryo 384

- failure to thrive 401
- fertilization 384
- fetal alcohol syndrome (FAS) 399
- fetus 385
- gestational diabetes 400
- gestational hypertension 400
- hypertensive disorders of pregnancy, or pregnancy-induced hypertension 400

- implantation 384
- infancy 401
- lactation 385
- large for gestational age 386
- let-down 412
- low birth weight 385
- morning sickness 387
- nursing bottle syndrome 406
- oxytocin 412

- pica 392
- placenta 384
- preeclampsia 400
- preterm, or premature 385
- prolactin 412
- small for gestational age 385
- teratogen 395
- trimester 385
- very low birth weight 385

Critical and Creative Thinking Questions

1. Keep a three-day diet record. Use iProfile to analyze the nutrient composition of your diet. Would your diet meet the energy, protein, and micronutrient needs of a 25-year-old pregnant woman who is 165 cm (5′5″) tall, weighed 59 kg (130 lb.) at the start of her pregnancy, and is now in her second trimester? If not, what foods or supplements should need to be added to meet these needs?

2. Many people object to infant formula manufacturers advertising their products in developing nations. Do you feel it is appropriate to promote the use of formula in developing nations? Why or why not?

3. HIV, the virus that causes AIDS, passes via breastfeeding to one out of seven infants born to HIV-infected mothers; yet, in developing countries, some HIV-positive women are advised to breastfeed. Explain this recommendation, considering what you have learned about the benefits of breastfeeding.

4. If an infant is born weighing 2.7 kg (6 lb.), what might the baby weigh at 4 months of age and at 12 months? Why?

5. Sia, a vegan woman, has just learned she is pregnant. What nutrient deficiencies are common for vegans? For pregnant women? What supplements would you recommend Sia take during her pregnancy?

6. Marina, a 16-year-old, is four months pregnant. She is 163 cm (5′4″) tall and weighed 50 kg (110 lb.) before she became pregnant. Her typical diet, which provided 1,800 kilocalories, 60 g of protein, and 15 mg of iron, met her needs before she became pregnant. What changes in the amounts of energy, protein, and iron would you recommend now that Marina is in her second trimester?

What is happening in this picture?

Ultrasound imaging, shown here, uses sound waves to visualize the embryo or fetus in the uterus. It can be used to assess the progress of the pregnancy and identify fetal and maternal health problems.

Think Critically

1. If the baby is larger than expected, what might be the cause?
2. If the baby is smaller than expected, what might be the cause?

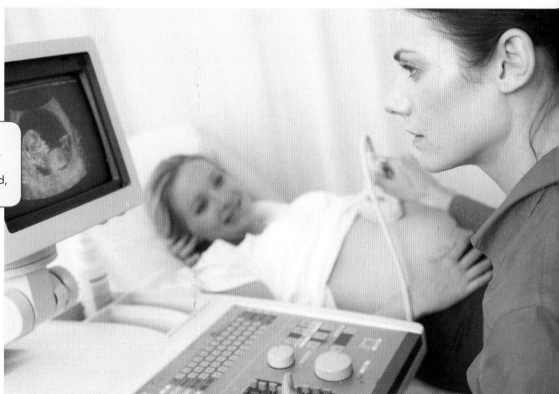

© Can Stock Photo Inc. / monkeybusiness

Self-Test

(Check your answers in Appendix J.)

1. An infant born at term, weighing 2 kg (4.5 lb.) at birth, is considered _____.
   a. large for gestational age
   b. premature
   c. very low birth weight
   d. low birth weight

2. Newborn infants receive an injection of _____ to prevent the possibility of hemorrhage.
   a. iron
   b. folate
   c. vitamin D
   d. vitamin K

3. Use the figure below to determine how much of the weight gained during pregnancy is due to an increase in body fluids.
   a. about 1.8 kg (4 lb.)
   b. about 900 g (2 lb.)
   c. as much as 4.5 kg (10 lb.)
   d. less than 1.8 kg (4 lb.)

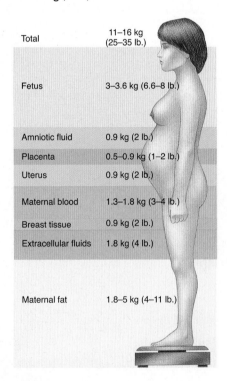

Total	11–16 kg (25–35 lb.)
Fetus	3–3.6 kg (6.6–8 lb.)
Amniotic fluid	0.9 kg (2 lb.)
Placenta	0.5–0.9 kg (1–2 lb.)
Uterus	0.9 kg (2 lb.)
Maternal blood	1.3–1.8 kg (3–4 lb.)
Breast tissue	0.9 kg (2 lb.)
Extracellular fluids	1.8 kg (4 lb.)
Maternal fat	1.8–5 kg (4–11 lb.)

4. A woman who enters pregnancy with excess weight (BMI > 30) should _____.
   a. lose about 2.3 to 4.5 kg (5 to 10 lb.) during her pregnancy
   b. gain about 5 to 9 kg (11 to 20 lb.) during her pregnancy
   c. not gain any additional weight during her pregnancy
   d. limit her intake to 1,200 Calories per day

5. According to *Eating Well with Canada's Food Guide*, how many extra daily food guide servings should a typical pregnant woman eat?
   a. 2-3
   b. 4-5
   c. 6-7
   d. 8-9

6. Which of the following is not associated with preeclampsia?
   a. high blood glucose
   b. a rise in blood pressure
   c. edema
   d. protein in the urine

7. The recommended intake for which of the following is not increased during pregnancy?
   a. calcium
   b. iron
   c. protein
   d. zinc

8. During which weeks of development is exposure to a teratogen most likely to result in a heart defect in the embryo or fetus?
   a. first 3 weeks
   b. about 3 to 7 weeks
   c. 7 to 8 weeks
   d. anytime after 9 weeks

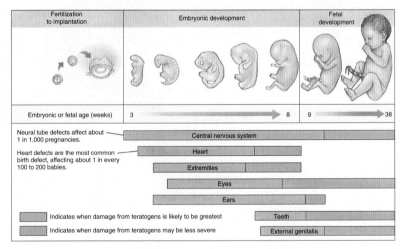

9. The hormone responsible for the let-down of milk is _____.
   a. estrogen
   b. prolactin
   c. progesterone
   d. oxytocin

10. When should solid food be introduced into an infant's diet?

    a. within two weeks of birth

    b. around 4 to 6 months of age

    c. at 9 months of age

    d. after one year

11. Which of the following statements comparing older and younger pregnant women is false?

    a. older pregnant women have different nutritional requirements than younger ones

    b. older pregnant women are more likely to develop gestational diabetes

    c. children born to older women are more likely to have chromosomal abnormalities

    d. older women are more likely to have pre-existing conditions that increase pregnancy-related risks

12. The leading cause of preventable birth defects and intellectual disability is _____ during pregnancy.

    a. coffee consumption

    b. tobacco use

    c. alcohol consumption

    d. cocaine use

13. During lactation, an infant consumes approximately _____ kcalories per day from breast milk.

    a. 200

    b. 500

    c. 850

    d. 1000

14. Colostrum is _____.

    a. a type of infant formula that is fortified with omega-3 fatty acids

    b. the first stool passed by the infant after delivery

    c. the first fluid produced by the breast after delivery

    d. the mature milk produced in the later part of a feeding

15. Which of the following statements about breast milk is false?

    a. It contains immune factors that protect the baby from infections.

    b. It provides about 50% of calories from fat.

    c. It contains a high concentration of iron.

    d. The proteins it contains are easily digested.

THE PLANNER ✓

Review your Chapter Planner on the chapter opener and check off your completed work.

Nutrition from 1 to 100

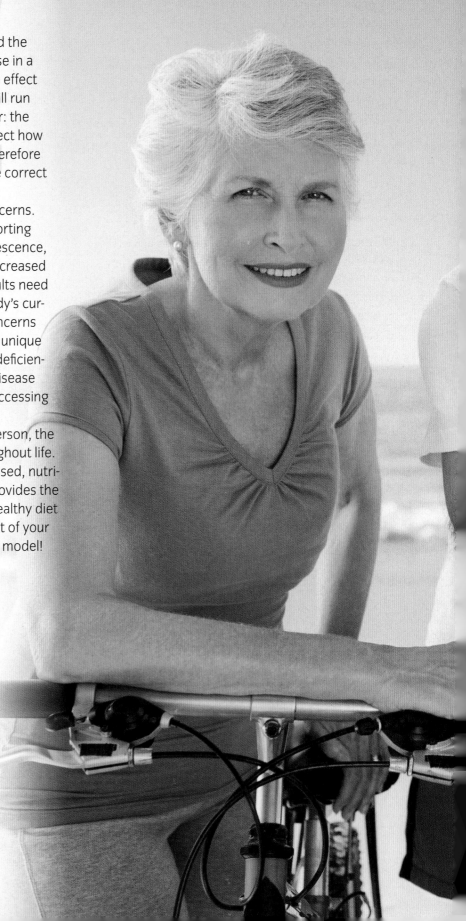

In the Chapter 3 opening story, we compared the human body to a car. The type of fuel you use in a car and the way you take care of it have a huge effect on how long that car will last and how well it will run throughout its life. The human body is like a car: the type and amount of nutrients we put into it affect how well it will work and how long it will last. It is therefore imperative that we provide our bodies with the correct blend of nutrients at every stage of life.

Each age group has its own nutritional concerns. Nutrition during childhood is focused on supporting proper growth and development. During adolescence, the drastic increase in growth rate brings an increased need for energy and nutrients. In contrast, adults need to get the proper nutrition to support their body's current state and reduce the risk of nutritional concerns and disease in later life. Older adults also have unique dietary concerns, often focusing on potential deficiencies, maintaining body structure, minimizing disease risk, managing disease symptoms, or simply accessing the foods they require.

While specific needs vary by age and by person, the basics of proper nutrition stay the same throughout life. A varied and balanced diet based on unprocessed, nutrient-dense options and eaten in moderation provides the best fuel and support to an aging body. This healthy diet helps ensure that you get the maximum life out of your body. After all, you can't trade it in for a newer model!

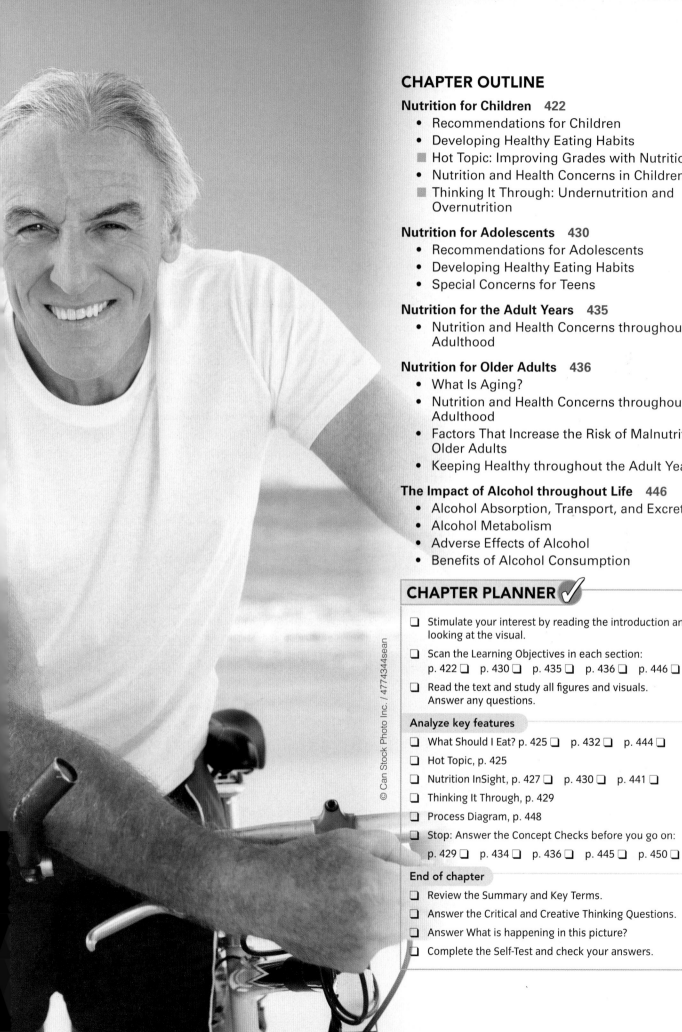

CHAPTER OUTLINE

© Can Stock Photo Inc. / 4774344sean

CHAPTER PLANNER ✓

- ☐ Stimulate your interest by reading the introduction and looking at the visual.
- ☐ Scan the Learning Objectives in each section:
  p. 422 ☐   p. 430 ☐   p. 435 ☐   p. 436 ☐   p. 446 ☐
- ☐ Read the text and study all figures and visuals. Answer any questions.

Analyze key features

- ☐ What Should I Eat? p. 425 ☐   p. 432 ☐   p. 444 ☐
- ☐ Hot Topic, p. 425
- ☐ Nutrition InSight, p. 427 ☐   p. 430 ☐   p. 441 ☐
- ☐ Thinking It Through, p. 429
- ☐ Process Diagram, p. 448
- ☐ Stop: Answer the Concept Checks before you go on:
  p. 429 ☐   p. 434 ☐   p. 436 ☐   p. 445 ☐   p. 450 ☐

End of chapter

- ☐ Review the Summary and Key Terms.
- ☐ Answer the Critical and Creative Thinking Questions.
- ☐ Answer What is happening in this picture?
- ☐ Complete the Self-Test and check your answers.

Nutrition for Children

LEARNING OBJECTIVES

1. **Describe** how children's nutrient needs change as they grow.

2. **Discuss** the role of the caregiver in developing children's eating habits.

3. **Explain** the impact of diet and lifestyle during childhood on the risk of chronic disease in adulthood.

4. **Relate** diet and nutrition to the incidence of dental caries and hyperactivity.

Childhood is the period between infancy and adolescence. Nutrient intake during this time affects health in adulthood. The foods offered to a child must supply the energy and nutrients needed for growth and development as well as for maintenance and activity. They must also be appropriate for the child's stage of physical development and suit his or her developing tastes. A nutritious, well-balanced eating pattern and an active lifestyle allow children to grow to their potential and can prevent or delay the onset of the chronic diseases that plague adults. Therefore, teaching healthy eating and exercise habits will benefit not only today's children but also tomorrow's adults.

Recommendations for Children

Much of what we choose to eat as adults depends on what we learned to eat as children. Caregivers are responsible for deciding what foods are offered to a child and when and where these foods are eaten. The child must then decide whether to eat, what foods to eat, and how much to consume.[1] As children grow older, their choices are increasingly affected by social activities, what they see at school, and what their friends are eating.

Fundamental nutritional principles are consistent throughout all age groups from 1 to 100. Children, like adults, should consume a balanced and varied diet that is adequate in energy and essential nutrients and meets their specific nutritional needs. The latest edition of Canada's Food Guide now outlines how dietary patterns change at different stages of childhood (ages 2–13) (**Figure 12.1**). Because children have smaller stomachs, their recommended daily servings from each food group are smaller than for adults. Canada's Food Guide illustrates that a healthy diet is based on nutritious meals and snacks containing whole grains, vegetables, fruits, adequate milk, high-quality protein, and healthy fats.[2] Children, like adults, should also consume enough water to satisfy their thirst.[3]

Energy and macronutrient needs of children As children grow and become more active, their requirements increase for energy and most nutrients. For example, the average 2-year-old needs about 1000 kilocalories and 13 g of protein/day, but by age 6, that child needs about 1600 kilocalories and 19 g of protein/day.[4] At age 12, if that child is a girl, she may require 1600 to 2600 kilocalories and 34 g of protein per day. If the child is a boy, he may require 1800 to 2800 kilocalories and 34 g of protein per day.[4] The exact number of kilocalories required can vary substantially, depending on body size, height, and activity level. The total amount of protein and energy needed continues to increase as children grow into adults; however,

Canada's Food Guide and children
• Figure 12.1

Eating Well with Canada's Food Guide now makes specific recommendations for the appropriate daily servings for children of varying ages. Note that the number of food guide servings increases moderately with increased age and that the recommendations are the same for both boys and girls.

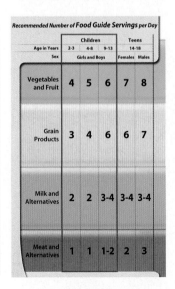

Recommended Number of *Food Guide Servings* per Day					
	Children			**Teens**	
Age in Years	2-3	4-8	9-13	14-18	
Sex	Girls and Boys			Females	Males
Vegetables and Fruit	4	5	6	7	8
Grain Products	3	4	6	6	7
Milk and Alternatives	2	2	3-4	3-4	3-4
Meat and Alternatives	1	1	1-2	2	3

Advice for different ages and stages...

Children

Following Canada's Food Guide helps children grow and thrive.

Young children have small appetites and need calories for growth and development.

- Serve small nutritious meals and snacks each day.

- Do not restrict nutritious foods because of their fat content. Offer a variety of foods from the four food groups.

- Most of all... be a good role model.

Energy needs • Figure 12.2

As children grow, their larger body size causes the total amount of energy they need to increase, but as growth slows, energy needs/kilogram of body weight decline.

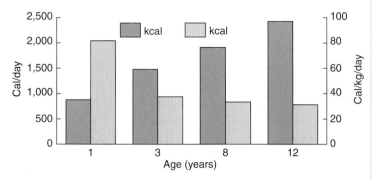

the amounts needed per kilogram of body weight decrease (**Figure 12.2**).

The recommended range of carbohydrate intake for children is the same as for adults: 45 to 65% of total energy intake. To provide enough energy to support rapid growth and development, the recommended range of fat intake is higher for children than for adults: 30 to 40% of total energy intake for 1- to 3-year-olds and 25 to 35% for 4- to 18-year-olds. As children grow, the recommended percentage of calories from fat decreases to avoid increasing their risk of chronic diseases.

In most situations, children can meet their fluid needs by drinking enough to satisfy thirst.[5] Fluid needs increase when there is illness, when the environmental temperature is high, and when activity increases sweat losses.

Because children are smaller than adolescents and adults, the recommended amounts of most micronutrients are also smaller (see inside cover). Like adults, children who consume a varied, nutrient-dense diet can meet all their vitamin and mineral requirements through food. However, in North America today, diets that frequently include fast-food meals and high-sugar and high-fat snacks put many children at risk for inadequate vitamin and mineral intake.[6] Deficiencies of calcium, vitamin D, and iron are of particular concern.

Calcium, vitamin D, and bone health Calcium intake in school-age children has been declining, primarily due to a decrease in the consumption of dairy products. Adequate calcium intake during childhood and regular weight-bearing exercises are essential for achieving maximum peak bone mass, which is critical for preventing os-

teoporosis later in life (see Chapter 8). The Recommended Dietary Allowance (RDA) for calcium is 700 mg/day for toddlers (ages 1 to 3), 1000 mg/day for young children (ages 4 to 8), and 1300 mg/day for older children (ages 9 to 13).[7]

Vitamin D, which is needed for calcium absorption, is also essential for bone health. Low intakes of milk combined with limited sun exposure may put many children at risk for vitamin D deficiency. The RDA is 15 μg/day for children, adolescents, and young adults.

Iron and anemia Children's iron needs are high because iron is required for growth. The RDA is 7 mg/day for toddlers and 10 mg/day for young children,[8] the latter being higher than the RDA for adult men. The high needs and finicky eating habits of young children often lead to iron deficiency anemia, a condition that can affect mood and impair learning ability, intellectual performance, and stamina.[9,10] When anemia is diagnosed, iron supplements are usually prescribed until the child's iron stores have been replenished. These supplements should be kept out of the reach of children to prevent iron toxicity from supplement overdoses (see Chapter 8).

Developing Healthy Eating Habits

Healthy eating habits are not just about *what* a child eats but also *how* a child eats. Healthy eating behaviours and food relationships start in childhood and can have a vital impact on future health. To be a good role model, parents and guardians are encouraged to have family dinners with their children, free from distraction. Also, children often model their behaviours after adults they respect. If a child sees an adult enjoying healthy foods, they may be more likely to also enjoy these foods. Food should rarely be used to regulate a child's mood, however, because using food in this way may lead to overconsumption in the future.[11]

Caregivers often face challenges when trying to persuade a child to eat a variety of foods from all the food groups, as Canada's Food Guide recommends. To increase variety, new foods should be introduced into a child's diet regularly and from a young age. Children's food preferences are learned through repeated exposure to foods; a new food may need to be offered 8 or 10 times before the child will accept it. Children are also more likely to eat a new food when three factors are present: when it is introduced at the beginning of a meal, when the child is hungry, and when the child sees his or her parents or peers also eating the food. Incorporating healthy foods into familiar dishes can also increase the variety of the diet. For example, vegetables can be added to soups and casseroles, and lean meats can be added to spaghetti sauce, stews, or pizza. Getting children to consume the recommended amount of fruit is usually not difficult, but most servings should come from fruit, with limited amounts from 100% juice, not from fruit drinks. The American Academy of Pediatrics recommends limiting juice to 113 to 170 mL (4 to 6 oz, or about a 1/2 cup to 3/4 of a cup) per day for children ages 1 to 6 and 226 to 355 mL (8 to 12 oz, or about 1 cup to 1.5 cups) per day for children age 7 and older (**Figure 12.3**).[12]

The setting in which a meal is consumed is also important. Children who eat dinner with their families have a higher-quality diet than those who don't.[13] Children learn by example; therefore, the eating patterns, attitudes, and feeding styles of their caregivers influence what they learn to eat. When meals are shared and caregivers make healthy food choices, children are likely to follow their example. Eating meals together also helps children connect with family and culture and is associated with better school performance and decreased risk of unhealthy weight loss practices and substance abuse. Children need companionship, conversation, and pleasant surroundings

Limiting juice consumption • Figure 12.3

Because of the sweet taste of juice, overconsumption is a concern. Drinking too much juice, even if it is 100% juice, can cause diarrhea, overnutrition or undernutrition, and dental caries. Furthermore, juice is typically low in nutrient density and high in calories. It may also suppress a child's appetite, promoting undernutrition. It is recommended that juice not be offered to children in containers that can be carried around, which encourages continuous sipping.[12]

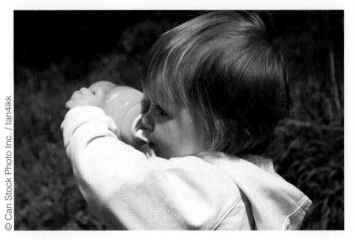

© Can Stock Photo Inc. / tan4ikk

at mealtimes. They should be given plenty of time to finish eating. Slow eaters are unlikely to finish eating if they are abandoned by siblings who run off to play or by adults who leave to wash dishes. Moreover, if mealtime is to be a nutritious, educational, and enjoyable experience, it should not be a battle zone. Food is not a reward or a punishment: It is simply nutrition.

No matter how erratic children's food intake may be, caregivers should continue to offer a variety of healthy foods at each meal and let children select what and how much they will eat. Children, like adults, tend to eat greater quantities when larger portions are provided.[14] When children are allowed to serve themselves, they eat more appropriate portions than when a large portion is put in front of them.

The best indicator that a child is receiving adequate nourishment, neither too little nor too much, is a normal growth pattern. Growth is most rapid in the first year of life, when an infant's length increases by 50%, or about 25 cm (10 in.). In the second year of life, children generally grow about 12.5 cm (5 in.); in the third year, 10 cm (4 in.); and thereafter, about 5 to 7.5 cm (2 to 3 in.) per year. Although growth often occurs in spurts, growth patterns are predictable and can be monitored by comparing a child's growth pattern with standard patterns shown on growth charts (Figure 11.14). The stature a child will eventually attain is affected by genetic, environmental, and lifestyle factors. For example, a child whose parents are 1.5 m (5 ft.) tall may not have the genetic potential to grow to 1.8 m (6 ft.).

When a child does not get enough to eat, weight gain slows, and if the deficiency continues, growth in height also slows. If food intake is excessive, a child is at risk for becoming obese and developing the chronic diseases that are increasingly common in Canadian adults (see *What Should I Eat?*).

When and where to offer meals and snacks

Because children have small stomachs and high nutrient needs, they need to consume small, nutrient-dense meals and snacks, ideally every two to three hours throughout the day. Establishing a consistent meal pattern is important because children thrive on routine and feel secure when they know what to expect. Starting the day with a good breakfast is particularly important; children who eat breakfast are more likely to meet their daily nutrient needs and to do better in school (see *Hot Topic*).[15] Snacks

WHAT SHOULD I EAT?
Childhood

Serve children frequent nutritious meals and snacks
- Smear peanut butter on a banana or an apple.
- Offer some sliced fruit with yogurt dip.
- Try to include at least four colours in every meal.
- Cut and arrange foods in interesting shapes.

Serve more fruits and vegetables
- Bake bananas and berries into breads and muffins.
- Add vegetables to soups, tacos, and casseroles.
- Blend fruit into shakes and smoothies.
- Mix extra vegetables into spaghetti sauce.

Include calcium where you can
- Make oatmeal with milk instead of water.
- Make soup creamier by adding milk.
- Serve pudding and custard.
- Offer nutritious breakfast cereals with milk.

Add iron
- Make your spaghetti sauce with meat.
- Cook your stew in an iron pot.
- Beef up your tacos and burritos.
- Serve iron-fortified breakfast cereal.

Use iProfile to find snacks that are high in iron.

HOT TOPIC

Improving grades with nutrition

This breakfast looks appealing, but regardless of what's on the table, many children and teens do not make time for breakfast; they are more likely to skip breakfast than to skip any other meal.[15] Eating breakfast has an impact on both nutritional status and school performance. Skipping breakfast may result in a span of 15 or more hours without food. Because breakfast provides energy and nutrients to the brain, children who skip this meal are more likely to have academic, emotional, and behavioural problems than those children who eat breakfast.[16] Studies have found that compared with children who do not eat breakfast, children who participate in school breakfast programs have better nutrient intakes, which are associated with improvements in academic performance, reductions in hyperactivity, better psychosocial behaviours, and fewer instances of absence and tardiness (see graph).[17]

Free school breakfast programs are found in many developed countries. Surprisingly, Canada is one of the only developed nations that lacks a national children's breakfast program, despite many believing that such a program is needed.

A two-year breakfast program trial was recently implemented in the Jane and Finch area of the Toronto School Board District to determine the potential benefits of such a program. Students who took part in the initiative were more able to stay on task during class, had a better attitude and attendance, and were more likely to be on track to graduate.[18] They also tended to perform better in mathematics and science. Although the program was a heralded as a success by the school and school board, the future of these programs in Canadian schools remains uncertain.

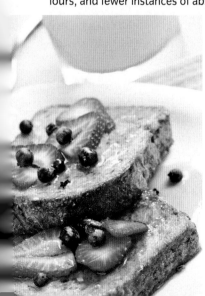

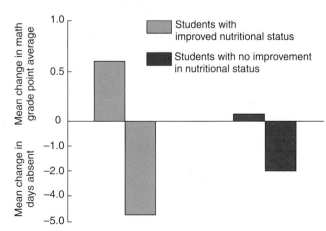

Mean change in math grade point average

Mean change in days absent

1.0
0.5
0
-1.0
-2.0
-4.0
-5.0

Students with improved nutritional status

Students with no improvement in nutritional status

Ask Yourself

In addition to enhancing learning by fuelling the brain after the overnight fast, in what other ways might breakfast contribute to better school performance?

© iStockphoto.com/Elena Elisseeva

Typical meal and snack patterns for 3- and 8-year-old children   Table 12.1

Food	Amount 3-year-old	8-year-old	Food	Amount 3-year-old	8-year-old
Breakfast			**Snack**		
Cereal	125 g (1/2 cup)	250 g (1 cup)	Yogurt	125 g (1/2 cup)	250 g (1 cup)
Milk, 2%	125 mL (1/2 cup)	250 mL (1 cup)	Berries	85 g (3/8 cup)	170 g (3/4 cup)
Banana	1/2 medium	1 medium			
			Dinner		
Snack			Rice	125 g (1/2 cup)	250 g (1 cup)
Peanut butter	30 mL (2 Tbsp)	30 mL (2 Tbsp)	Chicken drumsticks	1	2
Wheat crackers	5	5	Broccoli	4 florets	6 florets
			Milk, 2%	125 g (1/2 cup)	250 mL (1 cup)
Lunch					
Vegetable soup	125 mL (1/2 cup)	250 mL (1 cup)	**Snack**		
Grilled tuna sandwich	half	1	Graham crackers	1	2
Tomato	1/4 medium	1/2 medium	Milk	125 mL (1/2 cup)	125 mL (1/2 cup)
Orange	1/2 medium	1 medium			
Milk, 2%	125 mL (1/2 cup)	250 mL (1 cup)			

should be as nutritious as meals to ensure that nutrient needs are met (**Table 12.1**).

Nutrition and Health Concerns in Children

The diets of Canadian children today are not as healthy as they could be; as a result, children are not as healthy as they could be. Some nutrition and health concerns regarding children in Canada are related to their dietary and exercise patterns. Approximately 1 in 5 Canadian children consume more energy than they expend through physical activity.[19] The high-calorie, high-salt, high-fat diet and the low-activity lifestyle that contribute to obesity and chronic disease in adults are having the same effects in children. Another nutrition-related health concern in children is dental caries.

The rising rate of childhood obesity Approximately a quarter of Canadian children between the ages of 2 and 7 are overweight or obese.[20] Excessive weight can lead to several chronic conditions, including type-2 diabetes, high blood pressure, and elevated blood cholesterol, as well as social and psychological challenges (**Figure 12.4**).

Addressing the issue of excess weight in children requires changes in both eating and activity patterns. Because children are still growing, weight loss is rarely recommended, and the word *diet* should not be used to motivate change. Instead, overweight children should be encouraged to eat appropriately sized servings and

nutrient-dense foods and to enjoy various activities as they continue to grow taller. This eating and activity pattern will allow children to "grow into" their weight. A child who is at the 85th percentile for BMI at age 7 and gains only a kilogram or two a year may be at the 75th percentile by age 9. Focusing on losing weight instead of focusing on healthy weight-related behaviours is discouraged as it may promote disordered eating.

It can be difficult to modify a child's food consumption patterns. Denying food may promote further overeating because the child may feel that he or she will not obtain enough food to satisfy hunger. Thus, restrictions on food intake should be relatively mild, and the focus instead should be on offering nutrient-dense foods. The Canadian Physical Activity Guidelines and the Dietary Reference Intakes (DRIs) recommend that children be physically active for at least one hour per day. This extent of physical activity may be difficult for overweight children, who are often embarrassed by their bodies and may shy away from group activities.

Watching television has a major influence on children's energy balance because it affects both food intake and activity level (**Figure 12.5** and *Thinking It Through*). Sitting in front of the television encourages snacking and reduces activity. Television also affects the quality of the diet because commercials introduce children to foods they might otherwise not be aware of. Children who view food ads choose those food products more often than children who are not exposed to the ads.[22]

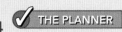
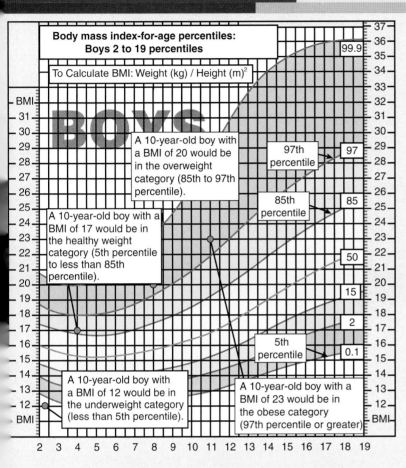

Body mass index-for-age percentiles: Boys 2 to 19 percentiles

To Calculate BMI: Weight (kg) / Height (m)^2

BOYS

A 10-year-old boy with a BMI of 20 would be in the overweight category (85th to 97th percentile).

A 10-year-old boy with a BMI of 17 would be in the healthy weight category (5th percentile to less than 85th percentile).

A 10-year-old boy with a BMI of 12 would be in the underweight category (less than 5th percentile).

A 10-year-old boy with a BMI of 23 would be in the obese category (97th percentile or greater)

97th percentile → 97
85th percentile → 85
50
15
2
5th percentile → 0.1
99.9

▲ A child's weight is assessed by determining his or her body mass index (BMI) and plotting it on a gender-specific BMI-for-age growth chart to determine his or her percentile (see Chapter 11). The BMI percentile is then used to classify the child as obese, overweight, healthy weight, or underweight.[21]

© Benedicte Desrus / Alamy

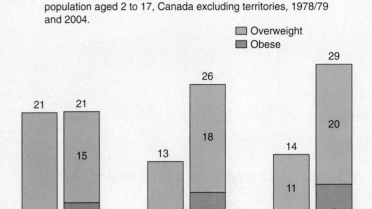

Percentage overweight or obese, by age group, household population aged 2 to 17, Canada excluding territories, 1978/79 and 2004.

■ Overweight
■ Obese

2 to 5 — 1978/79: 21 (15 / 6); 2004: 21 (15 / 6)
6 to 11 — 1978/79: 13; 2004: 26 (18 / 8)
12 to 17 — 1978/79: 14 (11 / 3); 2004: 29 (20 / 9)

Age group

▲ As in adults, the prevalence of overweight and obesity has increased significantly over the past three decades. An approximate twofold increase in the incidence of overweight and obesity is evidenced in older children and adolescents.

The social and psychological effects of obesity in children can be as damaging as the physical effects. Weight-associated bullying is one of the most common types of discrimination in both children and adults. Some people believe that ridiculing children about their weight may motivate them to change their weight-related behaviours. In actuality, people who experience bias because of their weight are more likely to binge eat and have higher BMIs than those who do not experience weight bias. Weight bias may result in a poor self-image, low self-esteem, and social isolation. Social isolation, in turn, may result in boredom, depression, inactivity, and withdrawal—all of which can increase eating and decrease activity, worsening the problem. ▼

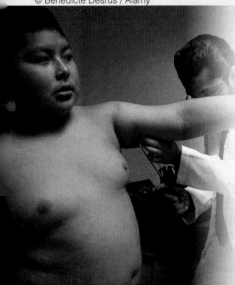

◄ Children whose blood pressure is at the high end of normal are more likely to develop high blood pressure as adults. As with adults, blood pressure can be affected by activity level, the amount of body fat, and the total pattern of dietary intake, including sodium intake.

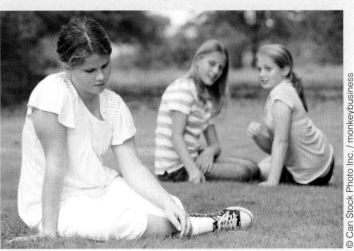

© Can Stock Photo Inc. / monkeybusiness

Television affects food intake and activity level • Figure 12.5

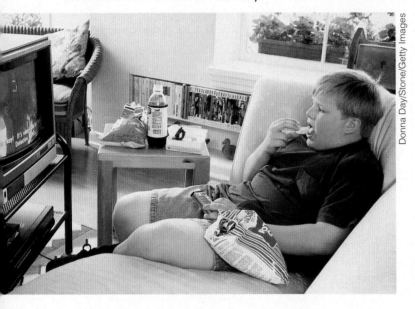

a. Hours spent watching television are hours when physical activity is at a minimum. Children who watch four or more hours of TV per day are 40% more likely to be overweight than those who watch an hour or less a day.[23]

Donna Day/Stone/Getty Images

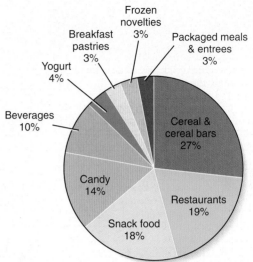

Frozen novelties 3%
Breakfast pastries 3%
Packaged meals & entrees 3%
Yogurt 4%
Cereal & cereal bars 27%
Beverages 10%
Candy 14%
Restaurants 19%
Snack food 18%

b. During children's television programming, food is the most frequently advertised product category. This pie chart, which illustrates the types of food advertised on Saturday morning children's television programming, shows that almost half of the commercials advertise candy, snack foods, beverages, and pastries.[24]

Food jags The importance of nutritional variety is promoted throughout this textbook, and this dietary variety is equally critical to support childhood development. Unfortunately, some children may refuse to eat new foods, perhaps because they have a fear of them. This refusal to eat new foods may result in a **food jag**, whereby a child wants to eat the same food meal after meal. Getting children to try new foods can be a difficult task for caregivers. Helpful suggestions include preparing colourful meals, introducing new tastes at an early age, and setting a good example by caregivers eating a variety of foods themselves. It may also be effective to implement the taste rule, telling a child: "You need to at least taste everything on your plate."

Preventing dental caries A diet that is high in sugary foods promotes the formation of dental caries (see Chapter 4). Because the primary teeth guide the growth of the permanent teeth, maintaining healthy primary teeth is just as important as preserving the permanent ones. Much of the added sugar in children's diets comes from soft drinks and other sweetened beverages; when these are sipped slowly between meals, the duration of the contact between sugar and bacteria on the surface of the teeth is prolonged, increasing the risk of tooth decay.

Hyperactivity Hyperactivity is a problem in 5 to 10% of school-age children, occurring more frequently in boys than in girls. Hyperactivity involves extreme physical activity, excitability, impulsiveness, distractibility, short attention span, and low tolerance for frustration. Hyperactive children have more difficulty learning but usually are of normal or above-average intelligence.

Hyperactivity is now considered part of a larger syndrome known as **attention-deficit/hyperactivity disorder (ADHD)**.

A popular misconception is that hyperactivity is caused by eating sugar, but research on the relationship between sugar intake and behaviour has failed to support this hypothesis.[25,26] The hyperactive behaviour observed after sugar consumption is more likely the result of situational factors. For example, the excitement of a birthday party rather than the sugar in the cake is most likely the cause of hyperactive behaviour.

Other possible causes of hyperactivity include caffeine consumption, lack of sleep, overstimulation, desire for more attention, and lack of physical activity. Specific foods and food additives have also been implicated as causes of hyperactivity. Numerous studies have failed to provide sufficient evidence for the efficacy of any dietary treatment for ADHD. However, some children are sensitive to specific additives and may benefit from a diet that eliminates them.[26]

> **attention-deficit/hyperactivity disorder (ADHD)** A condition characterized by a short attention span and a high level of activity, excitability, and distractibility.

THINKING IT THROUGH

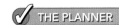

Undernutrition and Overnutrition

Luke is 10 years old and has gained 2.3 kg (5 lb.) in the past three months. His parents are worried because all Luke wants to do is watch TV. Because Luke's parents are both overweight, they are concerned that he will also have a weight problem, so they take him to see their pediatrician.

Based on this growth chart, how has Luke's BMI percentile changed over the past year?
▼

Your answer: _____

_____

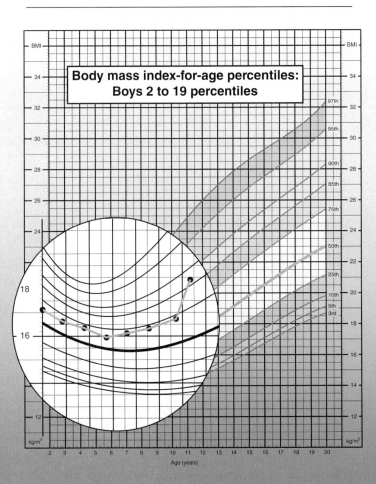

Body mass index-for-age percentiles: Boys 2 to 19 percentiles

Reviewing Luke's diet and exercise patterns, the doctor learns that Luke has been watching TV or playing video games for about six hours a day. A recall of his intake shows that he has doughnuts and milk for breakfast, eats a sandwich and a granola bar for lunch, and then snacks so much on chips and candy when he gets home from school that he doesn't really eat dinner. He likes fruit, refuses to eat vegetables, and drinks 1.1 to 1.3 L (5 to 6 cups) of whole milk daily.

What nutrients are likely to be excessive or deficient in Luke's dietary pattern?
▼

Your answer: _____

_____

A blood test reveals that Luke has iron deficiency anemia. The pediatrician prescribes an iron supplement and refers Luke and his parents to a dietitian. She recommends that the family switch to 1% milk to reduce Luke's energy and fat intake and introduce a fortified cereal for breakfast to increase his iron intake. She also suggests limiting Luke's after-school snacking to fruit so he can eat a better evening meal.

Why might excessive consumption of dairy products contribute to Luke's anemia?
▼

Your answer: _____

_____

How might Luke's iron deficiency have contributed to his weight gain?
▼

Your answer: _____

_____

(Check your answers in Appendix I.)

CONCEPT CHECK   🛑 STOP

1. **How do** children's energy and protein requirements change as they age?

2. **What** factors affect children's food choices?

3. **How** does television viewing affect eating and exercise patterns?

Nutrition for Adolescents

LEARNING OBJECTIVES

1. **Describe** how growth and body composition are affected by puberty.

2. **Compare** the energy needs of adolescents with those of children and adults.

3. **Explain** why iron and calcium are of particular concern during the teen years.

4. **Use** Canada's Food Guide to plan a day's diet that would appeal to a teenager.

A dolescents are a unique population in many ways, and they have unique nutritional needs. The physical, emotional, mental, and social changes of adolescence transform a child into an adult. Organ systems develop and grow, **puberty** occurs, body composition changes,

> **puberty** A period of rapid growth and physical changes that ends in the attainment of sexual maturity.

and the growth rates and nutritional requirements of boys and girls diverge (**Figure 12.6**). The physiological changes associated with sexual maturation affect nutrient requirements, and social and psychological changes that occur during adolescence influence nutrient intakes.

Nutrition InSight • Adolescent growth • Figure 12.6 ✓ THE PLANNER

The **adolescent growth spurt** is an 18- to 24-month period of peak growth velocity that begins at about ages 10 to 13 in girls and ages 12 to 15 in boys. During a one-year growth spurt, girls can gain 9 cm (3.5 in.) in height and boys, 10 cm (4 in.).

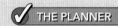

During the adolescent growth spurt, boys gain some fat but add so much lean mass as muscle and bone that their percentage of body fat actually decreases. Girls gain proportionately more body fat and less lean tissue than boys. By age 20, females have about twice as much adipose tissue as males and only about two-thirds as much lean tissue. ▼

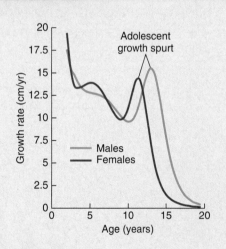

Tom Carter/PhotoEdit

◄ At age 14, some boys are physically still children, while others have matured sexually. Because of large individual variations in the age at which these growth and developmental changes occur, the stage of maturation is often a better indicator of nutritional requirements than is chronological age.

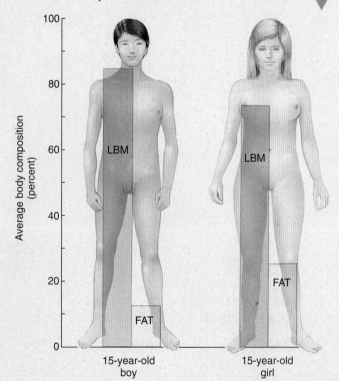

15-year-old boy
15-year-old girl

Recommendations for Adolescents

Eating Well with Canada's Food Guide provides recommendations for teens (ages 14–18) that reflect their increased nutritional needs compared with those of children (**Figure 12.7**). The DRIs also provide more specific recommendations for adolescents to further reflect their developmental needs. Separate recommendations are made for boys and girls because their needs begin to differ during the adolescent years.

Energy and macronutrient needs of adolescents

The percentages of calories from carbohydrate, fat, and protein recommended for adolescents are similar to those for adults, but the total amount of energy needed by teenagers usually exceeds adult needs. Boys require more energy than girls because they have more muscle and their bodies are larger. Energy recommendations for boys and girls can vary dramatically during this age group, especially at different levels of activity. For example, a sedentary 14-year-old boy may require 2000 kilocalories per day, while a very active 18-year-old boy may require up to 4000 kilocalories per day or more.[4] On the other hand, a 14-year-old sedentary girl may require 1700 kilocalories per day, while a very active 18-year-old girl may require up to 3000 kilocalories per day or more. The estimated energy requirements calculation (Chapter 2) can be used to better approximate the actual energy level required by considering the adolescent's gender, age, weight, height, and activity level. Protein requirements per kilogram of body weight are the same for boys and girls, but because boys are generally heavier, they require more total protein than do girls. Water is also essential at this and any age to support body structure and function.

Vitamins The need for most of the vitamins rises to adult levels during adolescence. The requirement for B vitamins, which are involved in energy metabolism, is much higher in adolescence than in childhood because of higher energy needs. The rapid growth of adolescence further increases the need for vitamin B_6, which is important for protein synthesis, and for folate and vitamin B_{12}, which are essential for cell division. The high calorie intakes of teens help them meet most of their vitamin needs, but inadequate intakes of vitamin A, specifically, may put some teens at risk for future complications. Vitamin A is a common deficiency in both adolescents and adults and may lead to vision problems in later life.

Iron The need for iron rises between childhood and adolescence. Iron is needed to synthesize hemoglobin for the expansion of blood volume and myoglobin for the increase in muscle mass. Because blood volume expands at a faster rate in boys than in girls, boys require more iron for tissue synthesis than do girls. However, in girls, the onset of menstruation increases their iron losses, making their total iron needs greater. The RDA is set at 11 mg/day for boys and 15 mg/day for girls ages 14 to 18.[8] Girls are more likely than boys to consume less than the recommended amount because they require more iron, tend to eat fewer iron-rich foods, and consume fewer overall calories.

Calcium The adolescent growth spurt increases both the length and mass of bones. Adequate calcium is essential for forming healthy bone. The RDA for calcium rises from 1000 mg/day in children ages 4 to 8 to 1300 mg/day during adolescence,[7] but intake is typically below these amounts in both sexes, raising concerns that teens may not be meeting their nutritional needs for this vital nutrient.[27] This low intake may reduce the level of peak bone mass achieved, increasing the risk of developing osteoporosis later in life.

Canada's Food Guide and adolescents
• Figure 12.7 ⎯⎯⎯⎯⎯⎯⎯⎯⎯⎯⎯⎯

The number of Canada's Food Guide servings recommended from each group increases in adolescence to reflect the increased nutritional needs required to promote adequate growth and development. For example, the recommended intake of milk and milk alternatives is higher in this age group than any other to promote the development of a strong skeleton.

Recommended Number of *Food Guide Servings* per Day

	Children			Teens		Adults			
Age in Years	2-3	4-8	9-13	14-18		19-50		51+	
Sex	Girls and Boys			Females	Males	Females	Males	Females	Males
Vegetables and Fruit	4	5	6	7	8	7-8	8-10	7	7
Grain Products	3	4	6	6	7	6-7	8	6	7
Milk and Alternatives	2	2	3-4	3-4	3-4	2	2	3	3
Meat and Alternatives	1	1	1-2	2	3	2	3	2	3

Milk and cheese, which are major sources of calcium in teen diets, can be high in fat, which should be further decreased in adolescent diets.[27] Adolescents are encouraged to consume low-fat dairy products, calcium-fortified cereals, and vegetable sources of calcium. One of the contributors to low calcium intake is the use of pop, rather than milk, as a beverage.

Developing Healthy Eating Habits

During adolescence, physiological changes dictate nutritional needs, but peer pressure may dictate food choices. Parents often have little control over what adolescents eat. They may skip meals, and having meals away from home is common. A food is more likely to be selected because it tastes good, is easy to grab, or friends are eating it, not because it is a healthy choice. No matter when foods are consumed throughout the day, an adolescent's diet should follow the recommendations of Canada's Food Guide for the appropriate age, gender, and activity level (see *What Should I Eat?*). The best indicators of adequate intake are satiety and a growth pattern that follows the curve of the growth charts.

Making fast food fit There is nothing wrong with an occasional fast-food meal, but a steady diet of burgers, fries, and tacos will likely contribute to an overall unhealthy diet. Fast food is typically high in kilocalories, fat, and sodium and low in fruits and vegetables. Most teens in Canada consume more than the recommended amounts of kilocalories, fat, and sodium and fewer fruits and vegetables than recommended. The lettuce and tomatoes that garnish a burger or sub are not enough to meet the serving recommendations for vegetables. French fries, which are high in fat and salt, are the most frequently consumed vegetable. To fit fast food into a healthy diet, make more nutrient-dense fast-food choices and ensure other meals and snacks supply the nutrients not obtained from fast food. Many fast-food franchises now offer fruit, salads, yogurt, and milk. And some of the old standbys are not bad choices. For example, a plain, single-patty hamburger provides much less fat and energy than a burger with two patties and a high-fat sauce. A chicken sandwich can be a healthy choice if it is grilled or barbecued, not breaded and fried (**Table 12.2**).

Choosing a vegetarian diet It is not uncommon for a teen to decide to consume a vegetarian diet even if the rest of the family does not. Some give up meat for health reasons or to lose weight, while others give up meat because they are concerned about animals and the environment. A vegetarian diet can be a healthy choice when it is carefully planned to meet nutrient needs, not just to eliminate meat.

WHAT SHOULD I EAT?

Adolescence

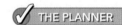

Balance unhealthy choices with healthy choices
- Have milk with your burger.
- Eat an extra vegetable with dinner.
- If you have a large, unhealthy lunch, have a smaller, nutritious dinner.
- Try fresh fruit for dessert.

Eat breakfast
- Have a quick bowl of whole grain cereal or oatmeal and top with some berries.
- Stick a granola bar or low-fat muffin in your backpack.
- Have a yogurt on the go.

Snack well
- Reach for an apple, a pear, or an orange before the cookies and chips.

- Dip your chips in salsa, guacamole, or hummus.
- Nibble on nuts and seeds.
- Snack on some baby carrots or sliced red peppers.

Count up your calcium
- Drink milk—low-fat milk has fewer calories and many more nutrients than pop.
- Put extra milk on your cereal.
- Make a shake by mixing yogurt and fruit in the blender.
- Remove the seeds from half a cantaloupe and fill it with cottage cheese.

Use iProfile to calculate the calcium content of your favourite fast-food meal.

Make healthier fast-food choices Table 12.2

Instead of . . .	Choose . . .
Double-patty hamburger with cheese, mayonnaise, special sauce, and bacon	Regular single-patty hamburger without mayonnaise, special sauce, and bacon
Breaded and fried chicken sandwich	Grilled chicken sandwich
Chicken nuggets or tenders	Grilled chicken strips
Large french fries	Baked potato, side salad, or small order of fries
Fried chicken wings	Broiled skinless wings
Crispy-shell chicken taco with extra cheese and sour cream	Grilled-chicken soft taco without sour cream
Nachos with cheese sauce	Tortilla chips with bean dip
30-cm (12-in.) meatball marinara sub	15-cm (6-in.) turkey breast sub with lots of vegetables
Thick-crust pizza with extra cheese, meat toppings, and stuffed crust	Thin-crust pizza with extra veggies

A poorly planned vegetarian diet will be no healthier than any other poorly planned diet. Adequate protein is generally not a problem, but meatless diets can be low in iron and zinc. Teenage vegans, who consume no animal products, may also be at risk for a vitamin B_{12} deficiency and inadequate calcium and vitamin D intake. We generally think of vegetarian diets as being low in fat, but any diet that relies on high-fat dairy products can be high in total fat, saturated fat, and cholesterol. Adolescents who choose to become vegetarians can consult a registered dietitian to ensure that they are meeting their nutritional needs during this important stage of life (**Figure 12.8**).

Special Concerns for Teens

Peer pressure to fit in and concern about physical appearance probably have a greater impact on behaviour during adolescence than at any other time in life. Many girls want to lose weight even if they are not overweight, and boys want to gain weight to achieve a strong, muscular appearance.

Eating disorders As discussed in Chapter 9, the excessive concerns about weight, low self-esteem, and poor body image that are common during the teenage years contribute to the development of eating disorders. These disorders can be fatal, but, even in less severe cases, the nutritional consequences of an eating disorder can affect growth and development during adolescence and have a lifelong impact on bone health. Obsessions with perfection, weight, and food in general can promote eating disorders and should be avoided.

Healthy vegetarian choices • Figure 12.8

Cheese pizza and ice cream combine to make a high-fat, high-calorie vegetarian choice. In contrast, whole-grain pita bread stuffed with chickpeas, corn, spinach, and tomatoes served with reduced-fat milk, is low in fat and calories, high in complex carbohydrate and fibre, and a good source of calcium and iron.

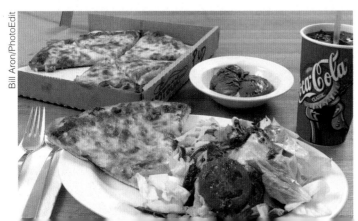

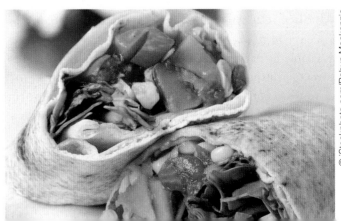

The impact of athletics Participation in competitive sports may affect adolescent nutrient needs and eating patterns. Like adult athletes, teen athletes have increased nutrient needs; they require more water, energy, protein, carbohydrate, and micronutrients than do their less active peers. Individuals involved in sports such as football that require the athlete to be large and heavy usually do not have trouble eating enough to meet these additional needs, but they may compromise their health by experimenting with anabolic steroids or other ergogenic supplements in an effort to "bulk up." As discussed in Chapter 10, steroids can stunt growth in adolescence and can lead to sexual and reproductive disorders, heart disease, liver damage, acne, and aggressive, violent behaviour. Teens participating in gymnastics and wrestling may restrict their food intake in their effort to stay light and lean. Weight restriction at this stage of life may affect nutritional status and maturation and may increase the risk of developing an eating disorder.[28] In female athletes, the combination of hard training and weight restriction can lead to the *female athlete triad* (see Chapter 10).[29]

Tobacco use In 1985, more than 25% of teens aged 15 to 19 smoked. In 2011, this rate dropped to 12% of teens, mainly as a result of the rising price of tobacco, decreases in tobacco advertising, and various health promotion campaigns.[30] Although this decrease is quite remarkable, a significant population of teens continue to smoke, thereby increasing their health risks, including their risk of early mortality. Smoking increases the risk of cardiovascular disease and lung cancer. Smoking can also limit appetite, and many teens start smoking in an effort to control their weight and then are reluctant to quit for fear they will gain weight.[31] Smoking may also affect nutrient intake; a study of smokers found that they eat more saturated fat and fewer fruits and vegetables than do nonsmokers.[32] This dietary pattern may increase the risk of developing heart disease and cancer. Furthermore, smokers have an increased need for vitamin C consumption due to the increased oxidative damage being inflicted on their body.

Alcohol use Although it is illegal to sell alcohol to adolescents in Canada, alcoholic beverages are commonly available at parties and social gatherings, and peer pressure to consume alcohol is strong. Approximately 75% of youth report having had at least one drink during the previous year and more than 20% report either frequent or infrequent heavy drinking, which could be considered binge drinking.[33] Alcohol is a drug that has short-term effects that occur soon after ingestion and long-term health consequences that are associated with overuse. It provides 7 kilocalories/gram but no nutrients, and alcohol is often consumed instead of consuming foods that are nutritious. Once alcohol has been ingested, it alters nutrient absorption and metabolism and affects overall health. These effects are discussed in greater depth in the last section of the chapter.

Nutrition and acne Acne is a problem for many teenagers. Not only can it be physically painful for some, it can also lead to insecurities about appearance and social isolation. A large body of evidence supports a relationship between diet and acne development.

Acne responds to hormones found in the body. Some people have a hormone profile that promotes the development of acne. When you factor in the typical Western diet, which can promote hormone imbalances, it is no surprise that many current teens suffer from acne-prone skin. Dietary intervention to reduce acne includes decreases in total energy intake, hyperglycemic carbohydrates, milk, and certain animal proteins.[34, 35] This recommendation poses a problem, however, because in adolescence, both Canada's Food Guide and the DRIs recommend an increased consumption of milk and milk alternatives. It is important to remember here that everyone's nutritional needs vary, and although it is recommended that most adolescents increase their milk and milk alternatives consumption, people who are prone to acne may want to choose milk alternatives, such as fortified almond milk and soy milk, to reduce their risk of acne.

CONCEPT CHECK	

1. **How** does puberty affect body composition in males and females?

2. **How** do the energy needs of teens compare with those of adults?

3. **What** factors contribute to low calcium intake in teens?

4. **What** could a teen choose at a fast-food restaurant to boost vegetable intake?

Nutrition for the Adult Years

LEARNING OBJECTIVES

1. **Compare** the energy and nutrient requirements of adults with the same requirements for adolescents.

2. **Discuss** how energy needs change during adulthood.

3. **Plan** a diet for a sedentary 40-year-old woman, based on recommendations from Canada's Food Guide.

The benefits of a healthy diet do not stop when you stop growing; in fact, the basic principles of a healthy diet carry on into adulthood. *Eating Well with Canada's Food Guide* recommends a fairly similar eating pattern from the ages of 19 to 50, compared with from ages 14 to 18 (**Figure 12.9**), but

Recommended number of food guide servings per day • Figure 12.9

Canada's Food Guide recommends a slight increase in the consumption of grain products and vegetables and fruit between the ages of 19 and 50. This increase is balanced by a decrease in the recommended consumption of milk and milk alternatives.

Recommended Number of *Food Guide* Servings per Day

	Children			Teens		Adults			
Age in Years	2-3	4-8	9-13	14-18		19-50		51+	
Sex	Girls and Boys			Females	Males	Females	Males	Females	Males
Vegetables and Fruit	4	5	6	7	8	7-8	8-10	7	7
Grain Products	3	4	6	6	7	6-7	8	6	7
Milk and Alternatives	2	2	3-4	3-4	3-4	2	2	3	3
Meat and Alternatives	1	1	1-2	2	3	2	3	2	3

our actual need for the energy-yielding nutrients will decrease as we age and our basal metabolic rate slows down.

Nutrition and Health Concerns throughout Adulthood

The physiological and health changes that accompany aging throughout adulthood can affect energy and nutrient requirements, how some nutrient requirements must be met, and the risk of malnutrition. To best recommend nutrient intakes for adults of all ages, the DRIs include two age categories for adults aged 19 to 50: young adulthood (ages 19 to 30) and middle age (ages 31 to 50). These recommendations are designed to meet the needs of the majority of healthy individuals in each age group.

Energy and energy-yielding nutrient recommendations Adult energy needs typically decline with age, due primarily to decreases in basal metabolic rate (BMR) and activity level. For instance, a typical, low-active 30-year-old woman with a healthy BMI requires approximately 2000 to 2200 kilocalories, whereas a typical low-active 30-year-old man requires 2200 to 2500 kilocalories per day.[4] By age 48, the daily caloric needs of these same low-active individuals respectively decrease to 1600 to 1900 and 1900 to 2300 kilocalories. The need for most nutrients does not change, however, so to meet nutrient needs without exceeding energy needs, adults must consume a nutrient-dense diet. For example, adult protein requirements do not change with age; therefore, compared with younger adults, older adults must consume a diet that is higher in protein relative to calories. A typical male requires 56 g of protein daily, while a typical female requires 46 g of protein daily, regardless of whether they are 19 or 85.[4] Recall, however, that a person's body weight, activity level, and pregnancy status can affect protein needs. These factors should also be considered when determining the appropriate consumption pattern for each individual.

The proportions of carbohydrate and fat recommended in the diet also remain the same in adults over the age of 18. To ensure adequate vitamin, mineral, and fibre intake, most dietary carbohydrate should come from unrefined sources. High-fibre diets may also be beneficial in the prevention and management of diabetes, cardiovascular disease, and obesity.

Sources of dietary fat should also be chosen with nutrient density in mind. A diet is recommended to include 20 to 35% of energy from fat that contains adequate amounts of the essential fatty acids and limits *trans* fat and saturated fat.

Calcium After the adolescent growth spurt, the recommendation for adult calcium consumption decreases from 1300 mg per day for a 14- to 18-year-old, to 1000 mg per day for men and women between the ages of 19 and 50.[7] To meet these needs, approximately two daily food guide servings of milk and milk alternatives are recommended.

Vitamin and mineral needs The DRIs have similar recommendations for both adults and adolescents for the amount of each micronutrient required. These needs do not change significantly throughout these ages. One significant change is a lower RDA for phosphorous, which is due to the decrease in bone mineralization rate evidenced after adolescence. Also, slightly higher intakes of vitamin K and vitamin C are recommended in adulthood compared with in adolescence, but most other micronutrient recommendations stay the same.

CONCEPT CHECK	

1. **How** do the serving recommendations from *Eating Well with Canada's Food Guide* differ between adult males and females?

2. **How** do the energy needs of adults change as they age?

3. **How** do calcium needs differ between teens and adults?

Nutrition for Older Adults

LEARNING OBJECTIVES

1. **Distinguish** life expectancy from health-adjusted life expectancy.

2. **Outline** the energy and nutrient requirements of older adults and seniors.

3. **Discuss** how the physical, mental, and social changes of aging increase nutritional risks.

G ood nutrition throughout your adult years can keep you healthy and active into your 80s and beyond. In Canada, life expectancy is 80.4 years: 78.0 years for men and 82.7 years for women.[36] However, **health-adjusted life expectancy** is only 68.3 years for men and 70.8 years for women.[37] In

other words, on average, the last 10 or so years of life are often restricted by disease and disability; but they do not have to be!

The goal of successful aging is to increase not only life expectancy but also healthy life expectancy. Achieving this goal is particularly important because we live in a nation with an aging population (**Figure 12.10a**). Keeping older adults healthy will benefit not only the aging individuals themselves but also

life expectancy
The average length of life for a particular population of individuals.

the family members who must find the time and resources to care for them and the public health programs that attempt to meet their needs. The increased medical needs of our aging population represent one of the reasons why the Canadian health care system faces concerns over budgetary sustainability. Although nutrition is not the key to immortality, a healthy diet can prevent malnutrition and delay the onset of chronic diseases that typically begin in middle age and reduce the quality of life in older adults (**Figure 12.10b**).

What Is Aging?

Aging is universal to all living things, but it is a process that we still don't fully understand. We know that as organisms grow older, the number of cells in their bodies decreases and the functioning of the remaining cells declines. This loss of cells and cell functions occurs throughout life, but the effects are not felt for many years because organisms start out life with more cells and cell functions than they need. This reserve capacity allows an organism to continue functioning normally despite a

aging The inevitable accumulation of changes associated with and responsible for an ever-increasing susceptibility to disease and death.

The number of older adults is rising • Figure 12.10

a. Approximately 15% of the Canadian population is 65 years of age or over; by 2041, this percentage is expected to reach more than 20%.[38] The **oldest old** (≥85 years) are one of the fastest-growing age groups. Compared with younger adults, they have more activity limitations and chronic conditions and require more public health dollars and services.[38]

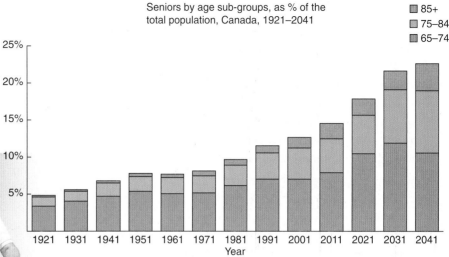

Seniors by age sub-groups, as % of the total population, Canada, 1921–2041

- 85+
- 75–84
- 65–74

b. Chronological age is not always the best indicator of a person's health. A person who is 75 may have the vigour and health of someone who is 55, or vice versa. Some older adults are healthy, independent, and active, while others are chronically ill, dependent, and at high risk for malnutrition. Proper nutrition and adequate physical activity *throughout* life can improve quality of life in older age.

decrease in the number and functions of cells. In young adults, the reserve capacity of organs is 4 to 10 times what is required to sustain life. As a person ages and the reserve capacity decreases, the effects of aging become evident in all body systems. With this loss of function comes a reduction in the ability to repair damage and resist infection, so older people may die from diseases that they could have easily recovered from when they were younger.

The human **life span** is about 120 years, but how long individuals live and the rate at which they age are determined by the genes they inherit, their lifestyle, and the extent to which they are able to avoid accidents, disease, and environmental toxins (**Figure 12.11**). A person with a family history of heart disease who eats a healthy diet and exercises regularly may never develop heart disease. In contrast, someone with no family history of heart disease who is inactive, smokes, and eats a poor diet may develop heart problems.

> **life span** The maximum age to which members of a species can live.

Factors that affect how fast we age • Figure 12.11

Although genes determine both the efficiency with which our cells are maintained and repaired and our susceptibility to age-related diseases, such as cardiovascular disease and cancer, lifestyle and environment also affect our rate of aging.

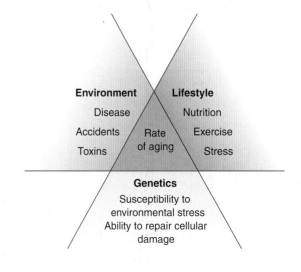

Nutrition and Health Concerns throughout Older Adulthood

Eating Well with Canada's Food Guide now makes specific recommendations for adults over the age of 50. In general, these recommendations reflect a decreased need for overall energy intake and an increased need for calcium and vitamin D (**Figure 12.12**). The DRIs further break down this age group into two age categories: adulthood (ages 51–70) and older adulthood (over age 70). Although the incidence of chronic diseases and disabilities increases with advancing age, these increases are not considered when making general nutrient intake recommendations. Individuals should tailor their diet based on basic dietary principles and their own individual needs.

Energy and energy-yielding nutrient recommendations

Basal metabolic rate declines even more in older age as the amount of lean body tissue decreases (**Figure 12.13**), and physical activity levels also typically decrease. Both these factors lead to a significantly decreased energy need over the age of 50. For instance, a typical healthy-weight, 75-year-old woman, who is only lightly active, requires between 1500 and 1700 kilocalories per day, while a similar typical man requires 1700 to 2000 kilocalories per day.

The acceptable macronutrient distribution ranges are the same for older adults. Adequate fibre, when consumed with adequate fluid, helps prevent constipation, hemorrhoids, and diverticulosis—conditions that are common in older adults. High-fibre diets may also be beneficial in the prevention and management of diabetes, cardiovascular disease, and obesity.

Meeting the water needs of older adults

The recommended water intake for older adults is the same as for younger adults, but meeting these needs may be more

Canada's Food Guide recommendations for older adults • Figure 12.12

Canada's Food Guide recommends that adults over the age of 50 decrease their overall number of food guide servings, while at the same time adding one more serving of milk and milk alternatives per day. This latter change reflects the importance of maintaining bone density in older age. The guide also specifically recommends taking a 10-μg supplement of vitamin D daily, which reflects the decreased ability to synthesize vitamin D in later life.

Men and women over 50

The need for **vitamin D** increases after the age of 50.

In addition to following *Canada's Food Guide*, everyone over the age of 50 should take a daily vitamin D supplement of 10 μg (400 IU).

Recommended Number of Food Guide Servings per Day

	Children			Teens		Adults			
Age in Years	2-3	4-8	9-13	14-18		19-50		51+	
Sex	Girls and Boys			Females	Males	Females	Males	Females	Males
Vegetables and Fruit	4	5	6	7	8	7-8	8-10	7	7
Grain Products	3	4	6	6	7	6-7	8	6	7
Milk and Alternatives	2	2	3-4	3-4	3-4	2	2	3	3
Meat and Alternatives	1	1	1-2	2	3	2	3	2	3

Body composition and energy needs[39]
• Figure 12.13

Some of the decline in energy needs in older adults is due to a decrease in lean body mass.[39] The less lean tissue a person has, the lower his or her BMR. The daily Estimated Energy Requirement (EER) for an 80-year-old man is almost 600 kilocalories less than for a 20-year-old man of the same size and activity level. For women, the difference in daily EER between an 80- and a 20-year-old of the same height, weight, and physical activity level is about 400 kilocalories.

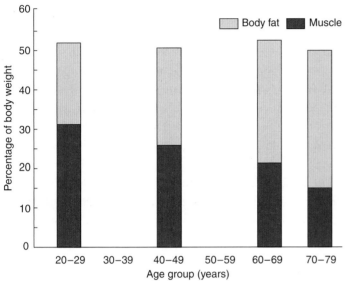

Adapted from Cohen, SH et al Compartmental body composition based on the body nitrogen, potassium, and calcium. American Journal of Physiology. 239: 192–200, 1980.

challenging in older adults. With age comes a reduction in the sense of thirst, which can decrease fluid intake. In addition, older adults are likely to have mobility limitations that may limit their access to beverages. The risk of dehydration is further increased in older adults because many have greater water losses. Their kidneys are less efficient at conserving water as they once were, and many older adults take medications that increase water loss.

Risk of vitamin and mineral deficiencies in older adults
The physiological changes of aging and the decrease in calorie needs put older adults at risk for deficiency of several vitamins and minerals. For some of these, recommended intakes are increased or special recommendations are made about how needs should be met (**Figure 12.14**).

The RDA for vitamin B_{12} is not increased in individuals over age 50, but it is recommended that they meet their RDA for vitamin B_{12} by consuming foods that are fortified with this vitamin or by taking a supplement containing vitamin B_{12}. This recommendation is made because food-bound vitamin B_{12} is not absorbed efficiently in many older adults due to *atrophic gastritis*, an inflammation of the stomach lining that causes a reduction in stomach acid

Vitamin and mineral needs of older adults • Figure 12.14

This graph illustrates the percentage increase in micronutrient recommendations for adults aged 51 and older compared with those of young adults aged 19 to 30. For all the other micronutrients not featured in the graph, the recommendations for younger and older adults are the same.

The RDA for vitamin D for adults over 70 is more than 30% higher than adults aged 19–70.

The RDA for vitamin B_6 is greater in adults ages 51 and older than for younger adults because higher dietary intakes are needed to maintain the same functional levels in the body.

Folate intake is a concern in older adults because deficiencies of folate alone or in combination with vitamin B_{12} and B_6 deficiency may contribute to the development of cancer, cardiovascular disease, and cognitive dysfunction.[51]

Although the decrease in estrogen that occurs at menopause causes bone loss, it cannot be prevented by increasing calcium intake, so the AIs for older men and women do not differ.

The RDA for iron for women over age 50 is reduced by more than 50%. Nevertheless, iron deficiency anemia does occur among women in this age group. Common causes are chronic blood loss from disease and medication and poor iron absorption due to low stomach acid and antacid use.

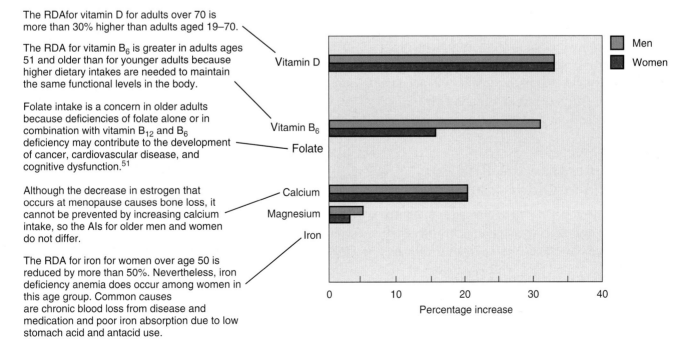

439

(see Chapter 7).[40,41] Reduced secretion of stomach acid also allows microbial overgrowth in the stomach and small intestine, and the greater number of microbes compete for available vitamin B_{12}, further reducing vitamin B_{12} absorption. The vitamin B_{12} in fortified foods and supplements is not bound to proteins, so it is absorbed even when stomach acid levels are low. Atrophic gastritis may also reduce the absorption of iron, folate, calcium, and vitamin K.

Calcium status is a problem in elderly people because calcium intake is low and intestinal absorption decreases with age. In general, most Canadians over age 50 receive less than the adequate intake for calcium. Without sufficient calcium, bone mass decreases, thereby increasing the risk of bone fractures due to osteoporosis. The reduction in estrogen that occurs with menopause also increases the risk of osteoporosis in women by increasing the rate of bone breakdown and decreasing the absorption of calcium from the intestine. The RDA for most adults over 50 is 1200 mg per day, with the exception of men between the ages of 51 and 70, whose RDA is 1000 mg. The higher recommendation for women in the 51 to 70 age group reflects their increased need for calcium during menopause.

Vitamin D, which is necessary for adequate calcium absorption, is also a concern in elderly individuals. Intake is often low, and synthesis in the skin is reduced due to limited exposure to sunlight and because the capacity to synthesize vitamin D in the skin decreases with age. The RDA for men and women ages 51 to 70 has recently been increased to 15 µg/day. For individuals over age 70, this recommendation is further increased to 20 µg/day. Canada's Food Guide also notes the increased need for vitamin D, by recommending a daily supplement of 10 µg/day for adults over age 50. As discussed in Chapter 7, some experts now believe that in the absence of adequate exposure to sunlight, 20 to 25 µg of vitamin D is needed per day in all adults and children.[42]

Factors That Increase the Risk of Malnutrition in Older Adults

The aging process itself usually does not cause malnutrition in healthy, active adults, but nutritional health can be compromised by the physical changes that occur with age, the presence of disease, and economic, psychological, and social circumstances.[44] These factors can increase the risk of malnutrition by altering nutrient needs and decreasing the motivation to eat and the ability to acquire and enjoy food. Malnutrition then exacerbates some of these factors, contributing to a downward health spiral from which it is difficult to recover (**Figure 12.15a**).

Physiological changes With age comes a decline in muscle size and strength (**Figure 12.15b**). This decline affects both the skeletal muscles needed to move the body and the heart and the respiratory muscles needed to deliver oxygen to the tissues. Some of this change is due to changes in hormone levels and muscle protein synthesis, but lack of exercise is also an important contributor.[45] The changes in muscle strength contribute not only to **physical frailty**, which is characterized by general weakness, impaired mobility and balance, and poor endurance, but also to the risk of falls and fractures. In the oldest old, those age 85 years and older, loss of muscle strength is the limiting factor determining whether they can continue to live independently. Incorporating physical activities, specifically weight-bearing activities, throughout life increases independence in older age and helps prolong the increase in frailty.

The immune system's ability to fight disease declines with age. With this decline come increases in the incidence of infections, cancers, and autoimmune diseases, and a decrease in the effectiveness of immunizations (**Figure 12.15c**).

In turn, increases in infections and chronic disease can lead to an increased use of medications that affect nutritional status (**Figure 12.15d**). Malnutrition exacerbates the decrease in immune function.[46]

Acute and chronic illness Most older adults experience some form of illness or disability, and the incidence increases with advancing age. These conditions affect the ability to maintain good nutritional health because they can change nutrient requirements, decrease the appeal of food, and impair the ability to obtain and prepare an adequate diet.

Some illnesses change the type of diet that is recommended. For instance, kidney failure reduces the ability to excrete protein waste products, leading to the need for a low-protein diet. Blood pressure can be affected by sodium intake, so a healthy, low-sodium diet, such as the DASH diet (Chapter 8), is recommended for individuals with high blood pressure. These types of dietary restrictions limit food choices and can affect the palatability of the diet, thereby contributing to malnutrition in elderly people.

a. Many of the physiological changes associated with age can affect nutritional status. This illustration shows how the decreases in muscle mass and immune function that occur with age contribute to malnutrition and how, in turn, malnutrition worsens these problems.

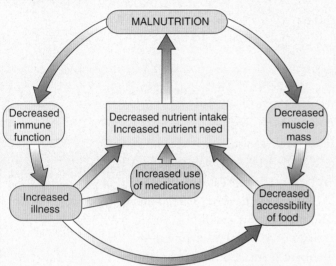

b. The thighs of this 25-year-old (at left) and 65-year-old (at right) are of similar size, but, in the older man, a significant amount of muscle has been replaced by fat (shown in white). In a malnourished individual, the loss of muscle mass and strength would be even greater. Loss of muscle can limit the ability to shop for and prepare food, and decreased intake contributes to further muscle loss.

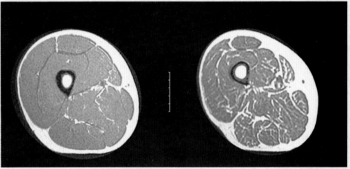

Courtesy S.A. Jubias and K.E. Conley, University of Washington Medical Center

c. The incidence of cancer increases with age.[43] One reason for the higher incidence is the decline in the immune system's ability to destroy cancer cells. Reduced immune function also increases the frequency of infectious diseases and reduces the ability to recover from these diseases.

Age-specific incidence rates (2007) for all cancers by sex, Canada

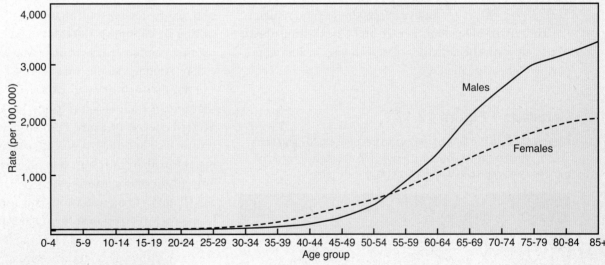

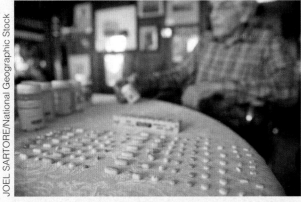

JOEL SARTORE/National Geographic Stock

d. It is common for older adults to take multiple medications. Shown here are the pills this 73-year-old man takes each week. Medications can affect nutritional status by interfering with taste, chewing, and swallowing; by causing loss of appetite, gastrointestinal upset, constipation, or nausea; and by increasing nutrient losses or decreasing nutrient absorption.

Osteoarthritis • Figure 12.16

Osteoarthritis, the most common form of arthritis, occurs when the cartilage that cushions the joints degenerates, allowing the bones to rub together and cause pain. Anti-inflammatory medications help reduce the pain. Supplements of glucosamine and chondroitin have also been found to improve symptoms and to slow the progression of the disease in some patients.[48]

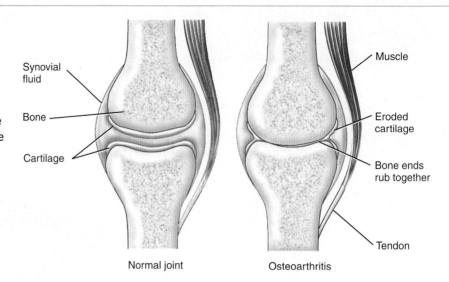

Synovial fluid

Bone

Cartilage

Muscle

Eroded cartilage

Bone ends rub together

Tendon

Normal joint   Osteoarthritis

Physical disabilities can also limit a person's ability to obtain and prepare food. The most common reason for physical disability among older adults is **arthritis**, a condition that causes pain in joints when they are moved (**Figure 12.16**). Arthritis affects more than 4 million Canadians and its incidence is almost 40% higher in females than in males.[47]

arthritis A disease characterized by inflammation of the joints, pain, and sometimes changes in structure.

Half of all individuals age 70 and older with arthritis need help with the activities of daily living, including preparing and eating meals.

Cataracts • Figure 12.17

Cataracts cause the lens of the eye to become cloudy and impair vision. When cataracts obscure vision, the affected lens can be removed and replaced with an artificial plastic lens.

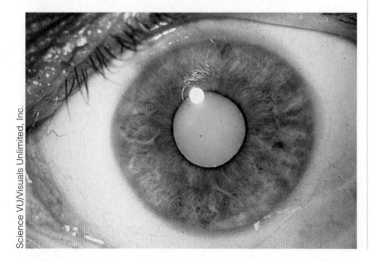

Science VU/Visuals Unlimited, Inc.

Visual disorders are also more common with age. **Macular degeneration** is the most common cause of blindness in older Canadians. The macula is a small area of the retina of the eye that distinguishes fine detail. If the number of viable cells in the macula is reduced, visual acuity declines, ultimately resulting in blindness. **Cataracts** are another common cause of declining vision. Among people who live to age 85, half will develop cataracts that impair their vision (**Figure 12.17**).[49] Oxidative damage is believed to cause both macular degeneration and cataracts. Therefore, a diet that is high in foods containing antioxidant nutrients and phytochemicals may slow or prevent these eye disorders.

macular degeneration Degeneration of a portion of the retina that results in loss of visual detail and eventually in blindness.

cataracts A disease of the eye that results in cloudy spots on the lens (and sometimes the cornea) that obscure vision.

Changes in mental status can affect nutrition by interfering with the response to hunger and the ability to eat, obtain, and prepare food. The incidence of **dementia** increases with age. Dementia involves impairment in memory, thinking, or judgement that is severe enough to cause personality changes and affect daily activities and relationships with others. Causes of dementia include multiple strokes, alcoholism, dehydration, side effects of medication, vitamin B_{12} deficiency, and **Alzheimer's disease**.

dementia A deterioration of mental state that results in impaired memory, thinking, and/or judgement.

Alzheimer's disease A disease that results in a relentless and irreversible loss of mental function.

Regardless of the cause, these neurological problems can affect the ability to consume a healthy diet.

Another cause of altered mental status in the elderly is depression. Social, psychological, and physical factors all contribute to the incidence of depression in elderly people. Retirement and the death and relocation of friends and family can cause social isolation, which contributes to depression. Physical disability causes loss of independence. The inability to engage in normal daily activities, easily visit with friends and family, and provide for personal needs contributes to depression. Depression can make meals less appetizing and decrease the quantity and quality of foods consumed, thereby increasing the risk of malnutrition.

Use of medications The higher frequency of acute and chronic illnesses in the elderly makes it likely that they will be taking multiple medications (see Figure 12.15d).[50] Medications can affect nutritional status, and nutritional status can alter the effectiveness of medications. The more medications are taken, the greater the chance of side effects that affect nutritional status, such as decreased appetite, changes in taste, and nausea. Diet can also change the effectiveness of medications. For example, vitamin K hinders the action of anticoagulants, which are taken to reduce the risk of blood clots. On the other hand, omega-3 fatty acids, such as those in fish oils, inhibit blood clotting and may intensify the effect of an anticoagulant drug and cause bleeding.

Keeping Healthy throughout the Adult Years

No secret dietary factor will bestow immortality, but good nutrition and an active lifestyle are major determinants of successful aging. A well-planned, nutritionally adequate diet can extend an individual's years of healthy life by preventing malnutrition and delaying the onset of chronic diseases. Regular exercise can help maintain muscle mass, bone strength, and cardiorespiratory function, helping to prolong independent living. For those with economic, social, or physical limitations, food assistance programs or assisted living can help prevent **food insecurity**.

food insecurity a situation in which people lack adequate physical, social, or economic access to sufficient, safe, nutritious food that meets their dietary needs.

Identifying older adults at risk

To adequately address the nutritional concerns of elderly individuals,

DETERMINE: A checklist of the warning signs of malnutrition Table 12.3	
Disease	Any disease, illness, or condition that causes changes in eating can predispose a person to malnutrition. Memory loss and depression can also interfere with nutrition if they affect food intake.
Eating poorly	Eating either too little or too much can lead to poor health.
Tooth loss/ mouth pain	Poor health of the mouth, teeth, and gums interferes with the ability to eat.
Economic hardship	Having to, or choosing to, spend less than $25 to $30 per person per week on food interferes with nutrient intake.
Reduced social support	Not having contact with people on a daily basis has a negative effect on morale, well-being, and eating.
Multiple medicines	The more medicines a person takes, the greater the chances of side effects such as weakness, drowsiness, diarrhea, changes in taste and appetite, nausea, and constipation.
Involuntary weight loss or gain	Unintentionally losing or gaining weight is a warning sign that should not be ignored. Being overweight or underweight also increases the risk of malnutrition.
Needs assistance in self-care	Difficulty walking, shopping, and cooking increases the risk of malnutrition.
Elder over age 80	The risks of frailty and health problems increase with increasing age.

those at risk for malnutrition must first be identified. The DETERMINE checklist (**Table 12.3**) may help identify these at-risk individuals. The checklist is based on an acronym for the physiological, medical, and socio-economic situations that increase the risk of malnutrition among elderly individuals. Elderly people themselves, as well as their family members and caregivers, can use this tool to determine when malnutrition is a potential problem.

Meeting nutrient needs Meeting the nutrient needs of older adults can be challenging (see *What Should I Eat?*). Because energy needs are reduced while most micronutrient needs remain the same or increase, food choices must be nutrient dense. In addition, the medical, social, and economic challenges that often accompany aging make it more difficult to meet these needs. Many older adults need supplements of vitamin D, vitamin B_{12}, and calcium to meet their nutrient needs. However, supplements should not take the place of a balanced, nutrient-dense diet that is high in whole

WHAT SHOULD I EAT?
Advancing Age

Consume plenty of fluids and fibre
- Drink a beverage with every meal.
- Keep a bottle of water handy and sip on it.
- Choose whole-wheat bread.
- Bake bran muffins.

Pay attention to vitamin B_{12}, calcium, and vitamin D
- Make sure your cereal is fortified with vitamin B_{12}.
- Drink milk; it gives you both calcium and vitamin D.
- Sit in the sun to get some vitamin D with no calories at all.
- Add some canned salmon to a salad for lunch.

Antioxidize
- Have a bowl of strawberries or blueberries.
- Choose colourful vegetables to boost your carotenoids.
- Use vegetable oils in cooking to supply vitamin E.
- Eat some nuts, but not too many—they are high in calories.

Work on your meals for one
- Ask the grocer to break up larger packages of eggs and meats.
- Buy in bulk and share with a friend.
- Make a whole pot of stew but freeze it in meal-size portions.
- Top a baked potato with leftover vegetables or sauces.

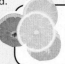

Use iProfile to find foods that are fortified with vitamin B_{12}.

---

grains, fruits, and vegetables (**Figure 12.18**). In addition to essential nutrients, these foods contain phytochemicals and other substances that may protect against disease.

Older adults who have physical limitations need to choose foods that they can easily prepare and consume. Those who have difficulty preparing foods can choose pre-cooked foods, frozen dinners, and canned soup or dry soup mixes to provide a meal with almost no preparation. Meal delivery programs such as Meals on Wheels can also be useful to these Canadians (see Figure 12.18). Medical nutritional products, such as Ensure or Boost, can also be used to supplement intake.

Meals on Wheels • Figure 12.18

As people age, they may encounter various limitations to getting around, including difficulty walking and the inability to drive. These problems may make it difficult for them to get to the grocery store or corner market to pick up groceries. Meals on Wheels is a service that brings inexpensive ready-to-eat meals to the homes of those who may face some of these limitations or any difficulty preparing their own meals. While the service is not limited to seniors, they make up the majority of the Meals on Wheels clientele. Since the first Canadian chapter opened in Brampton, Ontario, in 1963, Meals on Wheels has helped reduce nutritional concerns of seniors throughout the country.

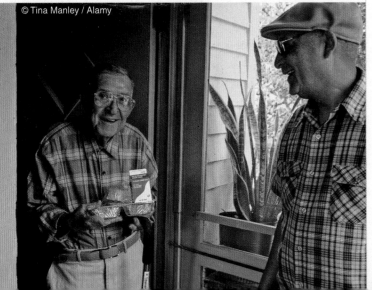
© Tina Manley / Alamy

Physical activity for older adults Regular physical activity can extend years of active, independent life, reduce the risk of disability, and improve the quality of life for older adults. Exercise also allows an increase in food intake without weight gain, so micronutrient needs are met more easily. A physical activity program for older adults should improve endurance, strength, flexibility, and balance and be tailored to their own needs and limitations.[51] Endurance activities such as walking, biking, and swimming provide protection against chronic disease (**Figure 12.19**). Strengthening exercises increase strength and lean body mass and slow the rate of bone loss. Flexibility makes the tasks of everyday life easier and reduces the risk of injuries. Improvements in strength, endurance, and flexibility all enhance balance, which reduces the risk of falls. Specific balance exercises such as those practised in tai chi and yoga can further improve balance.

Overcoming economic and social issues Overcoming economic limitations may involve providing education about economics and food preparation or providing assistance with shopping and food preparation. Options for people with limited incomes include reduced-cost meals at senior centres, food banks, and soup kitchens.

Physical activity for older adults
• Figure 12.19

Exercise classes and other group-based activities can be a good way for older adults to start an exercise program. Water activities such as water aerobics and swimming do not stress the joints and hence can be used to improve endurance in individuals with arthritis or other bone and joint disorders. Some weight-bearing exercise, such as walking, is encouraged to promote bone health.

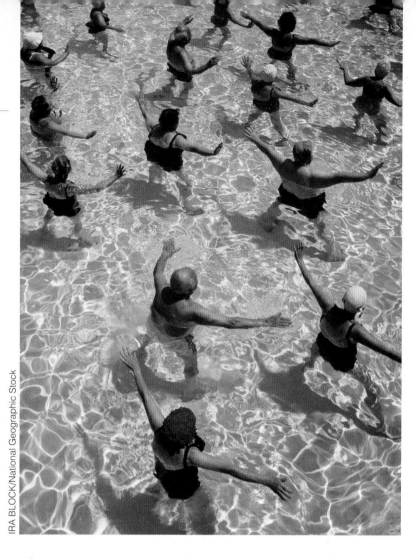

IRA BLOCK/National Geographic Stock

Another problem that contributes to poor nutrient intake in older adults is loneliness. Living, cooking, and eating alone can decrease interest in food. Programs that provide nutritious meals in communal settings promote social interaction and can improve nutrient intake. For those who are unable to attend communal meals, home-delivered meals are available. Studies have shown that compared with others, individuals who receive these meals have better-quality diets.[52]

Overcoming physical limitations: Assisted living The physical and psychological declines associated with aging eventually cause many people to require assistance in everyday living. Assisted living facilities allow individuals to live in their own apartments but provide help as needed with activities such as eating, bathing, dressing, housekeeping, and taking medications. These facilities provide an interim level of care for those who cannot live safely on their own but do not require the total care provided in a nursing home. Eventually, many older adults may need to live in a nursing home. Even though nursing homes provide access to food and medical care, their residents are at increased risk for malnutrition because they are more likely to have medical conditions that increase nutrient needs or interfere with food intake or nutrient absorption, and because they are dependent on others to provide for their care. Even when adequate meals are provided, many nursing home residents require assistance in eating and frequently do not consume all the food served. This increases their likelihood of developing deficits of energy, water, and other nutrients.[53]

CONCEPT CHECK 🛑 STOP

1. **What** is the goal of successful aging?

2. **What** nutrients have higher recommended intakes for older adults than for younger adults?

3. **Why** are older adults at risk for malnutrition?

4. **Where** can older adults get assistance in meeting their nutrient needs?

The Impact of Alcohol throughout Life

LEARNING OBJECTIVES

1. **Define** moderate alcohol consumption.

2. **Explain** how alcohol is absorbed and metabolized.

3. **Describe** the short- and long-term problems of excess alcohol consumption.

4. **Discuss** the potential benefits of moderate alcohol consumption.

Since the dawn of civilization, almost every human culture has produced and consumed some type of alcoholic beverage. Depending on the times and the culture, alcohol use has been touted, casually accepted, denounced, and even outlawed.

Whether alcohol consumption represents a risk to health or provides some benefits depends on who is drinking and how much is consumed. When consumed by a pregnant woman, alcohol can cause birth defects in the developing child. When consumed during childhood and adolescence,

Alcohol recommendations • Figure 12.20

Alcoholic beverages consist primarily of water, ethanol, and sugars, with few other nutrients. A drink, defined as about 140 mL (5 oz) of wine, 355 mL (12 oz) of beer, or 42 mL (1.5 oz) of distilled spirits, contains 12 to 14 g of alcohol, providing about 90 kilocalories (7 kilocalories/g). The remaining calories come from sugars. In moderation, alcohol may provide some health benefits, but high intakes can also have very negative effects on the human body. To address this issue, the Canadian Centre on Substance Abuse provides guidelines for moderating alcohol consumption. The guidelines also specifically detail what is considered an alcoholic serving depending on the type of alcohol that is being consumed.

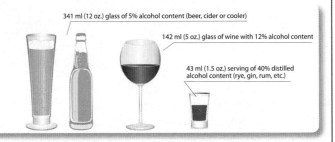

For these guidelines, "a drink" means:

341 ml (12 oz.) glass of 5% alcohol content (beer, cider or cooler)

142 ml (5 oz.) glass of wine with 12% alcohol content

43 ml (1.5 oz.) serving of 40% distilled alcohol content (rye, gin, rum, etc.)

▶ Your limits

Reduce your long-term health risks by drinking no more than:

- 10 drinks a week for women, with no more than 2 drinks a day most days
- 15 drinks a week for men, with no more than 3 drinks a day most days

Plan non-drinking days every week to avoid developing a habit

▶ Special occasions

Reduce your risk of injury and harm by drinking no more than 3 drinks (for women) or 4 drinks (for men) on any single occasion.

Plan to drink in a safe environment. Stay within the weekly limits outlined above in *Your limits*.

▶ When zero's the limit

Do not drink when you are:

- driving a vehicle or using machinery and tools
- taking medicine or other drugs that interact with alcohol
- doing any kind of dangerous physical activity
- living with mental or physical health problems
- living with alcohol dependence
- pregnant or planning to be pregnant
- responsible for the safety of others
- making important decisions

▶ Pregnant? Zero is safest

If you are pregnant or planning to become pregnant, or about to breastfeed, the safest choice is to drink no alcohol at all.

▶ Delay your drinking

Alcohol can harm the way the body and brain develop. Teens should speak with their parents about drinking. If they choose to drink, they should do so under parental guidance; never more than 1–2 drinks at a time, and never more than 1–2 times per week. They should plan ahead, follow local alcohol laws and consider the *Safer drinking tips* listed below.

Youth in their late teens to age 24 years should never exceed the daily and weekly limits outlined in *Your limits*.

Safer drinking tips

- Set limits for yourself and stick to them.
- Drink slowly. Have no more than 2 drinks in any 3 hours.
- For every drink of alcohol, have one non-alcoholic drink.
- Eat before and while you are drinking.

- Always consider your age, body weight and health problems that might suggest lower limits.
- While drinking may provide health benefits for certain groups of people, do not start to drink or increase your drinking for health benefits.

when the brain is still developing and changing, alcohol can cause permanent reductions in learning and memory.[54]

When excess alcohol is consumed by anyone, it has medical and social consequences that negatively affect drinkers and those around them. Alcohol consumption can reduce nutrient intake and affect the storage, mobilization, activation, and metabolism of nutrients. The breakdown of alcohol produces toxic compounds that damage tissues, particularly the liver.

However, when alcohol is consumed in moderation by healthy adults it provides some health advantages. To reflect both these advantages and the need to moderate alcohol use, the Canadian Centre on Substance Abuse now provides five guidelines for low-risk alcohol drinking[55] (**Figure 12.20**).

Alcohol Absorption, Transport, and Excretion

Chemically, any molecule that contains an OH group is an **alcohol**, but we usually use the term to refer to **ethanol** and often to any beverage that contains ethanol (**Figure 12.21**). Ethanol is a small molecule that is rapidly and almost completely absorbed in the upper gastrointestinal

> **ethanol** The alcohol in alcoholic beverages; it is produced by yeast fermentation of sugar.

The molecular structure of ethanol
• Figure 12.21

Ethanol is the type of alcohol found in wine, spirits, and beer.

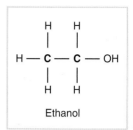

Ethanol

tract. Because some alcohol is absorbed directly from the stomach, its effects are almost immediate, especially when consumed on an empty stomach. If there is food in the stomach, absorption is slowed because food dilutes the alcohol in the stomach and slows the rate of stomach emptying.

After alcohol has been absorbed, it enters the bloodstream and is rapidly distributed throughout all body water. Peak blood alcohol concentrations are attained approximately one hour after ingestion. Many variables affect blood alcohol level, including the type and quantity of alcoholic beverage consumed, the speed at which the beverage is consumed, whether food is also consumed, the weight and gender of the consumer, and the activity of alcohol-metabolizing enzymes in the body (**Figure 12.22a**).

Blood alcohol levels • Figure 12.22

a. When men and women consume the same amount of alcohol, blood alcohol levels will be higher in women than in men. This discrepancy may be due to women having lower levels of the enzymes that break down alcohol or because women have less body water than men, so the alcohol they consume is distributed in a smaller amount of body water.

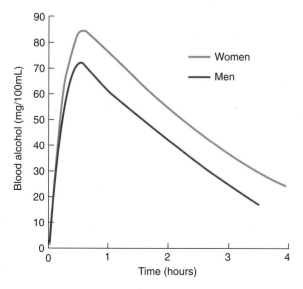

b. In the lungs, some alcohol diffuses out of the blood, into the air, and is exhaled. The amount of alcohol lost through the lungs is reliable enough to estimate blood alcohol level by using a Breathalyzer test.

© 67photo / Alamy

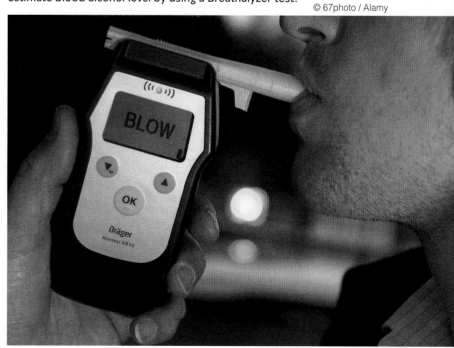

Because alcohol is a toxin and cannot be stored in the body, it must be eliminated quickly. Absorbed alcohol travels to the liver, where it is given metabolic priority and is therefore broken down before other molecules. About 90% of the alcohol is metabolized by the liver. The remainder is excreted through the urine or eliminated via the lungs during exhalation (**Figure 12.22b**). The alcohol that reaches the kidney acts as a diuretic, increasing fluid excretion. Therefore, excessive alcohol intake can contribute to dehydration.

Alcohol Metabolism

In people who occasionally consume moderate amounts of alcohol, most of the alcohol is broken down in the liver by the enzyme alcohol dehydrogenase (ADH) (**Figure 12.23**). This enzyme has also been found in all parts of the gastrointestinal tract.[56] When greater amounts of alcohol are consumed, a second pathway in the liver, called the microsomal ethanol-oxidizing system (MEOS), also metabolizes alcohol.[57] The rate at which ADH breaks down alcohol is fairly constant, but MEOS activity increases when more alcohol is consumed. MEOS also metabolizes other drugs, so as activity increases in response to high alcohol intake, it can alter the metabolism of other drugs.

Adverse Effects of Alcohol

The consumption of alcohol has short-term effects that interfere with organ function for several hours after inges-

PROCESS DIAGRAM

Alcohol metabolism • Figure 12.23

THE PLANNER

The alcohol dehydrogenase pathway predominates when small amounts of alcohol are consumed. The microsomal ethanol-oxidizing system (MEOS) becomes important when larger amounts are consumed. The MEOS reaction requires oxygen and the input of energy to break down alcohol. It also generates reactive oxygen molecules that can contribute to liver disease.

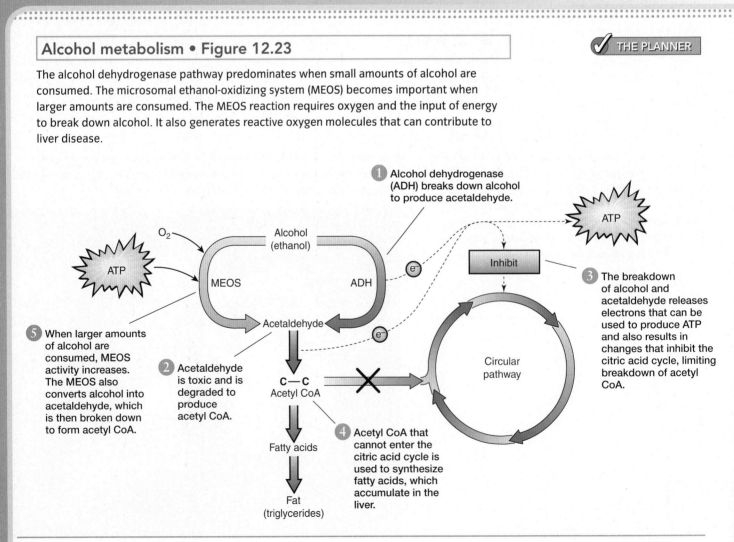

1 Alcohol dehydrogenase (ADH) breaks down alcohol to produce acetaldehyde.

2 Acetaldehyde is toxic and is degraded to produce acetyl CoA.

3 The breakdown of alcohol and acetaldehyde releases electrons that can be used to produce ATP and also results in changes that inhibit the citric acid cycle, limiting breakdown of acetyl CoA.

4 Acetyl CoA that cannot enter the citric acid cycle is used to synthesize fatty acids, which accumulate in the liver.

5 When larger amounts of alcohol are consumed, MEOS activity increases. The MEOS also converts alcohol into acetaldehyde, which is then broken down to form acetyl CoA.

tion. Chronic alcohol consumption has long-term effects that cause disease both because the alcohol interferes with nutritional status and because alcohol metabolism produces toxic compounds.

Short-term effects

When alcohol intake exceeds the liver's ability to break it down, the excess accumulates in the bloodstream. The circulating alcohol acts as a central nervous system depressant, impairing mental and physical abilities. First, alcohol affects reasoning; if drinking continues, the brain's vision and speech centres are affected. Next, large-muscle control becomes impaired, causing lack of coordination. Finally, if alcohol consumption continues, it can result in **alcohol poisoning**, a serious condition that can slow breathing, heart rate, and the gag reflex, and may lead to loss of consciousness, choking, coma, and even death. This condition most frequently occurs as a result of *binge drinking*. Even if an individual does not experience a loss of consciousness, excess drinking may still cause memory loss. Drinking enough alcohol to cause amnesia is called **blackout drinking**. Blackout drinking puts people at risk because they have no memory of events that occurred during the blackout. During alcohol-related memory blackouts, people may engage in risky behaviours such as having unprotected sexual intercourse, vandalizing property, or driving a car—and later have no memory of their actions.

The effects of alcohol on the central nervous system make it dangerous to drive while under the influence of alcohol. Alcohol affects reaction time, eye–hand coordination, accuracy, and balance. Not only does alcohol impair the ability to operate a motor vehicle but it also impairs one's judgement in making the decision to drive. Abuse of alcohol also contributes to domestic violence and is a factor in almost 40% of all traffic fatalities.[58]

Alcoholism

One risk associated with regular alcohol consumption is the possibility of alcohol dependence, or **alcoholism**. The risk of alcoholism is increased in individuals who begin drinking at a younger age. Alcoholism, like any other drug dependency, is a physiological and psychological condition that needs treatment. It is believed that alcoholism has a genetic component that makes some people more likely to become dependent, but environmental factors also play a significant role.[59] Thus, a person with a genetic predisposition toward alcoholism whose family and peers do not consume alcohol is much less likely to become addicted than someone with the same genes who drinks regularly with friends.

Alcoholic liver disease

The most significant physiological effects of chronic alcohol consumption occur in the liver. The metabolism of alcohol by alcohol dehydrogenase promotes fat synthesis (see Figure 12.23), which leads to the accumulation of fat in the liver. Metabolism by the microsomal ethanol-oxidizing system (MEOS) generates reactive oxygen molecules, which cause the oxidation of lipids, membrane damage, and altered enzyme activities. Whether alcohol is broken down by alcohol dehydrogenase or MEOS, toxic acetaldehyde is formed. Acetaldehyde binds to proteins and inhibits chemical reactions and mitochondrial function, allowing more acetaldehyde to accumulate and causing further liver damage.

Chronic alcohol consumption leads to three types of alcoholic liver disease. **Fatty liver** is the accumulation of fat in liver cells. It occurs in almost all people who drink heavily due to the increased synthesis and deposition of fat. If drinking continues, this condition may progress to **alcoholic hepatitis**. Both of these conditions are reversible if alcohol consumption is stopped and good nutritional and health practices are followed. If alcohol consumption continues, **cirrhosis** may develop (**Figure 12.24**).

> **alcoholic hepatitis** Inflammation of the liver caused by alcohol consumption.
>
> **cirrhosis** Chronic and irreversible liver disease characterized by loss of functioning liver cells and accumulation of fibrous connective tissue.

Alcohol, malnutrition, and other health problems

Malnutrition is one of the complications of long-term excessive alcohol consumption. Alcohol contributes energy —7 kilocalories/gram—but few nutrients; it may replace more nutrient-dense energy sources in the diet. In addition to decreasing nutrient intake, alcohol interferes with nutrient absorption. Alcohol causes inflammation of the stomach, pancreas, and intestine, which impairs digestion of food and absorption of nutrients into the blood. Deficiency of the B vitamin thiamin is a particular concern with chronic alcohol consumption. Alcohol also contributes to malnutrition by altering the storage, metabolism, and excretion of other vitamins and some minerals.

In addition to causing liver disease and malnutrition, heavy drinking is associated with cancer of the oral cavity, pharynx, esophagus, larynx, breast, liver, colon, rectum, and stomach.[60, 61] Even moderate alcohol consumption has

Alcoholic cirrhosis • Figure 12.24

The liver on the left is normal. The one on the right has cirrhosis. Cirrhosis is an irreversible condition in which fibrous deposits scar the liver and interfere with its functioning. Because the liver is the primary site of many metabolic reactions, including the detoxification of harmful substances that are ingested, cirrhosis is often fatal.

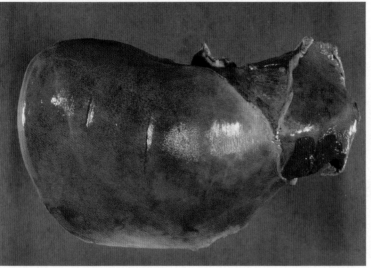

Martin M. Rotker / Science Source

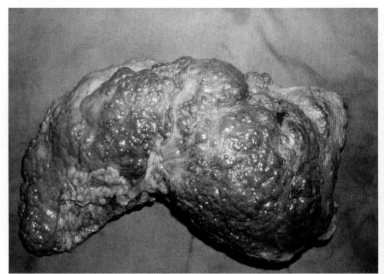

Biophoto Associates / Photo Researchers, Inc.

been found to increase the risk of certain cancers in women.[62] Alcohol use also increases the risk of hypertension, heart disease, and stroke.[62] Some of this effect relates to calories consumed as alcohol being more likely to be deposited as fat in the abdominal region, where excess fat increases the risk of high blood pressure, heart disease, and diabetes.

Benefits of Alcohol Consumption

For some adults, moderate alcohol consumption may have benefits. Consuming alcoholic beverages can stimulate appetite, improve mood, and enhance social interactions. Light to moderate drinking can also reduce the risk of heart disease and stroke. The primary mechanisms by which alcohol lowers cardiovascular risk are by raising blood levels of HDL cholesterol and by inhibiting the formation of blood clots. The phytochemicals in red wine are thought to make it more cardioprotective than other alcoholic beverages.[63]

Whether or not the benefits of alcohol consumption outweigh the risks, drinking is a personal decision that must take into account medical and social considerations.

But anyone who chooses to drink should do so in moderation. Alcohol should be consumed slowly; no more than one drink every 1.5 hours. Sipping, not gulping, allows the liver time to break down what has already been consumed. Also, shots should be consumed with caution as they may lead to overconsumption. Alternating nonalcoholic and alcoholic drinks may also slow the rate of alcohol intake and prevent dehydration. Alcohol absorption is most rapid on an empty stomach. Consuming alcohol with meals slows its absorption and may also enhance its protective effects on the cardiovascular system.

CONCEPT CHECK

1. **How** much beer per day constitutes moderate drinking for a man?

2. **How** can alcohol metabolism lead to fatty liver?

3. **What** are the symptoms of alcohol toxicity?

4. **How** does moderate alcohol intake reduce the risk of cardiovascular disease?

Summary

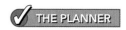

1 Nutrition for Children 422

- A child's diet should meet the child's current needs for growth, development, and activity and reduce the risk of chronic disease later in life. Energy and protein needs per kilogram of body weight decrease as children grow, but total needs increase. The acceptable range of fat intake is higher for young children than for adults. Calcium and iron intakes are often low in children's diets, putting them at risk for low bone density and anemia.

- To meet the nutrient needs of children and to develop nutritious habits, caregivers should offer a variety of healthy foods at meals and as snacks throughout the day. Children can then choose what and how much they consume.

- The typical diet of Canadian children contributes to their rising obesity rates and to an increasing incidence of diabetes, high blood cholesterol, and high blood pressure. Watching television contributes to childhood obesity by promoting the intake of foods that are high in calories, fat, and sugar and by reducing the amount of exercise children get. A diet high in sugary foods can increase the risk of dental caries, but no clear link has been established between sugary foods and **attention-deficit/hyperactivity disorder (ADHD)**. Children who experience **food jags** risk underconsuming the nutrients that are not found in the food they prefer to eat.

Energy needs • Figure 12.2

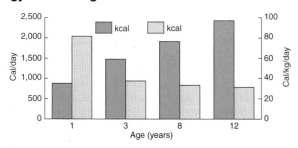

2 Nutrition for Adolescents 430

- During adolescence, the changes associated with **puberty**, especially the **adolescent growth spurt**, have an impact on nutrient requirements. Body composition and the nutritional requirements of boys and girls diverge. Energy and protein requirements are higher than in adulthood, and vitamin requirements increase to meet the needs of rapid growth. Calcium intake is often low in the adolescent diet, particularly when pop is consumed in place of milk. Iron deficiency anemia is common in adolescent girls due to low intake and iron losses through menstruation.

- The food choices of adolescents are usually determined not by nutrient needs but by social activities, peer pressure, and participation in athletics. Teens can improve their diets by making healthier fast-food choices. Poorly planned vegetarian diets may be low in iron, zinc, calcium, vitamin D, and vitamin B$_{12}$, and may be high in saturated fat and cholesterol.

- Psychological and social changes occurring during the adolescent years make eating disorders more common than at any other time. Adolescent nutritional status may also be affected by weight loss diets and supplements taken to enhance athletic performance and the use of cigarettes or alcohol.

Adolescent growth • Figure 12.6

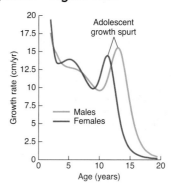

3 Nutrition for the Adult Years 435

- Nutrition recommendations are similar for adolescents and adults aged 19 to 50, but the amount of energy and macronutrients required will decrease with increasing age as basal metabolism and, possibly, physical activity slows. In the adult years, a healthy diet is one that supports the current needs of the individual and that does not increase the risk of chronic diseases in later life.

Recommended number of food guide servings per day • Figure 12.9

Recommended Number of Food Guide Servings per Day								
	Children			Teens		Adults		
				14-18		19-50		51+
Age in Years	2-3	4-8	9-13					
Sex	Girls and Boys			Females	Males	Females	Males	Females	Males
Vegetables and Fruit	4	5	6	7	8	7-8	8-10	7	7
Grain Products	3	4	6	6	7	6-7	8	6	7
Milk and Alternatives	2	2	3-4	3-4	3-4	2	2	3	3
Meat and Alternatives	1	1	1-2	2	3	2	3	2	3

4 Nutrition for Older Adults 436

- As a population, Canadians are living longer but not necessarily healthier lives. A typical Canadian's **life expectancy** is around 80 years of age, but the human **life span**, the maximum amount of time humans typically live, is around 120 years. While living a long life may be desirable to some, to others it is more important to have a long **health-adjusted life expectancy**, which takes into account how many years are spent free from chronic disease. How long and how well we live is determined by the genes we inherit, our diet, lifestyle, and other environmental factors. Currently, the Canadian population is an **aging** one, with the number of **oldest old**, those over the age of 85, increasing at a fast rate.

- Energy needs decrease with age, but the needs for protein, water, fibre, and most micronutrients remain the same. Older adults are at risk for deficiencies because aging can lead to decreases in nutrient intake and absorption and to changes in the metabolism or absorption of certain micronutrients, including vitamin B_{12}, vitamin D, and calcium. Iron requirements decrease in women after menopause, but many older adults are at risk for iron deficiency due to poor absorption or blood loss from disease or medications.

- Older adults are at risk for malnutrition due to the physiological changes that accompany aging, such as the decline in muscle mass and immune function. The decrease in muscle mass can promote **physical frailty**, which can limit an individual's ability to remain independent. Acute and chronic illnesses, which are more common in elderly people, may change nutrient requirements, decrease the appeal of food, and impair the ability to obtain and prepare an adequate diet. Medications to treat these diseases may also affect nutritional status. Physical disabilities that can limit quality of life include **arthritis**, **macular degeneration**, and the development of **cataracts**. Changes in mental status caused by depression or **Alzheimer's disease**, which can promote **dementia**, can further limit healthy aging.

- A nutrient-dense diet and regular exercise can prevent malnutrition, delay the chronic diseases associated with aging, and increase independence in older adults. Unfortunately, seniors are more likely than younger adults to suffer from **food insecurity**, increasing their risk of malnutrition. Economic or physical assistance may be required to meet nutritional needs.

5 The Impact of Alcohol Throughout Life 446

- **Alcohol**, which refers to **ethanol**, is absorbed rapidly, causing the blood alcohol level to rise and its effects to be felt almost immediately. Absorption is slowed when there is food in the stomach. Alcohol is metabolized primarily in the liver. Some is excreted in urine and exhaled in expired air.

- Moderate amounts of alcohol are broken down by the enzyme alcohol dehydrogenase. When greater amounts of alcohol are consumed, a second pathway in the liver, called the microsomal ethanol-oxidizing system (MEOS), also metabolizes alcohol. Alcohol metabolism increases fat synthesis in the liver and generates reactive oxygen molecules that can contribute to liver disease.

- In the short term, excess alcohol consumption causes **alcohol poisoning**, which interferes with brain function. **Blackout drinking** can affect the brain to a point where the memory of the drinking episode is erased. Chronic alcohol consumption can lead to **alcoholism** and can damage the liver, resulting in **fatty liver**, **alcoholic hepatitis**, and eventually **cirrhosis**. Excess alcohol consumption also increases the risks of malnutrition and of developing hypertension, heart disease, stroke, and some cancers.

- Moderate alcohol consumption can decrease the risk of heart disease by increasing HDL cholesterol and reducing blood clot formation.

Physical activity for older adults • Figure 12.19

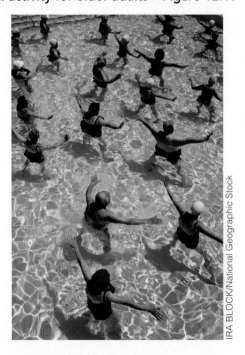

IRA BLOCK/National Geographic Stock

Alcoholic cirrhosis • Figure 12.24

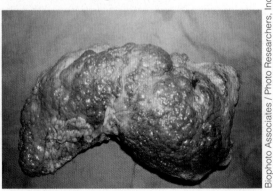

Biophoto Associates / Photo Researchers, Inc.

Key Terms

- adolescent growth spurt 430
- aging 436
- alcohol 447
- alcohol poisoning 449
- alcoholic hepatitis 449
- alcoholism 449
- Alzheimer's disease 442
- arthritis 442
- attention-deficit/hyperactivity disorder (ADHD) 428
- blackout drinking 449
- cataracts 442
- cirrhosis 449
- dementia 442
- ethanol 447
- fatty liver 449
- food insecurity 443
- food jag 428
- health-adjusted life expectancy 436
- life expectancy 436
- life span 437
- macular degeneration 442
- oldest old 452
- physical frailty 440
- puberty 430

Critical and Creative Thinking Questions

1. Plot these height and weight measurements that were recorded for a girl from age 6 to age 9 on a growth chart and discuss any problems this pattern suggests.

Age	Height in cm (in.)	Weight in kg (lb.)
6	114 (45)	20 (44)
7	122 (48)	24 (53)
8	127 (50)	35 (77)
9	132 (52)	44 (97)

2. Use Canada's Food Guide to design a day's menu for a 15-year-old boy who spends two hours a day playing soccer.

3. Use Canada's Food Guide to design a day's menu for a sedentary 70-year-old woman who must limit her sodium intake.

4. Use iProfile to look up the nutrient composition of your favourite fast-food meal. For this meal, determine the percentage of calories from carbohydrate, protein, and fat. Compare these percentages with the percentages of calories from carbohydrate, fat, and protein recommended for a 10-year-old boy. Assuming that he exercises for 30 to 60 minutes a day, would he be able to eat this meal and maintain his daily intake within the recommended percentages? Why or why not?

5. With age, there is a loss of smell and taste sensation. How might you design meals for a seniors' centre to compensate for these sensory losses?

6. Jared is 8 years old. He refuses to eat breakfast before leaving for school. How can Jared's parents ensure that he has a nutritious meal before school starts?

7. Laura is 55 years old and has a family history of heart disease. She eats a healthy diet that is high in whole grains, fruits, and vegetables, and she does not smoke or consume alcohol. She recently heard that moderate alcohol consumption can help reduce her risk of heart disease. Should she start consuming alcohol? Why or why not?

What is happening in this picture?

Clara Hughes is shown after receiving her sixth Olympic medal at the Vancouver Olympics in 2010. At age 38, which we consider middle age, she was twice the age of many of her competitors. Clara is one of the only athletes to have won multiple medals at both the summer and winter Olympics.

Kevork Djansezian/Staff/Getty Images Sport

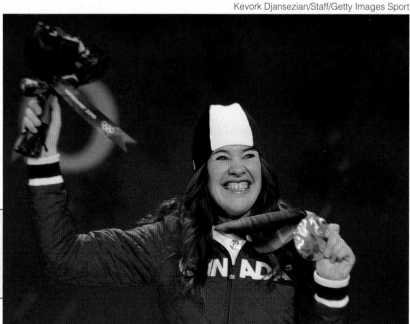

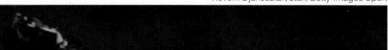

Think Critically

1. How does Clara's physiological age compare with her chronological age?
2. How do you think Clara's lean body mass compares with that of the average 38-year-old woman?

Self-Test

(Check your answers in Appendix J.)

1. Which of the following statements about childhood nutrition is correct?

   a. Childhood obesity rates have started to decline in Canada.

   b. Fat intake should be reduced in childhood to prevent obesity.

   c. Obese children should be put on a diet to promote weight loss.

   d. Children who are bullied about their weight are more likely to binge eat.

2. Which of the following is true about children and hyperactivity?

   a. Eating sugary treats makes children more hyperactive.

   b. Hyperactivity is more common in girls than boys.

   c. Children who are hyperactive perform better in school.

   d. No direct link has been found between diet and hyperactivity in children.

3. Television affects the nutritional status of children in all except which of the following ways?

   a. by helping them recognize the importance of fresh fruits and vegetables

   b. by exposing them to new snack foods

   c. by providing an environment that encourages snacking

   d. by reducing the time spent engaged in activity

4. Nutrients most likely to be deficient in an adolescent's diet are _____.

   a. sodium and selenium

   b. iodine and vitamin A

   c. iron and calcium

   d. protein and zinc

5. Which of the following statements about energy requirements is true?

   a. Total energy needs are higher in childhood than at any other time of life.

   b. Energy needs per kilogram of body weight increase as children grow.

   c. Energy needs are the same for adolescent boys and girls.

   d. Energy needs are lower in older adults than in younger adults.

6. Which of the following statements about iron is false?

   a. Iron deficiency is a risk in children, adolescents, and older adults.

   b. The RDA is higher in a 60-year-old woman than in a 20-year-old woman.

   c. Iron needs increase in adolescent males due to increases in muscle mass.

   d. Iron needs increase in adolescent females due to menstrual losses.

7. Which of the following can contribute to low calcium status in children and teens?

   a. spending too little time outdoors

   b. replacing milk with pop

   c. having lactose intolerance

   d. eating a vegan diet

   e. all of the above

8. The graph shows changes in body composition that occur from _____.

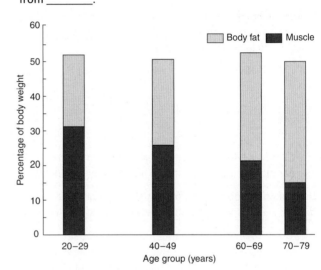

   a. infancy to childhood

   b. childhood to adolescence

   c. young adulthood to older adulthood

   d. moderate to excessive alcohol consumption

9. Life expectancy refers to _____.

   a. the average age to which people in a population live

   b. how long an individual will live

   c. the longest any person can live

   d. how long an individual remains healthy

10. Which of the following statements about vitamin B_{12} is false?

    a. Absorption from food is reduced in individuals with atrophic gastritis.

    b. Older adults are not at risk for vitamin B_{12} deficiency.

    c. It is recommended that older adults meet vitamin B_{12} needs with supplements and/or fortified foods.

    d. Vegan diets must include supplements or foods fortified with vitamin B_{12} to meet needs.

11. For which of the following nutrients is the recommended intake greater in older adults than in younger adults?

    a. vitamin D   c. vitamin A

    b. protein   d. vitamin C

12. In older adults, atrophic gastritis may lead to a _____ deficiency.

   a. vitamin D
   b. calcium
   c. vitamin B$_{12}$
   d. iron

13. _____ is a type of alcoholic liver disease that results in irreversible scaring.

   a. Fatty liver
   b. Alcohol poisoning
   c. Cirrhosis
   d. Alcoholic hepatitis

14. Which of the following statements about the Canadian population is illustrated by this graph?

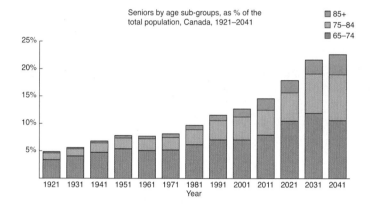

Seniors by age sub-groups, as % of the total population, Canada, 1921–2041

■ 85+
■ 75–84
■ 65–74

a. The number of people who are over age 65 is expected to more than double between 2011 and 2050.
b. By 2050, 20% of the population will be over age 85.
c. The life expectancy of the population is expected to increase between 2010 and 2050.
d. The average healthy life expectancy is expected to increase between 2010 and 2050.

15. Which of the following statements about alcohol is true?

   a. It is absorbed faster on a full stomach than on an empty stomach.
   b. It can contribute to malnutrition.
   c. Moderate alcohol consumption lowers HDL cholesterol levels.
   d. It can reduce the risk of cancer.

THE PLANNER ✓

Review your Chapter Planner on the chapter opener and check off your completed work.

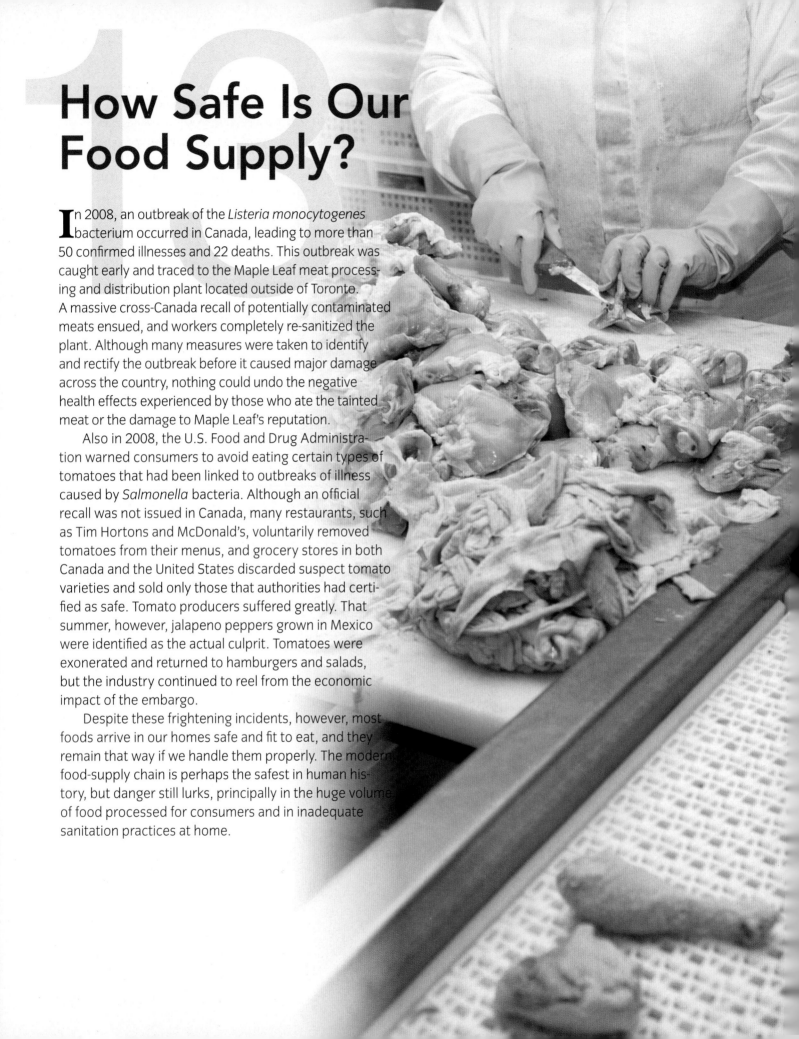

How Safe Is Our Food Supply?

In 2008, an outbreak of the *Listeria monocytogenes* bacterium occurred in Canada, leading to more than 50 confirmed illnesses and 22 deaths. This outbreak was caught early and traced to the Maple Leaf meat processing and distribution plant located outside of Toronto. A massive cross-Canada recall of potentially contaminated meats ensued, and workers completely re-sanitized the plant. Although many measures were taken to identify and rectify the outbreak before it caused major damage across the country, nothing could undo the negative health effects experienced by those who ate the tainted meat or the damage to Maple Leaf's reputation.

Also in 2008, the U.S. Food and Drug Administration warned consumers to avoid eating certain types of tomatoes that had been linked to outbreaks of illness caused by *Salmonella* bacteria. Although an official recall was not issued in Canada, many restaurants, such as Tim Hortons and McDonald's, voluntarily removed tomatoes from their menus, and grocery stores in both Canada and the United States discarded suspect tomato varieties and sold only those that authorities had certified as safe. Tomato producers suffered greatly. That summer, however, jalapeno peppers grown in Mexico were identified as the actual culprit. Tomatoes were exonerated and returned to hamburgers and salads, but the industry continued to reel from the economic impact of the embargo.

Despite these frightening incidents, however, most foods arrive in our homes safe and fit to eat, and they remain that way if we handle them properly. The modern food-supply chain is perhaps the safest in human history, but danger still lurks, principally in the huge volume of food processed for consumers and in inadequate sanitation practices at home.

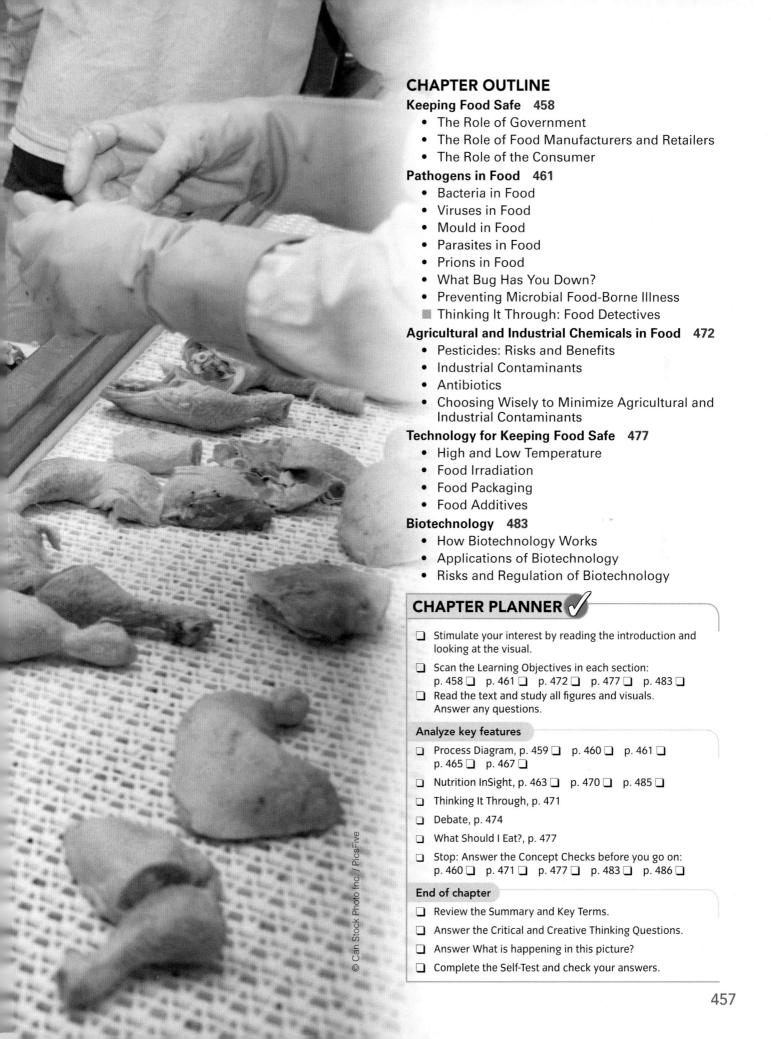

CHAPTER OUTLINE

Keeping Food Safe 458
- The Role of Government
- The Role of Food Manufacturers and Retailers
- The Role of the Consumer

Pathogens in Food 461
- Bacteria in Food
- Viruses in Food
- Mould in Food
- Parasites in Food
- Prions in Food
- What Bug Has You Down?
- Preventing Microbial Food-Borne Illness
- ■ Thinking It Through: Food Detectives

Agricultural and Industrial Chemicals in Food 472
- Pesticides: Risks and Benefits
- Industrial Contaminants
- Antibiotics
- Choosing Wisely to Minimize Agricultural and Industrial Contaminants

Technology for Keeping Food Safe 477
- High and Low Temperature
- Food Irradiation
- Food Packaging
- Food Additives

Biotechnology 483
- How Biotechnology Works
- Applications of Biotechnology
- Risks and Regulation of Biotechnology

CHAPTER PLANNER ✓

© Can Stock Photo Inc./ PicsFive

457

Keeping Food Safe

LEARNING OBJECTIVES

1. **Name** the primary cause of food-borne illness.

2. **Explain** why a contaminated food does not cause illness in everyone who eats it.

3. **Discuss** the roles of the federal agencies responsible for the safety of the Canadian food supply.

4. **Explain** how an HACCP system helps prevent food-borne illness.

Have you ever had food poisoning? Whether you know it or not, you probably have. Often, what we call the 24-hour flu is actually food poisoning, also called **food-borne illness**. Most food-borne illness is caused by consuming food that has been contaminated by **microbes**; occasionally it is caused by toxic chemicals or other contaminants that find their way into food.

Each year, there are approximately 11 million cases of food-borne illness in Canada.[1] Whether or not you get sick from eating a contaminated food depends on how potent the contaminant is, how much of it you consume, and how often you consume it; your age, size, and health also play a role. Some food contaminants cause harm even when minute amounts are consumed, and almost any substance can be toxic if a large enough amount is consumed. How well a substance is absorbed and how it is metabolized by the body affect its toxicity. Absorption is affected by dietary factors and nutritional status. For example, mercury, which is extremely toxic, is not absorbed well in a person whose diet is high in selenium, and lead absorption is decreased by the presence of iron and calcium in the diet. Contaminants that are stored in the body after being absorbed are more likely to be toxic because they accumulate over time, eventually causing symptoms of toxicity. Contaminants that are easily excreted from the body are less likely to cause toxicity.

An individual's size, immune function, and overall health and nutritional status affect the risk of food-borne illness. Infants and children are at greater risk than adults because their immune systems are immature and their small size means that a given amount of contaminant represents a greater percentage of body weight than it would in an adult. Elderly people, people with AIDS, and those receiving chemotherapy or other immunosuppressant drugs are at increased risk because their immune systems may be compromised. Pregnancy weakens the immune system, putting pregnant women and their unborn babies at risk. Poor nutritional status and chronic conditions such as diabetes and kidney disease may decrease the body's ability to detoxify harmful substances.

> **food-borne illness** An illness caused by consumption of contaminated food.
>
> **microbes** Microscopic organisms, or microorganisms, including bacteria, viruses, and fungi.

The Role of Government

The safety of the food supply is monitored by agencies at international, federal, provincial or territorial, and local levels. Federal agencies set standards and establish regulations both for the safe handling of food and water and for the information included on food labels. The Food Directorate, under Health Canada, created the Food and Drug Act to outline the proper and safe import, export, transport, and sale of food products across Canada. The specific regulations that keep our food safe are provided by the Food and Drug Regulations, which were created by Health Canada and based on the latest food safety research. The Canadian Food Inspection Agency is the federal body that uses these regulations to govern the use of additives, packaging materials, and agricultural chemicals; to inspect food processing and storage facilities; to monitor domestic and imported foods for contamination; and to investigate outbreaks of food-borne illness.

The Canadian Food Inspection Agency monitors food at different points in the supply chain—from where food is grown to where it is sold (**Figure 13.1**). Local municipalities oversee public health inspectors who routinely visit food and drink establishments to ensure they are operating according to the standards set by the Food and Drug Regulations. Should an establishment not meet the standards set, it will be forced to close until its conditions are sufficiently improved.

Keeping food safe from farm to table • Figure 13.1

☑ THE PLANNER

Keeping food safe involves identifying possible points of contamination along a food's journey from the farm to the dinner table and implementing controls to prevent or contain contamination.

1 Farm Crops can be contaminated with bacteria before they are even harvested. Good agricultural practices can minimize contamination during growing, harvesting, sorting, packing, and storage.

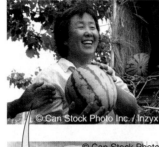

© Can Stock Photo Inc. / Inzyx

2 Processing Contamination of processing equipment can transfer microbes to food. To prevent contamination, processors must follow guidelines concerning cleanliness and training of workers. They must also follow a protocol that anticipates how biological, chemical, or physical hazards are most likely to occur and establish appropriate measures to prevent such hazards from occurring.

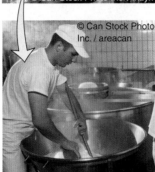

© Can Stock Photo Inc. / areacan

3 Transportation During transport, poor sanitation and inadequate refrigeration can contaminate food and allow microbes to grow. Clean containers and vehicles and proper refrigeration can prevent the growth of food-borne bacteria.

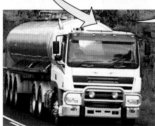
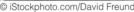

© iStockphoto.com/David Freund

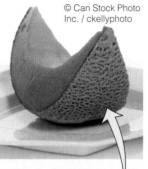

© Can Stock Photo Inc. / ckellyphoto

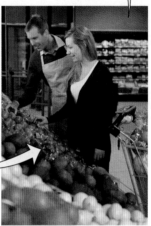

© Can Stock Photo Inc. / Leaf

5 Table Even a safe food can be contaminated in the home. Consumers can prevent food-borne illness at their table by learning to handle, store, and prepare food safely.

4 Retail Food can become contaminated during handling or storage in grocery stores or during preparation in restaurants. The Food and Drug Regulations provide recommendations for the handling and service of food in an effort to help owners and employees at retail establishments prevent food-borne illness. Local health inspections ensure compliance with appropriate levels of cleanliness and proper food-handling procedures.

The Role of Food Manufacturers and Retailers

The responsibility for providing safe food to the marketplace falls on the shoulders of food manufacturers, processors, and distributors. To meet this responsibility, they must establish and implement a **Hazard Analysis Critical Control Point (HACCP)** system. An HACCP system analyzes food production, processing, and transport, with the goal of identifying potential sources of contamination and points where measures can be taken to control contamination. These **critical control points** are monitored in an attempt to prevent and eliminate food contamination (**Figure 13.2**). Unlike traditional methods of protecting the food supply, which use visual spot checks and random testing to catch contamination after it occurs, HACCP systems are designed to *prevent* contamination.

Hazard Analysis Critical Control Point (HACCP)
A food safety system that focuses on identifying and preventing hazards that could cause food-borne illness.

The Role of the Consumer

Although government agencies, manufacturers, and retailers are involved in creating a safe food supply, consumers also need to assume responsibility for their food. Even a food that has been manufactured, packaged, and transported with great care can cause food-borne illness if it is not handled carefully at home. In fact, most cases of food-borne illness are caused by foods prepared at home.[2] Consumers can prevent most food-borne illness through careful food handling, storage, and preparation (discussed in depth later in the chapter). They can also protect themselves and others by reporting to the appropriate agencies any incidents involving unsanitary, unsafe, deceptive, or mislabelled food (**Table 13.1**).

PROCESS DIAGRAM

HACCP in liquid egg production • Figure 13.2

The scrambled eggs served in your cafeteria at school or work most likely came out of a carton rather than a shell. To produce this product, eggs are shelled, mixed together in large vats, heated to kill microbial contaminants, packaged, and either refrigerated or frozen. A contaminated batch could sicken hundreds of people. This example shows how an HACCP system might be used to prevent contaminated eggs from reaching the consumer.

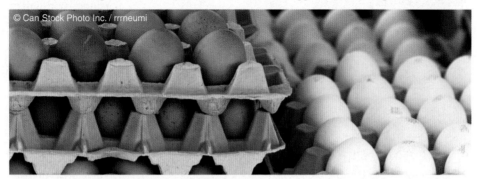

© Can Stock Photo Inc. / rrrneumi

65°C (150°F) 30 minutes

1. **Conduct a hazard analysis**
The manufacturer analyzes its processing steps for potential hazards and determines the preventive measures it can take. Eggs have a large potential for contamination from the *Salmonella* bacteria. Adequate heating is a preventive measure that can eliminate this hazard.

2. **Identify the critical control points**
Critical control points are the steps in a food's processing at which the hazard can be eliminated. In the case of egg processing, the critical control point is heating the shelled egg mixture in a large chamber.

3. **Establish critical limits**
Critical limits are the parameters that will prevent the hazard. In the case of these eggs, the critical limits are sufficient heating time and temperature to ensure that *Salmonella* bacteria are killed.

How to report food-related issues   Table 13.1

Before reporting a food-related problem, gather all the facts. Determine whether you have used the product as intended and according to the manufacturer's instruction. Check to see whether the item is past its expiration date. After these steps have been taken, report the incident to the appropriate agency.

- **Problems related to food safety:** A food-borne illness that affects the health of an individual should first be dealt with by a physician or a local health authority. The incident should then be reported to the Canadian Food Inspection Agency (CFIA) at cfiamaster@inspection.gc.ca or by telephone at 1-800-442-2342.

- **Restaurant food and sanitation problems:** Report issues relating to restaurant meals and cleanliness directly to your local or provincial health authority. A list of these authorities by province can be found at www.inspection.gc.ca/english/fssa/concen/restaure.shtml.

- **Products purchased at the grocery store:** Return the product to the store where it was purchased. Grocery stores are concerned with the safety of the foods they sell, and they will take responsibility for tracking down and correcting the problem. They will either refund your money or replace the product.

CONCEPT CHECK   STOP

1. **What** causes food-borne illness?
2. **Why** might the same food make one person sick but not another person?
3. **Who** is responsible for the safety of the food you eat?
4. **How** does HACCP differ from traditional visual food inspection?

PROCESS DIAGRAM

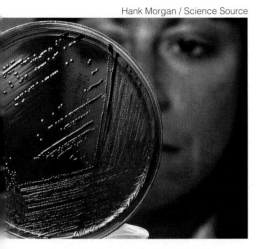

Hank Morgan / Science Source

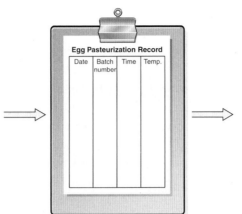

Egg Pasteurization Record

Date	Batch number	Time	Temp.

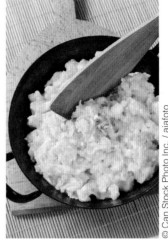

© Can Stock Photo Inc. / ajafoto

④ Establish monitoring procedures
Procedures need to be in place to continually monitor the critical control points. With egg processing, each batch is tested for the presence of *Salmonella*. If the temperature is not hot enough or the heating is not continued long enough, *Salmonella* can survive, as shown here by the growing bacterial colonies.

⑤ Establish corrective action
If a critical limit is not met, corrective action is necessary. Batches of eggs that are contaminated with *Salmonella* are discarded, and the temperature of the heat chamber is adjusted to ensure that *Salmonella* in the next batch will be killed.

⑥ Record keeping
Extensive records document the monitoring of critical control points, all verification activities, and the corrective actions taken. This documentation enables the manufacturer to trace the source of the problem in the event of an outbreak of food-borne illness.

⑦ Verification procedures
Reviewing the plans and records will help ensure that the HACCP plan is working and only safe eggs are reaching the consumer.

Pathogens in Food

LEARNING OBJECTIVES

1. **Distinguish** food-borne infection from food-borne intoxication.

2. **Discuss** three types of bacteria that commonly cause food-borne illness.

3. **Explain** how viruses, moulds, and parasites can make us sick.

4. **Describe** how careful food handling can prevent food-borne illness.

Most cases of food-borne illness in North America are caused by food that has been contaminated with **pathogens**. The pathogens that most commonly affect the food supply include bacteria, viruses, moulds, and parasites. A typical case of food-borne illness causes a short bout of flu-like symptoms, including abdominal pain, nausea, diarrhea, and vomiting. However, more severe symptoms sometimes occur, such as kidney failure, arthritis, paralysis, miscarriage, and even death.

pathogen A biological agent that causes disease.

Any food-borne illness caused by pathogens that multiply in the human body is called a **food-borne infection**. Contracting a food-borne infection usually involves consumption of a large number of pathogens that infect the body or produce toxins within the body. Any food-borne illness caused by consuming a food that contains toxins produced by pathogens is referred to as **food-borne intoxication**. Even food that contains only a few pathogens can cause food-borne intoxication if the pathogens have produced enough toxins. Avoiding food-borne illness—both infection and intoxication—requires knowing how to handle and store food in ways that will prevent contamination and prevent or minimize the growth of pathogens that may already be present in the food. Even a food that is contaminated with pathogens can be safe if it is prepared in a manner that destroys any pathogens or toxins that are present.

Bacteria in Food

Bacteria are present in the soil, on our skin, on most surfaces in our homes, and in the food we eat. Most bacteria are harmless, some are beneficial, and a few are pathogenic, causing food-borne infection or intoxication.

Bacterial food-borne infection

Each year, an estimated 6,000 to 12,000 Canadians become infected with the bacterium *Salmonella*.[3] Contaminated meat, dairy products, seafood, fresh produce, and cereal have caused outbreaks, but poultry and eggs are the foods most commonly contaminated with the bacterium (**Figure 13.3a** and **b**). Because *Salmonella* is killed by heat, foods that are likely to be contaminated should be cooked thoroughly.

Campylobacter jejuni is the leading cause of acute bacterial diarrhea in developed countries.[4] Common sources are undercooked chicken, unpasteurized milk, and untreated water (**Figure 13.3b** and **c**). This organism grows slowly in cold temperatures and is killed by heat, so thorough cooking and careful storage help prevent infection.

Escherichia coli, commonly called *E. coli*, is a bacterium that inhabits the gastrointestinal tracts of humans and other animals. It comes into contact with food through fecal contamination of water or unsanitary handling of food. Some strains of *E. coli* are harmless, but others can cause serious food-borne infection. One strain of *E. coli*, found in water contaminated by human or animal feces, is the cause of "travellers' diarrhea." Another strain, *E. coli* O157:H7, produces a toxin in the body that causes abdominal pain, bloody diarrhea, and, in severe cases, a potentially fatal form of kidney failure called hemolytic-uremic syndrome.[5]

E. coli O157:H7 entered the public spotlight in 1993, when it led to the deaths of several children who had consumed undercooked, contaminated hamburgers from a fast-food restaurant in the United States (**Figure 13.3d**). Thorough cooking of the hamburgers would have killed the bacteria that caused these deaths. *E. coli* can also contaminate produce such as lettuce, spinach, and green onions, causing illness if the produce is eaten raw.

Listeria became a household name in Canada following an outbreak in 2008. While that specific outbreak drew much public attention to the bacterium *Listeria monocytogenes*, infections by this bacterium affect hundreds of Canadians each year. *Listeria* infection causes flu-like symptoms, but in high-risk groups, such as children, pregnant women, and elderly people, it can cause meningitis and serious blood infections. *Listeria* is ubiquitous in the environment and can survive and grow at refrigerator temperatures. As a result, this bacterium can infect ready-to-eat foods, such as hot dogs and lunchmeats, even when they have been kept properly refrigerated. To prevent infection, ready-to-eat meats should be heated to the steaming point, and unpasteurized dairy products should be avoided.

The food-borne infection caused by the bacterium *Vibrio vulnificus* usually causes gastrointestinal upset but can be deadly in people with compromised immune systems. The most common way in which people become infected is by eating raw or undercooked shellfish, particularly oysters. *Vibrio* bacteria grow in warm seawater. The incidence of *Vibrio* infection is higher during the summer months, when warm water promotes its growth.

Bacterial food-borne intoxication

Staphylococcus aureus is a common cause of bacterial food-borne intoxication. These bacteria live in human nasal passages and can be transferred to food through coughing or sneezing. They can then grow on the food, producing a toxin that causes vomiting soon after ingestion. In buffet-style restaurants, sneeze guards help to protect food from these bacteria.

Another cause of food-borne intoxication is the bacterium *Clostridium perfringens*. It is often called "the cafeteria germ" because it grows in foods that are stored in large containers like those used in cafeterias. Little oxygen gets to the food at the centre of a large container, thus providing an excellent growth environment for these bacteria, which thrive in low-oxygen environments. *C. perfringens* are difficult to kill because they form heat-resistant **spores**. Spores are a stage of bacterial life that remains dormant until environmental conditions favour their growth. *C. perfringens* may cause illness through both infection and intoxication.

The deadliest of all bacterial food toxins is produced by *Clostridium botulinum*. Heat-resistant spores of *C. botulinum* are found in soil, water, and the intestinal tracts of animals. The toxin is produced when the spores begin to grow and develop. When consumed, the toxin blocks nerve function, resulting in vomiting, abdominal pain, double vision, and paralysis that leads to respiratory failure. If untreated, **botulism** is often fatal, but modern

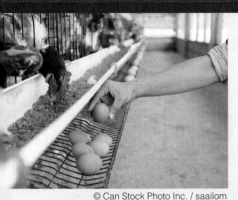

© Can Stock Photo Inc. / saailom

a. Because poultry farms house large numbers of chickens in close proximity, one infected chicken can infect thousands of others. *Salmonella* can infect the ovaries of hens and contaminate the eggs before the shells are formed, so that the bacteria are present inside the shell when the eggs are laid. Therefore, eggs should never be eaten raw.

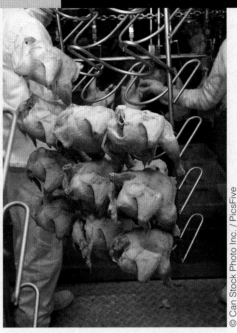

© Can Stock Photo Inc. / PicsFive

b. In processing plants, *Salmonella* and *Campylobacter* from infected birds can be transferred to the meat of healthy birds. Consumers should always handle raw chicken as if it contains pathogens.

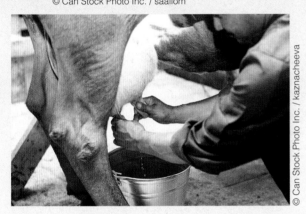

© Can Stock Photo Inc. / kaznacheeva

c. *Campylobacter* are often carried by healthy cattle and by flies on farms. As a result, the bacteria are commonly present in unpasteurized (raw) milk. Unpasteurized milk is also a common source of *Listeria*. During pasteurization, milk is heated to a temperature that is high enough to kill both *Campylobacter* and *Listeria*.

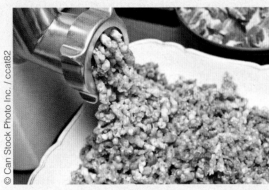

© Can Stock Photo Inc. / ccat82

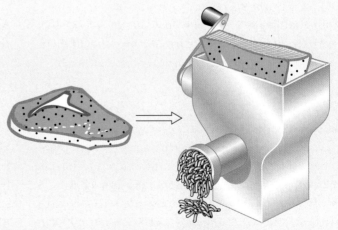

d. *E. coli* O157:H7 can live in the intestines of healthy cattle and contaminate the meat after slaughter. Ground beef contaminated with *E. coli* O157:H7 is a particular concern because the pathogens are mixed throughout during grinding rather than remaining on the surface, as they do on steaks and chops. The *E. coli* bacteria on the outside of the meat are quickly killed during cooking, but those in the interior survive if the meat is not cooked thoroughly. *E. coli*–contaminated meat that comes into contact with a grinder may contaminate hundreds of pounds of ground beef.

Canned foods and botulism • Figure 13.4

Because acid prevents the germination of *Clostridium botulinum* spores, foods that are low in acid, such as green beans, corn, peppers, asparagus, and mushrooms, are more likely to cause botulism than are acidic foods. To avoid botulism, discard bulging cans, which could indicate the presence of gas produced by the bacteria as they grow. Once the botulism toxin has formed, it can be destroyed by boiling for at least 10 minutes. However, when the safety of a food is in question, throw it away; even a taste of a food contaminated with botulism toxin can be deadly.

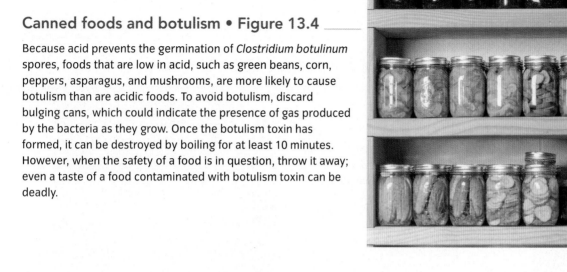

© Can Stock Photo Inc. / zigzagmtart

detection methods and the rapid administration of the appropriate antitoxin have reduced mortality rates. *C. botulinum* grows in low-oxygen, low-acid conditions, so improperly canned foods and foods such as potatoes or stew that are held in large containers with little exposure to oxygen provide optimal conditions for botulism spores to germinate (**Figure 13.4**).

Infant botulism is a type of botulism that is seen only in infants. Though rare, it occurs worldwide and is often undiagnosed.[6] It is caused by the ingestion of botulism spores. When ingested, the spores germinate in the infant's gastrointestinal tract, producing toxin. Some of the toxin is absorbed into the bloodstream, causing weakness, paralysis, and respiratory problems. In the absence of complications, infants generally recover. Only infants are affected because in adults, competing intestinal microflora prevent the spores from germinating. In Canada, contaminated honey is the only food known to be associated with the disease. Unpasteurized honey should therefore never be fed to infants younger than 1 year of age.

Viruses in Food

Unlike bacteria, the viruses that cause human diseases cannot grow and reproduce in foods. Human viruses can reproduce only inside human cells. They make us sick by turning our cells into virus-producing factories (**Figure 13.5**).

Noroviruses are a group of viruses that cause gastroenteritis, or what we commonly call "stomach flu." Norovirus illness is contracted either by eating food that is contaminated with the virus or by touching a contaminated surface and then putting your fingers in your mouth. Shellfish can be contaminated with norovirus if the water in which they live is polluted with human or animal feces. Cooking destroys noroviruses, so uncooked foods and water are the most common causes of norovirus food-borne illness. Norovirus infection can be spread from one infected person to another, so it spreads swiftly where many people congregate in a small area. You may have heard of it as a cause of food-borne illness aboard cruise ships. These outbreaks make headlines, but norovirus outbreaks are just as likely to occur in nursing homes, restaurants, hotels, and dormitories.

Hepatitis A is another viral infection that can be contracted from food or water that is contaminated with fecal matter. Hepatitis A infection causes liver inflammation, jaundice, fever, nausea, fatigue, and abdominal pain. The infection can require a recovery period of several months, but it does not typically require treatment or cause permanent liver damage. Hepatitis in drinking water is destroyed by chlorination. Cooking destroys the virus in food, and good sanitation can prevent its spread. A vaccine that protects against hepatitis A (and hepatitis B) infection is available in Canada and is sometimes required for those who work in the food or hospitality industry.

Mould in Food

Many types of **moulds** grow on foods such as bread, cheese, and fruit. Under certain conditions, these moulds produce toxins (**Figure 13.6**). More than 250 different mould toxins have been identified. Cooking and freezing will stop mould growth but will not destroy the toxins that have already been produced. If a food is mouldy, it should be discarded, the area where it was stored should be cleaned, and neighbouring foods should be checked for contamination.

> **mould** Multicellular fungi that form filamentous branching growths.

How viruses make us sick • Figure 13.5

Viruses make us sick by reproducing inside our cells. Viruses that cause food-borne illness enter the body through the gastrointestinal (GI) tract. Other types of viruses may enter the body through open cuts, the respiratory tract, or the genital tract. The sickness you feel when you are infected by a virus or another pathogen is often due to the actions taken by your body to eliminate it. Sneezing, coughing, mucus, tears, and high body temperatures are examples of our natural defences to infection, which help eliminate foreign invaders.

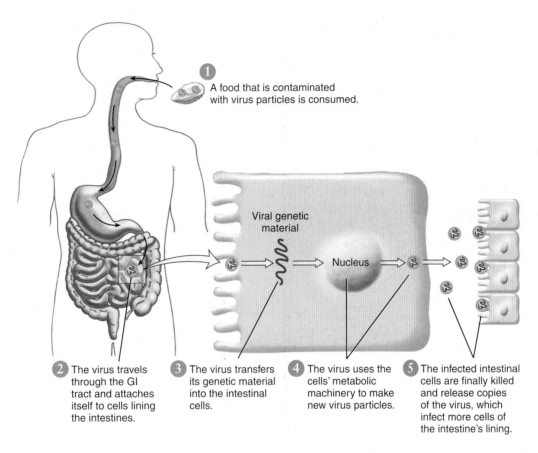

1 A food that is contaminated with virus particles is consumed.

Viral genetic material

Nucleus

2 The virus travels through the GI tract and attaches itself to cells lining the intestines.

3 The virus transfers its genetic material into the intestinal cells.

4 The virus uses the cells' metabolic machinery to make new virus particles.

5 The infected intestinal cells are finally killed and release copies of the virus, which infect more cells of the intestine's lining.

Parasites in Food

Some **parasites** are microscopic single-celled animals, while others are worms large enough to be seen with

parasites Organisms that live at the expense of others.

the naked eye. Parasites that are transmitted through consumption of contaminated food and water can cause food-borne illness.

Giardia lamblia is a single-celled parasite that is often contracted by hikers who drink untreated water from streams contaminated with animal feces. It causes the intestinal illness giardiasis, more commonly known as "beaver fever." *Giardia* infection is also a problem in daycare centres, where many diapers are changed and hands and surfac-

es may not always be thoroughly washed. *Cryptosporidium parvum* is another single-celled parasite that is commonly spread by contaminated water. Infection with either of these parasites can lead to diarrhea, abdominal cramps, abdominal gas, and headaches. Symptoms can appear a few days or few weeks after infection and can last up to a month.[8]

Trichinella spiralis is a parasite that is found in raw and undercooked pork and game meats. Once ingested, these small, wormlike organisms find their way to the muscles, where they grow, causing flu-like symptoms. Fish are another common source of parasitic infections because they carry the larvae of parasites such

Mould toxin and liver cancer • Figure 13.6

a. The filamentous growths seen in this electron micrograph belong to the mould *Aspergillus flavus*. It produces *aflatoxin*, which is among the most potent of the known carcinogens and mutagens. This mould commonly grows on corn, rice, wheat, peanuts, almonds, walnuts, sunflower seeds, and spices such as black pepper and coriander. The level of aflatoxin that may be present in foods in Canada is regulated to prevent toxicity.

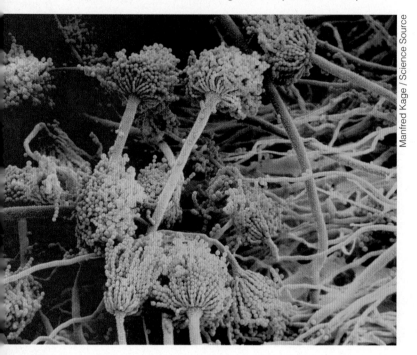

Manfred Kage / Science Source

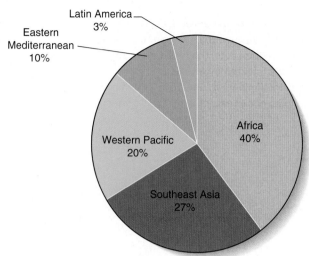

b. This figure shows the distribution of HCC cases attributable to aflatoxin in different regions of the world. Exposure to aflatoxin can lead to liver cancer. In fact, 4.6 to 28.2% of global cases of liver cancer are attributable to the toxin. Many regions with high rates of liver cancer also have high exposure to aflatoxin.[7] Regions not shown here, such as North America and Europe, do not account for a significant number of cases.

Think Critically

Which regions of the world have the highest proportions of aflatoxin-induced lung cancer? Why might rates be higher in these regions and lower in others?

Herring worm • Figure 13.7

The body cavity of this herring contains the larval form of the small roundworm *Anisakis* simplex, also called herring worm. When consumed in raw fish, these parasites invade the stomach and intestinal tract, causing *Anisakis* disease, which is characterized by severe abdominal pain. The fresher the fish is when it is eviscerated, the less likely it is to cause this disease because the larvae move from the fish's stomach to its flesh only after the fish dies.

Anilocra

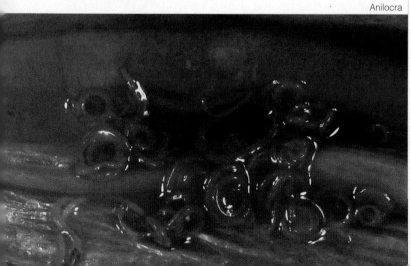

as roundworms, flatworms, flukes, and tapeworms (**Figure 13.7**). As the popularity of eating raw fish has increased, so has the incidence of parasitic infections from fish. Parasites, including those in fish, are killed by thorough cooking. If raw fish is consumed, parasitic infections can be avoided by eating fish that has been previously frozen.

Prions in Food

The strangest, scariest, yet rarest food-borne illness is caused not by a microbe but by a protein that has folded improperly, called a **prion**. Abnormal prions are believed to be the cause of the so-called mad cow disease, or **bovine spongiform encephalopathy (BSE)**, a deadly degenerative neurological disease that affects cattle.

> **prion** A pathogenic protein that is the cause of degenerative brain diseases called spongiform encephalopathies. *Prion* is short for *proteinaceous infectious particle.*

The human form of this disease is **variant Creutzfeldt-Jakob Disease (vCJD)**. People are believed to contract it by eating tissue from a cow infected with BSE, but the exact cause of vCJD is still under debate (**Figure 13.8**).[9] Symptoms of vCJD begin as mood swings and numbness and, within about 14 months, progress to dementia and death.

The disease vCJD is believed to be transmitted by consumption of the brain, nervous tissue, intestines, eyes, or tonsils of contaminated animals, but, thus far, meat (if free from central nervous system tissue) and milk have not been found to transmit either BSE or vCJD.[9] Although cooking does not destroy prions, the risk of acquiring vCJD is extremely small. To reduce the risk of Canadian cattle contracting BSE, the Canadian Food Inspection Agency has implemented safeguards, including restrictions on the ingredients that can be included in cattle feed, regulations for handling the nervous tissue and intestinal tissue of animals, and testing for BSE before meat is released into the food supply.[10]

In the late 1990s, contaminated beef lead to a small outbreak of vCJD in the United Kingdom. A man who frequently visited the United Kingdom became the first and only case of the disease in a Canadian. Although sales of Canadian beef suffered from the publicity of the disease, no one has ever developed vCJD from eating Canadian beef. A few cows with BSE were identified in Canada, but meat from these animals did not enter the food supply due to a highly regulated food inspection system.

What Bug Has You Down?

A wide variety of food-borne pathogens can make you sick (**Table 13.2**). Today, we can identify even more cases of food-borne illness than was possible a few years ago, as a result of recent improvements in governmental outbreak surveillance, attentiveness by health care professionals, and frequent and accurate testing. Increased public awareness of the problem and greater education on the safe handling of food should make food-borne illness much less frequent in the future.

Preventing Microbial Food-Borne Illness

Microbes in food multiply when they are presented with the right conditions for growth. The first step in preventing microbial food-borne illness is to minimize the presence of microbes by choosing food carefully (**Table 13.3**). Preparing food in a clean kitchen reduces cross-contamination. Storing food at refrigerator or freezer

> **cross-contamination** The transfer of contaminants from one food or object to another.

How prions multiply • Figure 13.8

☑ THE PLANNER

The abnormal prions that cause BSE differ from normal proteins in the way they are folded—that is, in their three-dimensional structure. When the improperly folded form of a prion is introduced into the brain after a person has eaten contaminated tissue, it can reproduce by corrupting neighbouring proteins, essentially changing their shape so that they, too, become abnormal prions. Because the abnormal prions are not degraded normally, they accumulate and form clumps called plaques, which cause deadly nervous tissue damage.

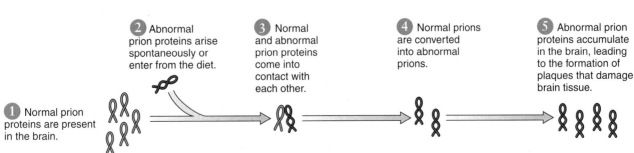

1 Normal prion proteins are present in the brain.

2 Abnormal prion proteins arise spontaneously or enter from the diet.

3 Normal and abnormal prion proteins come into contact with each other.

4 Normal prions are converted into abnormal prions.

5 Abnormal prion proteins accumulate in the brain, leading to the formation of plaques that damage brain tissue.

PROCESS DIAGRAM

Summary of bacterial, viral, and parasitic food-borne illnesses   Table 13.2

Microbe	Sources	Symptoms	Onset (time after consumption)	Duration
Bacteria				
Campylobacter jejuni	Unpasteurized milk, untreated water, undercooked meat and poultry	Fever, headache, diarrhea, abdominal pain	2–5 days	1–2 weeks
Clostridium botulinum	Improperly canned foods, deep casseroles, honey	Lassitude, weakness, vertigo, respiratory failure, paralysis	18–36 hours	10 days or longer (must administer antitoxin)
Clostridium perfringens	Fecal contamination, deep-dish casseroles	Nausea, diarrhea, abdominal pain	8–22 hours	6–24 hours
Escherichia coli O157:H7	Fecal contamination, undercooked ground beef	Abdominal pain, bloody diarrhea, kidney failure	5–48 hours	3 days–2 weeks or longer
Listeria monocytogenes	Raw milk products, soft ripened cheeses, deli meats and cold cuts, raw and undercooked poultry and meats, raw and smoked fish, raw vegetables	Fever, headache, stiff neck, chills, nausea, vomiting. May cause spontaneous abortion or stillbirth in pregnant women.	Days to weeks	Days to weeks
Salmonella	Fecal contamination, raw or undercooked eggs and meat, especially poultry	Nausea, abdominal pain, diarrhea, headache, fever	6–48 hours	1–2 days
Shigella	Fecal contamination of water or foods, especially salads such as chicken, tuna, shrimp, and potato salads	Diarrhea, abdominal pain, fever, vomiting	12–50 hours	5–6 days
Staphylococcus aureus	Human contamination from coughs and sneezes; eggs, meat, potato salads, and macaroni salads	Severe nausea, vomiting, diarrhea	2–8 hours	2–3 days
Vibrio vulnificus	Raw seafood from contaminated water	Cramps, abdominal pain, weakness, watery diarrhea, fever, chills	15–24 hours	2–4 days
Yersinia enterocolitica	Pork, dairy products, and produce	Diarrhea, vomiting, fever, abdominal pain; often mistaken for appendicitis	24–48 hours	Weeks
Viruses				
Hepatitis A	Human fecal contamination of food or water, raw shellfish	Jaundice, liver inflammation, fatigue, fever, nausea, anorexia, abdominal discomfort	10–50 days	1–2 weeks to several months
Norovirus	Fecal contamination of water or foods, especially shellfish and salad ingredients	Diarrhea, nausea, vomiting	1–2 days	2–6 days
Parasites				
Anisakis simplex	Raw fish	Severe abdominal pain	1 hour–2 weeks	3 weeks
Cryptosporidium parvum	Fecal contamination of food or water	Severe watery diarrhea	Hours	2–4 days, but sometimes weeks
Toxoplasma gondii	Meat, primarily pork	Toxoplasmosis (can cause central nervous system disorders, flu-like symptoms, and birth defects in the offspring of women exposed during pregnancy, see Chapter 11)	10–23 days	May become chronic

Safe grocery choices   Table 13.3

- Purchase food from reputable vendors.

- Make sure jars are closed, seals are unbroken, and safety "buttons" on jar lids have not popped.

- Reject cans that are rusted, dented, or bulging.

- Check that food packaging is secure.

- Select frozen foods from below the frost line in the freezer.

- Ensure frozen foods are solidly frozen and do not contain frost or ice crystals.

- Note the freshness dates and avoid foods with expired dates:

    - **Sell-by or pull-by date:** The date used by manufacturers to inform grocers when to remove the product from the shelves. You should buy the product before this date, but if the food has been handled and stored properly, it is usually still safe for consumption after that date. For example, milk is usually still good at least a week beyond its sell-by date if it has been properly refrigerated.

    - **Best before date:** The last date on which the product will retain maximum freshness, flavour, and texture. Beyond this date, the product's quality may diminish, but the food may still be safe if it has been handled and stored properly.

    - **Expiration date:** The last day on which a product should be eaten. The Food and Drug Regulations require that expiration dates be used on such products as formulated liquid diets, meal replacements, and nutritional supplements because after that date, the packaged contents may no longer meet the nutritional and compositional specifications listed on the product.

temperatures either limits or stops microbial growth. Heating foods to the recommended temperature kills microbes and destroys toxins (**Figure 13.9**). Foods that are served cold should be kept cold until they are served. Frozen foods should be kept frozen and then thawed in the refrigerator or microwave before cooking, not thawed at room temperature, which favours microbial growth. Cooked food should be handled with care and kept hot until it is served. When in doubt about the safety of a food, throw it out.

Cross-contamination can occur when uncooked foods containing live microbes come into contact with foods that have already been cooked. Therefore, cooked meat should never be returned to the same dish that held the raw meat, and sauces used to marinate uncooked foods should never be used as a sauce on cooked food. Cooked food should be refrigerated as soon as possible after it has been served. The temperature range that is most favourable for microbial growth is the range at which food usually sits between service and storage. Large portions of food should be divided before refrigeration so they will cool quickly. Most leftovers should be kept for only a few days.

Although most food-borne illness in Canada is caused by food prepared in homes, an outbreak in a commercial or institutional establishment usually involves more people and is more likely to be reported (see *Thinking It Through*). Food in retail establishments has many opportunities to be contaminated because of the large volume of food handled and the many people involved in its preparation. Consumers should choose restaurants with safety in mind. Restaurants should be clean, and cooked foods should be served hot. Cafeteria steam tables should be kept hot enough that the water is steaming and food is kept above 57°C (135°F). Cold foods, such as salad bar items, should be kept either refrigerated or on ice to keep the food at 5°C (41°F) or colder.

Picnics, potluck suppers, and other large events where food is served provide a prime opportunity for bacteria to flourish because food is often left at room temperature or in the sun for long periods before being consumed. When diners serve themselves, cross-contamination is possible from dirty hands or used plates and utensils. Unlike the food at a restaurant salad bar, the food at a family picnic is not sheltered under a sneeze guard to prevent contamination from coughs and sneezes. All food that is served outdoors at a family picnic or county fair should be approached with food safety in mind.

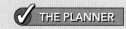
Be Food Safe is a national education campaign by the Canadian Partnership for Consumer Food Safety Education. The program focuses on educating the public about the four core food handling principles: Clean, Separate, Cook, and Chill (www.befoodsafe.ca).

Meats and casseroles should be cooked, and leftovers reheated, until they reach the internal temperatures shown here, which will ensure that microbes have been killed. Use a food thermometer to make sure that the food is cooked to a safe internal temperature; colour is not a good indicator of safety.

A clean kitchen is essential for food safety. Hands, countertops, cutting boards, and utensils should be washed with warm, soapy water before each step in food preparation.

be food safe.

clean. separate. cook. chill.

www.befoodsafe.ca

Canadian Partnership For Consumer Food Safety Education.

To prevent cross-contamination, foods that will be cooked should not be prepared on the same surface used to prepare foods that will be eaten raw.

SAFE COOKING TEMPERATURES
You can't tell by looking... use a food thermometer to be sure!

	Internal temperature
Ground Meat & Meat Mixtures	
Beef, Pork, Veal, Lamb	71°C (160°F)
Turkey, Chicken	74°C (165°F)
Fresh Beef, Veal, Lamb	
Medium Rare	63°C (145°F)
Medium	71°C (160°F)
Well Done	77°C (170°F)
Poultry	
Chicken & Turkey, whole	85°C (185°F)
Poultry parts	74°C (165°F)
Duck & Goose	74°C (165°F)
Stuffing (cooked alone or in bird)	74°C (165°F)
Fresh Pork	
Medium	71°C (160°F)
Ham	
Fresh (raw)	71°C (160°F)
Pre-cooked (to reheat)	74°C (165°F)
Eggs & Egg Dishes	
Egg dishes and casseroles	74°C (165°F)
Seafood	
Fin Fish	70°C (158°F)
	For one minute. Flesh is opaque
Shrimp, Lobster & Crabs	74°C (165°F)
	Flesh is pearly & opaque
Clams, Oysters & Mussels	Shells open during cooking
Scallops	Milky white or opaque & firm
Leftovers & Casseroles	74°C (165°F)

Source: Canadian Partnership For Consumer Food Safety Education, March 2010. Cooking temperatures provided by Health Canada.

121°C — Canning temperature for low-acid foods in pressure cooker.

100°C — Range of cooking temperatures to kill most bacteria. The amount of time needed decreases as the temperature increases.

75°C — Minimum temperature for reheating foods. Warming temperatures control growth but allow survival of some bacteria.

60°C / 52°C — Some growth may occur: Many bacteria survive.

Danger Zone
Temperatures in this zone allow rapid bacterial growth and production of bacterial toxins. Foods should only be allowed to remain in this temperature range for minimal amounts of time.

15°C — Some bacterial growth may occur in this zone.

4°C / 0°C — Cold temperatures allow slow growth for a few cold-tolerant organisms but stop the growth of most.

−18°C — Freezing temperatures prevent bacterial growth but some bacteria are able to survive.

Temperature is one of the best weapons consumers have for preventing food-borne illness. Low temperatures slow or stop microbial growth, and high temperatures kill microorganisms.

Fresh and frozen foods brought from the store should be refrigerated or frozen immediately. Fresh meat, poultry, and fish should be frozen if it will not be used within a day or two. Processed meats such as hot dogs and bologna should be refrigerated but can be kept longer than fresh meat. Freezers should be set to −18°C and refrigerators to less than 4°C.

THINKING IT THROUGH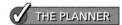
Food Detectives

On Friday, more than half of the 200 children enrolled at the local elementary school were either absent or went home sick sometime during the school day. Their symptoms included nausea and vomiting, diarrhea, abdominal pain, and fever. Food-borne illness was suspected, and the local health department was notified. Inspectors were able to trace the source of the outbreak to the Spring Celebration held at the school on Thursday. For this event, the grade one students made cupcakes, the grade two students made cookies, the grade three students made fruit salad, and the grade fours made frozen custard. All the children were interviewed about which of these foods they had eaten that day, and the information was used to compile the following graph:

Based on the graph, which food is the most likely cause of the illness? Why?
▼

Your answer: _____

_____

Physicians saw many of the sick children, and the bacterium *Salmonella enteritidis* was isolated from their stool samples. The health inspectors determined that the fourth-graders had used six grade-A raw eggs to make the frozen custard.

How can eggs become contaminated with *Salmonella*?
▼

Your answer: _____

_____

The cookie and cupcake recipes also called for eggs. Why are these eggs unlikely to be the cause of the problem?
▼

Your answer: _____

Suggest a reason why 20 children who consumed the frozen custard did not get ill.
▼

Your answer: _____

_____

What could the grade four students have done to avoid the risk of *Salmonella* in their frozen custard?
▼

Your answer: _____

_____

(Check your answers in Appendix I.)

CONCEPT CHECK STOP

1. **How** does *Clostridium botulinum* cause food-borne illness?

2. **What** pathogenic bacteria commonly contaminate chicken and eggs?

3. **How** do viruses make us sick?

4. **How** does refrigeration help prevent food-borne illness?

Agricultural and Industrial Chemicals in Food

LEARNING OBJECTIVES

1. **Illustrate** how contaminants move through the food chain and into our foods.

2. **Compare** the risks and benefits of using pesticides versus growing food organically.

3. **Describe** how to minimize the risks of exposure to chemical contaminants.

Industrial wastes and the chemicals used in agricultural production can contaminate the environment and find their way into the food supply. How harmful these chemicals are depends on how long they remain in the environment and whether they are stored in the organisms that consume them or can be broken down and excreted by these organisms. Some contaminants are eliminated from the environment quickly because they are broken down by microorganisms or chemical reactions. Others remain in the environment for very long periods, and when taken up by plants and small animals, they are neither metabolized nor excreted. When these plants or small animals are then consumed by larger animals and are, in turn, eaten by still larger animals, the contaminants accumulate, reaching higher concentrations at each level of the food chain (**Figure 13.10**). This process is called **bioaccumulation**. Because the toxins are not eliminated from the body, the greater the amount consumed, the greater the amount present in the body.

> **bioaccumulation** The process by which compounds accumulate or build up in an organism faster than they can be broken down or excreted.

Contamination throughout the food chain • Figure 13.10

Industrial pollutants and agricultural chemicals contaminate the water supply and accumulate as they progress through the food chain. Fat-soluble contaminants concentrate in body fat and cannot be excreted. An animal that occupies a higher level in the food chain has higher concentrations of these contaminants because it consumes all the contaminants that have been eaten by organisms at lower feeding levels.

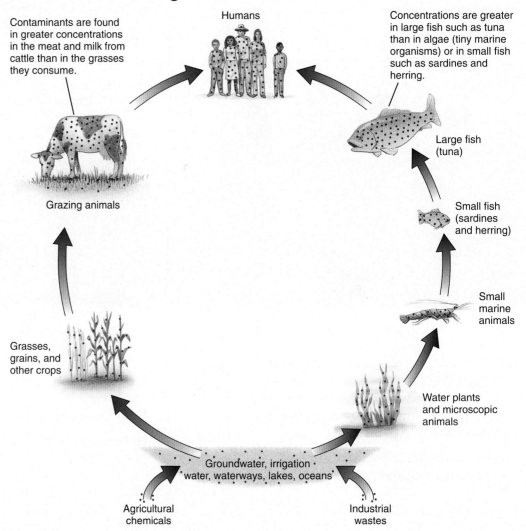

Contaminants are found in greater concentrations in the meat and milk from cattle than in the grasses they consume.

Concentrations are greater in large fish such as tuna than in algae (tiny marine organisms) or in small fish such as sardines and herring.

Humans

Large fish (tuna)

Small fish (sardines and herring)

Small marine animals

Water plants and microscopic animals

Groundwater, irrigation water, waterways, lakes, oceans

Grazing animals

Grasses, grains, and other crops

Agricultural chemicals

Industrial wastes

Pesticides: Risks and Benefits

Pesticides are used to prevent plant diseases and insect infestations. They are applied both to crops in the fields and to harvested produce in an effort to prevent spoilage and extend shelf life. Crops that are grown using pesticides generally produce higher yields and look more appealing because they have less insect damage. However, once pesticides have been applied, they can travel into water supplies, soil, and other parts of the environment. Because pesticides enter the environment, pesticide residues are found not only on the treated plants but also in meat, poultry, fish, and dairy products (see Figure 13.10).

For consumers, the potential risks from pesticides depend on an individual's size, age, and health and on the type and amount of pesticides consumed. To protect public health and the environment, the government regulates the types of pesticides that may be used on food crops, the frequency of their use, and the amount of residue remaining when foods are sold to consumers. The Pest Management Regulatory Agency (PMRA) of Health Canada approves and registers pesticides that are used in food production and establishes allowable limits, or **tolerances**, for both children and adults.[12] To establish tolerances for pesticides, the risk of toxicity is weighed against the pesticide's benefits. The risks are based on the known incidence of toxicity and the amount of the pesticide to which consumers are likely to be exposed. Tolerance levels are then set at the minimum amount of the pesticide needed to be effective; these levels are often several hundred times lower than the level that has been found to cause reactions in test animals.

The PMRA monitors pesticide residues in foods. In general, pesticide residue levels in both domestic and imported foods have been found to be well below federally permitted limits.[13] Although repeated consumption of large doses of any one pesticide could be harmful, such a situation is unlikely because most people consume a variety of foods that have been produced in many different locations.

Integrated pest management

One way to limit pesticide use is through **integrated pest management (IPM)**. IPM is a method of agricultural pest control that combines

> **integrated pest management (IPM)** A method of agricultural pest control that integrates nonchemical and chemical techniques.

chemical and nonchemical methods and emphasizes the use of natural toxins and more effective pesticide application. For example, increasing the use of naturally pest-resistant crop varieties that thrive without the use of pesticides can reduce costs

and minimize environmental damage. IPM programs use information about the life cycles of pests and their interaction with the environment to manage pest damage economically and with the least possible hazard to people, property, and the environment.

Organic food production

The sale and purchase of organic food has increased dramatically in Canada as consumers become more and more concerned about the quality of their food. The term *organic* simply implies that a substance contains carbon, which is a central component of all living things. Colloquially, the term *organic* refers to a food that has been produced through methods that are more natural and more environmentally friendly than many commercial methods. **Organic food** production emphasizes the recycling of resources and the conservation of soil and water to protect the environment. (See *Debate: Should You Go Organic?*) Organic food is produced without using most conventional pesticides, fertilizers made with synthetic ingredients, sewage sludge, genetically modified ingredients, irradiation, antibiotics, or growth hormones (**Figure 13.11**). Organic farming techniques reduce farm workers' exposure to pesticides and decrease the quantity of

> **organic food** Food that is produced, processed, and handled in accordance with the standards of the Organic Products Regulations.

Labelling organic foods • Figure 13.11

The Organic Products Regulations set standards regarding those substances that are approved for and prohibited from use in organic food production. Before a food can be labelled "organic," the farming and processing operations that produce and handle the food must be certified. Products that meet the definition of "100% organic" or "organic" may display the "organic" seal shown here.

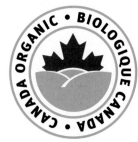

Canadian Food Inspection Agency (2012), Canada Organic Regime: A Certified Choice. Retrieved from http://www.inspection.gc.ca/food/organic-products/labelling-and-general-information/certified-choice/eng/1328082717777/1328082783032. Reproduced or adapted with the permission of the Minister of Public Works and Government Services Canada, 2012.

Labelling term	Meaning
100% organic	Contains 100% organically produced raw or processed ingredients.
Organic	Contains at least 95% organically produced raw or processed ingredients.
Made with organic ingredients	Contains at least 70% organically produced ingredients.

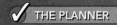
The Issue: As Canadians become more and more concerned about food safety, nutritional health, and the environment, they are turning to organic food. But is organic food necessarily more nutritious and more environmentally friendly than conventionally produced food?

In Canada, the growth and sale of organic foods is on the rise. From 2006 to 2008, the industry saw a 66% growth rate in retail sales.[15] The value of organic products sold in Canada through retail chains in 2008 was valued at approximately $2 billion.[15] Organic farming has also become far more common around the country, both for domestic use and for export. In 2009, an estimated 4,000 organic producers used almost 700 hectares (1,730 acres) of land to produce organic crops, mostly fruits and vegetables.[16]

Do organic production methods make these fruits and vegetables safer than traditional products? If *safer* is defined as containing fewer pesticides, the answer is clear. Organic foods are significantly lower in nitrates and pesticide residues than traditionally grown foods.[17] But, some argue there is little evidence that human health is at risk from the current levels of pesticide exposure from conventional produce. Other contamination risks are also associated with organic foods. For example, manure is often used for fertilizer. When the manure is not treated properly, it can contain pathogenic bacteria.[18]

Many consumers believe that organically produced food is not only safer but also more nutritious. *Nutritious* can mean that it is more effective at preventing nutrition-related diseases.[19] When consumption of organic food is compared with consumption of conventionally produced foods, the majority of studies do not show organic foods to be beneficial in terms of preventing nutrition-related diseases. Research data on the nutrient content of organically produced food are ambivalent. Some studies report that organically produced foods contain more nutrients than conventionally produced food, whereas other studies have found no consistent differences in nutrient content.[20] This confusion is not surprising because many factors affect the nutritional composition of fruits and vegetables, including growing conditions, the growing season, the fertilizer regime, and the methods used for crop protection (such as the use of pesticides and herbicides). Nutrient content is also affected by how the food is stored, transported, and processed prior to consumption.

What about the environment? It is hard to argue that organic farming is not better for the environment. Instead of using chemical pesticides and fertilizer, organic farming relies on crop rotation, compost, and cover crops to maintain the soil. The result is twofold: preservation of the soil, so crops can be grown far into the future, and reduction in the amounts of chemicals released into the environment. But organic growing still affects the environment because manure runoff can pollute waterways, and organic food is often shipped long distances, thereby consuming energy and polluting the environment.

Is a diet based on organic foods safer and more nutritious? We can assume that both conventional and organic foods sold in the Canada are generally safe. Whether organic is more nutritious depends not only on the individual foods but also on the consumer's diet as a whole. If your choices of organic foods are limited by availability or cost, then choosing only organic foods may limit your nutrient intake. Are organic foods better for the environment? They reduce pesticide and fertilizer use, but if organic foods are not available locally, the environmental cost of transporting them may outweigh those savings.

Think Critically

Are these organic onions that were shipped across the country a better environmental choice than conventionally grown onions from the farm across town?

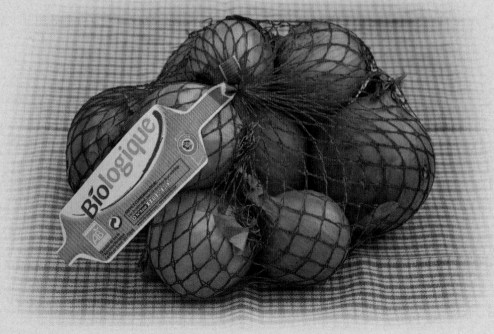

© Wrappers / Alamy

pesticides introduced into the food supply and the environment. However, organic foods are not risk free. Manure is often used to fertilize organic crops. However, if the manure is not treated properly, it can increase the risks of microbial food-borne illness, and its runoff can pollute lakes and streams. Organically grown food may also be exposed to traces of synthetic pesticides and other agricultural chemicals not approved for organic use, which may be introduced by irrigation water, rain, wind, and a variety of other sources. In Canada, for a product to be labelled organic, more than 95% of its content must be organic.[14]

Industrial Contaminants

Industrial chemicals that contaminate the environment can find their way into the food supply. For example, fish may accumulate substances from the water in which they live and feed, and shellfish may accumulate contaminants because they feed by passing large volumes of water through their bodies. Pollutants in the water can also contaminate crops and move through the food chain into meat and milk (see Figure 13.10).

One group of carcinogenic compounds that pollutes the environment is **polychlorinated biphenyls (PCBs)**. Prior to the 1970s, these chemicals were used in the manufacture of electrical capacitors and transformers, plasticizers, waxes, and paper. PCBs in runoff from manufacturing plants contaminated water, particularly near the Great Lakes. PCBs are no longer produced, but because they do not degrade, they are still in the environment and accumulate in fish caught in contaminated waters. PCBs are a particular problem for pregnant and lactating women because prenatal exposure to PCBs and consumption of contaminated breast milk can damage the fetal and infant nervous system and cause learning deficits. Pregnant and breastfeeding women should check with their local health department for recommendations regarding fish consumption.

Other contaminants from manufacturing, such as chlordane (used to control termites); radioactive substances, such as strontium-90; and toxic metals, such as cadmium, lead, arsenic, and mercury, have found their way into fish and shellfish. Cadmium and lead can interfere with the absorption of other minerals. Cadmium can cause kidney damage, and lead can impair brain development. Arsenic is believed to increase the risk of cancer. Mercury, which has been found in large fish, can damage nerve cells (**Figure 13.12**).[21] Health Canada therefore recommends

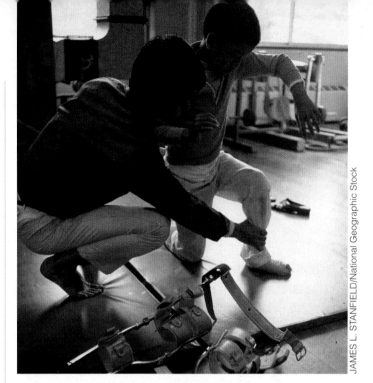

JAMES L. STANFIELD/National Geographic Stock

Mercury poisoning • Figure 13.12 _____

This Japanese boy has Minamata disease, a neurological syndrome caused by mercury poisoning. The disease first appeared in Minamata, Japan, in 1956 and was caused by the release of mercury into the water by a local chemical factory. The mercury accumulated in the fat of fish and shellfish that were eaten by the local population.

limiting the consumption of fresh and frozen tuna, shark, swordfish, and orange roughy to a combined total of 150 grams or less per week. Because mercury is more damaging during prenatal development, pregnant women are advised to consume less than 150 grams of these fish per month (see Chapter 11).[21]

Antibiotics

Antibiotics and hormones are administered to animals to improve health, increase growth, or otherwise enhance food production. To prevent these chemicals from being passed on to consumers, regulations address the types of drugs that can be used and when they can be administered; animal tissues are also monitored for drug residues.

Animals are treated with antibiotics when they are sick, and some animals are also given antibiotics to prevent disease and promote growth. This treatment increases the amount of meat produced and reduces costs, but if used improperly, antibiotic residues can remain in the meat. Another major concern is the creation of antibiotic-resistant bacteria. When exposed to an antibiotic, bacteria that are resistant to it will survive and produce offspring that are also resistant. If these antibiotic-resistant bacteria infect humans, the resulting illness cannot be treated with that antibiotic. This use of antibiotics is suspected of being a major contributor to the development of antibiotic-resistant strains of bacteria.[22] The Canadian Medical Association (CMA) argues that antibiotics are widely misused in Canada, thereby promoting antibiotic exposure and resistance. As a result, the CMA strongly urges that antibiotics only be given to livestock when prescribed by veterinarians.[23]

Choosing Wisely to Minimize Agricultural and Industrial Contaminants

Although most of us cannot detect chemical contaminants in our food, we can reduce the amounts of chemicals we consume by taking care in the selection and preparation of food. One of the easiest ways to reduce risk is to choose a wide variety of foods, thus avoiding excessive consumption of contaminants that may be present in any one food. To reduce exposure to pesticide residues in fruits and vegetables, consumers can choose organic foods or locally grown produce. Locally grown produce typically contains fewer chemicals because pesticides are not needed to prevent spoilage and extend the shelf life of shipped produce. Exposure to pesticide residues on conventionally grown produce can be minimized by washing and, in some cases, by peeling (**Figure 13.13a**). Pesticides and other toxins that are ingested by animals concentrate in fat, so intake can be reduced by trimming all fat from meat and removing the skin from poultry.

Intake of pesticides and other chemical pollutants from fish and seafood products can also be minimized by choosing wisely and consuming a variety of fish (**Figure 13.13b**). To minimize your consumption of contaminants, remove the skin, fatty material, and dark meat from fish. Use cooking methods such as broiling, poaching, boiling, and baking, which allow contaminants from the fatty portions of fish to drain. Do not eat the "tomale" in lobster. The tomale, a green paste inside the abdominal cavity of a cooked lobster, serves as the lobster's liver and pancreas and is the organ where toxins accumulate. The analogous organ in blue crabs, called the "mustard" because of its yellow colour, should also be avoided (see *What Should I Eat?*).

Reducing exposure to pesticides and pollutants • Figure 13.13 _____

a. Pesticide residues on fruits and vegetables can be removed or reduced by peeling or by washing with tap water and scrubbing with a brush, if appropriate. In the case of leafy vegetables, such as lettuce and cabbage, the outer leaves can be removed and discarded. Washing apples, cucumbers, eggplant, squash, and tomatoes may not remove all the pesticides because these fruits and vegetables are coated with wax to maintain freshness by sealing in moisture, but wax also seals in pesticides. The wax and pesticides can be removed by peeling, but removing the peel also eliminates fibre and some micronutrients.

b. Exposure to chemical contaminants can be minimized by choosing saltwater fish caught well offshore, away from polluted coastal waters. Fish that live near the shore or spend part of their life cycle in freshwater areas are more likely to contain contaminants. Smaller species of fish are safer because they are earlier in the food chain, and smaller fish within a species are safer because they are younger and hence have had less time to accumulate contaminants. Fresh and frozen fish such as tuna, shark, and swordfish should be consumed in moderation because they have a higher tendency to concentrate heavy metals such as mercury. Fortunately, fish that are more common in the Canadian diet, such as pollock, salmon, smelt, and rainbow trout, and shellfish such as mussels and clams tend to be relatively low in mercury (see Figure 13.10).

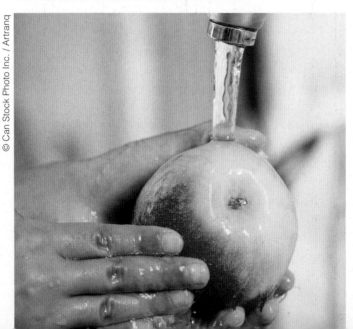

© Can Stock Photo Inc. / Artranq

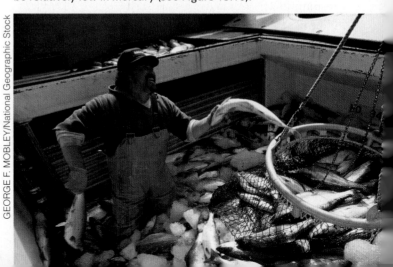

GEORGE F. MOBLEY/National Geographic Stock

WHAT SHOULD I EAT?
Food Safety

✔ THE PLANNER

- Make a salad after you have washed the lettuce or peeled off the outer leaves.
- Trim the fat and don't eat the skin of poultry and fish.
- Wash fruits and vegetables thoroughly before eating.

Avoid ingesting pathogenic microbes
- Make sure your burger is well done.
- Skip the runny eggs and have them scrambled.
- Pass on the dough! Treat yourself to chocolate chip cookies only after they come out of the oven.
- Slice up some melon, but make sure the knife, the cutting board, and the skin of the melon are clean before you begin slicing.

Reduce pesticides and pollutants in your food
- Buy locally grown produce.
- Look for the organic symbol.
- Opt for smaller species of fish.

 Use iProfile to compare the calories and grams of fat in a chicken breast with and without skin.

CONCEPT CHECK STOP

1. **How** can a pesticide used on broccoli plants end up in milk?

2. **How** can organic food cause food-borne illness?

3. **What** can you do to minimize PCBs in your diet?

Technology for Keeping Food Safe
LEARNING OBJECTIVES

1. **Describe** how temperature is used to prevent food spoilage.

2. **Discuss** how irradiation preserves food.

3. **Explain** how packaging protects food.

4. **Discuss** the risks and benefits of food additives.

Food spoils when its taste, texture, or nutritional value is changed, either by enzymes that are naturally present in the food or by microbes that grow on the food. For thousands of years, humans have treated food in their effort to prevent spoilage. Techniques that preserve food work by destroying enzymes present in the food, by killing microbes, or by slowing microbial growth (**Table 13.4**).

Most of the oldest methods of food preservation—heating, cooling, drying, smoking, and adding sugar or salt—are still used today. In addition, researchers have developed newer methods, such as irradiation and specialized packaging. While all these technologies offer benefits, they can also create risks. Some risk arises when substances find their way into food, either accidentally or as a normal part of the production process. Health Canada considers any substance that can be expected to become part of a food a **food additive** and regulates the types and amounts of food additives that may be present in a particular food.

> **food additive** A substance that is intentionally added to or can reasonably be expected to become a component of a food during processing.

High and Low Temperature

Cooking food is one of the oldest methods of ensuring that food is safe. Cooking kills disease-causing organisms and destroys most toxins. Other preservation techniques that rely on high temperature to kill microbes include **pasteurization**,

> **pasteurization** The process of heating food products to kill disease-causing organisms.

The acronym FAT TOM reminds us of the factors that affect microbial growth. Most food preservation techniques modify one or more of these factors to stop or slow microbial growth.

Food	Food provides the setting where the bacteria grow.
Acidity	Most bacteria grow best at a pH near neutral. Some food additives, such as citric acid and ascorbic acid (vitamin C), are acids, which prevent microbial growth by lowering the pH of food.
Time	The longer a food sits at an optimal growth temperature, the more bacteria it will contain. Preservation methods such as canning and pasteurization kill microbes by heating food to an appropriate temperature for the right amount of time.
Temperature	The high temperatures of canning, cooking, and pasteurization kill microbes, and the low temperatures of freezing and refrigeration slow or stop microbial growth.
Oxygen	Most bacteria need oxygen to grow, so packaging that eliminates oxygen prevents their growth.
Moisture	Bacteria need water to grow, so their growth can be prevented by preservation methods such as drying or using high concentrations of salt or sugar, which draw water away by osmosis.

aseptic processing The placement of sterilized food in a sterilized package using a sterile process.

sterilization, and **aseptic processing (Figure 13.14)**. Lowering the temperature of food by means of refrigeration or freezing does not kill microbes but preserves the food and protects consumers because it slows or stops microbial growth.

Preservation techniques that rely on temperature benefit consumers by providing appealing, safe foods, but these foods are not risk free, particularly when they are handled incorrectly. If foods are not heated long enough or to a high enough temperature, or if they are not kept cold enough, they can pose a risk of food-borne illness. In addition, some types of cooking can generate hazardous chemicals. Carcinogenic chemicals produced during the cooking of meats include **polycyclic aromatic hydrocarbons (PAHs)** and **heterocyclic amines (HCAs)**. PAHs are formed when fat drips on a grill and burns. They rise with the smoke and are deposited on the surface of the food. PAH formation can be minimized by selecting lower-fat meat and using a layer of aluminum foil to prevent fat from dripping on the coals. HCAs are produced by the burning of amino acids and other substances in meats and are formed during any type of high-temperature cooking. HCA formation can be reduced by precooking meat, marinating meat before cooking, cooking at lower temperatures, and reducing cooking time by using smaller pieces of meat and avoiding overcooking. The recommended cooking temperatures are designed to prevent microbial food-borne illness and minimize the production of PAHs and HCAs.

Another contaminant formed during food preparation is **acrylamide**. It is formed as a result of chemical reactions that occur during high-temperature baking or frying, particularly in carbohydrate-rich foods. The highest levels of acrylamide are found in French fries and snack chips. Smaller amounts are found in coffee and in foods made from grains, such as breakfast cereal and cookies. High doses can cause cancer and reproductive problems in experimental animals and act as a neurotoxin in humans. Thus far, dietary exposure to acrylamide has not been associated with cancer in humans, and more research is needed to determine whether long-term, low-level exposure has any cumulative effects.[24] Methods for reducing the amounts and potential toxicity of acrylamide in foods are being investigated.[25]

Aseptic processing • Figure 13.14

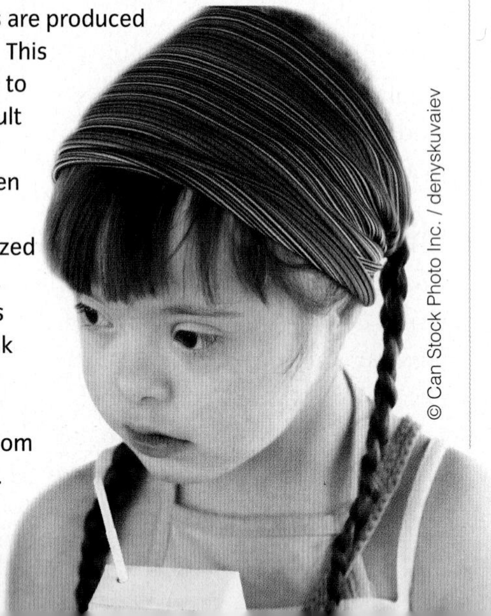

The juice boxes that fit so conveniently into school lunch bags are produced by aseptic processing. This technique heats foods to temperatures that result in sterilization. The sterilized foods are then placed in sterilized packages, using sterilized packaging equipment. If the package remains unopened, juice or milk packaged aseptically can remain free of microbial growth at room temperature for years.

© Can Stock Photo Inc. / denyskuvaiev

Food Irradiation

Food **irradiation**, also called cold pasteurization, is used in more than 40 countries to treat everything from frog legs

> **irradiation**
> A process that exposes foods to radiation for the purpose of killing contaminating organisms and retarding the ripening and spoilage of fruits and vegetables.

to rice. Irradiation exposes food to high doses of X-rays, gamma radiation, or high-energy electrons for the purpose of killing microbes and insects and inactivating enzymes that cause the germination and ripening of fruits and vegetables (**Figure 13.15**).[26] Because irradiation produces compounds that are not present in the original foods, it is treated as a food additive, and regulations limit the level of radiation that may be used. At the allowable levels of radiation, the amounts of these compounds produced are almost negligible and have not been found to pose a risk to consumers. Presently, Canada permits irradiation for onions, potatoes, wheat, flour, whole wheat flour, whole and ground spices, and dehydrated seasoning. Health Canada is currently considering the addition of more foods to the list, including frozen ground beef and chicken.[27]

Food irradiation is used relatively infrequently in Canada because of both a lack of irradiation facilities and public suspicion of the technology. The word *irradiation* fosters the belief that the food becomes radioactive. Opponents to food irradiation claim that it introduces carcinogens, depletes the nutritional value of food, and enables the sale of previously contaminated foods. In fact, irradiated food is not radioactive, and scientific studies conducted over the past 50 years have found that the benefits of irradiation outweigh the potential risks.[28] Irradiation can decrease the amounts of certain nutrients in foods, but these nutrient losses are similar to the losses incurred through canning or refrigerated storage.[27]

Because irradiation can be used in place of chemical treatments, it reduces consumers' exposure to chemical pesticides and preservatives. It is often promoted by individuals concerned with food safety because of its potential for improving the safety of food and reducing the incidence of food-borne illness.

Food Packaging

Packaging plays an important role in food preservation; it keeps moulds and bacteria out, keeps moisture in, and protects food from physical damage. An open package of refrigerated cheddar cheese will become mouldy in a few days, but an unopened package will stay fresh for weeks.

Food packaging is continually being improved. In the past two decades, for instance, consumer demand for fresh and easy-to-prepare foods has led manufacturers to offer partially cooked pasta, vegetables, seafood, fresh and cured meats, and dry products such as whole-bean and ground coffee in packaging that, if unopened, will keep

---

Irradiated foods • Figure 13.15

a. Irradiated foods must be labelled with the radura symbol shown here and the statement "treated with radiation," "treated by irradiation," or "irradiated." If a pre-packaged food includes an ingredient that has been irradiated, it will not be listed on the label unless it comprises more than 10% of the finished product.

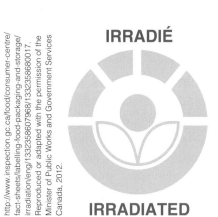

IRRADIÉ

IRRADIATED

Canadian Food Inspection Agency (2012), Food Irradiation. Retrieved from http://www.inspection.gc.ca/food/consumer-centre/fact-sheets/labelling-food-packaging-and-storage/irradiation/eng/1332358607968/1332358680017. Reproduced or adapted with the permission of the Minister of Public Works and Government Services Canada, 2012.

b. Irradiation increases the safety and shelf life of foods and does not significantly compromise nutritional quality or noticeably change food texture, taste, or appearance, as long as it is properly applied to a suitable product. After two weeks in cold storage, the strawberries on the left, which were treated by irradiation, remain free of mould, whereas the untreated strawberries on the right, which were picked at the same time, are covered with mould.

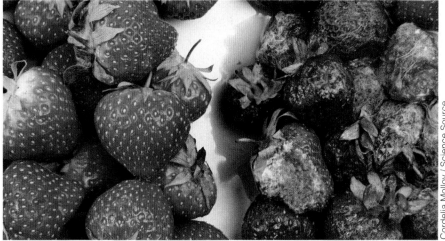

Cordelia Molloy / Science Source

perishable food fresh much longer than will conventional packaging. **Modified atmosphere packaging (MAP)** uses plastics or other packaging materials that are impermeable to oxygen. The air inside the package is vacuumed out to remove the oxygen. The product can then remain in a vacuum, or the package can be infused with another gas, such as carbon dioxide or nitrogen. The lack of oxygen prevents the growth of aerobic bacteria, slows the ripening of fruits and vegetables, and slows the oxidation reactions that cause discolouration in fruits and vegetables and rancidity in fats.

> **modified atmosphere packaging (MAP)** A preservation technique used to prolong the shelf life of processed or fresh food by changing the gases surrounding the food in the package.

MAP is often used to package cooked entrées such as pasta primavera or beef teriyaki. The raw ingredients are sealed in a plastic pouch, the air is vacuumed out, and the pouch and its contents are partially precooked and immediately refrigerated. This processing eliminates the need for the extreme cold of freezing or the extreme heat of canning, so flavour and nutrients are better preserved. Because these products are not heated to temperatures high enough to kill all bacteria and are not stored at temperatures low enough to prevent all bacteria from growing, they can pose a food safety risk. To ensure safety, fresh refrigerated foods should be purchased only from reputable vendors, used before the expiration date printed on the package, refrigerated until use, and heated according to the time and temperature directions on the package.

Packaging can protect food from spoilage, but even the best packaging can introduce risk if it becomes part of the food. A variety of substances found in paper and plastic containers and packaging, and even in dishes, can leach into food (**Figure 13.16**). Substances that are known to contaminate food are regulated by Health Canada and the Canadian Food Inspection Agency. However, these regulations apply only to the intended use of the product. When a product is used improperly, substances from its packaging can migrate into food. For instance, some plastics migrate into food when heated in a microwave oven. Thus, only containers designed for microwave cooking should be used when microwaving food.

Food Additives

What keeps bread from moulding, gives margarine its yellow colour, and keeps Parmesan cheese from clumping in

Bisphenol A from plastics • Figure 13.16

A topic of concern for many Canadians is the transfer of bisphenol A (BPA), a chemical found in the polycarbonate plastic used to manufacture hard, transparent water bottles; baby bottles; food containers; and found in the coating inside cans. However, the overall effects of BPA on humans are still unclear and under debate. The major concern with BPA is that it is associated with impaired neurological development in rodents and may mimic the hormone estrogen, a cancer promoter, in the human body. Due to BPA's controversial nature, and the higher levels of BPA exposure found in infants, in 2010, Canada became the first country to place BPA on its toxic chemicals lists.[29] Exposure to BPA can be minimized by eating fewer canned foods and drinking from containers made of glass or aluminum, rather than plastic.

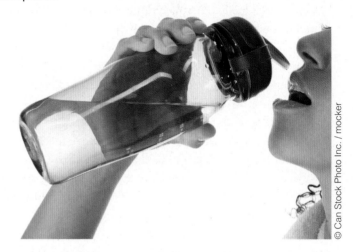

© Can Stock Photo Inc. / mocker

the shaker? The answer to all these questions is food additives. Substances that are intentionally added to foods are called **direct food additives**. Other substances that are added to food unintentionally—such as the oil used to lubricate food-processing machinery—are referred to as **indirect food additives**. Health Canada regulates the amounts and types of direct and indirect food additives in food.

> **direct food additives** Substances intentionally added to foods. Their use is regulated by Health Canada.
>
> **indirect food additives** Substances that are expected to unintentionally enter foods during manufacturing or from packaging.

Regulating food additives Food additives improve food quality and help protect us from disease, but if the wrong additive is used or the wrong amount is added, it can do more harm than good. Food additives are typically used to enhance the appearance, texture, or shelf life of a food. Any manufacturer that wants to use a new food additive must submit a petition to Health Canada describing the chemical composition of the additive, how it is manufactured, and how it is detected in food. The manufacturer must prove that the additive will be effective for its intended purpose at the proposed levels, that it is safe for its intended use, and that its use is necessary. Additives may not be used to disguise inferior products or deceive consumers. They cannot be used if they significantly destroy nutrients or if the same effect can be achieved through sound manufacturing processes.

Additives that are often of particular concern are nitrates and nitrites, which are used to retard the growth of *Clostridium botulinum* in cured meats. Their use has been controversial because they form carcinogenic **nitrosamines** in the digestive tract. They are still allowed in foods, however, because they prevent botulism, and there is little evidence they pose a serious risk in the amounts consumed in the human diet (**Figure 13.17**).[30]

Substances that are toxic at some level of consumption may be harmless at a lower level. To ensure that additives are safe, most of the allowable food additives can be added only at levels 100 times below the highest level that has been shown to have no harmful effects. This restriction provides a greater margin of safety than exists for many vitamins and other naturally occurring substances.

Identifying food additives Food additives are used to make food safer; maintain palatability and wholesomeness; improve colour, flavour, or texture; aid in process-ing; and enhance nutritional value (**Table 13.5**). The use of food additives ensures the availability of wholesome, appetizing, and affordable foods that meet consumer demands throughout the year. Health Canada's Food Additive Dictionary lists all the potential additives in Canadian-made foods and their typical uses.[31] Many of these additives, such as sugar and spices, are used in homes every day. Other additives may sound like a chemical soup: calcium propionate in bread, disodium EDTA in kidney beans, and BHA in potato chips. Understanding what these chemicals are used for can help make the ingredient list a source of information rather than a cause for concern.

Sensitivities to additives Some individuals are allergic or sensitive to certain food additives. For example, the flavour enhancer monosodium glutamate (MSG), commonly used in Chinese food, can cause adverse reactions known as *MSG symptom complex* in sensitive individuals (see Chapter 6). Sulphites can cause symptoms ranging from stomach ache and hives to severe asthma. Sulphites are used as preservatives in baked goods, canned foods, condiments, and dried fruits. Sensitive individuals can identify foods that contain sulphites by checking food labels. The forms of sulphites allowed in packaged foods include sulphur dioxide, sodium sulphite, sodium and potassium bisulphite, and sodium and potassium metabisulphite. Foods served in

Reducing nitrosamine risk • Figure 13.17

To minimize any risk posed by nitrosamines without increasing the risk of bacterial food-borne illness, Canada's Food and Drug Regulations limit the amount of nitrate and nitrite that can be added to food and require the addition of antioxidants such as vitamin C, which reduce nitrosamine formation, to foods that contain these additives. Consumers can reduce nitrosamine exposure by limiting their consumption of cured meat to 85 to 113 g (3 to 4 oz) per week and maintaining adequate intakes of the antioxidant vitamins C and E.

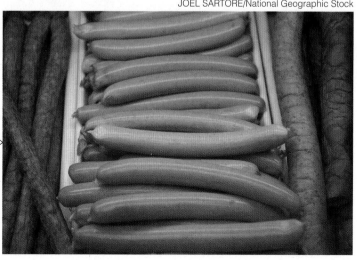

INGREDIENTS: MECHANICALLY SEPARATED CHICKEN, WATER, PORK, MODIFIED CORN STARCH, DEXTROSE, SALT, BEEF, CONTAINS 2% OR LESS OF THE FOLLOWING: CORN SYRUP, FLAVOURINGS, SODIUM PHOSPHATES, POTASSIUM LACTATE, SODIUM DIACETATE, SODIUM ASCORBATE (VITAMIN C), OLEO RESIN OF PAPRIKA, SODIUM NITRITE

Common food additives[32] Table 13.5

Type of additive	What's on the label	What they do	Where they are used
Anti-caking agents	Calcium silicate, iron ammonium citrate, silicon dioxide	Keep powdered foods free-flowing, prevent moisture absorption	Salt, baking powder, confectioners' sugar
Colour additives	FD&C blue nos. 1 and 2, FD&C green no. 3, FD&C red nos. 3 and 40, FD&C yellow nos. 5 and 6, orange B, citrus red no. 2, annatto extract, beta-carotene, grapeskin extract, cochineal extract or carmine, paprika oleoresin, caramel colour, fruit and vegetable juices, saffron, colourings or colour added	Prevent colour loss due to exposure to light, air, temperature extremes, and moisture; enhance colours; give colour to colourless and "fun" foods	Processed foods, candies, snack foods, margarine, cheese, soft drinks, jellies, puddings, pie fillings
Emulsifiers	Soy lecithin, mono- and diglycerides, egg yolks, polysorbates, sorbitan monostearate	Allow smooth mixing and prevent separation; reduce stickiness; control crystallization; keep ingredients dispersed	Salad dressings, peanut butter, chocolate, margarine, frozen desserts
Flavours, spices, and flavour enhancers	Natural flavouring, artificial flavour, spices, monosodium glutamate (MSG), hydrolyzed soy protein, autolyzed yeast extract, disodium guanylate or inosinate	Add specific flavours or enhance flavours already present in foods	Many processed foods, puddings and pie fillings, gelatin mixes, cake mixes, salad dressings, candies, soft drinks, ice cream, BBQ sauce
Humectants	Glycerin, sorbitol	Retain moisture	Shredded coconut, marshmallows, soft candies, confections
Leavening agents	Baking soda, monocalcium phosphate, calcium carbonate	Promote rising of baked goods	Breads and other baked goods
Nutrients	Thiamine hydrochloride, riboflavin (vitamin B_2), niacin, niacinamide, folate or folic acid, beta-carotene, potassium iodide, iron or ferrous sulfate, alpha-tocopherols, ascorbic acid, vitamin D, amino acids (L-tryptophan, L-lysine, L-leucine, L-methionine)	Replace vitamins and minerals lost in processing; add nutrients that may be lacking in the diet	Flour, breads, cereals, rice, pasta, margarine, salt, milk, fruit beverages, energy bars, breakfast drinks
pH control agents and acidulants	Lactic acid, citric acid, ammonium hydroxide, sodium carbonate	Control acidity and alkalinity, prevent spoilage	Beverages, frozen desserts, chocolate, low-acid canned foods, baking powder
Preservatives	Ascorbic acid, citric acid, sodium benzoate, calcium propionate, sodium erythorbate, sodium nitrite, calcium sorbate, potassium sorbate, BHA, BHT, EDTA, tocopherols	Maintain freshness; prevent spoilage caused by bacteria, moulds, fungi, or yeast; slow or prevent changes in colour, flavour or texture; delay rancidity	Jellies, beverages, baked goods, cured meats, oils and margarines, cereals, dressings, snack foods, fruits, vegetables
Stabilizers and thickeners, binders, and texturizers	Gelatin, pectin, guar gum, carrageenan, xanthan gum, whey	Produce uniform texture, improve "mouth-feel"	Frozen desserts, dairy products, cakes, pudding and gelatin mixes, dressings, jams and jellies, sauces
Sweeteners	Sucrose, glucose, fructose, sorbitol, mannitol, corn syrup, high-fructose corn syrup, saccharin, aspartame, sucralose, acesulfame potassium (acesulfame-K), neotame	Add sweetness with or without extra calories	Beverages, baked goods, table-top sweeteners, many processed foods

restaurants may also contain sulphites. For example, a restaurant's potato dish may have been prepared using potatoes that were peeled and soaked in a sulphite solution before cooking.

Colour additives can also cause adverse reactions. For example, FD&C yellow no. 5, which is listed on medicine labels as tartrazine, may cause itching and hives in sensitive people. It is found in beverages, desserts, and processed vegetables. Colour additives are listed in the ingredient list along with other food additives. Colours in foods are classified as certified or exempt. Certified colours are human-made, meet strict specifications for purity, and must be listed by name in the ingredient list. Colours that are exempt from certification include pigments from natural sources such as dehydrated beets and carotenoids; these may be listed collectively in the ingredient list as "artificial colour."

CONCEPT CHECK STOP

1. **What** is pasteurization?

2. **How** does irradiation help extend the shelf life of food?

3. **How** does modified atmosphere packaging prevent food spoilage?

4. **Why** are food additives regulated?

Biotechnology
LEARNING OBJECTIVES

1. **Explain** how genetic engineering introduces new traits into plants.

2. **List** ways in which genetic engineering is being used to enhance the food supply.

3. **Discuss** some potential risks associated with genetic engineering.

4. **Describe** how genetically modified foods and crops are regulated to ensure safety.

Biotechnology alters the characteristics of organisms by making selective changes in their DNA. The concept is not new. For centuries, farmers have selected seeds from plants with the most desirable characteristics to plant for the next year's crop, bred the animals that grew fastest or produced the most milk to improve the productivity of the next generation of animals, and cross-bred plant varieties to combine the desired traits of each. However, these traditional methods may require many generations to produce the desired results. Biotechnology uses **genetic engineering** to select genes for specific traits. Genetic engineering has significantly sped up the process of modifying the traits of organisms. Like all other new technologies, however, it may introduce new risks.

> **biotechnology**
> The process of manipulating life forms via genetic engineering for the purpose of providing desirable products for human use.

> **genetic engineering** A set of techniques used to manipulate DNA for the purpose of changing the characteristics of an organism or creating a new product.

How Biotechnology Works

Genetically modified (GM) crops are created through genetic engineering: A piece of DNA containing the gene for a desired characteristic is taken from plant, animal, or bacterial cells and transferred to plant cells (**Figure 13.18**).

The DNA is then referred to as recombinant DNA because the new DNA is a combination of the DNA from two organisms. The modified cells are then allowed to divide into more and more cells and eventually differentiate into the various types of cells that make up a whole plant. The new plant is a **transgenic** organism. Each cell in the new plant contains the transferred gene for the desired trait. This technique is used to introduce characteristics such as disease and drought resistance into plants. Genetic engineering is more difficult in animals because animal cells do not take up genes as easily as plant cells do, and making copies of these cells (clones) is also more difficult. However, these techniques have been used

> **transgenic** An organism with a gene or group of genes intentionally transferred from another species or breed.

Engineering a genetically modified plant • Figure 13.18

THE PLANNER

Crops developed by using the genetic engineering steps shown here are grown all over the world.

1. The desired gene is identified.

Nucleus

Plant cell wall

2. The gene is clipped out using DNA-cutting enzymes.

3. Various techniques are used to transfer the gene into the plant cell.

4. The gene migrates into the cell's nucleus and is integrated into the plant's DNA.

5. Modified plant cells are identified and placed into cell culture to multiply.

6. Special culture medium allows the cells to differentiate into the different cells that make up a whole plant.

7. Each mature plant carries the new gene and the trait for which it codes.

Think Critically Compare the number of genes transferred by genetic engineering with the number transferred by traditional plant breeding.

to produce cows that yield more milk, cattle and pigs that provide more meat, and sheep that grow more wool.[33]

Applications of Biotechnology

The techniques of biotechnology can be used in a variety of ways in food production to alter quantity, quality, cost, safety, and shelf life. By making plants resistant to herbicides, insects, and various plant diseases, this technology has increased crop yields and reduced damage from insects and plant diseases (**Figure 13.19a** and **c**). By altering enzyme activity and other traits, biotechnology is being used to increase the shelf life of fresh fruits and vegetables and to create products that have greater consumer appeal, such as seedless grapes and watermelons.

Biotechnology is also used in food processing. GM microbes now produce rennet, an enzyme used in cheese production; enzymes used in the production of high-fructose corn syrup; and the enzyme lactase, used to reduce the lactose content of milk.

Biotechnology also has great potential for addressing the problem of world hunger and malnutrition. Although world hunger is rooted in political, economic, and cultural issues that cannot be resolved by agricultural technology alone, GM crops are being developed to target some of the world's major nutritional deficiencies. For example, to address protein deficiency, researchers are developing new varieties of corn, soybeans, and sweet potatoes with enhanced levels of essential amino acids. To address iron deficiency, rice has been engineered to contain more iron.[36]

To address vitamin A deficiency, genes that code for the production of enzymes needed for the synthesis of the vitamin A precursor beta-carotene have been inserted into rice (**Figure 13.19b**).[37]

Currently, only four GM crops are grown in Canada: canola, corn, soy, and sugar beet. Canadians will also encounter imported GM foods such as papaya, squash, and some milk products.

Risks and Regulation of Biotechnology

The rapid advancement of biotechnology during the past decade has created the potential for health problems and environmental damage. Regulations are in place to control the use of genetic engineering and GM products. The National Academy of Sciences has concluded that the risks posed by biotechnology are the same as those posed by crops produced by traditional plant breeding.[38] Nevertheless, many consumers and scientists believe that these conclusions are premature and that the potential impact of this booming technology has not yet become apparent. They urge that this technology be used with caution to avoid health or environmental impacts that outweigh the benefits.

Consumer concerns Consumer safety concerns related to GM foods include the possibility that the nutrient content of a food may have been negatively affected or that an allergen or a toxin may have inadvertently been introduced into a food that was previously safe. For example, if DNA from fish or nuts—foods that commonly cause

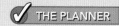
a. Insect-resistant corn is created by inserting a gene from the bacterium *Basillus thuringiensis* (or Bt). The gene produces a protein called Bt toxin that is toxic to certain insects, such as this European corn borer, but safe for humans and other animals. The presence of the new gene improves the crop yield and also reduces the amounts of chemical pesticides that need to be applied.

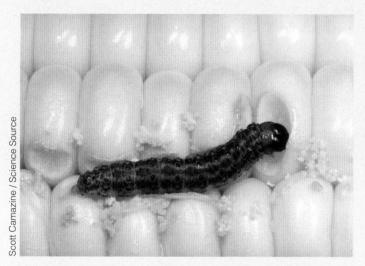

Scott Camazine / Science Source

b. Half the world's population depends on rice as a dietary staple, but rice is a poor source of vitamin A. Genetically modified rice, called golden rice (seen on the right, compared with white rice on the left) for the colour imparted by the beta-carotene pigment, has the potential to significantly increase vitamin A intake. One variety contains enough provitamin A in 125 g (1/2 cup) of dry rice to provide more than 50% of the RDA for a child.[35]

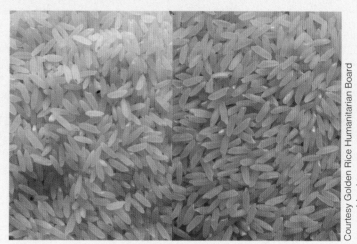

Courtesy Golden Rice Humanitarian Board
www.goldenrice.org

c. Genetically modified crops have increased substantially around the world and can be found on all of the continents, with the exception of Antarctica. Canada currently has the fifth highest yields of GM crops in the world, with 10.4 million hectares (25.7 million acres) of land being devoted to GM crops in 2011.[34] The United States has the highest yields worldwide, at almost seven times the Canadian level.

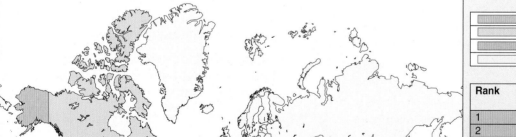

Data from ISAAA Brief 43-2012: Executive Summary, Global Status of Commercialized Biotech/GM Crops: 2012; http://www.isaaa.org/resources/publications/briefs/44/executivesummary/default.asp

	>25 million hectares
	1–24 million hectares
	0.1–0.9 million hectares
	<0.1 million hectares

Rank	Country	Area (million hectares)
1	USA	69.5
2	Brazil	166
3	Argentina	23.9
4	Canada	11.6
5	India	10.8
6	China	4.0
7	Paraguay	3.4
8	South Africa	2.9
9	Pakistan	2.8
10	Uruguay	1.4
11	Bolivia	1.0
12	Philippines	0.8
13	Australia	0.7
14	Burkina Faso	0.3
15	Myanmar	0.3
16	Mexico	0.2
17	Spain	0.1
18	Chile	<0.1

allergic reactions—were introduced into soybeans or corn, these foods would then be dangerous to individuals allergic to fish or nuts. To prevent the unintentional occurrence of this kind of situation, biotechnology companies have established systems for monitoring the allergenic potential of proteins used for plant genetic engineering.[39] In 1996, allergy testing successfully prevented soybeans containing a gene from a Brazil nut from entering the market.[40]

Environmental concerns An environmental concern about GM crops is that they will be used to the exclusion of other varieties, thereby reducing biodiversity. The ability of populations of organisms to adapt to new conditions, diseases, or other hazards depends on the presence of many different species and varieties that provide a diversity of genes. If farmers plant only GM insect-resistant, high-yielding crops, other species and varieties may eventually become extinct, and the genes for the traits they possess may be lost forever.

Another environmental issue is the possibility that GM crops will create "superweeds." Such plants might result, for example, if a trait such as increased rate of growth is introduced into a domesticated plant species and then is passed on to a related wild species. This process could produce a fast-growing weed, or superweed, that would compete with the domesticated species. As a safeguard, plant developers avoid introducing genes for traits that could increase a plant's competitiveness or other undesirable properties in weedy relatives.

Concern is also raised that crops that have been engineered to produce pesticides will promote the evolution of pesticide-resistant insects. An illustration is the case of insects that feed on plants modified to produce the Bt toxin (see Figure 13.19a). As more and more of the insects' food supply consists of plants that produce this pesticide, only insects that carry genes that make them resistant to the

Bt toxin survive and reproduce. The result is an increase in the number of Bt-resistant insects, which therefore reduces the effectiveness of the Bt toxin as a method of pest control. Pesticide-resistant insects may also evolve when pesticides are sprayed on crops.

Regulation of GM food products Health Canada has approved more than 100 GM foods for production and sale. Most Canadians don't recognize these foods as genetically modified because they appear no different from other foods, and food manufacturers are not required to provide special labelling unless the food is known to pose a potential risk.

Labelling of foods containing GM ingredients is required only when the nutritional composition of the food has been altered; the food contains potentially harmful allergens, toxins, pesticides, or herbicides; the food contains ingredients that are new to the food supply; or the food has been changed significantly enough that its traditional name no longer applies. Premarket approval is required when the new food contains a substance that is not commonly found in foods or when it contains a substance that does not have a history of safe use in foods. Typically, Health Canada takes seven to 10 years to approve a genetically modified food.[41]

CONCEPT CHECK

1. **Where** does the DNA introduced into GM plants come from?

2. **How** does biotechnology increase crop yields?

3. **Why** might a GM food cause an allergic reaction, whereas the unmodified version of the same food does not?

4. **What** types of GM foods carry special labels?

Summary

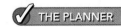

1 Keeping Food Safe   458

• Most **food-borne illness** is caused by food contaminated with disease-causing **microbes**; occasionally it can be caused by chemical contaminants in food. The harm caused by contaminants in the food supply depends on the type of toxin; its dose; the length of time over which

the contaminant is consumed; how it is metabolized and excreted; and the size, age, and health of the consumer.

• The food supply is monitored for safety by the Canadian Food Inspection Agency. This agency ensures that the food

Keeping food safe from farm to table
• Figure 13.1

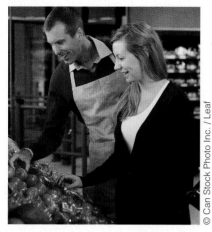

available for purchase meets the standards of the Food and Drug Regulations developed by Health Canada.

- Food manufacturers, processors, and distributors must establish and implement a **Hazard Analysis Critical Control Point (HACCP)** to prevent and eliminate food contamination rather than catch it after it occurs. This system helps identify **critical control points**, or steps in food handling where controls can be more effectively applied to prevent food contamination.

- Consumers can prevent most cases of food-borne illness by following safe food-handling and preparation guidelines.

2 Pathogens in Food   461

- The **pathogens** that affect the food supply include bacteria, viruses, moulds, parasites, and prions. Some bacteria cause **food-borne infection** because they are able to grow in the gastrointestinal tract when ingested. Others produce toxins in food, and consumption of the toxin causes **food-borne intoxication**.

Safe food handling, storage, and preparation
• Figure 13.9

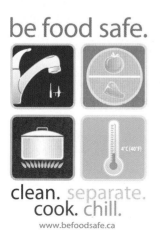

be food safe.

clean. separate.
cook. chill.

www.befoodsafe.ca

- Although most bacteria are harmless or beneficial, food-borne intoxication is often caused by pathogenic bacteria that damage cells by releasing toxins and enzymes. Most bacteria in food can be killed by heating food to recommended levels. Certain bacteria, such as *Clostridium perfringens*, form heat-resistant **spores** and are more difficult to kill, even when heated. The most fatal bacteria common to food cause **botulism**, which can lead to impaired nerve functions. Botulism is rarely fatal in Canadian adults because it is often detected and treated early. In Canada, **infant botulism** is typically related to the consumption of honey and can be fatal or lead to permanent disability if not detected early.

- Viruses do not grow on food, but when consumed in food, they can reproduce in human cells and cause food-borne illness.

- **Moulds** that grow on foods produce toxins that can harm consumers.

- **Parasites** include microscopic single-celled animals and worms that can be seen with the naked eye. They are consumed in contaminated water or food.

- Improperly folded **prion** proteins cause **bovine spongiform encephalopathy (BSE)** in cattle. The risk of acquiring **Creutzfeldt-Jakob Disease (vCJD)**, the human form of this deadly degenerative neurological disease, is extremely low.

- Bacteria, viruses, worms, and various other pathogens in food can cause food-borne illness. The Canadian government monitors the occurrence of outbreaks of these illnesses, so fewer Canadians feel their uncomfortable and potentially fatal effects. By increasing public awareness of proper food handling, future cases of food-borne illness may become even less frequent.

- The risk of food-borne illness can be decreased through proper food selection, preparation, and storage to kill pathogens or minimize their growth. For instance, using separate cutting boards and knives for meats and vegetables may help prevent **cross-contamination**.

3 Agricultural and Industrial Chemicals in Food   472

- Contaminants in the environment can find their way into the food supply. Contaminants that are deposited in the fatty tissue of animals are not eliminated, leading to **bioaccumulation** as they pass through the food chain.

- Pesticides help increase crop yields and the quality of produce. To decrease the risk of pesticide toxicity, **tolerances** are established, and foods are monitored for pesticide residues. Safer pesticides are being developed, and Canadian farmers are reducing the amounts applied by using **integrated pest management (IPM)** and **organic food** production methods.

Labelling organic foods
• Figure 13.11

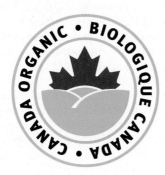

- Industrial pollutants such as **polychlorinated biphenyls (PCBs)** have contaminated some waterways and the fish and shellfish that live in them. Larger, longer-lived fish and those that live in contaminated waters have the highest concentrations.

- Antibiotics and hormones are used in conventional animal food production. The amounts entering the food supply pose little risk, but the use of antibiotics contributes to the development of antibiotic-resistant strains of bacteria.

- Consumers can reduce the amounts of pesticides and other environmental contaminants in food by carefully selecting and handling produce; selecting low-fat saltwater varieties of fish caught far offshore in unpolluted waters; and trimming fat from meat, poultry, and fish before cooking.

4 Technology for Keeping Food Safe 477

- **Food additives** are substances that are intentionally added to food to improve food quality, kill pathogens and/or add a desirable trait, such as a different colour, to a food.

- Heating foods to high temperatures; cooling them to low temperatures; and altering their levels of acidity, moisture, and oxygen prevent food spoilage and lengthen shelf life by killing microbes or slowing their growth. Both **pasteurization** and **aseptic processing** involve using high temperatures to ensure food safety. While these methods are generally safe, using temperature to ensure food safety also has risks. When meats are cooked, two substances that may cause cancer may be formed: **polycyclic aromatic hydrocarbons (PAHs)** and **heterocyclic amines (HCAs)**. **Acrylamide** is another carcinogen that may be formed, especially when carbohydrate-rich foods are cooked at high temperatures.

Irradiated foods • Figure 13.15

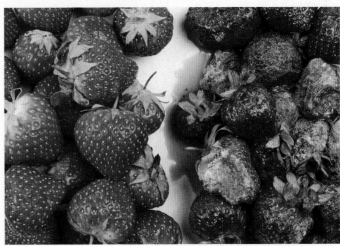

Cordelia Molloy / Science Source

- **Irradiation** preserves food by exposing it to radiation. This process kills microbes, destroys insects, and slows the germination and ripening of fruits and vegetables.

- Packaging keeps moulds and bacteria out of foods, keeps moisture in, and protects food from physical damage. **Modified atmosphere packaging (MAP)** reduces the oxygen available for microbial growth. The safety of packaging materials must be considered because components of packaging can leach into food.

- **Direct food additives** are used to preserve or enhance the appeal of food. **Indirect food additives** are substances known to find their way into food during cooking, processing, and packaging. Both are regulated. Accidental contaminants, which enter food when it is handled or prepared incorrectly, are not regulated. Just because an additive is regulated, its full safety cannot be ensured. An example is the use of nitrates and nitrites in cured meats. While their use helps prevent botulism, this process leads to the production of **nitrosamines**, known carcinogens, into food.

5 Biotechnology 483

- **Biotechnology** alters the characteristics of organisms by using **genetic engineering** to select genes for specific traits.

- Biotechnology produces **genetically modified (GM)** crops by transferring a gene for a desired characteristic from one organism to another. The result is a **transgenic** organism.

- Biotechnology has many different applications and is often employed to improve crop yield, reduce production costs, increase the nutrient quality of food, make foods safer, and extend shelf life.
- Biotechnology has the potential to improve the volume, safety, and quality of the food supply, but it also has the potential to introduce allergens or toxins into foods or to negatively affect nutrient content. Environmental concerns with the use of GM crops include reduction in biologic diversity, the creation of "superweeds," and the evolution of pesticide-resistant insects. Regulations are in place to control the use of genetic engineering and GM products.

Engineering a genetically modified plant
- **Figure 13.18**

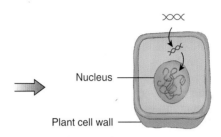

Nucleus

Plant cell wall

Key Terms

- acrylamide 478
- aseptic processing 478
- bioaccumulation 472
- biotechnology 483
- botulism 462
- bovine spongiform encephalopathy (BSE) 466
- critical control points 459
- cross-contamination 467
- direct food additives 480
- food additive 477
- food-borne illness 458
- food-borne infection 461
- food-borne intoxication 461

- genetically modified (GM) 483
- genetic engineering 483
- Hazard Analysis Critical Control Point (HACCP) 459
- heterocyclic amines (HCAs) 478
- indirect food additives 480
- infant botulism 464
- integrated pest management (IPM) 473
- irradiation 479
- microbes 458
- modified atmosphere packaging (MAP) 480
- mould 464
- nitrosamines 481

- organic food 473
- parasites 465
- pasteurization 477
- pathogen 461
- polychlorinated biphenyls (PCBs) 475
- polycyclic aromatic hydrocarbons (PAHs) 478
- prion 466
- spores 462
- tolerances 473
- transgenic 483
- variant Creutzfeldt-Jakob Disease (vCJD) 467

Critical and Creative Thinking Questions

1. After 67 people became ill from consuming food at a company picnic, investigators determined that the tossed green salad, the egg salad, and the turkey slices were all contaminated with the bacteria *Campylobacter*. Create a scenario to explain how all three foods might have become contaminated.

2. A restaurant decides not to replace an old dishwasher, even though it no longer heats the water to above 57°C (135°F). What are the potential risks associated with this decision? How else can the restaurant sanitize the dishes?

3. The chicken Simi brings home from the store is contaminated with *Salmonella* bacteria. She prepares a meal by grilling the chicken and making a salad. List the steps in the preparation of this meal that might result in cross-contamination and increase the likelihood of *Salmonella* infection. What steps can Simi take to prevent food-borne illness?

4. A town's voters decide that they can improve their own health and protect the environment by banning the production and sale of all but organically produced foods. What are the risks and benefits of this decision?

5. Fermentation, a process that uses microbes to convert carbohydrates into alcohols or acids, is used to produce alcoholic beverages and yogurt. Explain how fermentation converts milk into yogurt and why yogurt will keep longer than milk.

6. A train crash spills a load of industrial waste into a river that feeds into a local reservoir. Bottled water is provided to the residents of the community. How might this spill affect other segments of the food supply?

7. *Brassica* is a genus of plants that includes cabbage, broccoli, and several weeds. What risks might be associated with the use of a new genetically engineered variety of *Brassica* that grows faster and produces more seeds than traditional varieties?

What is happening in this picture?

These rye plants are infected with a fungus. When the grain is consumed, the fungal toxins cause a syndrome called ergotism. The symptoms include prickling skin sensations, facial distortions, incomprehensible speech, paralysis, hallucinations, convulsions, and dementia. Ergotism may have caused some of the symptoms exhibited by individuals who were supposedly cursed by the "witches" of 17th-century Salem, Massachusetts.[42]

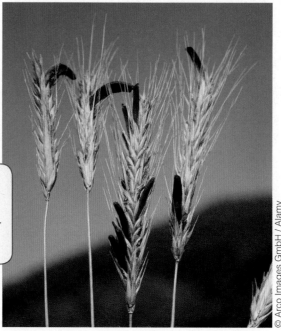

© Arco Images GmbH / Alamy

Think Critically

1. How could ergotism cause individuals to appear "bewitched"?
2. Why might mouldy rye have been more of a problem in the 17th century than it is today?
3. Why doesn't baking prevent this ailment?

Self-Test

(Check your answers in Appendix J.)

1. What is the major cause of food-borne illness in Canada today?
   a. pesticides
   b. microbes
   c. environmental toxins
   d. antibiotics

2. Which factor does not affect the likelihood that a contaminant will cause food-borne illness in an individual?
   a. body size
   b. immune status
   c. age
   d. dose of toxin
   e. time of year

3. Which of the following groups has the lowest risk of contracting a food-borne illness?
   a. Pregnant women
   b. Adolescent males
   c. The elderly
   d. AIDS patients

4. The foods that most frequently cause *Salmonella* infection are _____.
   a. beef and pork
   b. dairy products
   c. eggs and poultry
   d. shellfish

5. Pathogenic bacteria are killed by _____.
   a. freezing
   b. cooking
   c. refrigeration
   d. marinating

6. Below what temperature should food be refrigerated to reduce bacterial growth?
   a. A
   b. B
   c. C
   d. D

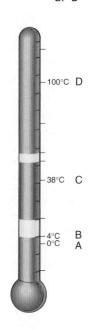

100°C D

38°C C

4°C B
0°C A

7. Which organism can cause food-borne intoxication and can be present in honey and home-canned foods?

   a. *Escherichia coli*

   b. *Clostridium perfringens*

   c. *Clostridium botulinum*

   d. *Salmonella*

8. Which of the following is most likely to be a concern in hamburger that is cooked to well done on a grill?

   a. polycyclic aromatic hydrocarbons (PAHs)

   b. *Escherichia coli*

   c. *Giardia*

   d. prions

9. Raw hamburger patties are taken to the grill on a platter. After being cooked, they are returned to the same platter and served. This is an example of _____.

   a. efficient use of kitchen equipment

   b. food intoxication

   c. cross-contamination

   d. an HACCP system

10. Glass that enters food from a broken jar is _____.

    a. regulated as an indirect food additive

    b. not regulated

    c. safe because it is sterilized

    d. regulated as an accidental contaminant

11. Which organism in the figure is most likely to contain the highest concentration of industrial contaminants?

    a. A

    b. B

    c. C

    d. D

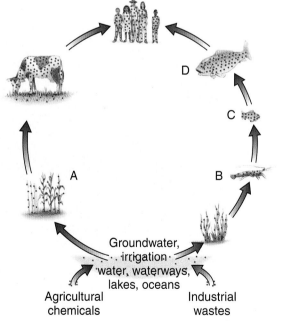

12. At what step in this process is recombinant DNA formed?

    a. 1   b. 3   c. 4   d. 6   e. 7

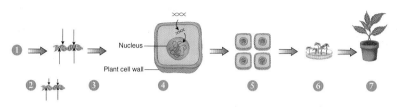

13. The potential benefits of biotechnology include all of the following except _____.

    a. increased biodiversity

    b. enhanced disease resistance

    c. improved crop yields

    d. reduced pesticide use

14. This insignia means the food _____.

    a. is not safe to eat

    b. has been irradiated

    c. is radioactive

    d. can safely be stored without refrigeration

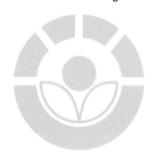

THE PLANNER ✓

Review your Chapter Planner on the chapter opener and check off your completed work.

Feeding the World

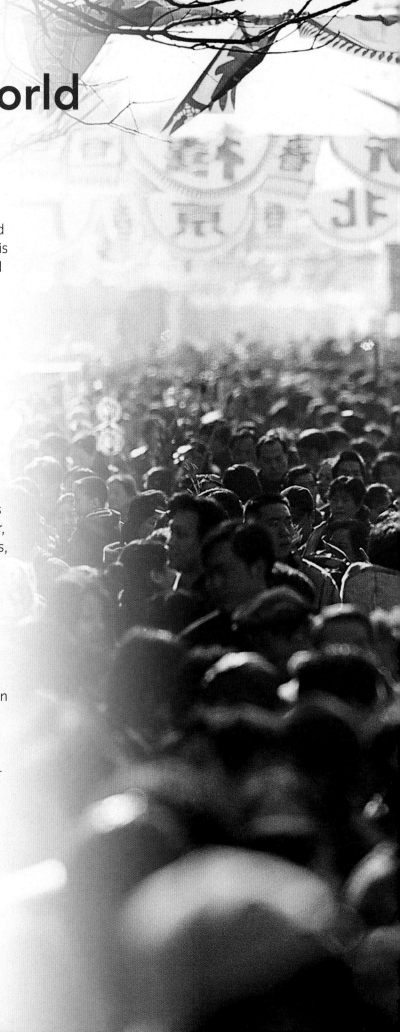

Between January 2007 and June 2008, global food prices soared and a major food crisis hit the world. The United Nations Food and Agriculture Organization (FAO) food price index rose by more than 60%, as prices for dietary staples, such as rice, wheat, corn, and soybeans, soared by 50 to 200%.[1] In many countries, this alarming trend led to food insecurity and economic and political instability, sometimes evidenced as rioting and outbreaks of violence.

In stark contrast, a wide variety of food is available in developed countries such as Canada, and access to food is rarely limited. Conversely, complications associated with overnutrition continue to dominate.

If having *too* much food is the main nutritional concern in Canada, why are many professionals in nutrition, agriculture, and economics concerned about the potential for major food shortages in both the near and distant future? The threat of global food shortages is associated with worldwide economic instability, the high price of oil, increased demand for biofuels, various natural disasters that affect food production and labour, unequal distribution of food, poor use of land resources, and unrealistic food prices that fail to reflect the true cost of producing food. Much of the developed world continues to overconsume, placing significant strain on land without considering future consequences.

Adding to these concerns, the world's population continues to grow. The world's population has skyrocketed from approximately 1 billion people in the early 1900s to 7 billion in 2011, and is projected to hit 9 billion by 2050.

The good news? We technically have enough food and agricultural potential to feed the world's growing population. But the bad news is we are not fully exploiting this potential and food is not being distributed equitably. Food scarcity is a complex issue, and no intervention can single-handedly reverse the current situation. Various economic, environmental, and social changes at multiple levels are needed before we can sustainably feed the world into the future.

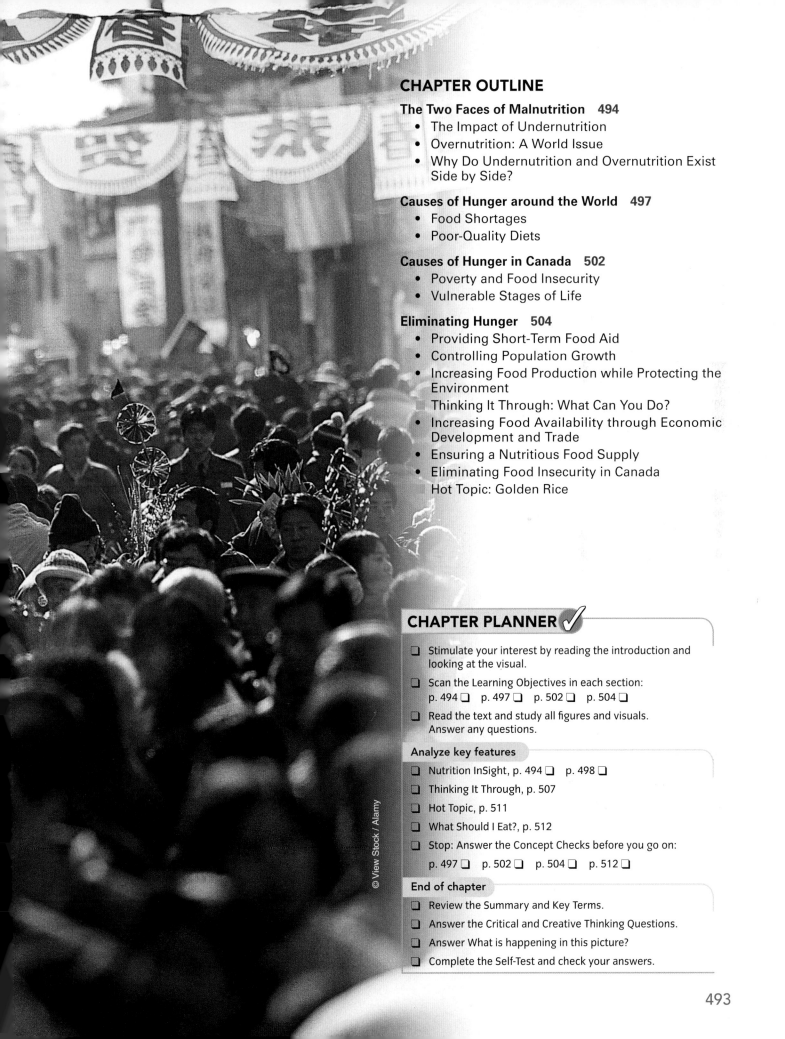

CHAPTER OUTLINE

CHAPTER PLANNER ✓

- ❑ Stimulate your interest by reading the introduction and looking at the visual.
- ❑ Scan the Learning Objectives in each section:
  p. 494 ❑   p. 497 ❑   p. 502 ❑   p. 504 ❑
- ❑ Read the text and study all figures and visuals. Answer any questions.

Analyze key features

- ❑ Nutrition InSight, p. 494 ❑   p. 498 ❑
- ❑ Thinking It Through, p. 507
- ❑ Hot Topic, p. 511
- ❑ What Should I Eat?, p. 512
- ❑ Stop: Answer the Concept Checks before you go on:
  p. 497 ❑   p. 502 ❑   p. 504 ❑   p. 512 ❑

End of chapter

- ❑ Review the Summary and Key Terms.
- ❑ Answer the Critical and Creative Thinking Questions.
- ❑ Answer What is happening in this picture?
- ❑ Complete the Self-Test and check your answers.

© View Stock / Alamy

493

The Two Faces of Malnutrition

LEARNING OBJECTIVES

1. **Compare** the problems of under- and overnutrition in the world today.

2. **Discuss** the impact of undernutrition throughout the life cycle.

3. **Explain** how nutrition transition affects the incidence of obesity.

When we think of malnutrition around the world, the image that comes to mind for most of us is one of undernutrition: **hunger** and **starvation**. This image is certainly valid because almost 900 million people around the world are chronically undernourished, and more than a third of all deaths in children under age 5 are due to undernutrition, which kills nearly 6 million children each year.[2-5] At the same time that health organizations are struggling with issues of undernutrition, however, rates of illness related to overnutrition are soaring. Those who are overweight and those who are undernourished both suffer from malnutrition and experience high levels of sickness and disability and lower levels of productivity. These two faces of malnutrition complicate the goal of solving the problem of malnutrition worldwide.

hunger Recurrent involuntary lack of food that over time may lead to malnutrition.

starvation A severe reduction in nutrient and energy intake that impairs health and eventually causes death. It is the most extreme form of malnutrition.

The Impact of Undernutrition

Populations where hunger is a chronic problem experience a **cycle of undernutrition** (**Figure 14.1a**). The cycle begins when women consume a nutrient-deficient diet during pregnancy. These women are more likely than others to give birth to low-birth-weight infants who are susceptible to illness and early death.

Nutrition InSight   The cycle of undernutrition • Figure 14.1

a. Undernutrition affects the health and productivity of individuals at every stage of life. It often begins in the womb, continues through infancy and childhood, and extends into adolescence and adulthood. Interruption of this cycle of undernutrition at any point can benefit both the individuals affected and their society. Healthy children can then grow into healthy adults who produce healthy offspring and can contribute fully to society.

b. Low-birth-weight infants are at increased risk for complications, illness, and early death. Survivors often suffer lifelong physical and cognitive disabilities. A higher number of low-birth-weight infants means a higher infant mortality rate. Every year, approximately one of every four children is born with low birth weight, and 96% of them live in developing countries.[7]

© Can Stock Photo Inc. / lucidwaters

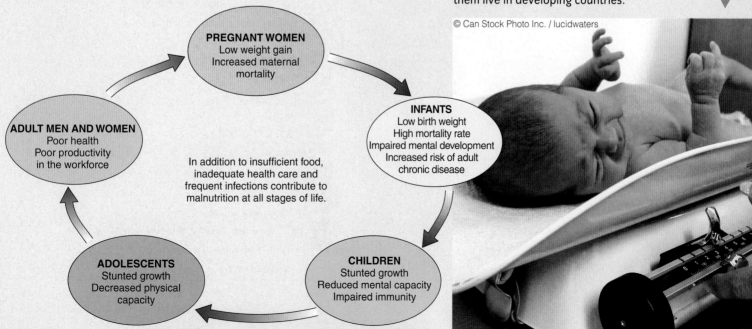

PREGNANT WOMEN
Low weight gain
Increased maternal mortality

INFANTS
Low birth weight
High mortality rate
Impaired mental development
Increased risk of adult chronic disease

ADULT MEN AND WOMEN
Poor health
Poor productivity in the workforce

In addition to insufficient food, inadequate health care and frequent infections contribute to malnutrition at all stages of life.

ADOLESCENTS
Stunted growth
Decreased physical capacity

CHILDREN
Stunted growth
Reduced mental capacity
Impaired immunity

The **infant mortality rate** and the number of low-birth-weight births are indicators of a population's health and nutritional status (**Figure 14.1b**). In most industrialized countries, the infant mortality rate is less than 6 per 1,000 live births; in developing countries, the rate is sometimes more than 100 per 1,000 live births.[6] Low-birth-weight infants who do survive require extra nutrients, which are often not available. Malnutrition in infancy and childhood has a profound effect on growth and development and on susceptibility to infectious disease. Infectious diseases are more common and more likely to be fatal in undernourished children, whereas the same infectious diseases are typically not life threatening in well-nourished children (**Figure 14.1c**).

Malnutrition in children causes **stunting** (**Figure 14.1d**), which is an indicator of undernutrition in a population's children. Stunting in childhood produces smaller adults who have a reduced work capacity and are unable to contribute optimally to their society's economic and social development. Stunted, malnourished women are more likely than others to give birth to low-birth-weight babies. In addition, those who have experienced a lower birth weight and early-childhood stunting are more likely to experience abdominal obesity in adulthood,[9] which increases their risk of morbidity from cardiovascular disease, hypertension, and diabetes.

> **infant mortality rate** The number of deaths during the first year of life, typically expressed per 1,000 live births.

> **stunting** A decrease in linear growth rate.

Overnutrition: A World Issue

For the first time in history, with nearly 1.5 billion overweight or obese adults worldwide, the number of overnourished people exceeds the number who are undernourished.[10,11] If recent trends continue, by 2030, more than 50% of the world's adult population will be either overweight or obese.[12] Because obesity increases the risk of cardiovascular disease, hypertension, stroke, type-2 diabetes, certain cancers, and arthritis, among other conditions, it is a major contributor to the global burden of chronic disease and disability.

THE PLANNER

c. Well over half of all deaths in children younger than 5 years of age are due to infectious disease.[5] Mortality from infections is increased among malnourished children. An estimated 35% of all deaths in children under age 5 result from undernutrition.[5] Immunizations against infectious disease are less effective in malnourished children because their immune systems cannot respond normally.

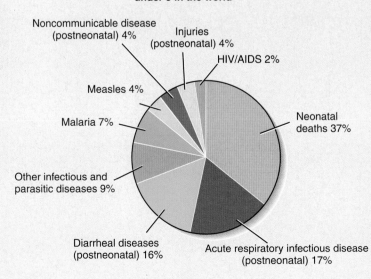

Causes of death in neonates and children under 5 in the world

Noncommunicable disease (postneonatal) 4%
Injuries (postneonatal) 4%
HIV/AIDS 2%
Measles 4%
Malaria 7%
Other infectious and parasitic diseases 9%
Neonatal deaths 37%
Diarrheal diseases (postneonatal) 16%
Acute respiratory infectious disease (postneonatal) 17%

d. In developing countries, more than 30% of children younger than 5 years of age suffer from stunting,[8] which may have resulted from prolonged infections and deficiencies of energy, protein, vitamin A, iodine, iron, and zinc.

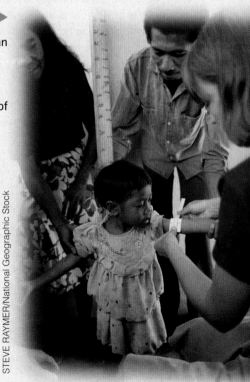

STEVE RAYMER/National Geographic Stock

The Two Faces of Malnutrition **495**

The prevalence of overweight and obesity is also growing among children worldwide.[12] More than 40 million preschool children are presently overweight, and more than 90 million are at future risk.[12] The percentage of overweight and obesity has increased by more than 50%, from 4.2% of the population in 1990 to 6.7% in 2010. At the current rate of increase, by 2020, an estimated 9% of preschool children will be overweight or obese.[13] In some countries, a high prevalence of overweight children exists alongside a high prevalence of undernourished children.

Why Do Undernutrition and Overnutrition Exist Side by Side?

Undernutrition and overnutrition exist side by side because diets and lifestyles change as economic conditions improve; but not everyone in a population improves equally or at all. Traditional diets in developing countries are based on a limited number of foods—primarily starchy root vegetables. Many poorer members of a community may still rely on these staples, but if food shortages hit, their ability to properly feed their family is compromised, and undernutrition results. On the other hand, as the incomes of other members of the population increase and food availability improves, the diets of some individuals become more varied and include more energy-dense foods such as meat, milk, fat, and sugar. Accompanying these dietary changes is often a decrease in activity due to occupations that are less physically demanding, greater access to transportation, more labour-saving technology, and more passive leisure time, all of which can lead to an increased risk of obesity (**Figure 14.2a**).

Some of the effects of this **nutrition transition** from undernutrition to overnutrition are positive: Life expectancy increases, and decreases are seen in the frequencies of low birth

> **nutrition transition** A series of changes in diet, physical activity, health, and nutrition that occurs as poor countries become more prosperous.

Nutrition transition • Figure 14.2

a. This schematic represents the dietary changes that occur as a result of nutrition transition and the health consequences associated with these changes.[14] The optimal diet for health falls between the traditional rural diet, which may be inadequate in energy, protein, or micronutrients, and the affluent Western diet, which meets nutrient needs but may be high in fat and sugar and low in fibre.

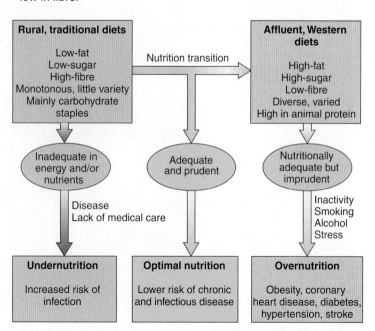

b. As countries develop economically, they face many of the nutrition-based problems that are common in industrialized countries, including obesity.[11] For example, in Argentina, Colombia, Mexico, Paraguay, Peru, and Uruguay, more than half of the population is overweight or obese.[15] Countries such as China and India, which have historically been plagued by undernutrition, must now also contend with overnutrition.[16,17] In some parts of Africa, obesity is now considered to be a major disease, along with AIDS and malnutrition.

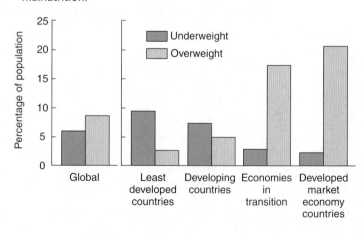

weight, infectious diseases, and nutrient deficiencies. However, at the same time, rates of heart disease, cancer, diabetes, and adult and childhood obesity may increase (**Figure 14.2b**).[14],[15] Increased reliance on animal proteins and refined and processed foods increases the amounts of energy and natural resources needed to produce the food, and, in the long term, these higher rates of consumption may damage the environment and deplete nonrenewable resources.

CONCEPT CHECK   STOP

1. **How** prevalent are undernutrition and overnutrition around the world?

2. **What** does a high incidence of stunting indicate?

3. **How** does nutrition transition affect a population's health?

Causes of Hunger around the World

LEARNING OBJECTIVES

1. **Explain** the concept of food insecurity.

2. **Discuss** the factors that cause food shortages for populations and individuals.

3. **Describe** the consequences of three nutrient deficiencies that are common worldwide.

T he specific reasons for hunger and **food insecurity** vary with time and location, but one of the main underlying causes is that the food that is available is not distributed equitably. For instance, in Canada, we have an overabundance of various kinds of food, whereas in developing countries, basic, nutritious staples, such as rice and wheat, are often scarce. To use a more local example, access to food for the majority of Canadians who live in the southern area of the country is rarely limited, while in Northern Canada, food insecurity is far more common. In developing countries, the inequitable distribution of food results in either a shortage of food or the wrong combination of foods to meet nutrient needs. This situation, in turn, results in protein-energy malnutrition and individual nutrient deficiencies.

food insecurity
A situation in which people lack adequate physical, social, or economic access to sufficient, safe, nutritious food that meets their dietary needs.

famine
A widespread lack of access to food due to a disaster that causes a collapse in the food production and marketing systems.

Food Shortages

The most obvious example of a food shortage is **famine**. Drought, floods, earthquakes, and crop destruction by diseases or pests are

natural causes of famines. Human causes include wars and civil conflicts (**Figure 14.3**).

Food shortages due to famine are very visible because they cause many deaths in an area during a short period, but chronic food shortages take a greater toll. Chronic shortages occur when economic inequities result in lack of

Famine • Figure 14.3

This girl awaits relief food in a nation beset by famine. Regions that produce barely enough food for survival under normal conditions are vulnerable to the disaster of famine. This situation is analogous to a man standing in water up to his nostrils: If all is calm, he can breathe, but if a ripple occurs, he will drown. When a ripple such as a natural or civil disaster occurs, it reduces the margin of survival and creates famine.

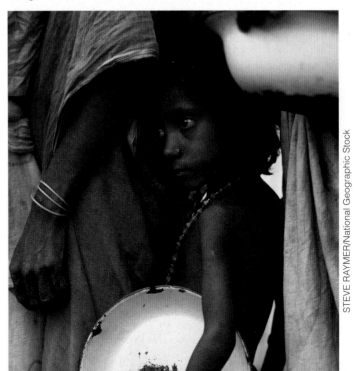

money, health care, and education for individuals or populations; when the population outgrows the food supply; when cultural and religious practices limit food choices; or when environmental damage limits the amount of food that can be produced.

Poverty Almost 1.4 billion people around the world live below the international poverty line, earning less than $1.25 per day.[18] Poverty is central to the problem of hunger and undernutrition (**Figure 14.4**). In addition to creating food insecurity, poverty also reduces access to health care, thereby increasing the prevalence of disease and disability. When diseases are untreated, nutrient needs are increased, a situation that further limits the ability to obtain an adequate diet and contributes to malnutrition. Those who are poor also have less access to education, which may contribute to their future undernutrition and disease and reduces their opportunities to escape poverty.

Nutrition InSight   The impact of poverty
• Figure 14.4

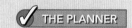 THE PLANNER

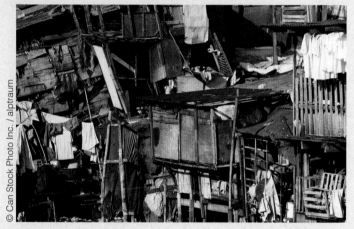
© Can Stock Photo Inc. / alptraum

▲ Nearly all (96%) of the world's undernourished people live in the developing world, where poverty is most prevalent.[19] In wealthy countries, social safety nets, such as soup kitchens, government food assistance programs, and job training programs, help those who are hungry to obtain food or the money to buy food. In poor countries, however, a family that cannot grow enough food or cannot earn enough money to buy food may have nowhere to turn for help.[20]

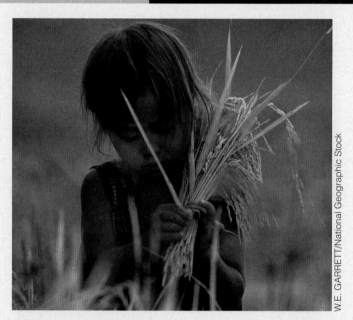
W.E. GARRETT/National Geographic Stock

▲ When young children must work in the fields with their parents, they are unlikely to attend school. Lack of education contributes to undernutrition and disease because it leads to inadequate care for infants, children, and pregnant women. Lack of education regarding food preparation and storage can affect food safety and the health of the household: Unsanitary food preparation increases the incidence of gastrointestinal diseases, which contribute to malnutrition.

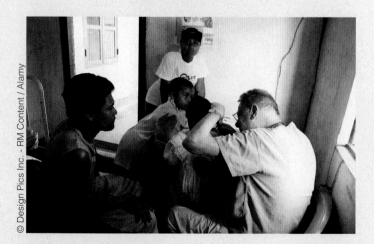
© Design Pics Inc. - RM Content / Alamy

◄ Clinics such as this one in Nicaragua are not accessible to many people in the developing world. Lack of immunizations and lack of treatment for infections and other illnesses can result in increased incidence and morbidity from infectious disease and a decrease in survival rates from chronic diseases such as cancer. Lack of health care also increases infant mortality and the incidence of low-birth-weight births.

Overpopulation Overpopulation exists when a region has more people than its natural resources can support. For example, a fertile river valley can support more people per hectare than can a desert environment. However, even in fertile regions of the world, when the number of people increases excessively, resources may be overwhelmed, leading to food shortages. When food is properly distributed, enough food is produced to prevent world hunger, but demand is rising. The human population is growing at a very rapid rate. In 1950, the world population was approximately 2.5 billion people. This number recently grew to approximately 7 billion people and is expected to rise to 9 billion by 2050 (**Figure 14.5**).[21] This population growth will be most pronounced in less developed countries, where issues of food insecurity already exist. In Canada, where we are rich in food and resources, our population is expected to increase 1.4 fold by 2050. In the same period of time, the populations of Niger, Angola, and Zambia, where resources are much scarcer, are expected to grow to three times their current sizes! These rates of growth could eventually outstrip the planet's ability to produce enough food to feed the world's population.

World population growth • Figure 14.5

About 90% of the world's population growth is occurring in less developed countries—and at an alarming rate. Developing countries cannot escape poverty because their economies cannot keep pace with such rapid population growth. Efforts to produce enough food can damage the soil and deplete environmental resources, further reducing the future capacity to produce food.

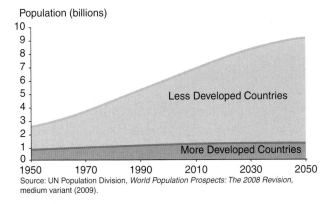

Source: UN Population Division, *World Population Prospects: The 2008 Revision*, medium variant (2009).

Ask Yourself

Since the 1950s, how has the population changed in developed countries compared with in less developed countries?

In addition, the demand for grain is increasing as a result of increased consumption of more grain-intensive livestock products and the recent sharp acceleration in the use of grain to produce ethanol to fuel cars.[22] The increased demand has contributed to dramatic increases in food prices, which were most dramatically evidenced during the food crisis of 2007–2008. These increases in prices make it even more challenging for low- and middle-income families worldwide to obtain enough food. The rising price of grain and fuel oil has also reduced the ability to distribute food aid, widening the gap between the amount of food available and the amount needed to meet nutritional needs.[23]

Climate change The majority of scientists and environmentalists agree that climate change is a very real and present threat to both the integrity of the earth and overall human health. Global surface temperatures have increased by approximately 0.5°C over the past two decades—a rate much higher than evidenced in previous years.[24] Most climate scientists agree that human-driven carbon dioxide emissions are one of the main contributors to this increase in global temperature.[25,26] While a hotter summer or less extreme winter may sound ideal to some Canadians, these shifts in weather patterns can lead to many negative effects on food availability and human health. If predictions are correct, and current practices aren't ameliorated, the earth may increase in temperature by another 4°C by the end of the century, resulting in disastrous effects on various plant and animal species. The warming effect can also, in turn, compromise agricultural yield, the availability of fresh water, and the quality of human health.

Cultural practices In some cultures, access to food may be limited for certain individuals within their households. For example, in cultures where women and girls are viewed as less important, they may receive less food than men and boys. How much food is available to an individual within a household may depend on gender, control of income, education, age, birth order, and genetic endowments.

The cultural acceptability or unacceptability of foods also contributes to food shortages and malnutrition. If available foods are culturally unacceptable, a food shortage may continue unless the population can be educated to accept the new food. For example, some cultures eat insects, which are an excellent source of protein, but other cultures view insects to be unacceptable as food.

Limited environmental resources The land and other resources available to produce food are limited. Some resources, such as minerals and fossil fuels, are present in finite amounts and are nonrenewable—that is, once they have been used, they cannot be replaced within a reasonable amount of time. Other resources, such as soil and water, are **renewable resources** because

> **renewable resources** Resources that are restored and replaced by natural processes and can therefore be used forever.

they will be available indefinitely if they are used at a rate at which the earth can restore them. For example, when agricultural land is used wisely—that is, when crops are rotated, erosion is prevented, and contamination is limited—it can be reused almost endlessly. However, when land is not used carefully, damage caused by soil erosion, nutrient depletion, and accumulation of pollutants may reduce the amount of usable land over the long term.

Modern mechanized agricultural methods have increased food production, but use more energy and resources and cause more environmental damage than does more traditional labour-intensive farming. In industrialized nations, about 17% of the energy used is employed in food production.[27]

In general, the environmental cost of producing plant-based foods is lower than the cost of producing animal products, but it may still be substantial. For example, modern large-scale farming can erode the soil and deplete its nutrients. Fertilizers and pesticides can contaminate groundwater and lead to polluted waterways. The environmental costs are increased even more when a plant product is shipped over long distances, requires refrigeration or freezing, or needs other types of processing.

Modern methods of raising cattle create both air pollution and water pollution. The animals themselves produce methane, a greenhouse gas, in their gastrointestinal tracts. More methane is produced when animal sewage is stored in ponds and heaps. In fact, livestock is responsible for 18% of greenhouse gas emissions, a larger share than is contributed by all the cars in the world combined. Livestock production also accounts for more than 8% of global human water use and releases nutrients, pathogens, and other pollutants into waterways.[28]

As more countries undergo nutrition transition, the demand for meat-based diets will increase, as will the use of natural resources and energy. It is not only the resources of the land that are at risk. Population growth has

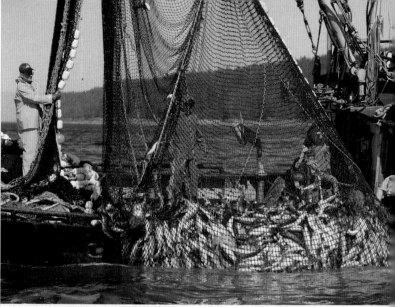

ALASKA STOCK IMAGES/National Geographic Stock

Environmental impact on the oceans • Figure 14.6

Overfishing has severely reduced the numbers of many marine species, leading to significant ecological and economic consequences. In 1992, the fisheries industry in Newfoundland and Labrador was rocked by cod overfishing, which led to the first fishing season marked by the ban on cod fishing, one of the driving forces of the industry. The ecosystem and economy of the province has yet to fully recover. Pollution also threatens the world's fishing grounds. Oil spills and deliberate dumping occur offshore; and sewage, pesticides, organic pollutants, and sediments from erosion wash into coastal waters, where most fish spend at least part of their lives. Even aquaculture, designed to increase fish production, produces wastes that can pollute ocean water and harm other marine organisms.

increased the demand for fish to the point that our oceans are being depleted of many species (**Figure 14.6**).

Poor-Quality Diets

Even when food is plentiful, malnutrition can occur when the quality of the diet is poor. The typical diet in developing countries is based on high-fibre grain products and has little variety. Adults who are able to consume a relatively large amount of this diet may be able to meet their nutrient needs. But some individuals are at risk for nutrient deficiencies, especially when food shortages hit. Populations at risk include those with high nutrient needs because they are ill or pregnant and those with limited capacity to consume this bulky grain diet, such as children and elderly individuals. Deficiencies of protein, iron, iodine, and vitamin A are common in those who consume poor-quality diets. The images in **Figure 14.7** will help you recall the information about these deficiencies discussed in earlier chapters.

Protein and micronutrient deficiencies • Figure 14.7

Protein-energy malnutrition is most common in children. A general lack of food can lead to the wasting associated with *marasmus*, and when the diet is limited to starchy grains and vegetables with minimal protein, *kwashiorkor*, characterized by a bloated belly, can predominate. Other factors, such as metabolic changes caused by infection, may also play a role in the development of kwashiorkor.

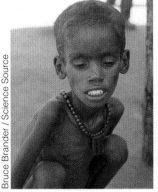
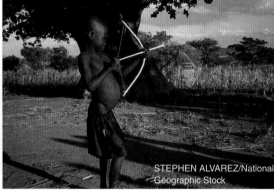

Marasmus   Kwashiorkor

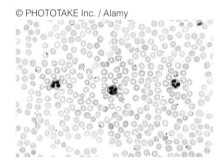

Normal red blood cells

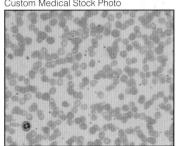

Iron deficiency anemia

More than 2 billion people worldwide suffer from iron deficiency anemia, which is characterized by small, pale red blood cells.[29] The lack of iron reduces the amount of hemoglobin produced, and the lack of hemoglobin lowers the blood's oxygen-carrying capacity. In developing countries, dietary iron deficiency is aggravated by intestinal parasites, which cause gastrointestinal blood loss, and acute and chronic infections, such as malaria. Iron deficiency can have a major impact on a population's health and productivity.

Although goiter, seen here, is a visible manifestation of iodine deficiency, the more subtle effects of a deficiency on mental performance and work capacity may have a greater impact on the population as a whole. Iodine-deficient children have lower IQs and impaired school performance.[30] Iodine deficiency in children and adults is associated with apathy and decreased initiative and decision-making capabilities.

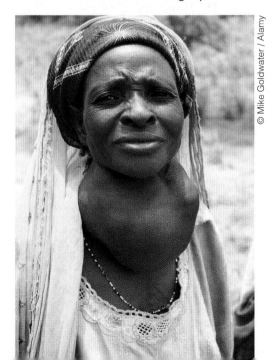

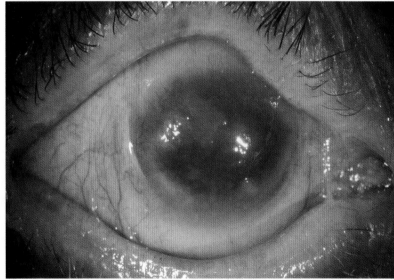

An estimated 250 million preschool children worldwide suffer from vitamin A deficiency.[31] Vitamin A deficiency can lead to *xerophthalmia*, shown here. Vitamin A deficiency is the leading cause of preventable blindness among children. It also depresses immune function, thus increasing the risk of illness and death from infections, particularly measles and diarrheal disease.

Causes of Hunger around the World **501**

Several other vitamin and mineral deficiencies have recently emerged or re-emerged as problems throughout the world. Beriberi, pellagra, and scurvy—diseases caused by deficiencies of thiamin, niacin, and vitamin C, respectively—are rare in the developed world but still occur among extremely poor and underprivileged people and in large refugee populations. In many parts of the world, folate deficiency causes megaloblastic anemia during pregnancy and often compounds existing iron deficiency anemia. Deficiencies of the minerals zinc, selenium, and calcium are also of concern.[32] Zinc deficiency affects about one-third of the world's population and is believed to cause as many deaths as vitamin A deficiency or iron deficiency.[33] Selenium deficiency has been identified in population groups in China, New Zealand, and the Russian Federation. Inadequate calcium intake is a worldwide concern due to its association with osteoporosis.

CONCEPT CHECK STOP

1. **What** causes food insecurity?

2. **How** can environmental damage lead to food shortages?

3. **Why** do children develop protein and micronutrient deficiencies more often than adults?

Causes of Hunger in Canada

LEARNING OBJECTIVES

1. **Discuss** the causes of food insecurity in Canada.

2. **Describe** factors that prevent people from escaping poverty.

3. **List** the population groups that are at greatest risk for undernutrition in Canada.

Most of the nutritional problems in Canada are related to overnutrition. Although news stories often focus on obesity, almost 8% of Canadian households experience food insecurity (**Figure 14.8**).[34] This situation is caused not by a general food shortage but by an inequitable distribution of food and money. For example, 32.5% of food-insecure Canadians have a household income of $10,000 or less.[34] The incidence of hunger and food insecurity is higher among Aboriginal people (20%), recent immigrants, women, infants, children, elderly individuals, and those who are poor, homeless, ill, or disabled. In Nunavut, the prevalence of food insecurity is more than four times the national average.[34] Although the majority of Canadians are food secure, a sudden decrease in income or an increase in living expenses can put anyone at risk for food insecurity.

Poverty and Food Insecurity

In Canada, as elsewhere in the world, poverty is the main cause of food insecurity. Poverty reduces access to food, education, and health care. Impoverished Canadians have less money to spend on food and often have less access to affordable food. Limited income also reduces the chances that healthier foods will be consumed. Choosing leaner meats and dairy products and whole grains costs more—about 35 to 40% of low-income consumers' food budgets.[35]

The high price of urban real estate has driven grocery stores into the suburbs, but because many low-income city families do not own cars, they must shop at the more

Food insecurity in Canada • Figure 14.8

In 2007–2008, approximately 92% of Canadian households were food secure, and approximately 8% of Canadians, or almost 2 million Canadians aged 12 or older, experienced food insecurity.[34]

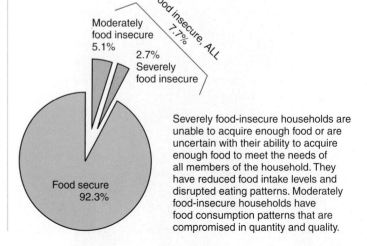

Severely food-insecure households are unable to acquire enough food or are uncertain with their ability to acquire enough food to meet the needs of all members of the household. They have reduced food intake levels and disrupted eating patterns. Moderately food-insecure households have food consumption patterns that are compromised in quantity and quality.

a. Income level in Canada is directly correlated with an individual's level of education.[37]

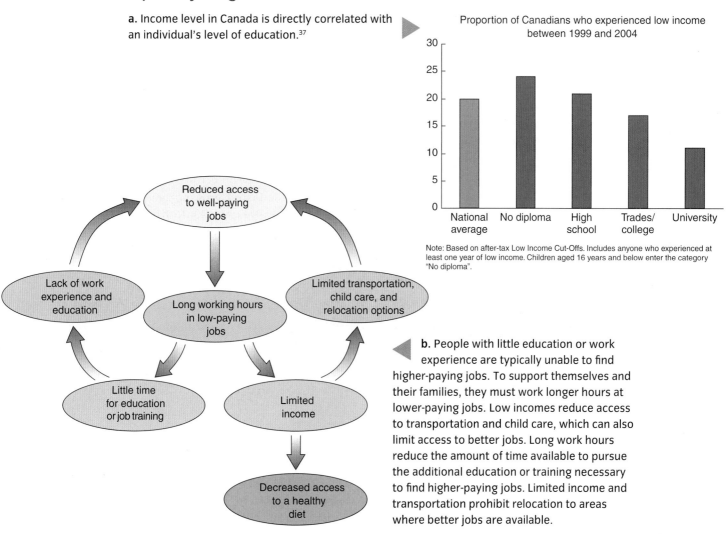

Proportion of Canadians who experienced low income between 1999 and 2004

Note: Based on after-tax Low Income Cut-Offs. Includes anyone who experienced at least one year of low income. Children aged 16 years and below enter the category "No diploma".

b. People with little education or work experience are typically unable to find higher-paying jobs. To support themselves and their families, they must work longer hours at lower-paying jobs. Low incomes reduce access to transportation and child care, which can also limit access to better jobs. Long work hours reduce the amount of time available to pursue the additional education or training necessary to find higher-paying jobs. Limited income and transportation prohibit relocation to areas where better jobs are available.

expensive cornerstores or pay cab fares to take advantage of lower prices at more distant, larger stores. People who live in rural areas may have limited access to food because they also live far from grocery stores. Furthermore, high rates of poverty and unemployment among Aboriginal people contribute to their food insecurity.[34]

As in developing nations, poverty is reflected in infant mortality rates. For instance, in some developing countries, the infant mortality rate is more than 100 per 1,000 live births. In contrast, the average infant mortality rate in Canada is about 4.9 per 1,000 live births, even lower than the American rate.[36] Although the infant mortality rate is relatively low in Canada as a whole, in Nunavut and the Northwest Territories, the rate is three times higher than the national average.[36] This alarming statistic is consistent with the high levels of food insecurity in the North.

Lack of education, which is both a cause and a consequence of poverty, also contributes to food insecurity

(Figure 14.9). For people living at or below the poverty level, educational opportunities are fewer and lower in quality than similar opportunities for people with higher incomes. In the short term, lack of knowledge about food selection, food safety, and home economics can contribute to malnutrition. Too little food may cause the diet to be deficient in energy or particular nutrients, but poor food choices also allow food insecurity to coexist with obesity. Lack of education about food safety can also increase the incidence of food-borne illness. In the long term, lack of education prevents people from gaining access to the higher-paying jobs that could allow them to escape poverty.

Poor families must use most of their income to pay for shelter, a situation that seriously reduces the likelihood that they will be adequately fed. The high cost of housing not only limits food budgets but also contributes to the problem of homelessness in Canada. An estimated 150,000 Canadians are currently homeless.[38] The actual level of homelessness is difficult to measure, however, since homeless people do not complete census surveys, and keeping track of this often transient population is challenging. Homelessness was previously found primarily in urban centres, such as Toronto, Vancouver, Calgary, and Montreal, but homelessness is increasingly evidenced in suburban areas.[38] One of the major health problems of the homeless population is malnutrition. Homeless people are at high risk of food insecurity because they lack not only money but also the proper facilities for food preparation and food storage.

Vulnerable Stages of Life

Because of their high nutrient needs, pregnant and lactating women and small children are at particular risk for undernutrition. Of all households comprising single women and their children, one-third live below the poverty line. Poverty and food insecurity place these women and children at risk for malnutrition, and their special nutritional needs magnify this risk. Because of their increased need for some nutrients, pregnant women, infants, and children may be malnourished even when the rest of the household is adequately fed. For example, the amount of iron in the family's diet may be enough to prevent anemia in all the family's members except a pregnant teenager.

Elderly individuals are vulnerable to food insecurity and undernutrition due to this population group's higher frequency of diseases and disabilities, which may limit their ability to purchase, prepare, and consume food. Greater nutritional risk among older adults is associated with more hospital admissions and hence higher health care costs. In 2001, approximately 1 in 8 Canadians was aged 65 or older. By 2026, that number is estimated to increase to 1 in 5 Canadians.[39] The fastest growing age group is those 85 or older, individuals who are at high risk of food insecurity.

| CONCEPT CHECK | STOP |

1. **Why** are some Canadians hungry in a land of plenty?

2. **How** are education and poverty related?

3. **Who** is at risk for undernutrition in Canada?

Eliminating Hunger

LEARNING OBJECTIVES

1. **Discuss** two strategies that can help reduce population growth.

2. **Discuss** the role of sustainable agriculture in maintaining the food supply.

3. **Explain** how international trade can help eliminate hunger.

Solving the problem of world hunger is a daunting task. In 1996, the World Food Summit set a goal of cutting world hunger in half by 2015. Some countries have seen positive advances toward this goal, but most gains preceded the global food shortage of 2007–2008, and, since then, little additional progress has been made.[40] Current estimates put the number of undernourished people in the world at 870 million, 25 million more than in the early 1990s, but 55 million less than in the early 2000s.[2]

Solutions to world hunger need to address population growth, ensure that the nutrient needs of a large and diverse population are met with culturally acceptable foods, and increase food production while maintaining the global ecosystem (**Figure 14.10**). Meeting these goals will require input from politicians, nutrition scientists, economists, and the food industry.

Economic policies, technical advances, education, and legislative measures must implement programs and policies that provide food in the short term; for the long term, they

Millennium development goals • Figure 14.10

These eight goals, to be achieved by 2015, were adopted by 189 nations during the United Nations (UN) Millennium Summit in September 2000. These goals correspond to the world's main development challenges. To achieve the first goal, stamping out hunger, most of the other goals must also be addressed.[41]

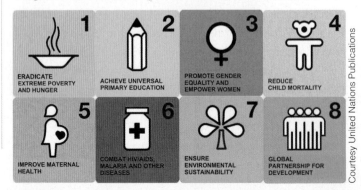

Courtesy United Nations Publications

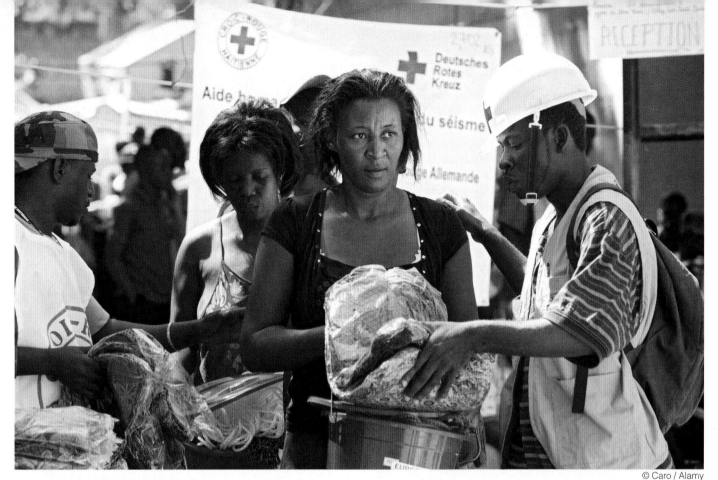

© Caro / Alamy

Emergency food relief • Figure 14.11

Many organizations are working to combat world hunger. The Canadian Red Cross, the American Red Cross, and the United Nations (UN) High Commissioner for Refugees all concentrate on famine relief. The UN Food and Agriculture Organization (FAO) works to improve the production, intake, and distribution of food worldwide. The World Health Organization (WHO) focuses on international health and emphasizes the prevention of nutrition problems, and the UN Children's Fund (UNICEF) targets education and vaccination and responds to crisis situations to improve the lives of children.

must establish sustainable programs to ensure the continued production and distribution of acceptable foods.

Providing Short-Term Food Aid

When people are starving, short-term food and medical aid must be provided immediately. The standard approach has been to bring food into stricken areas (**Figure 14.11**). This food generally consists of agricultural surpluses from other countries, and its nutrient content is often not well planned. Although this type of relief is necessary for a population to survive an immediate crisis such as famine, it does little to prevent future hunger.

Further complicating the ability to provide food aid is a region's political instability. For example, after massive droughts significantly compromised Somalia's food availability and led to widespread famine, the United Nations and various countries rallied to send aid to help those most affected. But the aid did not reach where it was most needed. For political reasons, the nation's rebel groups purposely blocked accessibility to food aid in some of the most devastated parts of the country, destroying ships and demanding bribes from those importing food. This region continues to face political instability and will produce more illness and deaths if food insecurity remains high and the famine continues.

Controlling Population Growth

In the long term, solving the problem of world hunger requires balancing the number of people with the amount of food produced. The world's population has increased dramatically since the middle of the 20th century, but population growth has recently begun to slow. The birth rate worldwide has declined—from five children per woman in 1950 to 2.6 in 2010.[42] This downward trend in population growth must continue to ensure that food production and natural resources can support the population. The birth rate can also be influenced by changes in cultural factors, economic factors, family planning, and government policies.

Education and birth rate • Figure 14.12

The large number of children in this impoverished Cambodian family is indicative of the uneven burden of population growth in the developing world. One of the reasons for the many children in this family is lack of education for women. The empowerment of women is often associated with better health outcomes for a population. Education builds job skills that enable women to join the workforce, which, in turn, means they are more likely to marry later in life, and have fewer children. Education increases the likelihood that women will have control over their fertility and provides them with knowledge that can be used to improve the family's health and economic situation. The graph shows that higher literacy among women is associated with lower birth rates.[44] Women who are better educated have options other than having numerous children.

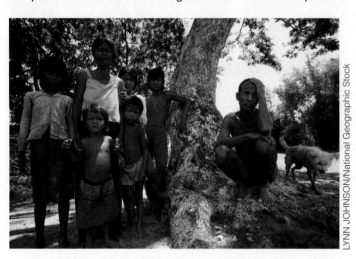

LYNN JOHNSON/National Geographic Stock

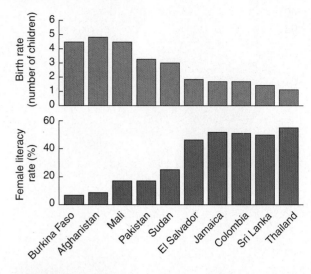

Ask Yourself

Imagine a graph that shows years of education versus birth rate in Canada. What would this graph look like?

Economic and cultural factors that affect birth rate In many cultures, a large family is expected. A major reason for this expectation is the high rate of infant and child mortality. When infant mortality rates are high, people choose to have many children in an effort to ensure that some will survive. Higher birth rates in some developing countries are also the result of children's economic and societal roles. For example, in some countries, children are needed to work the farms, support the elders, and otherwise contribute to the economic survival of the family. Programs that foster economic development and ensure access to food, shelter, and medical care have been shown to cause a decline in birth rates because people feel secure having fewer children. Economic development also reduces the need to employ children as workers.

Another cultural factor that influences birth rate is gender inequality. Girls are often kept at home to work rather than being sent to school. In most developing countries, the literacy rate is lower for women than men, and fewer women attend primary and secondary schools. This lack of education leaves women few options other than remaining home and having children. Providing education for girls has been shown to reduce birth rates (**Figure 14.12**).[43]

Family planning and government policies
Changes in cultural and economic factors may reduce the desire for large families, but achieving this goal depends on the availability of health and family planning services. To be successful, family planning must be acceptable to the population and compatible with cultural and religious beliefs. Governments around the world have used numerous approaches to decrease population growth, such as providing contraceptives, education, and economic incentives (**Figure 14.13**).

Increasing Food Production while Protecting the Environment

Advances in agricultural technology have allowed food production to keep pace with population growth. However, the use of energy-intensive modern agricultural techniques has contributed to serious environmental problems. Commercial inorganic fertilizers and pesticides and modern farm machinery increase food production but also pollute the air and water. Overuse of land causes deterioration of soil quality, which will limit food production in the future. For food production to continue to meet the needs of future generations, we must learn how to continue to increase food yields and food availability while conserving the world's natural resources (see *Thinking It Through*).

506 CHAPTER 14 Feeding the World

Access to birth control • Figure 14.13

A birth control vendor explains condoms to women at a market in the Ivory Coast. The birth rate in this West African country declined from nearly 7 children per woman in 1988 to 3.8 in 2012, due in part to increased use of modern methods of birth control. Increased knowledge and availability of contraceptives is linked to a decrease in birth rate.[45]

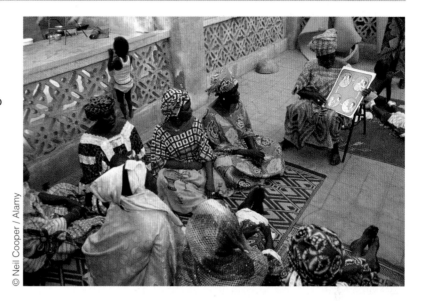

© Neil Cooper / Alamy

THINKING IT THROUGH ✓ THE PLANNER

What Can You Do?

Jean-Paul is concerned about the problems of hunger and malnutrition and the impact of his food choices on the environment. Although he is a university student who cannot afford to make monetary contributions to relief organizations, he would like his everyday choices to have a minimal impact on the environment.

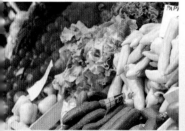

Stockphoto.com/Waltraud Ingerl

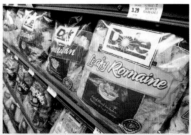

Justin Sullivan/Staff/Getty Images News

What are the advantages and disadvantages of these salad options in terms of convenience, food safety, and environmental impact?

▼

Your answer: _____

_____

The following are some inexpensive changes Jean-Paul can make to reduce his impact on the environment. What are the advantages and disadvantages of each?

Action	Advantages	Disadvantages
	Your answer:	*Your answer:*
Bike instead of drive on short trips around town.		
Buy a canvas bag to carry groceries.		
Pack juice in a thermos instead of buying it in a nonre-cyclable bottle.		
Compost vegetable scraps.		
Buy locally grown produce.		
Buy organically grown produce.		

(Check your answers in Appendix I.)

sustainable agriculture Agricultural methods that maintain soil productivity and a healthy ecological balance while having minimal long-term impacts.

Sustainable agriculture uses food production methods that prevent damage to the environment and allow the land to restore itself so that food can be produced indefinitely. For example, contour plowing and terracing help prevent erosion, keeping the soil available for future crops. Rotating the crops grown in a field prevents the depletion of nutrients in the soil, reducing the need for fertilizers. Sustainable agriculture uses environmentally friendly chemicals that degrade quickly and do not persist as residues in the environment. It also relies on diversification. This approach to farming maximizes the natural methods of pest control and fertilization and protects farmers from changes in the marketplace (**Figure 14.14**).

Sustainable agriculture is not a single program but involves choosing options that mesh well with the local soil, climate, and farming techniques. In some cases, a more sustainable option may be organic farming, which does not use synthetic pesticides, herbicides, and fertilizers (see Chapter 13). Organic farming techniques have a smaller environmental impact because they reduce both the use of agricultural chemicals and the release of pollutants into the environment. Organic farming is also advantageous in terms of soil quality and biodiversity, but it is a disadvantage when it comes to land use because crop yields are lower. A combination of organic and conventional techniques,

as is used with integrated pest management (see Chapter 13), might improve land use and protect the environment.

Other sustainable programs include agroforestry, in which techniques from forestry and agriculture are used together to restore degraded areas; natural systems agriculture, which attempts to develop agricultural systems that include many types of plants and therefore function like natural ecosystems; and the technique of reducing fertilizer use by matching nutrient resources with the demands of the particular crop being grown. Genetic engineering is a modern technology that may be integrated with sustainable systems. As we saw in Chapter 13, genetic engineering may also be a means to increase crop yields. Recall that plants may be more likely to thrive and their yields may be increased as a result of inserting genes that either improve the efficiency with which plants convert sunlight into food or make plants resistant to herbicides, insects, and plant diseases.

Increasing Food Availability through Economic Development and Trade

Hunger will exist as long as there is poverty. Even when food is plentiful, those who are poor do not have access to enough of the right foods to maintain their nutritional health. If hunger is to be eliminated, it is essential that economic development leads to safe and sanitary housing, access to health care and education, and the resources to acquire enough food. Government policies can help reduce

A sustainable farm • Figure 14.14

A sustainable farm consist of a total agricultural ecosystem rather than a single crop. It may include field crops, fruit- and nut-bearing trees, herds of livestock, and forests.

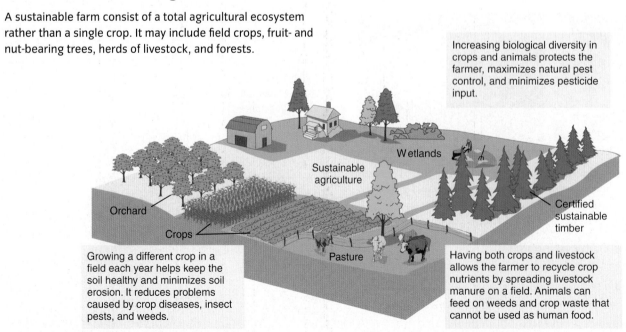

Increasing biological diversity in crops and animals protects the farmer, maximizes natural pest control, and minimizes pesticide input.

Wetlands

Sustainable agriculture

Orchard

Crops

Certified sustainable timber

Pasture

Growing a different crop in a field each year helps keep the soil healthy and minimizes soil erosion. It reduces problems caused by crop diseases, insect pests, and weeds.

Having both crops and livestock allows the farmer to recycle crop nutrients by spreading livestock manure on a field. Animals can feed on weeds and crop waste that cannot be used as human food.

poverty and improve food security by increasing the population's income, lowering food prices, or funding food programs for those who are poor.

Economic development in the form of industrialization can also help provide food for a country's population by increasing access to international trade. The newly industrialized countries of Asia, such as South Korea, rely on imported food to decrease the number of hungry people in their populations. In general, countries around the world are becoming more dependent on food imports—and on the exports of food and other goods to pay for the food they import. This trade can increase the availability of food for the world's population as a whole.

Whether a country's agricultural emphasis is on producing **subsistence crops** or **cash crops** influences the availability of food for its people. Shifting to cash crops improves the country's cash flow but uses local resources to produce crops for export. This shift, in turn, limits the ability of a country's people to produce enough food to feed their families. For example, when a large portion of the arable land in a country is used to grow cash crops, such as coffee and tea, then little agricultural land remains for growing grains and vegetables that nourish the local population. If, however, the cash from the crop is used to purchase nutritious foods from other countries, this decision may help alleviate undernutrition.

> **subsistence crop** Crops that are grown as food for the local population.
>
> **cash crop** Crops that are grown to be sold for monetary return rather than as food for the local population.

Ensuring a Nutritious Food Supply

To ensure the nutritional health of a population, the foods that are grown or imported must supply both sufficient energy and adequate amounts of all essential nutrients. If the diet does not provide enough of all the essential nutrients, either the dietary pattern must be changed, commonly consumed foods must be fortified, or supplements containing deficient nutrients must be provided. To make these changes effectively, consumers need to know how to choose foods that provide the needed nutrients and how to handle those foods safely.

Nutrition education Education can help improve nutrient intake by teaching consumers what foods to grow, which foods to choose, and how to prepare them safely.

Education is particularly important when introducing a new crop. No matter how nutritious a new plant variety may

be, it is not beneficial unless local farmers know how to grow it and the population accepts it as a food source and knows how to prepare it for consumption. For instance, white yams are common in some regions but are a poor source of beta-carotene, which the body can use to make vitamin A. If the yellow yam, which is rich in beta-carotene, became an acceptable choice, the amount of vitamin A available to the population would increase. For this strategy to be effective, however, local farmers would need to know how to grow yellow yam and people must be willing to buy and eat it.

Food safety is also a concern when changing traditional dietary practices. For example, introducing papaya to the diet as a source of vitamin A will not improve nutritional status if it is washed in unsanitary water and causes dysentery among the people it is meant to nourish.

Education to encourage breastfeeding can also improve nutritional status and health (**Figure 14.15**). To achieve optimal growth, development, and health, WHO recommends that infants be exclusively breastfed for the first six months

Nutritional and health benefits of breastfeeding • Figure 14.15

Breast milk provides infants with optimal nutrition and immune factors that reduce the risk of infectious diseases. In developing nations, where infant mortality from infectious disease is high, mothers are advised to breastfeed even if they are HIV-positive because the risk of the baby dying of malnutrition and other infections outweighs the risk of transmitting the virus in the milk.[47] When infants are not breastfed, education about nutritious substitutes for breast milk and safe preparation of formulas is essential.

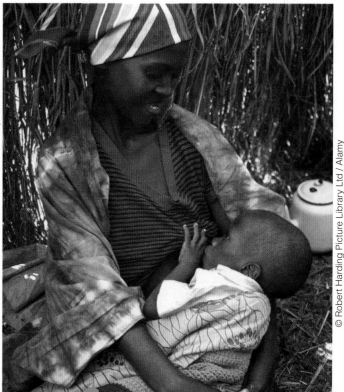

of life. After that, other foods should be offered, while breast-feeding continues for up to two years of age or beyond.[46]

Fortifying the food supply Although food fortification will not provide energy for a hungry population, it can increase the protein quality of the diet and eliminate micronutrient deficiencies. To solve a nutritional problem in a population, fortification must be implemented wisely. Fortification works only when the vulnerable groups consume centrally processed foods. The foods selected for fortification should be among those that are consistently consumed by the majority of the population, which will avoid the need for extensive promotion and re-education to encourage consumption of that food. The nutrient should be added uniformly and in a form that optimizes its utilization.

Fortification has been used successfully in preventing health problems in Canada. For example, cow's milk fortified to increase vitamin D intake was a major factor in the elimination of infantile rickets, and the enrichment of grains with niacin helped eliminate pellagra. Fortification of salt with iodine has been used successfully to eliminate iodine deficiency diseases in countries around the world (**Figure 14.16**).

An alternative to traditional fortification is biofortification. In this technique, plants are bred to select for higher amounts of specific nutrients. As an example, a type of corn has been bred to contain higher amounts of

Iodized salt • Figure 14.16 _____

Over the past decade, the number of countries with salt iodization programs has increased dramatically. It is estimated that 66% of households worldwide now have access to iodized salt.[30] As a result, the number of countries where iodine deficiency disorders are a public health problem has been cut in half.

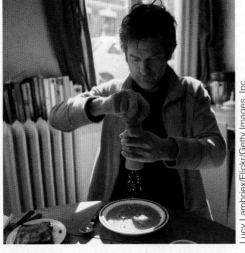

Lucy Lambriex/Flickr/Getty Images, Inc.

beta-carotene than traditional rice. For this strategy to be effective, farmers must want to grow biofortified crops, and consumers must want to buy them (see *Hot Topic: Golden Rice*).

Providing supplements Supplementing specific nutrients for at-risk segments of the population can help reduce the prevalence of malnutrition. Of all countries where vitamin A deficiency is a public health problem, about three-quarters have policies supporting regular vitamin A supplementation in children. Many have also adopted WHO's recommendation to provide all breast-feeding women with a high-dose supplement of vitamin A within eight weeks of delivery. This supplementation improves maternal vitamin A status and raises the amount of vitamin A that is present in breast milk and is therefore passed to the infant.

Many countries have adopted programs to supplement children older than 6 months with iron and pregnant women with iron and folate.

Eliminating Food Insecurity in Canada

As with world hunger, eliminating hunger in Canada involves improving economic security, keeping food affordable, providing food aid to the hungry, and offering education about healthy diets that will meet nutrient needs and reduce diseases related to overconsumption.

The nutrition safety net Federal programs that provide access to affordable food and promote healthy eating have been referred to as a nutrition safety net for the Canadian population. A large proportion of food assistance comes from the various food bank programs throughout the country. Canada has more than 900 food banks, and their use has increased significantly over time.[54] Nationally, food bank usage has increased 19% from 2000 to 2010. Two-fifths of those who use food banks are children and youth, and half all food bank users currently receive social assistance benefits. Unfortunately, the increase in demand for food banks has not been matched by an increase in delivery effectiveness. Currently, 27% of food banks lack adequate funding, and 31% do not have sufficient food to meet demand.[54]

Nutrition education People who consume healthier diets are generally people who have more nutrition information and a greater awareness of the relationship between diet and health. Healthy diets improve current health by optimizing growth, productivity, and well-being and are

HOT TOPIC

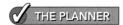

Golden rice

Micronutrient deficiencies are far less common in Canada than they once were. Unfortunately, they continue to be a major concern in developing countries where food is often scarce. An example of this concern is vitamin A deficiency, the leading cause of preventable blindness in the world.[31] To combat this deficiency in at-risk populations, a genetically modified (GM) form of rice, called Golden Rice, has been engineered to provide high levels of vitamin A. By introducing this micronutrient into a more affordable staple crop, scientists had hoped to lower the risk of vitamin A deficiency. Due to the controversy surrounding this crop, we still do not know how effective this strategy would be if fully implemented.

Initial concerns about Golden Rice focused on whether it would provide enough vitamin A to combat symptoms of deficiency. The initial strain did not supply enough vitamin A in a reasonable serving, but a newer variety is able to provide more than half the RDA for this micronutrient in a 125-mL (1/2 cup) portion.[48] Even if children were to consume this rice, some argue that it would prevent only some of their many nutritional deficiencies. That is, although Golden Rice may increase vitamin A intake, it would not change the intake of protein, fat, or zinc, which are needed for the efficient use of vitamin A.[49,50]

So should we continue to spend resources developing Golden Rice? Opponents argue that in the decade since Golden Rice was developed, it has done nothing to prevent vitamin A deficiency, and it has diverted resources from proven programs that address multiple nutrient deficiencies. Proponents contend that the problem is not the rice but rather the regulatory climate that has prevented it from being introduced; Golden Rice was developed in 1999 but will probably not be commercialized for some time.[51,52] The development costs of Golden Rice have been high, but it is predicted to be cost-effective in the long term because once it is introduced, recurrent costs should be low.[53]

Some concern has also been expressed that introducing GM rice is not safe for the environment. The worry is that its use will decrease the diversity of rice varieties grown. Reducing diversity increases the risk of crop destruction resulting from insects and disease.[49] Proponents of GM crops argue that this concern occurs whenever a new crop that is preferred by farmers is introduced.

GM crops such as Golden Rice are not substitutes for traditional solutions to malnutrition but can be used to complement such solutions. Supplementation may be necessary for those in immediate need. Fortification and supplementation may work better in urban settings; Golden Rice may be better at reaching isolated rural populations. In the long term, the goal is to use whatever means are available to solve the problem of vitamin A deficiency and other types of malnutrition.

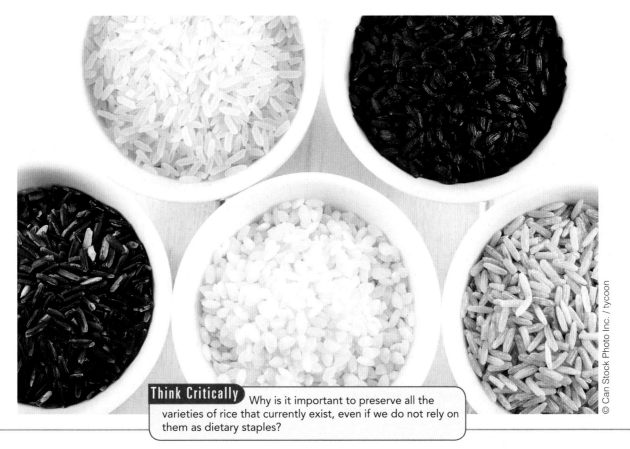

© Can Stock Photo Inc. / tycoon

Think Critically Why is it important to preserve all the varieties of rice that currently exist, even if we do not rely on them as dietary staples?

WHAT SHOULD I EAT?
Environmental Impact

Make your meals green
- Reduce the amount of meat in your meal.
- Eat vegetarian at least some of the time.
- Buy in bulk to cut down on packaging.
- Use reusable bags to take your groceries home.
- Choose foods that are locally grown or organically produced.
- Eat lower on the food chain—more plant foods and small fish.
- Cook from scratch—use fewer processed foods.
- Grow and eat some of your own vegetables.

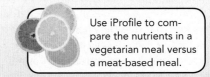

Use iProfile to compare the nutrients in a vegetarian meal versus a meat-based meal.

essential for preventing chronic diseases. Increasing our knowledge about nutrition can reduce our medical costs and improve our quality of life.

Education can help individuals with lower incomes stretch their limited food dollars by making wise choices at the store and reducing food waste at home. Education can also promote the use of community gardens to increase the availability of seasonal vegetables. People can be taught how to prepare foods received from commodity distribution programs and food banks and the safe methods for food handling and preparation. Knowing which foods to choose and how to handle them safely is as important in preventing malnutrition as having the money to buy enough food. *Eating Well with Canada's Food Guide* and

food labels educate the general public about making wise food choices (see *What Should I Eat?*).

CONCEPT CHECK	STOP

1. **How** does educating women help control population growth?

2. **What** impact does sustainable agriculture have on the world's food supply?

3. **How** can growing cash crops improve a nation's food supply?

4. **What** is the nutrition safety net?

Summary

1 The Two Faces of Malnutrition   494

- **Hunger** and **starvation** have historically been the faces of malnutrition, but they represent only one side of malnutrition: undernutrition. The world also faces an alarming rise in the number of cases and the negative health impacts of both undernutrition and overnutrition.

- In poorly nourished populations, a **cycle of undernutrition** exists, whereby poorly nourished women give birth to low-birth-weight infants who are at risk for disease and early death. If these children survive, they grow into adults who are physically unable to fully contribute to society. In populations where malnutrition is prevalent, low birth weight, a high **infant mortality rate**, **stunting**, and infections are more common.

Nutrition transition
• Figure 14.2

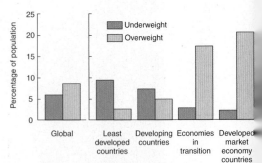

- For the first time in history, the cases of overnutrition in the world now exceed those of undernutrition. Overnutrition is one of the main driving forces behind the rising obesity epidemic, which is associated with increased risk of heart disease, type-2 diabetes, and cancer.

- As a country's economic conditions improve, a **nutrition transition** to a more Western diet and lifestyle patterns can contribute to the growing problem of overnutrition.

2 Causes of Hunger around the World 497

- The underlying cause of hunger and **food insecurity** is the inequitable distribution of the world's available food.

- **Famine** results from natural and human-caused disasters that temporarily disrupt food production and distribution. Chronic food shortage occurs when economic inequities result in lack of money, health care, and education; when overpopulation and limited natural resources create a situation in which there are more people than food; when cultural practices limit food choices; and when **renewable resources** are misused, limiting the ability to continue to produce food.

Famine • Figure 14.3

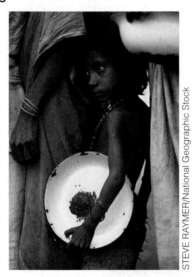

STEVE RAYMER/National Geographic Stock

- Deficiencies of protein, iron, iodine, and vitamin A are common worldwide when the quality of the diet is poor. Pregnant women, children, elderly individuals, and those who are ill may not be able to meet their nutrient needs with the available diet.

3 Causes of Hunger in Canada 502

- Both undernutrition and overnutrition are problems in Canada. As in developing nations, undernutrition and food insecurity are associated with poverty, which limits education and access to health care and adequate housing.

- High nutrient needs increase the risk of malnutrition in women and children, and disease and disability increase risk in elderly individuals.

Education and poverty • Figure 14.9

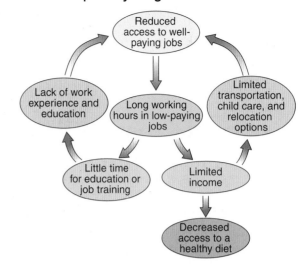

4 Eliminating Hunger 504

- Short-term solutions to hunger provide food through relief at the local, national, and international levels.

- Eliminating world hunger in the long term requires controlling population growth, which can be addressed by improving economic conditions; providing education, particularly for women; and ensuring access to family planning services.

- **Sustainable agriculture** helps eliminate hunger by allowing food to be produced without damaging the environment.

- Economic development helps prevent hunger by eliminating poverty and ensuring access to health care and education. It also increases access to international trade, which can be used to import food or to export **cash crops** to bring more money into the country. Some countries favour **subsistence crops**, which are used to feed the people that produce them, but aren't meant for export.

- Food fortification and dietary supplementation can be used to increase protein quality and eliminate micronutrient deficiencies, thereby improving the overall quality of the diet.

- Nutrition programs in Canada focus on maintaining a nutrition safety net that provides access to affordable food and education to promote healthy eating.

Nutritional and health benefits of breastfeeding • Figure 14.15

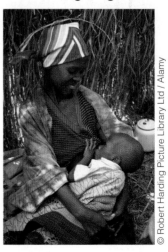

© Robert Harding Picture Library Ltd / Alamy

Key Terms

- cash crops 509
- cycle of undernutrition 494
- famine 497
- food insecurity 497
- hunger 494
- infant mortality rate 495
- nutrition transition 496
- renewable resources 500
- starvation 494
- stunting 495
- subsistence crops 509
- sustainable agriculture 508

Critical and Creative Thinking Questions

1. Describe the living conditions of the people and regions of the world that are most likely to be affected by undernutrition and the living conditions of the people and regions of the world that are most likely to be affected by overnutrition.

2. In Canada, particularly in the West, the growing of corn for ethanol biofuel has significantly increased over the past decade. How might this increase in corn crops impact food insecurity in North America and around the world?

3. Record how much money you spend on food in a day and use this information to estimate your monthly food costs. Would you be able to meet the recommendations of Canada's Food Guide on a budget of $3 a day? Which food groups contain the most expensive choices?

4. Compare the cost of a single-serving bottle of orange juice with the same size serving poured from a 1-litre container. Compare the costs of these two products from a large grocery store and from a convenience store. Explain why some consumers might pay the higher prices for orange juice.

5. The diet in a developing country is deficient in iodine. To correct this deficiency, the government imports iodized salt, but iodine deficiency continues to be a problem. Why might the iodine deficiency still be present?

6. Research one area of the world where hunger and undernutrition are major problems. What is the cause of undernutrition in this area? What solutions are in place, or what solutions have been proposed to solve these problems?

What is happening in this picture?

This 250-fold magnification shows the mouth of a hookworm, which it uses to attach to the lining of the small intestine and feed on blood. Hookworm larvae penetrate the skin, infecting people when they walk barefoot in contaminated soil. Hookworm infection affects 740 million people in tropical developing countries.[55]

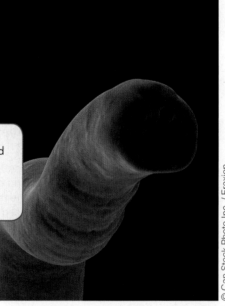

© Can Stock Photo Inc. / Eraxion

Think Critically

1. Why is this infection more common in poor tropical and subtropical regions than elsewhere?
2. How does hookworm infection affect iron status?
3. How does hookworm infection affect a population's productivity?

Self-Test

(Check your answers in Appendix J.)

1. The cycle of malnutrition can be broken by _____.
   a. providing better health care to children
   b. increasing the availability of nutritious foods for adults
   c. providing better health care and nutrition for women during pregnancy
   d. any of the above

2. Which of the following statements about overweight and underweight is not supported by the graph?
   a. Underweight is less of a problem in developed than in developing countries.
   b. Overweight occurs in developing and developed countries.

c. In developed countries, underweight is a problem only among children.

d. As a country develops economically, the incidence of overweight increases.

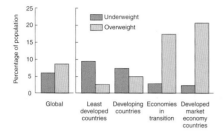

3. Which of the following statements is true of stunting?

a. It is an indicator of the health and well-being of populations of children.

b. It is an indicator of the health and well-being of adults.

c. It is measured with body mass index.

d. It is highest in well-nourished populations.

4. Which of the following dietary changes is not associated with nutrition transition?

a. consumption of a wider variety of foods

b. an increase in the fat and sugar content of the diet

c. an increase in the consumption of animal products

d. an increase in the fibre content of the diet

5. What proportion of the world's undernourished people live in the developing world?

a. half

b. one-third

c. more than 90%

d. less than a quarter

6. The yellow section of this graph of population growth most likely represents population growth in _____.

a. developed countries

b. the entire world

c. less-developed countries

d. North America

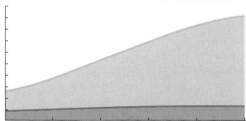

7. Which of the following statements is true of population growth?

a. Population growth parallels economic growth.

b. Education and economic growth slow population growth.

c. Education increases population growth.

d. Economic growth and education do not affect population growth.

8. Deficiencies of which three micronutrients are major world health problems?

a. vitamins A, K, and D

b. iodine, vitamin A, and iron

c. iodine, iron, and chromium

d. iron, biotin, and vitamin E

9. Crops that are grown and consumed locally are _____.

a. sustainable crops

b. cash crops

c. subsistence crops

d. renewable crops

10. Which product is not made from a renewable resource?

a. paper towels

b. plastic bags

c. bread

d. wooden crates

11. Fortifying _____ will be most likely to eliminate a nutrient deficiency in a country's population.

a. commonly eaten foods

b. locally grown foods

c. foods eaten seasonally

d. expensive foods

12. Which of the following statements is not supported by the information in the pie chart?

a. In 2.7% of households, food intake was reduced.

b. Food insecurity is highest among women and children.

c. Food insecurity is a problem for approximately 8% of Canadian households.

d. Most Canadian households are food secure.

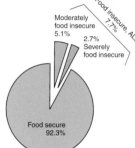

13. Which of the following statements about breastfeeding is true?

a. It decreases risk of malnutrition in infants.

b. It is important only for the first 6 months of life.

c. It is not recommended in poor countries.

d. It is never recommended for women who are HIV-positive.

14. Which of the following people are at the lowest risk for undernutrition?

a. pregnant women

b. small children

c. older adults

d. adolescent males

15. Which of the following statements about Golden Rice is false?

a. It is a genetically modified form of rice.

b. It provides more vitamin A than regular rice.

c. It is readily available in Canadian grocery stores.

d. It is a controversial food.

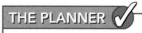

THE PLANNER ✓

Review your Chapter Planner on the chapter opener and check off your completed work.

Appendices

DRI tables for Vitamins and for Minerals are on the front and back covers of this text.

Dietary Reference Intakes: Recommended Intakes for Individuals: Carbohydrates, Fibre, Fat, Fatty Acids, Protein, and Water

Life Stage Group	Carbohydrate (g/day)	Fibre (g/day)[a]	Fat (g/day)[a]	Linoleic Acid (g/day)[a]	α-Linoleic Acid (g/day)[a]	Protein (g/kg/day)[e]	Protein (g/day)	Water[f] (litres)[a]
Infants								
0–6 mo	60[a]	ND[b]	31	4.4[c]	0.5[d]	1.52[a]	9.1[a]	0.7
6–12 mo	95[a]	ND	30	4.6[c]	0.5[d]	1.50	11.0	0.8
Children								
1–3 y	130	19	ND	7	0.7	1.10	13	1.3
4–8 y	130	25	ND	10	0.9	0.95	19	1.7
Males								
9–13 y	130	31	ND	12	1.2	0.95	34	2.4
14–18 y	130	38	ND	16	1.6	0.85	52	3.3
19–30 y	130	38	ND	17	1.6	0.80	56	3.7
31–50 y	130	38	ND	17	1.6*	0.80	56	3.7
51–70 y	130	30	ND	14	1.6	0.80	56	3.7
>70 y	130	30	ND	14	1.6	0.80	56	3.7
Females								
9–13 y	130	26	ND	10	1.0	0.95	34	2.1
14–18 y	130	26	ND	11	1.1	0.85	46	2.1
19–30 y	130	25	ND	12	1.1	0.80	46	2.3
31–50 y	130	25	ND	12	1.1	0.80	46	2.7
51–70 y	130	21	ND	11	1.1	0.80	46	2.7
>70 y	130	21	ND	11	1.1	0.80	46	2.7
Pregnancy	175	28	ND	13	1.4	1.10	71	3.0
Lactation	210	29	ND	13	1.3	1.10	71	3.8

[a]Values are AI (Adequate Intakes).
[b]ND = not determined.
[c]Refers to all ω-6 polyunsaturated fatty acids.
[d]Refers to all ω-3 polyunsaturated fatty acids.
[e]Based on g protein per kg of body weight for the reference body weight, e.g., for adults 0.8g/kg body weight for the reference body weight.
[f]Total water includes all water contained in food, beverages, and drinking water.

Source: Dietary Reference Intakes: The Essential Guide to Nutrient Requirements. Reprinted with permission from National Academies Press, Copyright 2006, National Academy of Sciences.

Dietary Reference Intakes: Tolerable Upper Intake Levels (UL[a]): Vitamins

Life Stage Group	Vitamin A (μg/day)[b]	Vitamin C (mg/day)	Vitamin D (μg/day)	Vitamin E (mg/day)[c,d]	Vitamin K	Thiamin	Riboflavin	Niacin (mg/day)[d]	Vitamin B6 (mg/day)[d]	Folate (μg/day)[d]	Vitamin B12	Pantothenic Acid	Biotin	Choline (mg/day)	Carotenoids[e]
Infants															
0–6 mo	600	ND[f]	25	ND	ND	ND	ND	ND	ND	ND	ND	ND	ND	ND	ND
6–12 mo	600	ND	25	ND	ND	ND	ND	ND	ND	ND	ND	ND	ND	ND	ND
Children															
1–3 y	600	400	50	200	ND	ND	ND	10	30	300	ND	ND	ND	1.0	ND
4–8 y	900	650	50	300	ND	ND	ND	15	40	400	ND	ND	ND	1.0	ND
Males, Females															
9–13 y	1,700	1,200	50	600	ND	ND	ND	20	60	600	ND	ND	ND	2.0	ND
14–18 y	2,800	1,800	50	800	ND	ND	ND	30	80	800	ND	ND	ND	3.0	ND
19–70 y	3,000	2,000	50	1,000	ND	ND	ND	35	100	1,000	ND	ND	ND	3.5	ND
>70 y	3,000	2,000	50	1,000	ND	ND	ND	35	100	1,000	ND	ND	ND	3.5	ND
Pregnancy															
14–18 y	2,800	1,800	50	800	ND	ND	ND	30	80	800	ND	ND	ND	3.0	ND
19–50 y	3,000	2,000	50	1,000	ND	ND	ND	35	100	1,000	ND	ND	ND	3.5	ND
Lactation															
14–18 y	2,800	1,800	50	800	ND	ND	ND	30	80	800	ND	ND	ND	3.0	ND
19–50 y	3,000	2,000	50	1,000	ND	ND	ND	35	100	1,000	ND	ND	ND	3.5	ND

[a] UL = The maximum level of daily nutrient intake that is likely to pose no risk of adverse effects. Unless otherwise specified, the UL represents total intake from food, water, and supplements. Due to lack of suitable data, ULs could not be established for vitamin K, thiamin, riboflavin, vitamin B12, pantothenic acid, biotin, or carotenoids. In the absence of ULs, extra caution may be warranted in consuming levels above recommended intakes.

[b] As preformed vitamin A only.

[c] As α-tocopherol; applies to any form of supplemental α-tocopherol.

[d] The ULs for vitamin E, niacin, and folate apply to synthetic forms obtained from supplements, fortified foods, or a combination of the two.

[e] β-Carotene supplements are advised only to serve as a provitamin A source for individuals at risk of vitamin A deficiency.

[f] ND = Not determinable due to lack of data of adverse effects in this age group and concern with regard to lack of ability to handle excess amounts. Source of intakes should be from food only to prevent high levels of intake.

Source: Dietary Reference Intakes: The Essential Guide to Nutrient Requirements. Reprinted with permission from National Academies Press, Copyright 2006, National Academy of Sciences.

Dietary Reference Intakes: Tolerable Upper Intake Levels (UL[a]): Minerals

Life Stage Group	Arsenic[b] (mg/day)	Boron (mg/day)	Calcium (g/day)	Chromium	Copper (µg/day)	Fluoride (mg/day)	Iodine (µg/day)	Iron (mg/day)	Magnesium (mg/day)[c]	Manganese (mg/day)	Molybdenum (µg/day)	Nickel (mg/day)	Phosphorus (g/day)	Selenium (µg/day)	Silicon[d]	Vanadium (mg/day)[e]	Zinc (mg/day)	Sodium (g/day)	Chloride (g/day)	Potassium
Infants																				
0–6 mo	ND[f]	ND	ND	ND	ND	0.7	ND	40	ND	ND	ND	ND	ND	45	ND	ND	4	ND	ND	ND
6–12 mo	ND	ND	ND	ND	ND	0.9	ND	40	ND	ND	ND	ND	ND	60	ND	ND	5	ND	ND	ND
Children																				
1–3 y	ND	3	2.5	ND	1,000	1.3	200	40	65	2	300	0.2	3	90	ND	ND	7	1.5	2.3	ND
4–8 y	ND	6	2.5	ND	3,000	2.2	300	40	110	3	600	0.3	3	150	ND	ND	12	1.9	2.9	ND
Males, Females																				
9–13 y	ND	11	2.5	ND	5,000	10	600	40	350	6	1,100	0.6	4	280	ND	ND	23	2.2	3.4	ND
14–18 y	ND	17	2.5	ND	8,000	10	900	45	350	9	1,700	1.0	4	400	ND	ND	34	2.3	3.6	ND
19–30 y	ND	20	2.5	ND	10,000	10	1,100	45	350	11	2,000	1.0	4	400	ND	1.8	40	2.3	3.6	ND
31–50 y	ND	20	2.5	ND	10,000	10	1,100	45	350	11	2,000	1.0	4	400	ND	1.8	40	2.3	3.6	ND
51–70 y	ND	20	2.0	ND	10,000	10	1,100	45	350	11	2,000	1.0	4	400	ND	1.8	40	2.3	3.6	ND
>70 y	ND	20	2.5	ND	10,000	10	1,100	45	350	11	2,000	1.0	3	400	ND	1.8	40	2.3	3.6	ND
Pregnancy																				
14–18 y	ND	17	3.0	ND	8,000	10	900	45	350	9	1,700	1.0	3.5	400	ND	ND	34	2.3	3.6	ND
19–50 y	ND	20	2.5	ND	10,000	10	1,100	45	350	11	2,000	1.0	3.5	400	ND	ND	40	2.3	3.6	ND
Lactation																				
14–18 y	ND	17	3.0	ND	8,000	10	900	45	350	9	1,700	1.0	4	400	ND	ND	34	2.3	3.6	ND
19–50 y	ND	20	2.5	ND	10,000	10	1,100	45	350	11	2,000	1.0	4	400	ND	ND	40	2.3	3.6	ND

[a]UL = the maximum level of daily nutrient intake that is likely to pose no risk of adverse effects. Unless otherwise specified, the UL represents total intake from food, water, and supplements. Due to lack of suitable data, ULs could not be established for arsenic, chromium, silicon, and potassium. In the absence of ULs, extra caution may be warranted in consuming levels above recommended intakes.

[b]Although the UL was not determined for arsenic, there is no justification for adding arsenic to food or supplements.

[c]The ULs for magnesium represent intake from a pharmacological agent only and do not include intake from food and water.

[d]Although silicon has not been shown to cause adverse effects in humans, there is no justification for adding silicon to supplements.

[e]Although vanadium in food has not been shown to cause adverse effects in laboratory animals and this data could be used to set a UL for adults but not children and adolescents, there is no justification for adding vanadium to food and vanadium supplements should be used with caution. The UL is based on adverse effects in laboratory animals and this data could be used to set a UL for adults but not children and adolescents.

[f]ND = Not determinable due to lack of data of adverse effects in this age group and concern with regard to lack of ability to handle excess amounts. Source of intake should be from food only to prevent high levels of intake.

Source: Dietary Reference Intakes: The Essential Guide to Nutrient Requirements. Reprinted with permission from National Academies Press, Copyright 2006, National Academy of Sciences.

Dietary Reference Intake Values for Energy: Total Energy Expenditure (TEE) Equations for Overweight and Obese Individuals

Life Stage Group	TEE Prediction Equation (Cal/day)	PA Values
Overweight boys aged 3–18 years	TEE = 114 − (50.9 × age in yrs) + PA [(19.5 × weight in kg) + (1,161.4 × height in m)]	Sedentary = 1.00 Low active = 1.12 Active = 1.24 Very active = 1.45
Overweight girls aged 3–18 years	TEE = 389 − (41.2 × age in yrs) + PA [(15.0 × weight in kg) + (701.6 × height in m)]	Sedentary = 1.00 Low active = 1.18 Active = 1.35 Very active = 1.60
Overweight and obese men aged 19 years and older	TEE = 1,086 − (10.1 × age in yrs) + PA [(13.7 × weight in kg) + (416 × height in m)]	Sedentary = 1.00 Low active = 1.12 Active = 1.29 Very active = 1.59
Overweight and obese women aged 19 years and older	TEE = 448 − (7.95 × age in yrs) + PA [(11.4 × weight in kg) + (619 × height in m)]	Sedentary = 1.00 Low active = 1.16 Active = 1.27 Very active = 1.44

Source: Institute of Medicine, Food and Nutrition Board, "Dietary Reference Intakes for Energy, Carbohydrate, Fiber, Fat, Fatty Acids, Cholesterol, Protein, and Amino Acids," Washington, DC: National Academy Press, 2002, 2005.

WHO GROWTH CHARTS FOR CANADA

GIRLS

BIRTH TO 24 MONTHS: GIRLS
Length-for-age and Weight-for-age percentiles

NAME: _____

DOB: _____ RECORD # _____

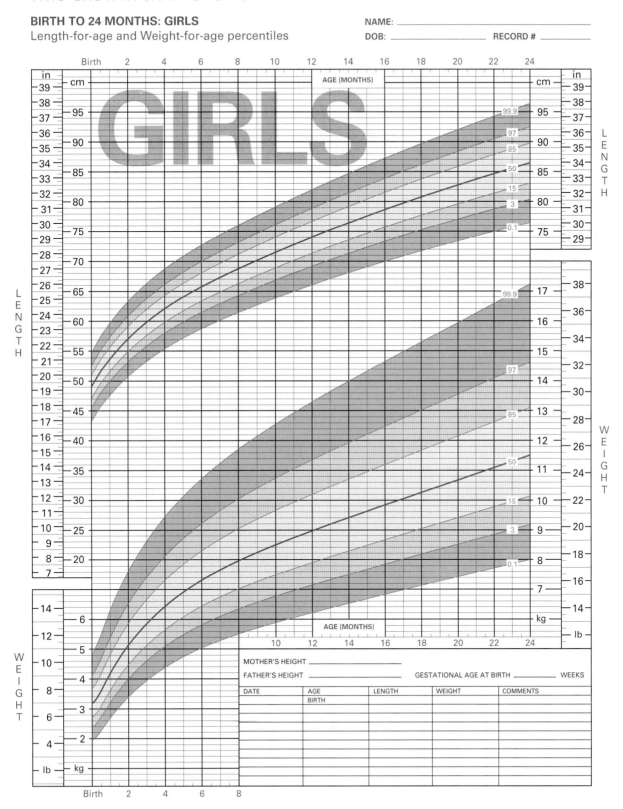

SOURCE: Based on the World Health Organization (WHO) Child Growth Standards (2006) and adapted for Canada by Dietitians of Canada, Canadian Paediatric Society, the College of Family Physicians of Canada and Community Health Nurses of Canada.

© Dietitians of Canada. 2010. May be reproduced in its entirety (i.e. no changes) for educational purposes only.
www.dietitians.ca/growthcharts

WHO GROWTH CHARTS FOR CANADA

BOYS

BIRTH TO 24 MONTHS: BOYS
Length-for-age and Weight-for-age percentiles

NAME: _____

DOB: _____ RECORD # _____

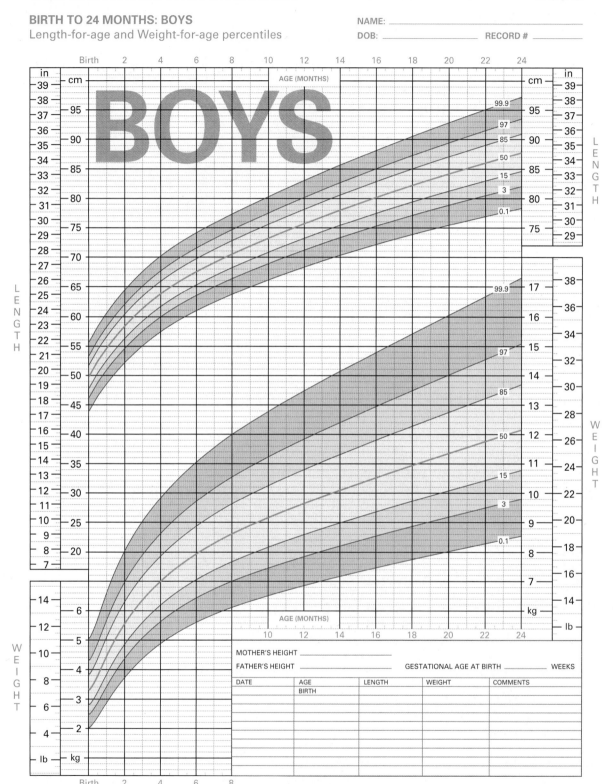

MOTHER'S HEIGHT _____

FATHER'S HEIGHT _____ GESTATIONAL AGE AT BIRTH _____ WEEKS

DATE	AGE	LENGTH	WEIGHT	COMMENTS
	BIRTH			

SOURCE: Based on the World Health Organization (WHO) Child Growth Standards (2006) and adapted for Canada by Dietitians of Canada, Canadian Paediatric Society, the College of Family Physicians of Canada and Community Health Nurses of Canada.

© Dietitians of Canada. 2010. May be reproduced in its entirety (i.e. no changes) for educational purposes only.
www.dietitians.ca/growthcharts

WHO GROWTH CHARTS FOR CANADA

GIRLS

2 TO 19 YEARS: GIRLS
Height-for-age and Weight-for-age percentiles

NAME: _____

DOB: _____ RECORD # _____

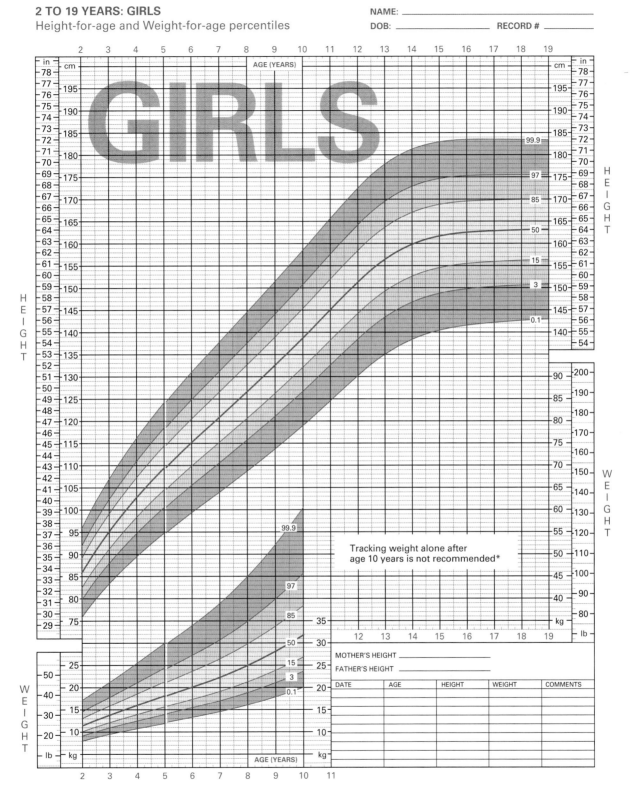

MOTHER'S HEIGHT _____

FATHER'S HEIGHT _____

DATE	AGE	HEIGHT	WEIGHT	COMMENTS

Tracking weight alone after age 10 years is not recommended*

SOURCE: Based on the World Health Organization (WHO) Child Growth Standards (2006) and WHO Reference (2007) adapted for Canada by Dietitians of Canada, Canadian Paediatric Society, the College of Family Physicians of Canada and Community Health Nurses of Canada.

© Dietitians of Canada. 2010. May be reproduced in its entirety (i.e. no changes) for educational purposes only. www.dietitians.ca/growthcharts
*BMI is a better measure due to variable age of puberty.

2 TO 19 YEARS: BOYS
Height-for-age and Weight-for-age percentiles

NAME: _____

DOB: _____ RECORD # _____

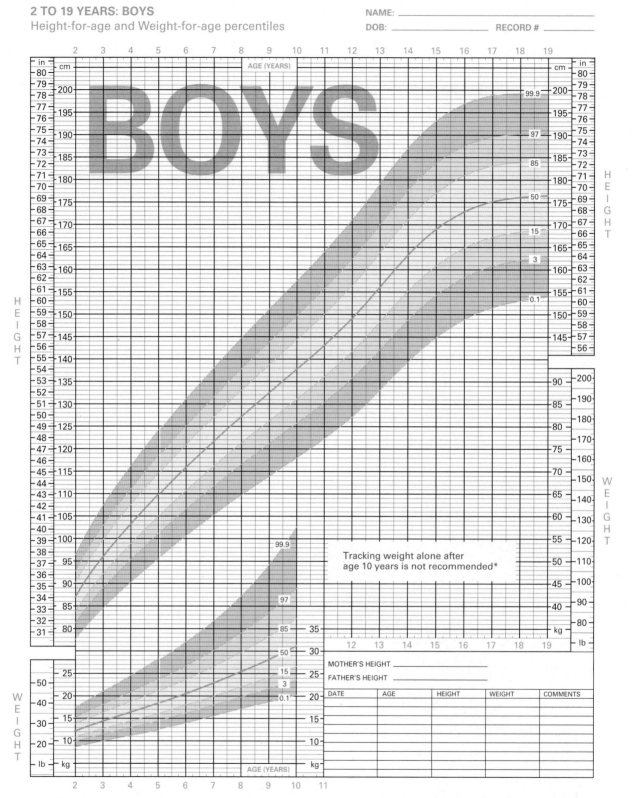

Tracking weight alone after
age 10 years is not recommended*

MOTHER'S HEIGHT _____
FATHER'S HEIGHT _____

DATE	AGE	HEIGHT	WEIGHT	COMMENTS

SOURCE: Based on the World Health Organization (WHO) Child Growth Standards (2006) and WHO Reference (2007) adapted for Canada by Dietitians of Canada, Canadian Paediatric Society, the College of Family Physicians of Canada and Community Health Nurses of Canada.

© Dietitians of Canada. 2010. May be reproduced in its entirety (i.e. no changes) for educational purposes only. www.dietitians.ca/growthcharts
*BMI is a better measure due to variable age of puberty.

Red blood cells
    Men $4.5\text{-}6.5 \times 10^{12}/L^a$

Red blood cells	
Men	$4.5\text{-}6.5 \times 10^{12}/L^a$
Women	$4.0\text{-}5.6 \times 10^{12}/L^a$
White blood cells	$4.0\text{-}10.0 \times 10^{9}/L^a$
Hematocrit	
Men	0.43-0.522
Women	0.37-0.462
Hemoglobin	
Men	140-174 g/L[b]
Women	123-157 g/L[b]
Ferritin	10-250 µg/L[a]
Calcium	2.15-2.55 mmol/L[a]
Iodine	0.24-0.63 µmol/L[a]
Iron	7-36 nmol/L[b]
Zinc	9.8-20.2 µmol/L[b]
Magnesium	0.65-1.05 mmol/L[b]
Potassium	3.5-5.0 mmol/L[b]
Sodium	135-145 mmol/L[b]
Chloride	98-107 mmol/L[b]
Vitamin A	1.2-2.8 µmol/L[b]
Vitamin B_{12}	200-672 pmol/L[b]
Vitamin C	$\geq$25 µmol/L[b]
Carotene	0.9-4.7 µmol/L[b]
Folate (red cells)	634-1792 nmol/L[b]
pH	7.35-7.45[a]
Total protein	64-83 g/L[b]
Albumin	35-52 g/L[b]
Cholesterol	<5.2 mmol/L[a]
LDL cholesterol	<3.5 mmol/L[c]*
HDL cholesterol	>1.0 mmol/L[c]*
Total cholesterol/HDL cholesterol	<5.0 mmol/L[c]*
Triglycerides	<1.7 mol/L[c]*
Glucose (serum)	3.3-5.8 mmol/L[a]

*These numbers may vary from individual to individual, depending on other risk factors (e.g., hypertension, diabetes).

Sources:

[a]Laboratory Test Information Guide. London Laboratory Services Group, London, Ontario, 2010. Available online at http://www.lhsc.on.ca/cgibin/view_labtest.pl. Accessed August 5, 2011.

[b]The Medical Council of Canada 2011 Clinical Laboratory Test. Normal Values. Available online at http://www.mcc.ca/objectives_online/objectives.pl?lang=english&loc=values. Accessed August 5, 2011.

[c]McPherson, R., Frohlich, J., Fodor, G., and Genest, J., Canadian Cardiovascular Society. Canadian Cardiovascular Society position statement–recommendations for the diagnosis and treatment of dyslipidemia and prevention of cardiovascular disease. Can J Cardiol 22(11):913–27, 2006.

Major Risk Factors (Exclusive of LDL Cholesterol) that Increase Heart Disease Risk

Risk Factors You Can Control	Risk Factors You Cannot Control
High blood pressure (BP ≥140/90mmHg)	Age
High blood cholesterol	Gender
Diabetes	Family history
Being overweight (waist circumference in men >102 cm or in women >88 cm; or BMI > 25kg/m²)	Ethnicity
Excessive alcohol consumption	History of stroke
Physical inactivity	
Smoking	
Stress	

Source: The Heart and Stroke Foundation. Prevention of Risk Factors. March 2010. Available online at http://www.heartandstroke.com/site/c.iklQLcMWJtE/b.3483919/k.F2CA/Heart_disease__Prevention_of_Risk_Factors.htm. Accessed August 5, 2012.

High Blood Pressure (Hypertension) Guidelines

Category	Systolic/Diastolic
Normal	120–129/80–84
High-normal	130–139/85–89
High blood pressure	140/90 or higher
High blood pressure for people with diabetes or kidney disease	130/80 or higher

Source: Heart and Stroke Foundation of Canada. High blood pressure. Available online at http://www.heartandstroke.com/site/c.iklQLcMWJtE/b.3484023/k.2174/Heart_disease__High_blood_pressure.htm. Accessed August 5, 2012.

This discussion of the Canadian Diabetes Association's *Beyond the Basics: Meal Planning for Healthy Eating, Diabetes Prevention and Management* consists of two parts:

- Part 1 is a detailed description of *Beyond the Basics* included as part of a case study.
- Part 2 is a comparison of Canada's Food Guide and *Beyond the Basics*.

Part 1: Case Study

Samantha is a registered dietitian and certified diabetes educator. The endocrinologist at the diabetes clinic where she works has asked her to meet with Robert to discuss a meal plan. Robert has been diagnosed with type-2 diabetes for three years and was previously taught Just the Basics for diabetes meal planning to help manage his condition (see Chapter 4). Samantha's dietary assessment shows that Robert has inconsistent carbohydrate intake from day to day and poor carbohydrate distribution throughout the day, which can lead to poor glycemic control (i.e., fluctuations in his blood glucose levels). He also tends to consume a lot of high glycemic index (GI) foods (see Chapter 4 for a discussion of GI). Robert has a BMI of 33, is physically active, and is motivated to make changes to his diet and lose weight, but requires a more advanced knowledge of nutrition management of diabetes. Samantha decides that the appropriate next step for education on nutrition management of diabetes for Robert is the Canadian Diabetes Association's tool *Beyond the Basics*.

After reading this appendix about *Beyond the Basics*, you will be able to understand this tool and its use for counselling individuals with type-2 diabetes.

Introduction to *Beyond the Basics*

Beyond the Basics: Meal Planning for Healthy Eating, Diabetes Prevention and Management was created to help primarily the adult with type-2 diabetes, but all forms of diabetes were considered when it was developed. It is a tool, in the form of a poster, to help Canadians control blood glucose levels, maintain a healthy weight, and meet daily nutritional needs, while navigating different eating situations and including ethnoculturally appropriate foods. It is based on current thinking around carbohydrate counting and reflects scientific evidence around heart health and glycemic index. Carbohydrate counting is a method of meal planning that is based on the premise that carbohydrate-containing foods increase blood glucose levels; it entails keeping track of the total carbohydrate consumed throughout the day to help control blood glucose levels. *Beyond the Basics* can be used as a progression from the Canadian Diabetes Association's *Just the Basics* tool or as a standalone resource. It is described in detail on the Canadian Diabetes Association website, at www.diabetes.ca/for-professionals/resources/nutrition/beyond-basics.

Components of *Beyond the Basics*

Figure D.1 shows the layout of the *Beyond the Basics* poster. Foods are divided into seven groups. Four food groups, which are rich in carbohydrates, are found on the left-hand side of the poster under the heading Carbohydrate-Containing Foods and include (**Figure D.2**):

- Grains and Starches
- Fruits
- Milk and Alternatives
- Other Choices

Three food groups, containing foods with little or no carbohydrates, are found on the righthand side of the poster (**Figure D.3**) and include:

- Vegetables
- Meat and Alternatives
- Fats

Figure D.1

Layout of the *Beyond the Basics* tool

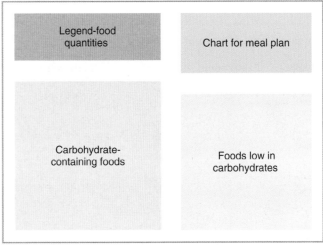

Source: Canadian Diabetes Association: Beyond the Basics. Available online at http://www.diabetes.ca/for-professionals/resources/nutrition/beyond-basics/. Accessed April 6, 2013.

Within each of the food groups, there are several features to note:

- The Legend (**Table D.1**) provides portion sizes for each of the illustrated foods.

- Portions of carbohydrate-containing foods are based on a serving that will provide approximately 15 g of available carbohydrate. Available carbohydrate = (total carbohydrate) - (total fibre) because fibre does not increase blood glucose levels. *Beyond the Basics* uses household measures to identify portion sizes; therefore, carbohydrate content in individual servings is approximate.

- All foods have been placed in a green or yellow box, with a green or yellow triangle in the upper-left corner of the box. Foods to "choose more often" are shown in green boxes; these foods are higher in vitamins, minerals, and fibre, have lower GI values, and/or lower fat content. Foods to "choose less often" are shown in yellow boxes; these foods may have a high fat or sugar content or may be low in fibre or other essential nutrients.

- The back page of the *Beyond the Basics* poster has a space for goal setting and a Nutrition Facts Table label-reading exercise for people with diabetes.

- The *Beyond the Basics* poster contains a limited number of foods under each category due to space restrictions. Complete food lists can be found on the Canadian Diabetes Association website and allow for greater variety and flexibility in meal planning.

The *Beyond the Basics* Food Groups

Food Groups that Contain Carbohydrate-Rich Foods

Figure D.2 illustrates the four food groups that contain carbohydrate-rich foods: Grains and Starches, Fruits, Milk and Alternatives, and Other Choices. One serving of these foods is equal to 15 g of available carbohydrates or 1 carbohydrate choice.

Grains and Starches This category includes grains, bread, pasta, rice, and starchy vegetables such as potatoes, plantains, and corn. These foods are considered a good source of carbohydrate, fibre, vitamins, minerals, and energy. People need a minimum of 4 servings per day, depending on age, sex, activity, and weight; however, excessive amounts should not be consumed because it will result in elevated blood glucose. "Choose more often" items found in green boxes are typically higher in fibre and vitamins and minerals, and lower in total and saturated fat compared to "choose less often" items.

Additional messages that can be included in the counselling session include:

- Choose whole grains, such as brown rice, quinoa, and whole wheat pasta, more often.

- Emphasize the natural taste of grain products by limiting spreads and sauces.

- Read the ingredient lists to find whole grain starches with maximum amounts of fibre.

- Choose low or medium GI foods. These will not raise blood glucose as much as high GI foods.

Fruits Fresh, frozen, canned, and dried fruit, as well as fruit juices and applesauce, are included in this food group. Fruits are a good source of carbohydrates, fibre, vitamins, minerals, and energy. Consuming 2–3 servings of fruit per day is sufficient. Most fruits are categorized as "choose more often" items. "Choose less often" items have been categorized as such because of their dramatic impact on blood glucose levels and in order to emphasize portion control.

Points to emphasize include:

- Try to choose whole fruit and fruit with skins to increase fibre content.

Legend Items of *Beyond the Basics* Tool   Table D.1

Symbol	Explanation	Symbol	Explanation
🥛	1 cup (250 mL)	🥄	1 tsp (5 mL)
🥛	½ cup (125 mL)	▮	1 ounce (30 grams) by weight
🥛	¼ cup (60 mL)	🔥	Measure after cooking
🥄	1 Tbsp (15 mL)		

Source: Used with permission from Canadian Diabetes Association: Beyond the Basics. Available online at http://www.diabetes.ca/for-professionals/resources/nutrition/beyond-basics/. Accessed April 1, 2013.

Figure D.2

Carbohydrate-containing foods. These include Grains and Starches, Fruits, Milk and Alternatives, and Other Choices.

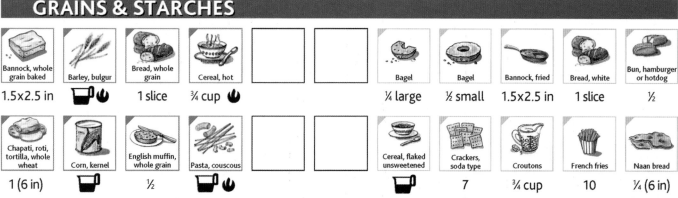

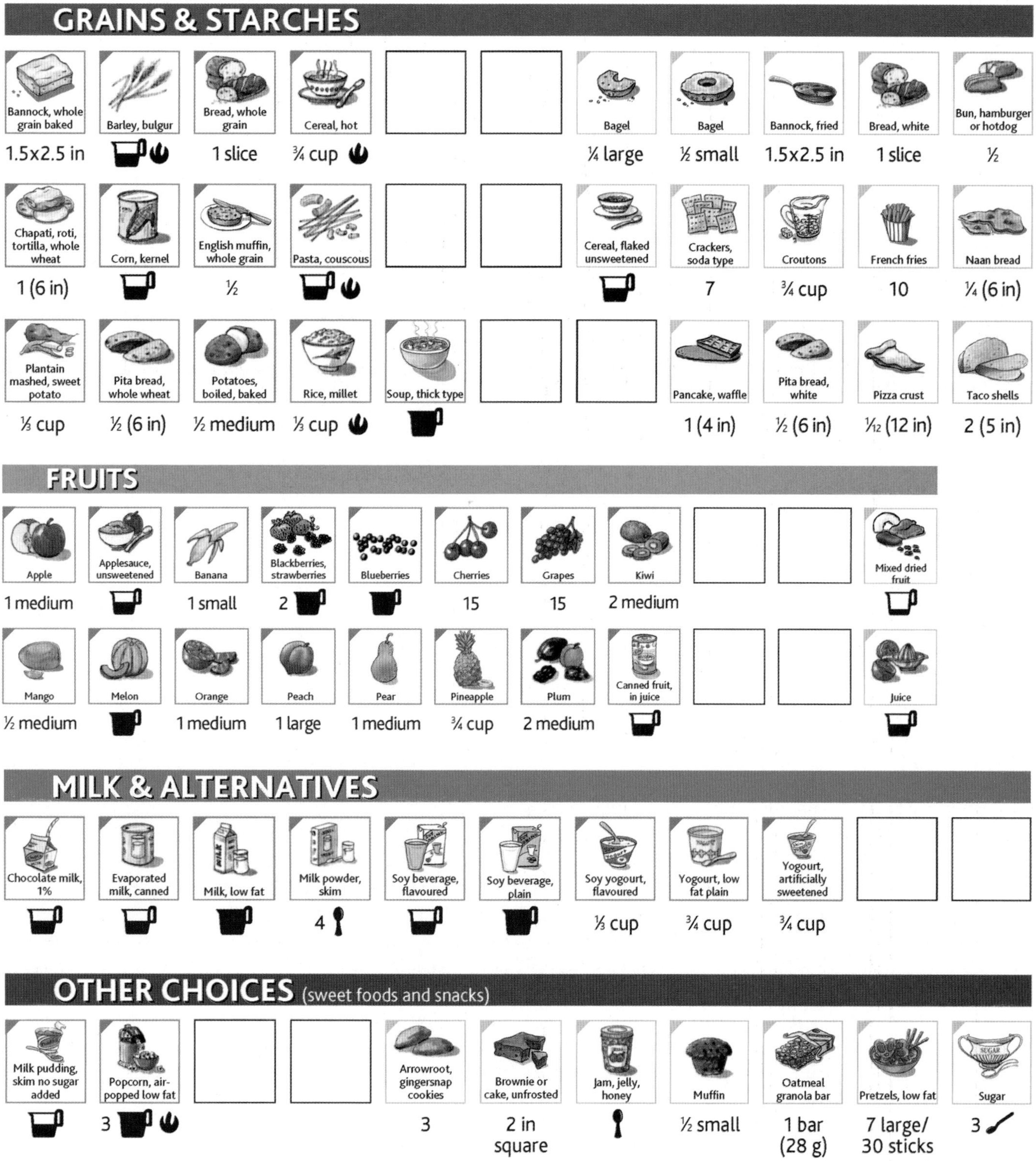

GRAINS & STARCHES

Bannock, whole grain baked	Barley, bulgur	Bread, whole grain	Cereal, hot			Bagel	Bagel	Bannock, fried	Bread, white	Bun, hamburger or hotdog
1.5x2.5 in		1 slice	¾ cup			¼ large	½ small	1.5x2.5 in	1 slice	½

Chapati, roti, tortilla, whole wheat	Corn, kernel	English muffin, whole grain	Pasta, couscous			Cereal, flaked unsweetened	Crackers, soda type	Croutons	French fries	Naan bread
1 (6 in)		½					7	¾ cup	10	¼ (6 in)

Plantain mashed, sweet potato	Pita bread, whole wheat	Potatoes, boiled, baked	Rice, millet	Soup, thick type			Pancake, waffle	Pita bread, white	Pizza crust	Taco shells
⅓ cup	½ (6 in)	½ medium	⅓ cup				1 (4 in)	½ (6 in)	1/12 (12 in)	2 (5 in)

FRUITS

Apple	Applesauce, unsweetened	Banana	Blackberries, strawberries	Blueberries	Cherries	Grapes	Kiwi			Mixed dried fruit
1 medium		1 small	2		15	15	2 medium			

Mango	Melon	Orange	Peach	Pear	Pineapple	Plum	Canned fruit, in juice			Juice
½ medium		1 medium	1 large	1 medium	¾ cup	2 medium				

MILK & ALTERNATIVES

Chocolate milk, 1%	Evaporated milk, canned	Milk, low fat	Milk powder, skim	Soy beverage, flavoured	Soy beverage, plain	Soy yogurt, flavoured	Yogourt, low fat plain	Yogourt, artificially sweetened		
			4			⅓ cup	¾ cup	¾ cup		

OTHER CHOICES (sweet foods and snacks)

Milk pudding, skim no sugar added	Popcorn, air-popped low fat			Arrowroot, gingersnap cookies	Brownie or cake, unfrosted	Jam, jelly, honey	Muffin	Oatmeal granola bar	Pretzels, low fat	Sugar
	3			3	2 in square		½ small	1 bar (28 g)	7 large/ 30 sticks	3

Source: With permission from Canadian Diabetes Association: Beyond the Basics. Available online at http://www.diabetes.ca/for-professionals/resources/nutrition/beyond-basics/. Accessed April 6, 2013.

- Try to spread fruit consumption across meals and snacks throughout the day.
- Canned fruit: read the label to see if it is preserved in sugar syrup. Rinse the fruit from the sugary syrup or adjust the amount eaten to follow your meal plan.

Milk and Alternatives This category includes cow's milk, fortified soy beverages, flavoured yogurts, and chocolate milk. "Choose more often" items are lower in fat (skim, 1%, 2%) and contain calcium and vitamin D. Milk products and yogurts can vary considerably in their carbohydrate, fat, and protein contents so label reading is particularly important with this food group.

Other choices (sweet foods and snacks) The "Other Choices" category covers a wide array of sweet foods and snacks, including popcorn, pudding, jams, cookies, and pretzels. These foods are typically lower in nutrients and higher in fat, sugar, salt, and calories and therefore should be eaten only occasionally. Most of these products are "choose less often" items except for plain popcorn and skim, no added sugar milk pudding. The "choose less often" items do not have to be eliminated from the diet; however, portions should be limited to the serving guide suggested in *Beyond the Basics*.

Food Groups that Contain Little or No Carbohydrates

The *Beyond the Basics* food groups that have little or no carbohydrates are vegetables, meat and alternatives, and fats. These are found in Figure D.3.

Vegetables Vegetables are nutritionally dense; they provide fibre, vitamins, and minerals. Non-starchy vegetables found in this category are illustrated in Figure D.3 and are considered "free items" (that is, people with diabetes can consume as many as they would like) to encourage increased consumption of this nutritious group. It is recommended that people with diabetes consume 4–5 servings a day (a serving is 125 mL (½ cup) cooked or 250 mL (1 cup) raw vegetables).

Most of the vegetables listed in this category have 2 g of protein and less than 5 g of carbohydrate per choice. However, 250 mL (1 cup) of squash, peas, and/or parsnips provides 15 g of available carbohydrate. Carrots and beets contain less carbohydrate than popularly believed due to their high fibre content (e.g., 22 miniature carrots contain 15 g of available carbohydrate). Tips to emphasize in the counselling session include:

- When preparing, limit cooking time to ensure vitamin retention.
- Choose vegetables that are prepared with little or no added fat, sugar, and salt.

Meat and Alternatives Items listed in this category have at least 7 g of protein and 3–5 g of fat per choice. Most of the items listed have no (0 g) carbohydrate per serving. Legumes contain carbohydrates but also have considerable amounts of fibre, which helps to decrease the absorption of glucose and therefore minimizes the blood glucose elevation. Cheese is found in the Meat and Alternatives category (rather than Milk and Alternatives) because it has 0 g of available carbohydrate and it is a source of protein. Cheese has a higher fat content, so lower-fat cheeses (< 20% milk fat) are recommended.

The Meat and Alternatives category is divided into "choose more often" and "choose less often" based on fat content (total and/or saturated) to encourage healthy eating, heart health, and weight control. Tips to include during the counselling session are:

- Choose lower-sodium items and lean cuts of meats. Trimming the visible fat is also recommended.
- Consume protein at meals and snacks to provide extra satiation.
- Emphasize vegetarian options such as legumes (beans, lentils, chickpeas).
- Watch portion control: 1 oz (30 g) = size of thumb; 3 oz (90 g) = palm of hand.
- Consume 2 servings of fatty fish per week, consistent with *Eating Well with Canada's Food Guide*.

Fats Fat choices contain 5 g of fat per choice and no carbohydrate, and therefore do not increase blood glucose levels. All of the items listed in the fats category are written in yellow boxes for "choose less often" because of their high calorie content and/or because they are an unhealthy type of fat. Nuts are incorporated into this category because of their high monounsaturated and polyunsaturated fat content. Refer to Figure D.3 for the complete *Beyond the Basics* poster section on fats. Additional messages to include in the counselling session are:

- The amount and type of fat are important to watch; unsaturated fats should be emphasized.
- Try to use foods that have less than 2 g of saturated and *trans* fat per serving.

Figure D.3

Foods that contain little or no carbohydrates. These include Vegetables, Meat and Alternatives, and Fats.

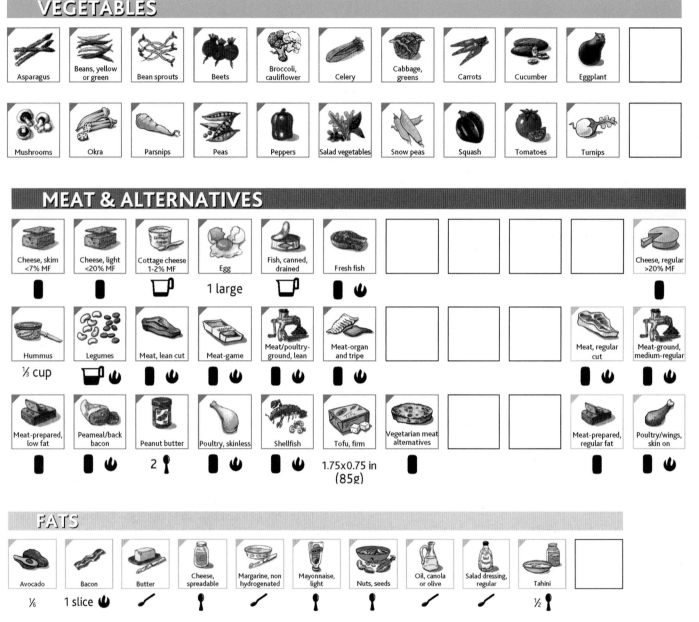

Source: With permission from Canadian Diabetes Association: Beyond the Basics. Available online at http://www.diabetes.ca/forprofessionals/resources/nutrition/beyond-basics/. Accessed April 6, 2013.

Meal Planning with *Beyond the Basics*

The simplest way to conduct meal planning with *Beyond the Basics* is to fill in **Table D.2** using the guidelines detailed in this appendix.

Carbohydrates

The main focus of meal planning for people with diabetes is the amount and type of carbohydrate they consume from the following groups: grains and starches, fruits, milk and alternatives, and other choices.

Meal Plan Framework   Table D.2

Meal Plan							
Time							
Carbohydrates (grams/choices)							
Grains & Starches							
Fruits							
Milk & Alternatives							
Other Choices							
Vegetables							
Meat & Alternatives							
Fats							

Source: Used with permission from Canadian Diabetes Association: Beyond the Basics. Available online at http://www.diabetes.ca/files/Meal%20plan%20web.pdf. Accessed April 6, 2013.

Amount of carbohydrates As per the *Beyond the Basics* poster, 1 portion is approximately 15 g of available carbohydrate, or 1 carbohydrate choice, regardless of the type of carbohydrate containing food consumed (fruit, grains, etc.). Typical quantities of carbohydrate choices per person per meal or snack are found in **Table D.3**.

Type of carbohydrates People with diabetes should aim to consume a variety of foods from each food group and more of the "choose more often" items.

Vegetables Vegetables should be consumed at each meal. These items are considered "free" as they are nutritious and do not increase blood glucose levels.

Meat and Alternatives Meat and alternatives can be consumed throughout the day, as these items do not increase blood glucose levels. The following serving sizes will help meet protein needs: 30–60 g (1–2 oz). for smaller meals and snacks (if desired), and 90–120 g (3–4 oz) (smaller appetites) or 150–180 g (5–6 oz) (bigger appetites) for main meals.

Fats Fats should be used in moderation. Consuming too much fat can lead to weight gain, which makes it harder for the body to control blood glucose levels.

Case Study Outcome

In the counselling session, Samantha, the diabetes educator, has gained an understanding of Robert's typical meals through the assessment process. She has also described the components of and food groups within *Beyond the Basics* to Robert. Now it is time to develop an individualized meal plan for Robert.

Typical Quantities of Carbohydrate Choices per Person per Meal or Snack   Table D.3

Men/Women	Meal/Snack	Number of Carbohydrate Choices*	Grams of Carbohydrates*
Men	Meal	3–5	45–75 g
Women	Meal	2–4	30–60 g
Men and women	Snack**	1–2	15–30 g

* Depending on physical activity level, age, size, and weight loss/maintenance goals
** Optional throughout day

Robert's Meal Plan   Table D.4

Time	Breakfast	Snack	Lunch	Snack	Dinner	Snack
Carbohydrates (grams/choices)	45 – 75 g	15 – 30 g	45 – 75 g	15 – 30 g	45 – 75 g	15 – 30 g
Grains & Starches Fruits Milk & Alternatives Other Choices	3 – 5 choices	1 – 2 choices	3 – 5 choices	1 – 2 choices	3 – 5 choices	1 – 2 choices
Vegetables	✓	✓	✓	✓	✓	✓
Meat & Alternatives	As is*					
Fats	Use in Moderation					

✓ Means "eat freely."

* Meat and Alternatives can be consumed as per usual, that is, consumed "as is," with a focus on watching portion size, meaning eating Canada's Food Guide servings of 75 g (the size of a deck of cards or the palm of the hand) and consuming "choose more often" items (e.g., lean meats).

As demonstrated in Robert's meal plan in **Table D.4**, he should aim for 3–5 carbohydrate choices (45–75 g of carbohydrate) per meal, and 1–2 choices (15–30 g of carbohydrate) per snack, when he chooses to eat snacks. These carbohydrate choices can fall within the different carbohydrate-containing food groups; however, variety within groups should be emphasized. Vegetables can be consumed freely throughout the day as indicated by the check mark in Table D.4. Portion sizes of Meat and Alternatives should be watched, with a focus on "choose more often" items. Fats should be consumed in moderation.

Here is a sample meal plan that Samantha prepared for Robert:

Breakfast: 2 slices of toasted whole grain bread, 1 cup (250 mL) 1% milk, ¾ cup (175 mL) yogurt, 2 poached eggs, 3 tomato slices, 1 Tbsp (15 mL) tub margarine, and tea or coffee with artificial sweetener → 4 choices, 60 g

Lunch: 2 cups (500 mL) thick soup, ½ small bagel, 2 oz (60 g) skim mozzarella cheese, baby carrots, sliced peppers, 1 orange → 4 choices, 60 g

P.M. snack: 7 whole wheat soda crackers, 1 cup (250 mL) low fat milk, 2 Tbsp (60 mL) peanut butter → 2 choices, 30 g

Dinner: 1 medium baked potato with melted cheese, mixed vegetables (carrots, green beans) with margarine, 5 oz. (150 g) roasted chicken, ½ cup (125 mL) corn, 1 cup (250 mL) cantaloupe, ½ cup (125 mL) cranberry juice → 5 choices, 75 g

Evening snack: 1 medium apple → 1 choice, 15 g

A follow-up appointment indicated that Robert, with the help of *Beyond the Basics*, was able to consume a more nutritionally balanced diet, stabilize his inconsistent carbohydrate intake, and improve his poor carbohydrate distribution, which led to improved blood glucose control. He also made some progress toward his weight loss goal.

Part 2: Comparison of Canada's Food Guide and *Beyond the Basics*

Eating Well with Canada's Food Guide and *Beyond the Basics* are meal planning guides to help Canadians make healthier dietary choices. Canada's Food Guide was developed with healthy Canadians in mind; however, concepts of Canada's Food Guide were incorporated in the development of *Beyond the Basics*. Although *Beyond the Basics* is targeted to people with diabetes, it also can be used by Canadians without diabetes to plan their meals. These two guides are compared in **Table D.5**.

Comparison of *Beyond the Basics* and *Eating Well with Canada's Food Guide* Table D.5

Item Of Comparison	Beyond The Basics	Canada's Food Guide
Target Audience	People with diabetes	All Canadians
Item classification	Meal planning tool to assist with healthy eating	Healthy eating guidelines
Developed by	Canadian Diabetes Association	Health Canada
Aim of tool or guidelines	Using the *Beyond the Basics* meal planning tool will help Canadians: • Control blood glucose levels • Maintain a healthy weight • Meet daily nutritional needs • Navigate different eating situations	Following *Canada's Food Guide* will help Canadians: • Meet nutrient needs • Reduce risk for developing obesity, type-2 diabetes, heart disease, osteoporosis, and certain types of cancer • Contribute to overall health and vitality
How foods are categorized within the tool	Foods are classified as: Carbohydrate-containing foods: Grains and Starches, Fruits, Milk and Alternatives, Other Choices Foods that contain little or no carbohydrate: Vegetables, Meat and Alternatives, Fats Items that do not obviously belong in a specific food group are classified based on most common usage (e.g., legumes) and botanical classification (e.g., corn)	Foods are classified into the four Food Groups (Vegetables and Fruit, Grain Products, Milk and Alternatives, Meat and Alternatives) based on the following criteria: • Foods originating from the same agricultural base • How foods traditionally have been classified • How people use foods
Serving sizes	½ cup (125 mL) cooked pasta or couscous	½ cup (125 mL) cooked pasta or couscous
	⅓ cup (80 mL) cooked rice	½ cup (125 mL) cooked rice
	1 slice bread, ½ small bagel	1 slice bread, ½ bagel (45 g)
	¾ cup (175 mL) cooked hot cereal	¾ cup (175 mL) hot cereal
	½ medium potato	½ cup (125 mL) potatoes
	1 medium apple or pear 2 medium kiwis or plums	1 fruit
	2 cups (500 mL) blackberries or strawberries 15 grapes or cherries ½ cup (125 mL) fruit juice ¼ cup (60 mL) dried fruit	½ cup (125 mL) fresh, frozen, canned fruit or fruit juice
	½ cup (125 mL) chocolate milk or flavoured soy beverage 1 cup (250 mL) low fat milk or plain soy beverage	1 cup (250 mL) chocolate or low fat milk, or fortified soy beverage
	¾ cup (175 mL) yogurt	¾ cup (175 g) yogurt
	1 oz (30 g) cheese	1 ½ oz (50 g) cheese
	½ cup (125 mL) cooked or 1 cup (250 mL) raw vegetables	½ cup (125 mL) fresh, frozen, canned vegetables or cooked leafy vegetables 1 cup (250 mL) raw leafy vegetables
	½ cup (125 mL) cooked legumes	¾ cup (175 mL) cooked legumes
	1 oz (30 g) cooked fresh fish or lean meat, poultry	2.5 oz (75 g) cooked fish, lean meat, poultry
	1 Tbsp (50 mL) nuts, seeds	¼ cup (60 mL) shelled nuts and seeds

Number of recommended servings/choices	Grains and Starches	Minimum of 4 servings per day	Females 19-50: 6–7 servings Males 19–50: 8 servings
		Adults should consume 1–2 servings of carbohydrate foods at snacks, and either 3–5 servings (males) or 2–4 servings (females) at meals	Females 51+: 6 servings Males 51+: 7 servings
	Fruit	2–3 servings, spread throughout the day	Grouped with "Vegetables"
		Adults should consume 1–2 servings of carbohydrate foods at snacks, and either 3–5 servings (males) or 2–4 servings (females) at meals	*Vegetables and Fruit:* Females 19–50: 7–8 servings Males 19–50: 8–10 servings Females 51+: 7 servings Males 51+: 7 servings
	Milk and Alternatives	Adults should consume 1–2 servings of carbohydrate foods at snacks, and either 3–5 servings (males) or 2–4 servings (females) at meals	Females 19–50: 2 servings Males 19–50: 2 servings Females 51+: 3 servings Males 51+: 3 servings
	Other Choices	Adults should consume 1–2 servings of carbohydrate foods at snacks, and either 3–5 servings (males) or 2–4 servings (females) at meals	No Food Group for "Other Choices"
	Vegetables	"Free"	Grouped with "Fruits" *Vegetables and Fruit:* Females 19–50: 7–8 servings Males 19–50: 8–10 servings Females 51+: 7 servings Males 51+: 7 servings
	Meat and Alternatives	"As is"	Females 19–50: 2 servings Males 19–50: 3 servings Females 51+: 2 servings Males 51+: 3 servings
	Fats	"Consume in Moderation"	Referred to as "Oils and Fats" Include small amount 30–45 mL (2 to 3 Tbsp) of unsaturated fat each day Limit saturated and *trans* fats
Food item classification	Cheese	Classified under "Meat and Alternatives"	Classified under "Milk and Alternatives"
	Potato, Corn, Sweet Potato, Plantains	Classified under "Grains and Starches"	Classified under "Vegetables and Fruit"
	Nuts	Classified under "Fats"	Classified under "Meat and Alternatives"
	Avocado	Classified under "Fats"	Classified under "Vegetables and Fruit"

We humans are creatures of habit. We may know that our excess food consumption and lack of physical activity pose risks to our health, but that doesn't mean we will change our ways.[1] One intervention strategy takes this aspect of human nature into account and has shown promising results at the individual level: motivational interviewing (MI). The use of MI, supported by appropriate counselling, has been effective in promoting behaviour changes that lead to lower body mass indexes (BMIs).[2]

In this practice, a health care practitioner leads a patient through a set of questions to identify a patient's readiness for change, the importance of that change to the patient, and the barriers that are limiting that change. The ultimate goal is for patients to understand how they can change and why they should change, in a manner that is personally relevant to them.

The questions shown in **Figure E.1** can be tailored to more adequately address patients' individual needs. During MI, practitioners are advised to provide constructive feedback to a patient's responses and further insight regarding both the personal benefits of making healthier decisions and how patients can lower the barriers they face. Practitioners can also offer advice on ways to promote success and provide various options that a patient can choose from. A main goal of MI is to emphasize that patients have the responsibility and freedom to make healthier decisions and that they are, in fact, capable of making those changes. This information needs to be communicated in an empathetic manner that avoids judging or condemning the individual.

Open-ended questions that may be asked during a motivational interview • Figure E.1

- How ready do you feel to change your eating patterns and/or lifestyle?
- How does your current weight affect your daily life?
- How would you like your health to be different?
- What are the most important things to you? What impact does your weight have on them?
- What barriers might limit your success? (e.g., child care, transportation, distance, cost, accessibility)
- What would have to happen before you seriously decided to change?
- What strategies have you used in the past to change your eating, and what has worked?
- Some people talk about part of them wanting to change their eating/activity levels while another part doesn't want to change. Is this true for you?
- What was your life like before your weight increased?
- If you changed, what would your life be like?
- What makes you feel like you can continue to make progress if you decide to make lifestyle changes?
- What are your hopes for the future if you are able to become healthier?
- How can I or others help you succeed?
- What practical things do you need to succeed?
- What are the short-term and long-term benefits and drawbacks of making these changes?

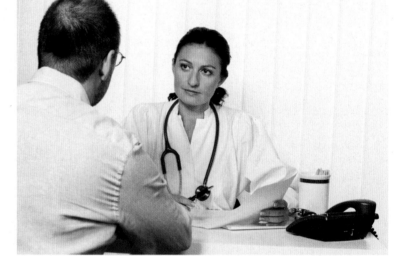

Can Stock Photo Inc./Gina Sanders

Source: Questions adapted from Yale Rudd Center for Food Policy and Obesity. Motivational interviewing for diet/exercise and obesity. Available online at ttp://www.yaleruddcenter.org/resources/bias_toolkit/toolkit/Module-2/2-07-MotivationalStrategies.pdf. Accessed March 10, 2013.

[1]Bundy, C. Changing behaviour: using motivational interviewing techniques. *J R Soc Med* 97: S43–S47, 2004.

[2]Rodin, R.L., Alexander, M.H., Guillory, V.J., et al. Physician counseling to prevent overweight in children and adolescents: American College of Preventative Medicine position statement. *J Public Health Manag Pract* 13:655–661, 2007.

While MI has successfully been used to motivate behaviour change, it is not readily available to all those who may benefit from it. For MI to be available to everyone would require training a new group of practitioners and locating facilities where MI can be carried out. Proponents of MI argue that it can be done in a few minutes following a meeting with a health care practitioner. Unfortunately, Canadian doctors may not have the time, knowledge, or skills to perform motivational interviewing for all of their clients. Also, one session may not be sufficient to properly motivate change, further increasing costs to our health care system. However, if MI can promote increased physical activity and better nutrition throughout the population, the lifestyle-related health complications suffered by Canadians would also likely decrease, as would the associated medical attention that is both expensive and time-consuming. For more information on motivational interviewing questions and strategies, visit the website for Yale University's Rudd Center for Food Policy and Obesity.[3]

[3]Yale Rudd Center for Food Policy and Obesity. *Motivational interviewing for diet/exercise and obesity*. Available online at http://www.yaleruddcenter.org/resources/bias_toolkit/toolkit/Module-2/2-07-MotivationalStrategies.pdf. Accessed March 10, 2013.

The Population Nutrient Goals from WHO

Dietary Factor	Goal (% of total energy intake, unless otherwise stated)
Total dietary fat	15–30
Saturated fatty acids (SFA)	<10
Polyunsaturated fatty acids (PUFA)	6–10
omega-6 PUFA	5–8
omega-3 PUFA	1–2
Trans fatty acids (TFA)	<1%
Monounsaturated fatty acids	(total dietary fat − [SFA + PUFA + TFA])
Total carbohydrate	55–75
Free sugars (all monosaccharides and disaccharides added during processing + monosaccharides and disaccharides present in honey, syrups, and fruit juices)	<10
Protein	10–15
Cholesterol	<300 mg/day
Sodium chloride (sodium)—salt should be iodized	<5 g/day (<2 g/day)
Vegetables and fruit	>400 g/day
Total dietary fibre (obtained from whole grain cereals, vegetables, fruit)	>25 g/day
Non-starch polysaccharides (NSP) (obtained from whole grain cereals, vegetables, fruit)	>20 g/day

Source: World Health Organization. Diet, Nutrition, and the Prevention of Chronic Diseases. WHO Technical Report Series 916, 2003. Available online at http://whqlibdoc.who.int/trs/who_trs_916.pdf. Accessed August 5, 2012.

Type of Activity	Kcalories per Hour (by body weight)				
	45 kg/ 100 lb	55 kg/ 120 lb	68 kg/ 150 lb	82 kg/ 180 lb	90 kg/ 200 lb
Aerobics, high impact	318	381	476	572	635
Aerobics, low impact	227	272	340	408	454
Backpacking, general	318	381	476	572	635
Ballroom dancing, fast (disco, folk, square)	249	299	374	449	499
Ballroom dancing, slow (waltz, foxtrot)	136	163	204	245	272
Badminton, social singles and doubles, general	204	245	306	367	408
Baseball, playing catch	113	136	170	204	227
Basketball, game, structured	363	435	544	653	726
Basketball, shooting baskets	204	245	306	367	408
Basketball, wheelchair	295	354	442	531	590
Boxing, punching bag	272	327	408	490	544
Boxing, sparring	408	490	612	735	816
Bowling	136	163	204	245	272
Calisthenics, heavy, vigorous (pushups, pullups)	363	435	544	653	726
Calisthenics, light/moderate	159	191	238	286	318
Circuit training, general	363	435	544	653	726
Cleaning, heavy (wash car, wash windows, mop)	136	163	204	245	272
Cycling, <16 km/h (<10 mph), leisurely	181	218	272	327	363
Cycling, 16–19 km/h (10–12 mph), light	272	327	408	490	544
Cycling, 19–23 km/h (12–14 mph), moderate	363	435	544	653	726
Dancing, general	204	245	306	367	408
Fencing	272	327	408	490	544
Fishing, general	136	163	204	245	272
Football, competition	408	490	612	735	816
Football, playing catch	113	136	170	204	227
Golf, pulling clubs	227	272	340	408	454
Golf, using power cart	159	191	238	286	318
Gymnastics, general	181	218	272	327	363
Hacky sack	181	218	272	327	363
Handball, general	544	653	816	980	1,089
Hiking, cross country	272	327	408	490	544
Horseback riding, trotting	295	354	442	531	590
Ice hockey	363	435	544	653	726
Ice or in-line skating, general	318	381	476	572	635
Ice or in-line skating, speed, competition	680	816	1,021	1,225	1,361
Jai alai	544	653	816	980	1,089

Continued

Type of Activity	Kcalories per Hour (by body weight)				
	45 kg/ 100 lb	55 kg/ 120 lb	68 kg/ 150 lb	82 kg/ 180 lb	90 kg/ 200 lb
Jog/walk combination	272	327	408	490	544
Jumping rope, moderate, general	454	544	680	816	907
Kayaking	227	272	340	408	454
Mowing lawn, general	249	299	374	449	499
Playing with children, heavy (walk/run)	227	272	340	408	454
Playing with children, light (standing)	127	152	191	229	254
Racquetball, casual, general	318	381	476	572	635
Rowing or canoeing, 6.4–10 km/h (4.0–5.9 mph)	318	381	476	572	635
Running, 12 km/h (7.5 mph)	567	680	850	1,021	1,134
Running, 14 km/h (8.6 mph)	635	762	953	1,143	1,270
Running, 16 km/h (10 mph)	726	871	1,089	1,306	1,451
Sailing, Sunfish/Laser/Hobie Cat, keel boat, ocean	136	163	204	245	272
Skateboarding	227	272	340	408	454
Skiing, cross country, vigorous downhill	363	435	544	653	726
Skiing, downhill, moderate effort	272	327	408	490	544
Soccer, casual, general	318	381	476	572	635
Softball, fast or slow pitch	227	272	340	408	454
Surfing, body or board	136	163	204	245	272
Swimming, laps, freestyle, fast	454	544	680	816	907
Swimming, laps, freestyle, slow	363	435	544	653	726
Table tennis (ping pong)	181	218	272	327	363
Tae kwan do, judo, juijitsu, karate, kick boxing	454	544	680	816	907
Tai chi	181	218	272	327	363
Tennis, general	318	381	476	572	635
Volleyball, noncompetitive, general	136	163	204	245	272
Walking, 4 km/h (2.5 mph), firm surface	136	163	204	245	272
Walking, 6.4 km/h (4 mph), level, firm surface	227	272	340	408	454
Weight lifting, free or machine	272	327	408	490	544
Yoga, hatha	113	136	170	204	227

From N-Squared Computing. First Databank Division of the Hearst Corporation.

Weights and Measures

Measure	Abbreviation	Equivalent
1 gram	g	1000 milligrams
1 milligram	mg	1000 micrograms
1 microgram	mcg/μg	1/1000000 of a gram
1 nanogram	ng	1/1000000000 of a gram
1 picogram	pg	1/1000000000000 of a gram
1 kilogram	kg	1000 grams
		2.2 pounds
1 pound	lb.	454 grams
		16 ounces
1 teaspoon	tsp	approximately 5 grams
1 tablespoon	Tbsp	3 teaspoons
1 ounce	oz	28.4 grams
1 cup	c	8 fluid ounces
		16 tablespoons
1 pint	pt	2 cups
		16 fluid ounces
1 quart	qt	2 pints
		32 fluid ounces
1 gallon	gal	128 fluid ounces
		4 quarts
1 litre	l	1.06 quarts
		1000 millilitres
1 millilitre	mL	1000 microlitres
1 decilitre	dl	100 millilitres
1 kilocalorie	kcal, Cal	1000 calories
		4.167 kilojoules
1 kilojoule	kJ	1000 joules

Chapter 1: What's Wrong with this Diet?

What's wrong with Brandi's diet? Brandi needs to increase the variety in her diet. Not only is she choosing the same foods every day, but she is not choosing foods from all of the food groups. She doesn't eat any fruit, and her only vegetable is lettuce. Increasing the variety of her diet will ensure she is meeting her nutrient needs and consuming a variety of phytochemicals. She can still stick with a routine, but have a different type of cereal every morning, topped with a variety of fresh and dried fruit. She can have sandwiches for lunch but make them using different types of breads and different fillings. For dinner, she can try different grains and a variety of vegetables rather than always having rice and a salad. When she has a salad, she can include a variety of greens, fruit, nuts, and seeds to add nutrients, texture, and taste.

Based on this photo, what might be wrong with Loretta's diet? Loretta's diet is varied, but based on this photograph, she is short on moderation. Her portions are large. If she does not balance the calories she consumes with sufficient exercise, she will gain weight.

Chapter 2: Using Food Labels to Make Healthy Choices

Refer to the labels shown here. Are they equivalent in terms of the amounts of saturated fat and added sugar? Which has more unsaturated fat? The old fashioned oats are much lower in saturated fat, providing only 0.5 gram per serving, 3% of the Daily Value, compared with the granola's 3.5 grams of saturated fat, 18% of the Daily Value. The granola also contains 1 gram of *trans* fat, whereas the old fashioned oats have no *trans* fat. Canada's Food Guide recommends limiting both saturated fat and *trans* fat in the diet. The granola is higher in sugars at 16 grams compared with 0 gram per serving in the old fashioned oats.

Which choice provides more vitamin C? The orange juice provides more vitamin C: 120% of the Daily Value, compared with 100% of the Daily Value for the juice drink.

Other than water, what is the most abundant ingredient, by weight, in the juice drink? In the orange juice? Glucose/fructose is the most abundant ingredient (other than water) in the juice drink. In the orange juice, the most abundant ingredient is concentrated orange juice.

The added vitamin C increases the nutrient density of the juice drink, but does that make it a better choice than the orange juice? No. The juice drink provides less vitamin C than the orange juice, and it contains more total sugar, much of which has been added. The sugar in the orange juice is from the oranges used to make the juice and comes with the other nutrients and phytochemicals that are present in these oranges. These nutrients increase the nutrient density of the orange juice. The high-fructose corn syrup used to sweeten the juice drink adds nothing but calories. Some of the sugar in the juice drink comes from fruit juice concentrates, which do add nutrients, but their placement in the ingredient list tells us that, by weight, the fruit juice concentrates are present in smaller amounts than the high-fructose corn syrup.

What advice would you give Scott when choosing between more- and less-processed products? Choosing less-processed products usually means they are lower in added sugars (and salt—discussed in Chapter 8) and contain more of the nutrients present in the original plant or animal product.

Chapter 3: How Do Changes in the GI Tract Affect Health?

What effect might this side effect of medication have on his nutrition and health? If he doesn't have enough saliva, he will have difficulty swallowing and tasting his food, which will decrease the appeal of food and may reduce his food intake. Also, because saliva helps protect the teeth, he will be more likely to develop cavities.

How might her poorly fitting dentures affect the digestion and absorption of nutrients contained in the carrots? If she can't chew the carrots thoroughly, the enzymes needed to digest the carrots will not be able to access all of the carrot. As a result, carrot pieces will remain undigested and will pass through the GI tract. The vitamins and minerals contained in the undigested carrot will not be available for absorption.

How does this surgery affect the amount of fluid she needs to consume? Much of the water that enters the large intestine is absorbed there. Because most of her large intestine has been removed, she will lose much more water and will need to consume more fluid than before to prevent dehydration.

What foods should he avoid and why? He should avoid fatty foods. Bile is needed for fat absorption. Fat entering the small intestine causes the gallbladder to contract and release bile. A low-fat diet will minimize gallbladder contraction and the pain caused by the contraction.

Why can't she eat as much food as before or absorb all the nutrients from the food she eats? The surgery reduces the size of her stomach so she can consume only small amounts of food at any one time. Small meals are also necessary because the surgery bypasses the sphincter that regulates the entry of food into the small intestine. A large meal would allow too much material to enter the small intestine too rapidly, causing diarrhea. She does not absorb all the nutrients from her food because a section of the small intestine has been bypassed, reducing the area available for absorption. In addition, her smaller stomach may reduce the efficiency of both mechanical and chemical digestion in the stomach. Undigested food cannot be absorbed.

Chapter 4: Becoming Less Refined

How does her intake compare with the recommended amounts of carbohydrate and fibre? Lucia consumes more than the minimum recommended amount of carbohydrate and approximately 60% of her calories come from carbohydrates, which is within the AMDR. She consumes less than half of the recommended amount of daily fibre.

How does her intake of grains, fruits, and vegetables compare with *Eating Well with Canada's Food Guide*? Canada's Food Guide recommends she consume 6 to 7 servings of grains, half of which should be whole grains, and 7 to 8 servings of vegetables and fruit. She therefore consumes the recommended amount of grains, but only about half the recommended servings of vegetables and fruit.

Choose a combination of fruits and vegetables from this list that will add at least 13 grams of fibre to Lucia's diet. Many possible answers are correct. For example, consuming 125 mL (½ cup) of black beans, 250 mL (1 cup) of asparagus, and an apple will provide 14 grams of fibre. Another option is consuming 250 mL (1 cup) of broccoli, two kiwis, and an orange, which will provide almost 13 grams of fibre.

What are the carbohydrate pros and cons of these two choices? Neither the dried apricots nor the granola bar is a good source of fibre, as each provides only 8% of the Daily Value. The fibre in the granola bar comes from whole grain oats, the first ingredient in the list. Both choices are fairly high in sugar; 15 grams of sugars in the apricots and 11 grams in the granola bar. All of the sugar in the dried apricots comes from the fruit, whereas the sugar in the granola bar comes from added sugar (the second ingredient in the ingredient list), with smaller amounts from honey and brown sugar syrup.

Chapter 5: Improving Heart Health

Which of the factors listed above increase Tony's risk of developing cardiovascular disease? Tony has a family history of heart disease because his mother died of a heart attack before the age of 65. He is a smoker and is inactive, so his lifestyle further increases his risk. His blood pressure is elevated, and his total blood cholesterol of 5.4 mmol/L is over the recommended maximum of 5.2 mmol/L. His LDL cholesterol of 4.2 mmol/L is also above the recommended maximum of 2.6 mmol/L, and his HDL cholesterol is less than the recommended minimum 1.6 mmol/L. His triglycerides are in the healthy range.

What could he choose at his favourite fast-food restaurants to reduce his intake of saturated fat? Tony can choose a grilled chicken sandwich, which would be lower in saturated fat than a cheeseburger. A vegetarian pizza would also be lower than a triple-meat pizza. Also, a chicken taco would be lower in saturated fat than a burrito filled with beef and cheese.

Which of the following snack choices is the most heart healthy? Give two reasons. The dried fruit and nut mix is the more heart-healthy choice because nuts are a good source of monounsaturated fatty acids and low in saturated fat. A serving provides 3.5 grams of monounsaturated fat, only 1 gram of saturated fat, and no *trans* fat. The cheese sandwich crackers have 14 grams of total fat per serving, of which 3.5 grams is saturated fat, 4 grams is *trans* fat, and only 1 gram is monounsaturated fat. The cheese sandwich crackers are low in cholesterol, at only 5 mg, but the dried fruit and nut mix has no cholesterol. The dried fruit and nut mix is also a better choice when it comes to fibre, providing 2 grams of fibre per serving compared with less than 1 gram in the cheese sandwich crackers.

Chapter 6: Is a Vegetarian Diet Always Healthy?

What is the RDA for protein for someone of Jeremy's age and weight? The RDA is 0.8 grams of protein per kilogram of body weight. Jeremy weighs 70 kg; therefore, his recommended protein intake is 56 g per day (70 kg × 0.8 g/kg = 56 g).

This is a photo of Jeremy's typical lunch. Why is it high in saturated fat? Whole fat dairy products are high in total fat and saturated fat. The cheese provides about 4 grams of saturated fat per 28 grams. Therefore, the 56 grams of cheese on this sandwich would include about 8 grams of saturated fat. If butter was used to grill the sandwich, it would add about 7 grams of saturated fat per 15 mL.

Is this diet providing all the health benefits of a vegetarian diet? No. Jeremy may not be eating meat, but he is consuming many high-fat dairy products. Since these are animal products, they are likely high in saturated fat and cholesterol. His diet is also low in fruits and vegetables. He eats cereal for breakfast, which might be a whole grain, but the pizza or lasagna he has for dinner is probably not made with whole grains. So, he is not benefiting from a high intake of whole grains, fruits, and vegetables, and the low saturated fat and cholesterol content typical of a healthy vegetarian diet.

What could be included in Jeremy's vegan diet to meet his needs for calcium and vitamin D? To increase his calcium intake, Jeremy could eat more leafy green vegetables and legumes, which are a good source of calcium. He can also use calcium-fortified products, such as orange juice, soy milk, and breakfast cereal. To ensure he gets enough vitamin D, he could spend plenty of time outdoors in the sun to boost vitamin D synthesis in his skin and eat breakfast cereal and soy milk fortified with vitamin D.

Suggest a sandwich Jeremy could have for lunch that makes use of complementary plant proteins. Peanut butter (legumes) and bread (grains) provide complementary proteins. Another option is spreading bread with hummus, which is made from chickpeas (a legume).

Chapter 7: How Much Vitamin A Is in Your Fast-Food Meal?

Which of the meals shown here is higher in vitamin A? Which ingredients are sources of vitamin A? The pizza is higher in vitamin A because it has cheese, which is a source of preformed vitamin A, and tomato sauce, tomatoes, and peppers, which provide provitamin A. The beef, bun, and fries in the other meal are all poor sources of vitamin A.

How could John change his breakfast and lunch so they are higher in vitamin A? John can boost his provitamin A intake by adding a carotenoid-rich fruit, such as cantaloupe, mango, or apricots, to his breakfast. He can increase his intake of preformed vitamin A by replacing the pop he has at lunch with a glass of milk. He can add some high-carotenoid vegetables to his lunch. For example, he can add sweet red peppers and spinach to his sandwich and take a bag of baby carrots to snack on.

John's meals are also low in vitamin C. What can he add to his breakfast and lunch to increase his intake of vitamin C? The key to increasing vitamin C intake is increasing fruit and vegetable intake. Adding fruits such as strawberries or a glass of orange juice at breakfast and an orange or kiwis at lunch will add vitamin C. Including some sliced sweet peppers or raw broccoli florets with his lunch will provide a vegetable source of vitamin C.

Chapter 8: Avoiding Anemia

What puts Jodie at risk for iron deficiency anemia? Jodie is a lacto-ovo vegetarian so she does not consume highly absorbable heme iron. She is a menstruating female so her iron losses are high.

What does the blood test reveal about Jodie's iron status? Is her tiredness due to iron deficiency anemia? Why or why not? The blood test results show that Jodie's iron stores are depleted and the iron levels in her plasma are low. Because the amount of iron in her red blood cells is normal, her symptoms of tiredness are not due to iron deficiency anemia.

Name three dietary factors that put Jodie at risk for iron deficiency. Jodie's overall iron intake is low, and she consumes only non-heme iron, which is poorly absorbed. Her diet is high in whole grains, which reduce iron absorption because they are high in phytates. Also, she drinks a lot of tea, which is high in tannins, which inhibit iron absorption.

What can Jodie do to increase the absorption of the non-heme iron in her diet? Jodie can include a source of vitamin C, such as an orange, with meals that contain iron.

Chapter 9: Balancing Energy: Genetics and Lifestyle

What is her BMI? Is it in the healthy range? What does BMI not tell us? Lucia is 163 cm (5′4″) tall and weighs 70 kg (155 lb.):

Her BMI is equal to 70 kg ÷ (1.63 m)^2 = 26.3 kg/m^2, which is in the overweight range. Her BMI does not tell us how healthy her body composition is.

What is her EER? Lucia is 1.63 m (5′4″) tall and weighs 70 kg (155 lb.):

Lucia is in the low active activity category, so PA = 1.12

Using the equation in Table 9.1 Lucia's EER is equal to:

EER = 354 − (6.91 × 23 yrs) + 1.12 [(9.36 × 70 kg) + (726 × 1.63 m)] = 2,254 kilocalories

Note: This answer uses the EER equations in Table 9.1. Because Lucia is overweight, it is more accurate to use the equations in Appendix A for calculating the total energy expenditure of individuals who are overweight or obese:

TEE = 448 − (7.95 × 23 yrs) + 1.16 [(11.4 × 70.4 kg) + (619 × 1.63 m)] = 2,367 kilocalories

How does Lucia's EER compare with her intake? Is she in energy balance? Lucia consumes about 2,450 kilocalories per day but is expending only 2,254 kilocalories per day, so she is not in energy balance. She is consuming 196 kilocalories per day more than she is expending.

How can Meal B have fewer calories even though it looks like more food? The meal on the left is much higher is fat (9 kilocalories/gram), making it more energy dense. The vegetables in the sandwich and the fruit in the meal on the right are high in fibre and water, which add bulk and volume to the meal, but provide few calories.

Why might Meal B satisfy hunger just as well as or better than Meal A? The high fat content of the meal on the left provides satiety. In the meal on the right, the fibre in the whole grain bread and the fibre and fluid in the apple and vegetables help fill up the stomach and provide satiety.

If Lucia adds an additional 30 minutes of moderate-intensity exercise every day, by how much will her EER increase? This exercise will boost Lucia into the active physical activity category, and her EER will increase as follows:

EER = 354 − (6.91 × 23 yrs) + 1.27 [(9.36 × 70 kg) + (726 × 1.63 m)] = 2,530 kilocalories

If the equation from Appendix A for calculating the total energy expenditure of individuals who are overweight or obese is used:

TEE = 448 − (7.95 × 23 yrs) + 1.27 [(11.4 × 70 kg) + (619 × 1.63 m)] = 2,560 kilocalories

Do you think Lucia is destined to be overweight? Explain your answer. Lucia is not destined to be overweight, but to maintain her weight in a healthy range she probably needs to monitor her energy intake more carefully and to exercise more than an individual with no genetic tendency to store excess body fat. If she makes changes in her diet and exercise patterns that she can stick with, she is more likely to succeed.

Chapter 10: What Are You Getting from That Sports Bar?

What are the advantages and disadvantages of sports bars? The biggest advantage of sports bars is their convenience. They are pre-portioned, ready to eat, and transportable. They may also provide a psychological edge if the consumer believes consuming them will enhance performance. A disadvantage is that they are expensive and do not provide everything you get from food. The overall quality of the diet may suffer if sports bars take the place of the whole grains, fresh vegetables and fruits, low-fat dairy products, and lean meats or meat substitutes that make up a healthy diet. They also don't provide fluid—an essential during any activity. If you choose to consume sports bars, wash them down with plenty of water. They do provide calories, generally about 200 to 300 per bar. Even though they are eaten to support activity, they still add to your overall energy intake and can contribute to weight gain if consumed in excess.

Based on the labels shown here, how do sports bars differ from chocolate bars? Typically, sports bars are lower in total fat, saturated fat, cholesterol, and sugar; higher in fibre and protein; and contain more vitamins and minerals than chocolate bars.

Suggest a snack for Brad that is nutritionally comparable to a sports bar but less expensive. Some less pricey options are granola or cereal bars, fruit-filled cookies, fresh or dried fruit, a sandwich, a bagel, and trail mix.

Chapter 11: Nutrient Needs for a Successful Pregnancy

Based on the graph below, how much weight would you recommend that Erin gain? Why would gaining only 9 kg (20 lb.) or as much as 23 kg (50 lb.) put the baby at risk? The graph illustrates that the incidence of low-birth-weight babies increases as maternal weight gain decreases, but as maternal weight gain increases the incidence of large-for-gestational-age babies increases. Based on this graph, to minimize having a high- or low-birth-weight baby, Erin should gain between 9 and 16 kilograms (20 and 35 lb.).

How should the amounts of food from each food group be changed so that Erin meets her needs during the second trimester of her pregnancy? Based on Erin's age, *Eating Well with Canada's Food Guide* recommends that she consume 7 to 8 servings of vegetables and fruit, 6 to 7 servings of grain products, 2 servings of milk or milk alternatives and 2 servings of meat or meat alternatives. For her age group, she consumes enough meat and meat alternatives, and milk and milk alternatives, but she should consume another 2 to 3 servings of grains and 2 to 3 servings of vegetables and fruits to meet basic recommendations. Since she is also pregnant, Canada's Food Guide recommends an additional 2 to 3 servings of food per day. While Canada's Food Guide does not specify which groups these servings should come from, she should ensure that her choices are nutrient dense and are from more than one food group.

Suggest some foods that Erin can include in her diet so she consumes an additional 13.5 mg of iron. Red meat is the best source of absorbable heme iron. Fortified breakfast cereals, legumes, and leafy greens are good sources of non-heme iron.

Is it reasonable for Erin to consume 27 mg of iron each day from her diet alone? Why or why not? No, it is not reasonable to consume that much iron from diet alone. Even if she chose all of the foods listed above in one day, she would still not consume enough.

Chapter 12: Undernutrition and Overnutrition

Based on this growth chart, how has Luke's BMI percentile changed over the past year? Luke's BMI has gone from about the 65th percentile to the 87th percentile in just a few months. The increase in BMI indicates that his weight gain was not accompanied by a corresponding increase in height. This weight gain moves Luke from the healthy weight range into the overweight range.

What nutrients are likely to be excessive or deficient in Luke's dietary pattern? The diet is high in added sugar and fat from the doughnuts, candy, and chips he consumes. The whole milk Luke drinks adds calcium, total fat, saturated fat, and cholesterol. His intake from all the food groups except milk and possibly grains is low so he is likely to consume less than the recommended amounts of vitamin C, vitamin A, and iron.

Why might excessive consumption of dairy products contribute to Luke's anemia? Calcium interferes with iron absorption. Luke seems to have milk with every meal. The calcium in the milk he drinks reduces his body's absorption of the iron in his meals.

How might Luke's iron deficiency have contributed to his weight gain? Iron deficiency causes fatigue and lethargy, which would have caused a decrease in his activity level, shifting his energy balance toward weight gain.

Chapter 13: Food Detectives

Based on the graph, which food is the most likely cause of the illness? Why? The frozen custard is most likely to be the cause because of all the foods, more people who ate the custard became ill.

How can eggs become contaminated with *Salmonella*? The outside of the eggs can become contaminated with *Salmonella* when it comes in contact with fecal material in the chicken coop. The inside of the egg can be contaminated with *Salmonella* before the shell is formed if the hen is infected with *Salmonella*. Therefore, raw eggs can cause *Salmonella* food-borne illness even if the shell is clean.

The cookie and cupcake recipes also called for eggs. Why are these unlikely to be the cause of the problem? After the eggs were added, both of these foods were cooked at temperatures high enough to kill the bacteria.

Suggest a reason why 20 children who consumed the frozen custard did not get ill. The children who did not become ill may have consumed smaller amounts of custard. Their immune systems may be stronger than the other children's. Also, they may have been larger children. More bacteria is needed to make a larger person ill than a smaller person.

What could the fourth-graders have done to avoid the risk of *Salmonella* in their frozen custard? They could have used an ice cream recipe that did not call for eggs, or they could have used pasteurized liquid eggs instead of whole eggs from the shell.

Chapter 14: What Can You Do?

What are the advantages and disadvantages of these salad options in terms of convenience, food safety, and environmental impact? The prepackaged lettuce in the grocery store is more convenient. It is pre-washed and just needs to be poured into a bowl. The disadvantage is that once opened, it deteriorates more quickly. Also, more energy is used to produce the prepackaged salad, and it generates plastic waste from the bags. The unpackaged produce requires more washing and other preparation to make a salad but consumes fewer of the earth's resources.

The following are some inexpensive changes Jean-Paul can make to reduce his impact on the environment. What are the advantages and disadvantages of each?

Action	Advantages	Disadvantages
Bike instead of drive on short trips around town.	Uses no gas so saves money, reduces fossil fuel use, reduces pollution, and increases Jean-Paul's fitness level.	Difficult to carry heavy or bulky items, more time required for each errand.
Buy a canvas bag to carry groceries.	Reduces the number of plastic grocery bags that must be disposed of.	Small monetary cost of the bags.
Pack juice in a thermos instead of buying it in a nonrecyclable bottle.	Reduces the amount of material that ends up in landfills, saves money because juice can be purchased in more economical sizes and packaged down.	Must be washed after each use, requiring time and using energy to heat water and generating waste water.
Compost vegetable scraps.	Reduces the amount of material that ends up in landfills and generates fertile material that can be added to a garden.	Cost and time needed to set up and maintain a composting bin.
Buy locally grown produce.	Contains fewer pesticides. Likely to be fresher because it is purchased soon after harvest.	Limited variety. Not everything is available at all times of the year.
Buy organically grown produce.	Reduces the pesticides on food. Reduces the environmental damage associated with food production.	Costs more. Occasionally has more insect damage.

Chapter 1:
1. b; 2. d; 3. a; 4. b; 5. c; 6. c; 7. d; 8. a; 9. d; 10. d; 11. a; 12. c; 13. c; 14. b; 15. a

Chapter 2:
1. d; 2. c; 3. d; 4. a; 5. b; 6. d; 7. a; 8. c; 9. b; 10. c; 11. e; 12. a; 13. b; 14. d; 15. c

Chapter 3:
1. c; 2. e; 3. a; 4. d; 5. c; 6. c; 7. b; 8. a; 9. c; 10. b; 11. c; 12. b; 13. c; 14. a; 15. b

Chapter 4:
1. c; 2. b; 3. b; 4. a; 5. d; 6. b; 7. b; 8. d; 9. c; 10. c; 11. b; 12. a; 13. a; 14. a; 15. d

Chapter 5:
1. d; 2. d; 3. a; 4. e; 5. d; 6. b; 7. c; 8. e; 9. e; 10. e; 11. c; 12. a; 13. c; 14. a; 15. a

Chapter 6:
1. d; 2. a; 3. c; 4. e; 5. a; 6. b; 7. c; 8. a; 9. b; 10. d; 11. c; 12. b; 13. d; 14. b; 15. a

Chapter 7:
1. d; 2. a; 3. b; 4. c; 5. d; 6. d; 7. c; 8. e; 9. a; 10. c; 11. b; 12. c; 13. e; 14. b; 15. c

Chapter 8:
1. d; 2. e; 3. b; 4. e; 5. d; 6. a; 7. b; 8. a; 9. c; 10. e; 11. b; 12. e; 13. b; 14. a; 15. c

Chapter 9:
1. b; 2. e; 3. a; 4. d; 5. e; 6. d; 7. d; 8. c; 9. b; 10. c; 11.a; 12. b; 13. b; 14. e; 15. b

Chapter 10:
1. a; 2. e; 3. d; 4. a; 5. a; 6. b; 7. c; 8. b; 9. a; 10. d; 11. a; 12. c; 13. a; 14. b

Chapter 11:
1. d; 2. d; 3. c; 4. b; 5. a; 6. a; 7. a; 8. b; 9. d; 10. b; 11. a; 12. c; 13. b; 14. c; 15. c

Chapter 12:
1. d; 2. d; 3. a; 4. c; 5. d; 6. b; 7. e; 8. c; 9. a; 10. b; 11. a; 12. c; 13. c; 14. c; 15. b

Chapter 13:
1. b; 2. e; 3. b; 4. a; 5. c; 6. b; 7. b; 8. c; 9. a; 10. c; 11. b; 12. d; 13. c; 14. a; 15. b

Chapter 14:
1. d; 2. c; 3. a; 4. d; 5. c; 6. c; 7. d; 8. b; 9. c; 10. b; 11. a; 12. b; 13. a; 14. d; 15. c.

Glossary

absorption The process of taking substances from the gastrointestinal tract into the interior of the body.

Acceptable Macronutrient Distribution Ranges (AMDRs) Healthy ranges of intake for carbohydrate, fat, and protein, expressed as percentages of total energy intake.

active transport The transport of substances across a cell membrane with the aid of a protein carrier and the expenditure of energy.

adenosine triphosphate (ATP) A high-energy molecule that the body uses to power activities that require energy.

Adequate Intakes (AIs) Nutrient intakes that should be used as a goal when no RDA exists. AI values are an approximation of the nutrient intake that sustains health.

adipocytes Cells that store fat.

adjustable gastric banding A surgical procedure in which an adjustable band is placed around the upper portion of the stomach to limit the volume that the stomach can hold and the rate of stomach emptying.

aerobic capacity The maximum amount of oxygen that can be consumed by the tissues during exercise. Also called *maximal oxygen consumption*, or *VO₂ max*.

aerobic exercise Endurance exercise that increases heart rate and uses oxygen to produce energy as ATP.

aerobic metabolism Metabolism in the presence of oxygen. It can completely break down glucose to yield carbon dioxide, water, and energy in the form of ATP.

age-related bone loss The bone loss that occurs in both men and women as they advance in age.

aging The inevitable accumulation of changes associated with and responsible for an ever-increasing susceptibility to disease and death.

alcoholic hepatitis Inflammation of the liver caused by alcohol consumption.

allergen A substance that causes an allergic reaction.

Alzheimer's disease A disease that results in a relentless and irreversible loss of mental function.

amenorrhea Delayed onset of menstruation or the absence of three or more consecutive menstrual cycles.

amino acid pool All the amino acids in body tissues and fluids that are available for use by the body.

amino acids The building blocks of proteins. Each contains an amino group, an acid group, and a unique side chain.

anabolic steroids Synthetic fat-soluble hormones that mimic testosterone and are used to increase muscle strength and mass.

anaerobic metabolism Metabolism in the absence of oxygen.

anorexia nervosa An eating disorder typically characterized by self-starvation, a distorted body image, and abnormally low body weight.

antibodies Proteins, released by a type of lymphocyte, that interact with antigens and promote the removal of foreign invaders from the body.

antigen A protein found on disease-causing agents that identifies them as foreign from the body's cells. When introduced into the body, it stimulates an immune response.

antioxidants Substances that are able to neutralize reactive oxygen molecules and thereby prevent cell damage.

appetite The *psychological* drive to consume food that is independent of hunger.

arthritis A disease characterized by inflammation of the joints, pain, and sometimes changes in structure.

aseptic processing The placement of sterilized food in a sterilized package using a sterile process.

atherosclerosis A type of cardiovascular disease that involves the buildup of fatty material in the artery walls.

atherosclerotic plaque Cholesterol-rich material that is deposited in the arteries of individuals with atherosclerosis. It consists of cholesterol, smooth muscle cells, fibrous tissue, and eventually calcium.

atoms The smallest units of an element that retain the properties of the element.

ATP (adenosine triphosphate) A high-energy molecule that the body uses to power activities that require energy.

atrophic gastritis An inflammation of the stomach lining that results in reduced secretion of stomach acid, microbial overgrowth, and, in severe cases, a reduction in the production of intrinsic factor.

attention-deficit/hyperactivity disorder (ADHD) A condition characterized by a short attention span and a high level of activity, excitability, and distractibility.

autoimmune disease A disease that results from immune reactions that destroy normal body cells.

basal metabolic rate (BMR) The rate of energy expenditure under resting conditions. It is measured after 12 hours without food or exercise.

basal metabolism The energy expended to maintain an awake, resting body that is not digesting food or being physically active.

beriberi A thiamin deficiency disease that causes weakness, nerve degeneration, and, in some cases, heart changes.

bile A digestive fluid made in the liver and stored in the gallbladder that is released into the small intestine, where it aids in fat digestion and absorption.

binge-eating disorder An eating disorder characterized by recurrent episodes of binge eating in the absence of compensatory behaviour such as purging or over-exercising.

bioaccumulation The process by which compounds accumulate or build up in an organism faster than they can be broken down or excreted.

bioavailability The extent to which the body can absorb and use a nutrient.

biotechnology The process of manipulating life forms via genetic engineering for the purpose of providing desirable products for human use.

blood pressure The amount of force exerted by the blood against the walls of arteries.

body image The way a person perceives and imagines his or her body.

body mass index (BMI) A measure of body weight relative to height that is used to compare body size with a standard.

bone remodelling A continuous process in which small amounts of bone are removed and replaced by new bone.

bulimia nervosa An eating disorder characterized by the consumption of a large amount of food at one time (binge eating) followed by purging behaviours such as self-induced vomiting to prevent weight gain.

calorie A unit of measure used to express the amount of energy provided by food. 1 kilocalorie = 1 Calorie = 1,000 calories.

capillaries Small, thin-walled blood vessels through which blood and the body's cells exchange gases and nutrients.

carbohydrates A class of nutrients that includes sugars, starches, and fibres. Chemically, they all contain carbon, hydrogen, and oxygen, in the same proportions as in water (H_2O).

cardiorespiratory endurance The efficiency with which the body delivers to cells the oxygen and nutrients needed for muscular activity and transports waste products from cells.

carotenoids Natural pigments synthesized by plants and many microorganisms. They give yellow and red-orange fruits and vegetables their colour.

cash crops Crops that are grown to be sold for monetary return rather than as food for the local population.

cataracts A disease of the eye that results in cloudy spots on the lens (and sometimes the cornea) that obscure vision.

celiac disease A disorder that causes damage to the intestines when the protein gluten is eaten.

cells The basic structural and functional units of living things.

cholesterol A sterol produced by the liver and consumed in the diet that is needed to build cell membranes and make hormones and other essential molecules. High blood levels increase the risk of heart disease.

chronic diseases Long-term diseases such as heart disease or obesity that often negatively affect physical and mental health and increase risk of early mortality.

chylomicrons Lipoproteins that transport lipids from the mucosal cells of the small intestine and deliver triglycerides to other body cells.

cirrhosis Chronic and irreversible liver disease characterized by loss of functioning liver cells and accumulation of fibrous connective tissue.

coenzymes Organic non-protein substances that bind to enzymes to promote their activity.

cofactors Inorganic ions or coenzymes that are required for enzyme activity.

colostrum The first milk, produced by the breast late in pregnancy and for up to a week after delivery. Compared with mature milk, it contains less fat and more water, protein, immune factors, minerals, and vitamins.

condensation A reaction in which two structural units combine to create a larger molecule, typically resulting in the loss of a water molecule.

control group In a scientific experiment, the group of participants used as a basis of comparison. They are similar to the participants in the experimental group but do not receive the treatment being tested.

creatine phosphate A compound stored in muscle that can be broken down quickly to make ATP.

cretinism A condition resulting from poor maternal iodine intake during pregnancy that impairs mental development and growth in the offspring.

cross-contamination The transfer of contaminants from one food or object to another.

Daily Value A reference value for the intake of nutrients used on food labels to help consumers see how a given food fits into their overall diet.

dehydration A state that occurs when not enough water is present to meet the body's needs.

dementia A deterioration of mental state that results in impaired memory, thinking, and/or judgement.

denaturation Alteration of a protein's three-dimensional structure.

diabetes mellitus A disease characterized by elevated blood glucose due to either insufficient production of insulin or decreased sensitivity of cells to insulin.

dietary supplements Products sold to supplement the diet; may include nutrients (vitamins, minerals, amino acids, fatty acids), enzymes, herbs, or other substances.

digestion The process by which food is broken down into components small enough to be absorbed into the blood stream.

direct food additives Substances intentionally added to foods. Their use is regulated by Health Canada.

disaccharide A carbohydrate made up of two sugar units.

diuretic A substance that increases the amount of urine passed from the body.

diverticulosis A condition in which outpouches (or sacs) form in the wall of the large intestine.

eating disorder A psychological illness characterized by specific abnormal eating behaviours, often intended to control weight.

eclampsia Convulsions or seizures brought on by seriously high blood pressure during pregnancy (preeclampsia). Untreated, it can lead to coma or death.

eicosanoids Regulatory molecules that can be synthesized from omega-3 and omega-6 fatty acids.

electrolytes Positively and negatively charged ions that conduct an electrical current in solution. Commonly refers to sodium, potassium, and chloride.

embryo The developing human from two through eight weeks after fertilization.

empty calories Energy with few additional nutrients.

endorphins Compounds that cause a natural euphoria and reduce the perception of pain under certain stressful conditions.

energy balance The amount of energy consumed in the diet compared with the amount of energy expended by the body over a given period.

enrichment The addition of specific amounts of thiamin, riboflavin, niacin, and iron to refined grains. Since 1998, folic acid has also been added to enriched grains.

enzymes Protein molecules that accelerate the rate of specific chemical reactions without being changed themselves.

epidemiology The branch of science that studies health and disease trends and patterns in populations. In epidemiological studies, observations are made without the manipulation of variable.

epiglottis A piece of elastic connective tissue that covers the opening to the lungs during swallowing.

ergogenic aid A substance, appliance, or procedure that improves athletic performance.

essential amino acids or **indispensable amino acids** Amino acids that cannot be synthesized by the body in sufficient amounts to meet its needs and therefore must be included in the diet.

essential fatty acids Fatty acids that must be consumed in the diet because they cannot be made by the body or cannot be made in sufficient quantities to meet needs.

essential nutrients Nutrients that the body cannot make itself and, as a result, humans must consume to maintain health.

Estimated Average Requirements (EARs) Nutrient intakes estimated to meet the needs of 50% of the healthy individuals in a given gender and life-stage group.

Estimated Energy Requirements (EERs) Average energy intake values predicted to maintain body weight in healthy individuals.

ethanol The alcohol in alcoholic beverages; it is produced by yeast fermentation of sugar.

experimental group In a scientific experiment, the group of participants who undergo the treatment being tested.

facilitated diffusion The assisted diffusion of a substance across the cell membrane with the help of a protein carrier.

failure to thrive Inability of a child's growth to keep up with normal growth curves.

famine A widespread lack of access to food due to a disaster that causes a collapse in the food production and marketing systems.

fatigue The inability to continue an activity at an optimal level.

fatty acids Molecules made up of a chain of carbons linked to hydrogen, with an acid group at one end of the chain.

feces Body waste, including unabsorbed food residue, bacteria, mucus, and dead cells, which is eliminated from the gastro-intestinal tract by way of the anus.

fertilization The union of a sperm and an egg.

fetal alcohol syndrome (FAS) A characteristic group of physical and mental abnormalities in an infant resulting from maternal alcohol consumption during pregnancy.

fetus A developing human from the ninth week after fertilization to birth.

fibre A type of carbohydrate that cannot be digested by human enzymes.

fitness A set of attributes related to the ability to perform routine physical activities without undue fatigue.

fluorosis A condition caused by chronic overconsumption of fluoride, characterized by black and brown stains and cracking and pitting of the teeth.

folic acid An easily absorbed form of the vitamin folate that is present in dietary supplements and fortified foods.

food additive A substance that is intentionally added to or can reasonably be expected to become a component of a food during processing.

food allergy An adverse immune response to a specific food protein.

food-borne illness An illness caused by consumption of contaminated food.

food insecurity A situation in which people lack adequate physical, social, or economic access to sufficient, safe, nutritious food that meets their dietary needs.

food intolerance or **food sensitivity** An adverse reaction to a food that does not involve the production of antibodies by the immune system.

fortification The addition of nutrients to foods.

fortified foods Foods to which one or more nutrients have been added.

free radicals One type of highly reactive atom or molecule that causes oxidative damage.

functional foods Foods that have health-promoting and/or disease-preventing properties beyond basic nutritional functions.

gastric bypass A surgical procedure that reduces the size of the stomach and bypasses a portion of the small intestine.

gastroesophageal reflux disease (GERD) A chronic condition in which acidic stomach contents leak into the esophagus, causing pain and damaging the esophagus.

gene A length of DNA that contains the information needed to synthesize a specific polypeptide chain; responsible for inherited traits.

gene expression The events of protein synthesis in which the information coded in a gene is used to synthesize a protein.

genetic engineering A set of techniques used to manipulate DNA for the purpose of changing the characteristics of an organism or creating a new product.

gestational diabetes A condition characterized by high blood glucose levels that develop during pregnancy.

glucagon A hormone made in the pancreas that raises blood glucose levels by stimulating the breakdown of liver glycogen and the synthesis of glucose.

glucose A six-carbon monosaccharide that is the primary form of carbohydrate used to provide energy in the body.

glutathione peroxidase A selenium-containing enzyme that protects cells from oxidative damage by neutralizing peroxides.

glycemic response The rate, magnitude, and duration of the rise in blood glucose that occurs after food is consumed.

glycogen The storage form of carbohydrate in animals, made up of many glucose molecules linked together in a highly branched structure.

glycogen super-compensation or **carbohydrate loading** A regimen designed to increase muscle glycogen stores beyond their usual capacity.

glycolysis An anaerobic metabolic pathway that splits glucose into two three-carbon pyruvate molecules; the energy released from one glucose molecule is used to make two molecules of ATP.

goiter An enlargement of the thyroid gland caused by a deficiency of iodine.

Hazard Analysis Critical Control Point (HACCP) A food safety system that focuses on identifying and preventing hazards that could cause food-borne illness.

healthy weight The weight that minimizes health risks and promotes overall health.

heartburn A burning sensation in the chest or throat caused when acidic stomach contents leak back into the esophagus.

heat-related illnesses Health conditions, including heat cramps, heat exhaustion, and heat stroke, that can occur due to an unfavourable combination of exercise, hydration status, and climatic conditions.

heme iron A readily absorbable form of iron that is chemically associated with certain proteins and is found in meat, fish, and poultry.

hemochromatosis An inherited disorder that results in increased iron absorption.

high-density lipoproteins (HDL) Lipoproteins that pick up cholesterol from cells and transport it to the liver so that it can be eliminated from the body. They are not consumed from the diet; they are made by the body.

hormones A *physiological* desire to consume food that is triggered by internal physiological signals or the recurrent involuntary lack of food that over time may lead to malnutrition.

hydrogenation A process whereby hydrogen atoms are added to the carbon–carbon double bonds of unsaturated fatty acids, making them more saturated.

hydrolysis A reaction that uses water to break down larger molecules into their structural units.

hypercarotenemia A condition caused by the accumulation of carotenoids in the adipose tissue, causing the skin to appear yellow-orange.

hypertension Blood pressure that is consistently elevated to 140/90 mm mercury or greater.

hypoglycemia Abnormally low blood glucose levels.

hypotheses Proposed explanations for an observation or a scientific problem that can be tested through experimentation.

implantation The process through which a developing embryo embeds itself in the uterine lining.

indirect food additives Substances that are expected to unintentionally enter foods during manufacturing or from packaging.

infant mortality rate The number of deaths during the first year of life, typically expressed per 1,000 live births.

insoluble fibre Fibre that, for the most part, does not dissolve in water and cannot be broken down by bacteria in the large intestine. Insoluble fibre includes cellulose, some hemicelluloses, and lignin, which can all be found in the cell walls of plants.

insulin A hormone made in the pancreas that allows glucose to enter cells, where it stimulates the synthesis of protein, fat, and liver and muscle glycogen.

integrated pest management (IPM) A method of agricultural pest control that integrates nonchemical and chemical techniques.

intrinsic factor A protein produced in the stomach that is needed for the absorption of adequate amounts of vitamin B12.

iodized salt Table salt to which a small amount of sodium iodide or potassium iodide has been added for the purpose of supplementing the iodine content of the diet.

ions Atoms or groups of atoms that carry an electrical charge.

irradiation A process that exposes foods to radiation for the purpose of killing contaminating organisms and retarding the ripening and spoilage of fruits and vegetables.

ketones or **ketone bodies** Acidic molecules formed when the body has insufficient carbohydrate to completely metabolize the acetyl CoA produced from fatty acid breakdown.

ketosis High levels of ketones in the blood.

kwashiorkor A form of protein-energy malnutrition in which only protein is deficient.

lactation Production and secretion of milk.

lacteals Lymph vessels in the villi of the small intestine that pick up particles containing the products of fat digestion.

lactose intolerance The inability to digest lactose due to a reduction in the levels of the enzyme lactase.

large for gestational age Weighing more than 4 kg (8.8 lb.) at birth.

lean body mass Body mass attributed to nonfat body components such as bone, muscle, and internal organs. Also called *fat-free mass*.

legumes The starchy seeds of plants that produce bean pods, including peas, peanuts, beans, soybeans, and lentils.

let-down The release of milk from the milk-producing glands and its movement through the ducts and storage sinuses.

life expectancy The average length of life for a particular population of individuals.

life span The maximum age to which members of a species can live.

limiting amino acid The essential amino acid that is available in the lowest concentration relative to the body's needs.

lipids A class of nutrients often referred to as fats. Chemically, they contain carbon, hydrogen, and oxygen, and most do not dissolve in water. They include fatty acids, triglycerides, phospholipids, and sterols.

lipoproteins Particles that transport lipids in the blood.

low birth weight A birth weight less than 2.5 kg (5.5 lb.).

low-density lipoproteins (LDLs) Lipoproteins that transport cholesterol to cells. They are not consumed from the diet; they are made by the body.

macrocytic anemia or **megaloblastic anemia** A reduction in the blood's capacity to carry oxygen that is characterized by abnormally large immature and mature red blood cells.

macular degeneration Degeneration of a portion of the retina that results in loss of visual detail and eventually in blindness.

major minerals Minerals that are required in the diet in amounts greater than 100 mg/day or are present in the body in amounts greater than 0.01% of body weight.

malnutrition A condition resulting from an energy or nutrient intake either above or below that which is optimal.

marasmus A form of protein-energy malnutrition in which a deficiency of energy in the diet causes severe body wasting.

maximum heart rate The maximum number of beats per minute that the heart can attain.

menopause The time in a woman's life when the menstrual cycle ends.

micelles Particles that are formed in the small intestine when the products of fat digestion are surrounded by bile. They are an aggregation of lipid molecules as a droplet that facilitates the absorption of lipids.

microbes Microscopic organisms, or microorganisms, including bacteria, viruses, and fungi.

minerals In nutrition, elements needed by the body in small amounts to maintain structure and regulate chemical reactions and body processes.

modified atmosphere packaging (MAP) A preservation technique used to prolong the shelf life of processed or fresh food by changing the gases surrounding the food in the package.

molecules Units of two or more atoms of the same or different elements bonded together.

monosaccharide A carbohydrate made up of a single sugar unit.

mould Multicellular fungi that form filamentous branching growths.

mucus A viscous fluid secreted by glands in the digestive tract and other parts of the body. It lubricates, moistens, and protects cells from harsh environments.

muscle endurance The ability of a muscle group to continue muscle movement at a sub-maximal intensity over time.

muscle strength The amount of force that can be produced by a single contraction of a muscle.

neural tube defects Abnormalities in the brain or spinal cord that result from errors that occur during prenatal development.

neurotransmitter A chemical substance produced by a nerve cell that can stimulate or inhibit another cell.

nitrogen balance The amount of nitrogen consumed in the diet compared with the amount excreted over a given period.

nonexercise activity thermogenesis (NEAT) The energy expended for everything we do other than sleeping, eating, or sports-like exercise.

nutrient density A measure of the nutrients provided by a food relative to its calorie content.

nutrients Substances in food that humans need to live and grow. They provide energy and structure to the body and regulate body processes.

nutrition transition A series of changes in diet, physical activity, health, and nutrition that occurs as poor countries become more prosperous.

nutritional genomics or **nutrigenomics** The study of how diet affects our genes and how individual genetic variation can affect the impact of nutrients or other food components on health.

nutritional status An individual's health, as it is influenced by the intake and utilization of nutrients.

obese Having excess body fat. Obesity is defined as having a body mass index (ratio of weight to height squared) of 30 kg/m^2 or greater.

obesogenic environment A setting that promotes excessive energy intake and low levels of physical activity, resulting in an increase in obesity rates.

oligosaccharides Short carbohydrate chains containing 3 to 10 sugar units.

organic compounds Substances that contain carbon bonded to hydrogen in their molecular structure.

organs Discrete structures composed of more than one tissue that perform a specialized function.

osmosis The unassisted diffusion of water across the cell membrane.

osteomalacia A vitamin D deficiency disease in adults, characterized by loss of minerals from bone, bone pain, muscle aches, and an increase in bone fractures.

osteoporosis A bone disorder characterized by reduced bone mass, increased bone fragility, and increased risk of fractures.

overload principle The concept that the body adapts to the stresses placed on it.

overtraining syndrome A collection of emotional, behavioural, and physical symptoms that occurs when the mount and intensity of exercise exceeds an athlete's capacity to recover.

overweight Being too heavy for one's height, usually due to an excess of body fat. Overweight is defined as having a body mass index (ratio of weight to height squared) of 25 to 29.9 kg/m^2.

parasites Organisms that live at the expense of others.

parathyroid hormone (PTH) A hormone released by the parathyroid gland that acts to increase blood calcium levels.

pasteurization The process of heating food products in order to kill disease-causing organisms.

pathogen A biological agent that causes disease.

peak bone mass The maximum bone density attained at any time in life, usually occurring in young adulthood.

pellagra A disease resulting from niacin deficiency, which causes dermatitis, diarrhea, dementia, and, if not treated, death.

peptic ulcers Open sores in the lining of the stomach, esophagus, or upper small intestine.

peristalsis Coordinated muscular contractions that move material through the GI tract.

pernicious anemia A macrocytic anemia resulting from vitamin B_{12} deficiency that occurs when dietary vitamin B_{12} cannot be absorbed due to a lack of intrinsic factor.

phenylketonuria (PKU) A genetic disease in which the amino acid phenylalanine cannot be metabolized normally, causing it to build up in the blood. If untreated, the condition results in brain damage.

phospholipids Types of lipids whose structure includes a phosphorus atom.

phytochemicals Substances found in plant foods that are not essential nutrients but may have health-promoting properties.

pica An abnormal craving for and ingestion of non-food substances that have little or no nutritional value.

placenta An organ produced from maternal and embryonic tissues. It secretes hormones, transfers nutrients and oxygen from the mother's blood to the fetus, and removes metabolic wastes.

polypeptide A chain of amino acids linked by peptide bonds that is part of the structure of a protein.

polysaccharide A carbohydrate made up of many sugar units linked together.

postmenopausal bone loss The accelerated bone loss that occurs in women for about five years after the menstrual cycle stops.

preeclampsia A condition characterized by elevated blood pressure, a rapid increase in body weight, protein in the urine, and edema. Also called *toxemia*.

prion A pathogenic protein that is the cause of degenerative brain diseases called spongiform encephalopathies. *Prion* is short for *proteinaceous infectious particle*.

proteins A class of nutrients that includes molecules made up of one or more intertwining chains of amino acids. They contain carbon, hydrogen, oxygen, and nitrogen. They promote the growth and development of the body.

protein complementation The process of combining proteins from different sources so that they collectively provide the proportions of amino acids required to meet the body's needs.

protein-energy malnutrition (PEM) A condition characterized by loss of muscle and fat mass and an increased susceptibility to infection that results from the long-term consumption of insufficient amounts of energy and/or protein to meet the body's needs.

provitamin or vitamin precursor A compound that can be converted into the active form of a vitamin in the body.

puberty A period of rapid growth and physical changes that ends in the attainment of sexual maturity.

Recommended Dietary Allowances (RDAs) Nutrient intakes that are sufficient to meet the needs of almost all healthy people in a specific gender and life-stage group.

refined Refers to foods that have undergone processing to remove the coarse parts of the original food.

renewable resources Resources that are restored and replaced by natural processes and can therefore be used forever.

resistant starch Starch that escapes digestion in the small intestine.

retinoids The chemical forms of preformed vitamin A: retinol, retinal, and retinoic acid.

rickets A vitamin D deficiency disease in children, characterized by poor bone development resulting from inadequate calcium absorption.

saliva A watery fluid that is produced and secreted into the mouth by the salivary glands. It contains lubricants, enzymes, and other substances.

satiation While eating, the feeling of fullness and satisfaction that eliminates the desire to continue eating.

satiety After a meal has been consumed, the feeling of fullness that determines the length of time before the desire to eat returns.

saturated fats Lipids that contain no double bonds in their structure. They are most abundant in solid animal fats and may be associated with an increased risk of heart disease.

saturated fatty acid A fatty acid in which the carbon atoms are bonded to as many hydrogen atoms as possible; it therefore contains no carbon–carbon double bonds.

scurvy A vitamin C deficiency disease characterized by bleeding gums, tooth loss, joint pain, bleeding into the skin and mucous membranes, and fatigue.

segmentation Coordinated, periodic muscular contractions that aid in digestion and absorption, but do not significantly propel chyme forward.

self-efficacy An individual's belief in his or her ability to achieve a certain outcome.

simple diffusion The unassisted diffusion of a substance across the cell membrane.

soluble fibre Fibre that dissolves in water or absorbs water and can be broken down by intestinal microbiota. It includes pectins, gums, and some hemicelluloses.

starch A carbohydrate found in plants, made up of many glucose molecules linked in straight or branched chains.

starvation A severe reduction in nutrient and energy intake that impairs health and eventually causes death. It is the most extreme form of malnutrition.

sterols Types of lipids with a structure composed of multiple chemical rings.

strength-training exercise or **resistance-training exercise** Activities that are specifically designed to increase muscle strength, endurance, and size.

stunting A decrease in linear growth rate.

subsistence crops Crops that are grown as food for the local population.

sugar unit A sugar molecule that cannot be broken down to yield other sugars.

sustainable agriculture Agricultural methods that maintain soil productivity and a healthy ecological balance while having minimal long-term impacts.

theories Formal explanations of an observed phenomenon made after a hypothesis has been repeatedly supported and tested through experimentation.

thermic effect of food (TEF) or **diet-induced thermogenesis** The energy required for the digestion of food and absorption, metabolism, and storage of nutrients.

Tolerable Upper Intake Levels (ULs) Maximum daily intake levels that are unlikely to pose risks of adverse health effects to almost all individuals in a given gender and life-stage group.

trace minerals Minerals required in the diet in amounts of 100 mg or less/day or present in the body in amounts of 0.01% of body weight or less.

transamination The process by which an amino group from one amino acid is transferred to a carbon compound to form a new amino acid.

transgenic An organism with a gene or group of genes intentionally transferred from another species or breed.

triglycerides The major form of lipids in food and the body; consist of three fatty acids attached to a glycerol molecule.

type-1 diabetes The form of diabetes caused by autoimmune destruction of insulin-producing cells in the pancreas, usually leading to absolute insulin deficiency.

type-2 diabetes The form of diabetes characterized by insulin resistance and relative (rather than absolute) insulin deficiency.

unsaturated fats Lipids that contain one or more double bonds in their structure. They are most abundant in plant oils and may be associated with a reduced risk of heart disease.

unsaturated fatty acid A fatty acid that contains one or more carbon–carbon double bonds; may be either monounsaturated or polyunsaturated.

vegan diets Plant-based diets that eliminate all animal products.

vegetarian diets Diets that include plant-based foods and eliminate some or all foods of animal origin.

very low birth weight A birth weight less than 1.5 kg (3.3 lb.).

waist circumference A measurement of the tendency for visceral fat deposition. A waist circumference higher than 102 cm for men and 88 cm for women is associated with a greater risk of disease.

water intoxication A condition that occurs when a person drinks enough water to significantly lower the concentration of sodium in the blood.

weight bias Negative attitudes toward overweight or obese individuals that affect social interactions.

xerophthalmia A spectrum of eye conditions resulting from vitamin A deficiency that may lead to blindness.

References

Chapter 1

1. Wansink, B., and Sobal, J. Mindless eating: the 200 daily food decisions we overlook. *Environ Behav* 39:106–123, 2007.
2. American Dietetic Association. Position of the American Dietetic Association: fortification and nutritional supplements. *J Am Diet Assoc* 105:1300–1311, 2005.
3. Galeone, C., Pelucchi, C., Levi, F., et al. Onion and garlic use and human cancer. *Am J Clin Nutr* 84:1027–1032, 2006.
4. Gullett, N.P., Ruhul Amin, A.R., Bayraktar, S., et al. Cancer prevention with natural compounds. *Semin Oncol* 37:258–281, 2010.
5. Rice, S., and Whitehead, S.A. Phytoestrogens and oestrogen synthesis and breast cancer. *J. Sterois Biochem Mol Biol* 108:186–195, 2008.
6. Sacks, F.M., Lichtenstein, A., Van Horn, L., et al. Soy protein, isoflavones, and cardiovascular health: an American Heart Association science advisory for professionals from the nutrition committee. *Circulation* 113:1034–1044, 2006.
7. Cassidy, A., and Hooper, L. Phytoestrogens and cardiovascular disease. *J Br Menopause Soc* 12:49–56, 2006.
8. Rao, A.V., and Rao, L.G. Carotenoids and human health. *Pharmacol Res* 5:207–216, 2007.
9. Crozier, A., Jaganath, I.B. and Cliffors, M.N. Dietary phenolics: chemistry, bioavailability and effects on health. *Nat Prod Rep* 26: 1001–1043, 2009.
10. Basu, A., Rhone, M., and Lyons, T.J. Berries: emerging impact on cardiovascular health. *Nutr Rev* 68:168–177, 2010.
11. Seeram, N.P. Recent trends and advances in berry health benefits research. *J Agri Food Chem* 58:3869–3870, 2012.
12. Prasad, K. Flaxseed and cardiovascular health. *J Cardiovasc Pharmacol* 54:369–377, 2009.
13. Grassi, D., Desideri, G., and Ferri, C. Blood pressure and cardiovascular risk: what about cocoa and chocolate? *Arch Biochem Biophysi* 501:112–115, 2010.
14. Butt, M.S., Sultan, M.T., Butt, M.S., et al. Garlic: nature's protection against physiological threats. *Crit Rev Food* 49:538–551, 2009.
15. Carpentier, S., Knaus, M., and Suh, M. Associations between lutein, zeaxanthin, and age-related macular degeneration: an overview. *Crit Rev Sci Nutr* 49:313–326, 2009.
16. Sanclemente, T., Marues-Lopes, I., Puzo, J., et al. Role of naturally occurring plant sterols on intestinal cholesterol absorption and plasmatic levels. *J Physiol Biochem* 65:87–98, 2009.
17. Bolling, B.W., McKay, D.L., and Blumbers, J.B. The phytochemical composition and antioxidant actions of tree nuts. *Asia Pac J Clin Nutr* 19:117–123, 2010.
18. Sadiq Butt, M., Tahir-Nadeem, M., Khan, M.K., et al. Oat: unique among the cereals. *Eur J Nutr* 47:68–79, 2008.
19. Manerba, A., Vizzardi, E., Metra, M., et al. n-3 PUFAs and cardiovascular disease prevention. *Future Cardiol* 6:343–350, 2010.
20. Lambert, J.D., and Elia, R.J. The antioxidant and pro-oxidant activities of green tea polyphenols: a role in cancer prevention. *Arch Biochem Biophys* 501:65–72, 2010.
21. Fardet, A. New hypotheses for the health-protective mechanisms of wholegrain cereals: what is beyond fibre? *Nutr Res Rev* 23:65–134, 2010.
22. Tjepkema, M. Adult obesity in Canada: measured height and weight. Statistics Canada-Cat. No. 82-620-MWE, 2005.
23. World Health Organization. *Diet, Nutrition and the Prevention of Chronic Diseases* (Technical Report Series no. 916). Available online at www.who.int/dietphysicalactivity/publications/trs916/download/en/index.html. Accessed January 13, 2013.
24. Statistics Canada. *Overweight and obesity in children and adolescents: results from the 2009 to 2011 Canadian Health Measures Survey.* Available online at http://www.statcan.gc.ca/pub/82-003-x/2012003/article/11706-eng.htm. Accessed January 13, 2013.
25. Statistics Canada. Ranking and number of deaths for the 10 leading causes, Canada, 2000 and 2009. Available online at http://www.statcan.gc.ca/pub/84-215-x/2012001/table-tableau/tbl001-eng.htm. Accessed January 13, 2013.
26. Kaput, J. Nutrigenomics—2006 update. *Clin Chem Lab Med* 45:279–287, 2007.
27. Public Health Agency of Canada and the Canadian Institute for Health Information. *Obesity in Canada: a joint report from the Public Health Agency of Canada and the Canadian Institute for Health Information*, June 2011. Available online at http://www.phac-aspc.gc.ca/hp-ps/hl-mvs/oic-oac/index-eng.php. Accessed February 6, 2013.
28. Vaitheeswaran, V. Economist debates food policy. *Economist*, December 8, 2009. Available online at http://www.economist.com/debate/days/view/427. Accessed January 13, 2013.
29. Tirtha, D., and Baylis, K. Fast-food consumption and the ban on advertising targeting children: the Quebec experience. *J Mark Res* 48:799–813, 2011.

Chapter 2

1. Health Canada. *Canada's Food Guides from 1942 to 1992.* Available online at http://dsp-psd.pwgsc.gc.ca/Collection/H39-651-2002E.pdf. Accessed December 27, 2010.
2. Statistics Canada. *Heart Health and Cholesterol Levels of Canadians, 2007 to 2009.* Available online at http://www.statcan.gc.ca/pub/82-625-x/2010001/article/11136-eng.htm. Accessed April 22, 2012.
3. Health Canada. *Articles on Canadians' Food and Nutrient Intakes—Canadian Community Health Survey, Cycle 2.2, Nutrition (2004).* Available online at http://www.hc-sc.gc.ca/fn-an/surveill/nutrition/commun/art-nutr-eng.php. Accessed December 20, 2010.
4. Health Canada. *Dietary Reference Intakes.* Available online at http://www.hc-sc.gc.ca/fn-an/nutrition/reference/index-eng.php. Accessed December 27, 2010.
5. Health Canada. *Do Canadian Adults Meet Their Nutrient Requirements through Food Intake Alone?* Available online at http://www.hc-sc.gc.ca/fn-an/surveill/nutrition/commun/art-nutr-adult-eng.php#a332. Accessed January 4, 2010.
6. Health Canada. *Dietary Reference Intakes Tables.* Available online at http://hc-sc.gc.ca/fn-an/nutrition/reference/table/index-eng.php#eeer. Accessed December 27, 2010.
7. CTV News. New "Canada Food Guide" dishes out fresh advice, February 5, 2007. Available online at http://www.ctv.ca/servlet/ArticleNews/story/CTVNews/20070205/food_guide_070205/20070205?hub=TopStories. Accessed January 4, 2011.
8. Health Canada. *Eating Well with Canada's Food Guide.* Available online at http://www.hc-sc.gc.ca/fn-an/alt_formats/hpfb-dgpsa/pdf/food-guide-aliment/view_eat-well_vue_bienmang-eng.pdf. Accessed December 27, 2010.
9. Katamay, S., Esslinger, K., Vigneault, M., et al. Eating well with Canada's Food Guide (2007): development of the food intake pattern. *Nutr Rev* 65:155–166, 2007.
10. Hu, F.B., and Malik, V.S. Sugar-sweetened beverages and risk of obesity and type 2 diabetes: epidemiologic evidence. *Physiol Behav* 100:47–54, 2010.
11. Pan, A., Sun, Q., Bernstein, A., et al. Red meat consumption and mortality. *Arch Intern Med* 172:555–563, 2012.
12. Health Canada. Consumption advice: making informed choices about fish. Available online at http://www.hc-sc.gc.ca/fn-an/securit/chem-chim/environ/

mercur/cons-adv-etud-eng.php. Accessed December 20, 2010.

[13] Canadian Food Inspection Agency. *Guide to Food Labelling and Advertising.* Available online at http://www.inspection.gc.ca/english/fssa/labeti/guide/toce.shtml. Accessed December 28, 2010.

[14] Health Canada. *Status of Disease Risk Reduction Claims in Canada.* Available online at http://www.hc-sc.gc.ca/fn-an/label-etiquet/claims-reclam/permitted_claims-allegations_autorisees-eng.php. Accessed January 2, 2013.

[15] Roberto, C., Agnew, H., and Brownell, K. An observational study of consumers' accessing of nutrition information in chain restaurants. *Am J Pub Health* 99: 820–821, 2009.

[16] Chandon, P., and Wansink, B. The biasing health halos of fast-food restaurant health claims: lower calorie estimates and higher side-dish consumption intentions. *J Consumer Res* 34:301–314, 2007.

[17] Burton, S., Creyer, E., Kees, J., et al. Attacking the obesity epidemic: the potential health benefits of providing nutrition information in restaurants. *Am J Pub Health* 96:1669–1675, 2006.

Chapter 3

[1] Guarner, F., and Malagelada, J.R. Gut flora in health and disease. *Lancet* 361:512–519, 2003.

[2] Gill, H., and Prasad, J. Probiotics, immunomodulation, and health benefits. *Adv Exp Med Biol* 606:423–454, 2008.

[3] Isolauri, E., and Salminen, S. Probiotics: use in allergic disorders: a Nutrition, Allergy, Mucosal Immunology, and Intestinal Microbiota (NAMI) Research Group Report. *J Clin Gastroenterol* 42(Suppl 2):S91–S96, 2008.

[4] Rescigno, M. The pathogenic role of intestinal flora in IBD and colon cancer. *Curr Drug Targets* 9:395–403, 2008.

[5] Bäckhed, F., Ding, H., Wang, T., et al. The gut microbiota as an environmental factor that regulates fat storage. *Proc Natl Acad Sci USA* 101:18–23, 2004.

[6] Health Canada. Guidance Document— *The Use of Probiotic Microorganisms in Food,* April 2009. Available online at http://www.hc-sc.gc.ca/fn-an/legislation/guide-ld/probiotics_guidance-orientation_pro-biotiques-eng.php. Accessed September 6, 2012.

[7] Soller, L., Ben-Shoshan, M., Harington, D.W., et al. Overall prevalence of self-reported food allergy in Canada. *J Allergy Clin Immunol.* Available online at http://www.medicine.mcgill.ca/epidemiology/Joseph/publications/Medical/Soller2012.pdf. Accessed September 6, 2012.

[8] Canadian Celiac Association. *About Celiac Disease,* 2011. Available online at http://www.celiac.ca/index.php/about-celiac-disease-2/symptoms-treatment-cd/. Accessed September 1, 2012.

[9] Health Canada. *Celiac Disease,* 2012. Available online at http://www.hc-sc.gc.ca/fn-an/securit/allerg/cel-coe/index-eng.php. Accessed September 1, 2012.

[10] Konturek, S.J., Konturek, P.C., Konturek, J.W., et al. *Helicobacter pylori* and its involvement in gastritis and peptic ulcer formation. *J Physiol Pharmacol* 57(Suppl 3):29–50, 2006.

[11] Lynch, N.A. *Helicobacter pylori* and ulcers: a paradigm revisited. Available online at http://opa.faseb.org/pdf/pylori.pdf. Accessed December 20, 2008.

[12] Marieb, E.N., and Hoehn, K. *Human Anatomy and Physiology,* 7th ed. Menlo Park, CA: Benjamin Cummings, 2007.

Chapter 4

[1] Canadian Digestive Health Foundation. *Digestive Disorder Statistics,* 2009. Available online at http://www.cdhf.ca/digestive-disorders/statistics.shtml. Accessed January 28, 2011.

[2] Heaney, R.P., and Rafferty, K. The settling problem in calcium-fortified soybean drinks. *J Am Diet Assoc* 106:1753–1754, 2006.

[3] Blaut, M. Relationship of prebiotics and food to intestinal microflora. *Eur J Nutr* 41 (Suppl 1):111–116, 2002.

[4] Topping, D.L., Fukushima, M., and Bird, A.R. Resistant starch as a prebiotic and synbiotic: state of the art. *Proc Nutr Soc* 62:171–176, 2003.

[5] Andoh, A., Tsujikawa, T., Fujiyama, Y. Role of dietary fiber and short-chain fatty acids in the colon. *Curr Pharm Des* 9:347–358, 2003.

[6] Canadian Diabetes Association. *The Glycemic Index,* 2008. Available online at http://www.diabetes.ca/files/Diabetes_GL_FINAL2_CPG03.pdf. Accessed September 8, 2012.

[7] Canadian Diabetes Association. *The Prevalence and Costs of Diabetes,* 2011. Available online at http://www.diabetes.ca/diabetes-and-you/what/prevalence/. Accessed January 28, 2011.

[8] Public Health Agency of Canada. *Report from the National Diabetes Surveillance System: Diabetes in Canada, 2009.* Available online at http://www.phac-aspc.gc.ca/publicat/2009/ndssdic-snsddac-09/index-eng.php. Accessed January 7, 2013.

[9] Canadian Diabetes Association. *Type I Diabetes: The Basics,* 2011. Available online at http://www.diabetes.ca/diabetes-and-you/living/just-diagnosed/type1/. Accessed January 27, 2011.

[10] American Diabetes Association. Nutrition recommendations and interventions for diabetes. A position statement of the American Diabetes Association. *Diabetes Care* 31:S61–S78, 2008.

[11] Hayes, C., and Kriska, A. Role of physical activity in diabetes management and prevention. *J Am Diet Assoc* 108 (4 Suppl 1):S19–S23, 2008.

[12] Knowler, W.C., Barrett-Conner, E., Fowler, S.E., et al. Reduction in the incidence of type 2 diabetes with lifestyle intervention or metformin. *N Engl J Med* 346:393–403, 2002.

[13] Canadian Broadcasting Corporation. *The 50 Inventions,* 2010. Available online at http://www.cbc.ca/inventions/inventions.html. Accessed February 7, 2011.

[14] Gross, L.S., Li, L., Ford, E.S., et al. Increased consumption of refined carbohydrates and the epidemic of type 2 diabetes in the United States: an ecologic assessment. *Am J Clin Nutr* 79:774–779, 2004.

[15] Riccardi, G., Rivellese, A.A., and Giacco, R. Role of glycemic index and glycemic load in the healthy state, in prediabetes, and in diabetes. *Am J Clin Nutr* 87:269S–274S, 2008.

[16] Villegas, R., Liu, S., Gao, Y.T., et al. Prospective study of dietary carbohydrates, glycemic index, glycemic load, and incidence of type 2 diabetes mellitus in middle-aged Chinese women. *Arch Intern Med* 167:2310–2316, 2007.

[17] Krishnan, S., Rosenberg, L., Singer, M., et al. Glycemic index, glycemic load, and cereal fiber intake and risk of type 2 diabetes in US black women. *Arch Intern Med* 167:2304–2309, 2007.

[18] Canadian Dental Association. CDA position on use of fluorides in caries prevention. (no date) Available online at http://www.cda-adc.ca/_files/position_statements/Fluorides-English-2010-06-08.pdf. Accessed February 1, 2011

[19] van Dam, R.M., and Seidell, J.C. Carbohydrate intake and obesity. *Eur J Clin Nutr* 61 (Suppl 1):S75–S99, 2007.

[20] Westman, E.C., Feinman, R.D., and Mavropoulos, J.C. Low-carbohydrate nutrition and metabolism. *Am J Clin Nutr* 86:276–284, 2007.

[21] Health Canada. *Sugar Substitutes,* 2010. Available online at http://www.hc-sc.gc.ca/fn-an/securit/addit/sweeten-edul-cor/index-eng.php. Accessed January 27, 2011.

22 Stevia sweetener gets US FDA go-ahead, December 18, 2008. Available online at www.foodnavigator-usa.com/Legislation/Stevia-sweetener-gets-US-FDA-go-ahead. Accessed January 12, 2009.

23 Health Canada. *Frequently Asked Questions "FAQs" on Stevia*, 2010. Available online at http://www.hc-sc.gc.ca/fn-an/securit/addit/sweeten-edulcor/stevia-faq-eng.php. Accessed February 2, 2011.

24 Fried, S.K., and Rao, S.P. Sugars, hypertriglyceridemia, and cardiovascular disease. *Am J Clin Nutr* 78:873S–880S, 2003.

25 Van Horn, L., McCoin, M., Kris-Etherton, P.M., et al. The evidence for dietary prevention and treatment of cardiovascular disease. *J Am Diet Assoc* 108:287–331, 2008.

26 Marlett, J.A. Dietary fiber and cardiovascular disease. In Cho, S.S., Dreher, L.L. (eds.). *Handbook of Dietary Fiber*. New York: Marcel Dekker, 2001, pp. 17–25.

27 Anderson, J.W. Whole grains protect against atherosclerotic cardiovascular disease. *Proc Nutr Soc* 62:135–142, 2003.

28 The Heart & Stroke Foundation of BC & Yukon. Low carbohydrate diets and heart disease and stroke, 2004. Available online at http://www.heartandstroke.bc.ca/site/c.kpIPKXOyFmG/b.4027795/k.59D4/Position_Statements__Low_Carb_Diets.htm. Accessed February 8, 2011.

29 Peters, U., Sinha, R., Chatterjee, N., et al. Dietary fibre and colorectal adenoma in a colorectal cancer early detection programme. *Lancet* 361:1491–1495, 2003.

30 Bingham, S.A., Day, N.E., Luben, R., et al. Dietary fibre in food and protection against colorectal cancer in the European Prospective Investigation into Cancer and Nutrition (EPIC): An observational study. *Lancet* 361:1496–1501, 2003.

31 Schatzkin, A., Mouw, T., Park, Y., et al. Dietary fiber and whole-grain consumption in relation to colorectal cancer in the NIH-AARP Diet and Health Study. *Am J Clin Nutr* 85:1353–1360, 2007.

32 Park, Y., Hunter, D.J., Spiegelman, D., et al. Dietary fiber intake and colorectal cancer: a pooled analysis of prospective cohort studies. *JAMA* 294:2849–2857, 2005.

33 Institute of Medicine, Food and Nutrition Board. *Dietary Reference Intakes for Energy, Carbohydrates, Fiber, Fat, Protein and Amino Acids*. Washington, DC: National Academies Press, 2002.

34 Canadian Sugar Institute. *Carbohydrate News—Dietary Reference Intakes for Sugars*, Winter 2004. Available online at http://www.sugar.ca/english/healthprofessionals/carboIssue9.cfm. Accessed January 24, 2011.

Chapter 5

1 Statistics Canada. *Food Statistics*, 2009. Catalogue no. 21-020-x. Available online at http://www.statcan.gc.ca/pub/21-020-x/21-020-x2009001-eng.pdf. Accessed July 23, 2012.

2 Garriguet, D. More fruit, less fat: Canadians' eating habits. *Transitions* 37: 7–10, 2007. Available from http://www.vifamily.ca/media/node/296/attachments/More_fruit_less_fat_canadians_eating_habits.pdf. Accessed January 31, 2011.

3 Willet, W.C. Dietary fats and coronary artery disease. *J Int Med* 272:13–24, 2012.

4 Baum, S.J., Kris-Etherton, P.M., Willet, W.C., et al. Fatty acids in cardiovascular health and disease: a comprehensive review. *J Clin Lipid* 6:216–234, 2012.

5 Health Canada. *Eating Well with Canada's Food Guide*. Available online at http://www.hc-sc.gc.ca/fn-an/alt_formats/hpfb-dgpsa/pdf/food-guide-aliment/view_eat-well_vue_bienmang-eng.pdf. Accessed December 27, 2010.

6 Ratnayake, W.M., L'Abbe, M.R., Farnworth, S., et al. Trans fatty acids: current contents in Canadian foods and estimated intake levels for the Canadian population. *J AOAC Int* 92:1258–1276, 2009.

7 Libby, P. Inflammation and cardiovascular disease mechanisms. *Am J Clin Nutr* 83:456S–460S, 2006.

8 Kher, N., and Marsh, J.D. Pathobiology of atherosclerosis—a brief review. *Semin Thromb Hemost* 30:665–672, 2004.

9 Public Health Agency of Canada. *Tracking Heart Disease and Stroke in Canada: Report Highlights*, 2009. Available from http://www.phac-aspc.gc.ca/publicat/2009/cvd-avc/report-rapport-eng.php. Accessed January 31, 2011.

10 Van Horn, L., McCoin, M., Kris-Etherton, P.M., et al. The evidence for dietary prevention and treatment of cardiovascular disease. *J Am Diet Assoc* 108:287–331, 2008.

11 Constance, C. The good and the bad: what researchers have learned about dietary cholesterol, lipid management and cardiovascular disease risk since the Harvard Egg Study. *Int J Clin Pract Suppl* 163: 9–14, 27–43, 2009.

12 Anand, S.S., Yusuf, S., Vuksan, V., et al. Differences in risk factors, atherosclerosis, and cardiovascular disease between ethnic groups in Canada: the Study of Health Assessment and Risk in Ethnic groups (SHARE). *Lancet* 356:279–284, 2000.

13 Breslow, J.L. n-3 fatty acids and cardiovascular disease. *Am J Clin Nutr* 83(6 Suppl): 1477S–1482S, 2006.

14 Bruckdorfer, K.R. Antioxidants and CVD. *Proc Nutr Soc* 67:214–222, 2008.

15 Humphrey, L.L., Fu, R., Rogers, K., et al. Homocysteine level and coronary heart disease incidence: a systematic review and meta-analysis. *Mayo Clin Proc* 83:1203–1212, 2008.

16 Jenkins, D.A., Jones, P.J., Lamarche, B., et al. Effect of a dietary portfolio of cholesterol-lowering foods given at 2 levels of intensity of dietary advice on serum lipids in hyperlipidemia: a randomized controlled trial. *JAMA* 306:831–839, 2011.

17 Hibbeln, J.R., Nieminen, L.R., Blasbalg, T.L., et al. Healthy intakes of n-3 and n-6 fatty acids: estimations considering worldwide diversity. *Am J Clin Nutr* 83 (6 Suppl):1483S–1493S, 2006.

18 Griel, A.E., Cao, Y., Bagshaw, D.D., et al. A macadamia nut–rich diet reduces total and LDL-cholesterol in mildly hypercholesterolemic men and women. *J Nutr* 138:761–767, 2008.

19 Ros, E., Nunez, I., Perez-Heras, A., et al. A walnut diet improves endothelial function in hypercholesterolemic subjects: a randomized crossover trial. *Circulation* 109:1609–1614, 2004.

20 Fung, T.T., Chiuve, S.E., McCullough. M.L., et al. Adherence to a DASH-style diet and risk of coronary heart disease and stroke in women. *Arch Intern Med* 168:713–720, 2008.

21 Fernandez, M.L. Rethinking dietary cholesterol. *Curr Opin Clin Metab Care* 15:117–121, 2012.

22 Kritchevsky, S.B. A review of scientific research and recommendations regarding eggs. *J Am Coll Nutr* 23 (6 Suppl): 596S–600S, 2004.

23 Djousse, L., and Gaziano, J.M. Egg consumption and cardiovascular disease and mortality the Physicians' Health Study. *Am J Clin Nutr* 87:964–969, 2008.

24 Djousse, L., and Gaziano, J.M. Egg consumption and risk of heart failure in the Physician Health Study. *Circulation* 177:512–516, 2008.

25 Ratliff, J., Leite, J.O., de Ogburn, R., et al. Consuming eggs from breakfast influences plasma ghrelin, while reducing energy intake during the next 24 hours in adult men. *Nutr Res*, 30:96–103, 2010.

26 Statistics Canada. *Mortality, summary list of causes*, 2010. Available from http://www.statcan.gc.ca/daily-quotidien/101116/dq101116d-eng.htm. Accessed February 6, 2011.

[27] World Cancer Research Fund/American Institute for Cancer Research (AICR). *Food, Nutrition, Physical Activity, and the Prevention of Cancer: A Global Perspective.* Washington DC: AICR, 2007.

[28] Schulz, M., Hoffmann, K., Weikert, C., et al. Identification of a dietary pattern characterized by high-fat food choices associated with increased risk of breast cancer: the European Prospective Investigation into Cancer and Nutrition (EPIC)-Potsdam Study. *Br J Nutr* 100:942–946, 2008.

[29] Smith, B.K., Robinson, L.E., Nam, R., et al. Trans-fatty acids and cancer: a mini-review. *Br J Nutr* 102:1254–1266, 2009.

[30] Hall, M.N., Chavarro, J.E., Lee, I.M., et al. A 22-year prospective study of fish, n-3 fatty acid intake, and colorectal cancer risk in men. *Cancer Epidemiol Biomarkers Prev* 17:1136–1143, 2008.

[31] Devitt, A.A., and Mattes, R.D. Effects of food unit size and energy density on intake in humans. *Appetite* 42:213–220, 2004.

[32] Ledikwe, J.H., Blanck, H.M., Kettel Khan, L., et al. Dietary energy density is associated with energy intake and weight status in US adults. *Am J Clin Nutr* 83:1362–1368, 2006.

[33] Willett, W.C., and Leibel, R.L. Dietary fat is not a major determinant of body fat. *Am J Med* 113:47S–59S, 2002.

[34] Hill, J.O. Understanding and addressing the epidemic of obesity: an energy balance perspective. *Endocr Rev* 27:750–761, 2006.

[35] Institute of Medicine, Food and Nutrition Board. *Dietary Reference Intakes for Energy, Carbohydrates, Fiber, Fat, Protein, and Amino Acids.* Washington, DC: National Academies Press, 2002.

[36] Gidding, S.S., Dennison, B.A., Birch, L.L., et al. Dietary recommendations for children and adolescents: a guide for practitioners: consensus statement from the American Heart Association. *Circulation* 112:2061–2075, 2005.

[37] Health Canada. *Do Canadian Adults Meet Their Nutrient Requirements through Food Intake Alone?* 2012. Available online at http://www.hc-sc.gc.ca/fn-an/surveill/nutrition/commun/art-nutr-adult-eng.php#a322. Accessed October 15, 2012.

[38] Ratnayake, W.M., Hollywood, R., O'Grady, E., et al. Fatty acids in some common food items in Canada. *J Am Coll Nutr* 12:651–660, 1993.

[39] American Dietetic Association. Position of the American Dietetic Association: fat replacers. *J Am Diet Assoc* 105:266–275, 2005.

Chapter 6

[1] Williams, C.D. Kwashiorkor: nutritional disease of children associated with maize diet. *Lancet* 2:1151–1154, 1935.

[2] Alebiosu, C.O. An update on "progression promoters" in renal diseases. *J Natl Med Assoc* 95:30–42, 2003.

[3] Institute of Medicine, Food and Nutrition Board. *Dietary Reference Intakes for Energy, Carbohydrates, Fiber, Fat, Protein and Amino Acids.* Washington, DC: National Academies Press, 2002.

[4] Heaney, R.P., and Layman, D.K. Amount and type of protein influences bone health. *Am J Clin Nutr* 87:1567S–1570S, 2008.

[5] Kerstetter, J., O'Brien, K., and Insogna, K. Dietary protein, calcium metabolism, and skeletal homeostasis revisited. *Am J Clin Nutr* 78(Suppl): S584–S592, 2003.

[6] Weikert, C., Walter, D., Hoffmann, K., et al. The relation between dietary protein, calcium and bone health in women: results from the EPIC-Potsdam cohort. *Ann Nutr Metab* 49:312–318, 2005.

[7] Siener, R. Impact of dietary habits on stone incidence. *Urol Res* 34:131–133, 2006.

[8] van't Veer, P., Jansen, M.C., Klerk, M., et al. Fruits and vegetables in the prevention of cancer and cardiovascular disease. *Public Health Nutr* 3:103–107, 2000.

[9] MMA News. Brock Lesnar says high-protein diet to blame for ailment, vows permanent change. Available online at http://www.mmanews.com/forums/general-mma-forum/40136-brock-lesnar-says-high-protein-diet-blame-ailment-vows-permanent-change.html. Accessed February 8, 2011.

[10] Health Canada, Bureau of Chemical Safety, Food Directorate. *Health Canada Reviews and Answers Comments Received on Regulatory Project 1220—Enhanced Labelling for Food Allergens, Gluten Sources and Added Sulphites*, May 31, 2008. Available online at http://www.hc-sc.gc.ca/fn-an/label-etiquet/allergen/proj1220-comment-eng.php. Accessed on January 26, 2011.

[11] U.S. Department of Health and Human Services, U.S. Food and Drug Administration. *FDA and Monosodium Glutamate (MSG) FDA Backgrounder*, August 31, 1995. Available online at http://vm.cfsan.fda.gov/~lrd/msg.html. Accessed February 16, 2009.

[12] Health Canada. *Monosodium glutamate (MSG) – Questions and Answers*, June 27, 2006. Available online at http://www.hc-sc.gc.ca/fn-an/securit/addit/msg_qa-qr-eng.php. Accessed January 26, 2011.

[13] Canadian Celiac Association. *Celiac Disease Definition*. Available online at http://www.celiac.ca/celiac.php. Accessed February 8, 2011.

[14] Clifton, P.M., Noakes, M., Keogh, J., et al. Effect of an energy reduced high protein red meat diet on weight loss and metabolic parameters in obese women. *Asia Pac J Clin Nutr* 12: Suppl. S10, 2003.

[15] Johnstone, A. Safety and efficacy of high-protein diets for weight loss. *Proc Nutr Soc* 71: 339-349, 2012.

[16] Luhovyy, B., Akhava, T., and Anderson, H. Whey proteins in the regulation of food intake and satiety. *J Am Coll Nutr* 26: 7045-7125, 2007.

[17] Statistics Canada. Table 3: Canadian nutrient intake from food consumption, per person/per day. Catalogue No. 21-020-XIE. Available online at http://publications.gc.ca/Collection/Statcan/21-020-X/21-020-XIE2004001.pdf. Accessed January 21, 2013.

[18] American Dietetic Association. Position of the American Dietetic Association, Dietitians of Canada, and American College of Sports Medicine: nutrition and athletic performance. *J Am Diet Assoc* 109:509–527, 2009.

[19] Stipanuk, M.H. Protein and amino acid requirements. In Stipanuk, M.H. (ed.) *Biochemical, Physiological and Molecular Aspects of Human Nutrition*, 2nd ed. St. Louis: Saunders Elsevier, 2006, pp. 419–448.

[20] Xiao, C.W. Health effects of soy protein and isoflavones in humans. *J Nutr* 138:1244S–1249S, 2008.

[21] Soyfoods Association of North America. *Soyfood Sales and Trends*. Available online at http://www.soyfoods.or/products/sales-and-trens. Accessed January 14, 2011.

[22] Dorff, E. The soybean, agriculture's jack-of-all-trades, is gaining ground in Canada. *In Agriculture At A Glance*, Statistics Canada, Cat. No. 96-325-XWE, April 9, 2009. Available online at http://www.statcan.gc.ca/pub/96-325-x/2007000/article/10369-eng.htm. Accessed August 20, 2012.

[23] Sacks, F.M., Lichtenstein, A., Van Horn, L., et al. Soy protein, isoflavones, and cardiovascular health: an American Heart Association Science Advisory for professionals from the Nutrition Committee. *Circulation* 113:1034–1044, 2006.

[24] Messina, M., and Redmond, G. Effects of soy protein and soybean isoflavones on thyroid function in healthy adults and hypothyroid patients: a review of the relevant literature. *Thyroid* 16:249–258, 2006.

[25] Taku, K., Melby, M.K., Takebayashi, J., et al. Effect of soy isoflavone extract supplements on bone mineral in menopausal women: meta-analysis of randomized

controlled trials. *Asia Pac J Clin Nutr* 19:33–42, 2010.

[26] Hilakivi-Clark, L., Andrade, J.E., and Helferich, W. Is soy consumption good or bad for the breast? *J Nutr* 140:2326S–2334S, 2010.

[27] Craig, W.J., Mangels, A.R., and American Dietetic Association. Position of the American Dietetic Association: Vegetarian diets. *J Am Diet Assoc* 109:1266-1282, 2009

[28] Leitzmann, C. Vegetarian diets: what are the advantages? *Forum Nutr* 57:147–156, 2005.

[29] Berkow, S.E., and Barnard, N. Vegetarian diets and weight status. *Nutr Rev* 64:175–188, 2006.

Chapter 7

[1] De Wals, P., Tiarou, F., Van Allen, M.I., et al. Reduction in neural-tube defects after folic acid fortification in Canada. *N Engl J Med* 357:135–142, 2007.

[2] Centers for Disease Control and Prevention. Spina bifida and anencephaly before and after folic acid mandate—United States, 1995–1996 and 1999–2000. *MMWR Morb Mortal Wkly Rep* 17:362–365, 2004. Available online at www.cdc.gov/MMWR/preview/mmwrhtml/mm5317a3.htm. Accessed April 17, 2008.

[3] Miller, D.F. Enrichment programs: helping Mother Nature along. *Food Prod Dev* 12:30–38, 1978.

[4] Health Canada. *Addition of Vitamins and Minerals to Foods*, 2005. Available online at http://www.hc-sc.gc.ca/fn-an/nutrition/vitamin/fortification_final_doc_1-eng.php. Accessed September 25, 2012.

[5] Sacco, J.E. and Tarasuk, V. Health Canada's proposed discretionary fortification policy is misaligned with the nutritional needs of Canadians. *J Nutr* 139: 1980–1986. Available online at http://jn.nutrition.org/content/early/2009/08/19/jn.109.109637.full.pdf+html. Accessed September 20, 2012.

[6] Briefel, R., Hanson, C., Fox, M.K., et al. Feeding infants and toddlers study: do vitamin and mineral supplements contribute to nutrient adequacy or excess among US infants and toddlers? *J Am Diet Assoc* 106:S52–S65, 2006.

[7] Arsenault, J.E., and Brown, K.H. Zinc intake of US preschool children exceeds new dietary reference intakes. *Am J Clin Nutr* 78:1011–1017, 2003.

[8] Food and Nutrition Board, Institute of Medicine. *Dietary Reference Intakes for Vitamin C, Vitamin E, Selenium, and Carotenoids*. Washington, DC: National Academies Press, 2000.

[9] Valko, M., Leibfritz, D. Moncol, J., et al. Free radicals and antioxidants in normal physiological functions and human disease. *Int J Biochem Cell Biol* 39:44–84, 2007.

[10] Karasu, C. Glycoxidative stress and cardiovascular complications in experimentally-induced diabetes: effects of antioxidant treatment. *Open Cardiovasc Med J* 4:240–256, 2010.

[11] Institute of Medicine, Food and Nutrition Board. *Dietary Reference Intakes for Thiamin, Riboflavin, Niacin, Vitamin B-6, Folate, Vitamin B-12, Pantothenic Acid, Biotin, and Choline*. Washington, DC: National Academies Press, 1998.

[12] Saffert, A., Pieper, G., and Jetten, J. Effect of package light transmittance on vitamin content of milk. *Technology and Science* 21:47–55, 2008.

[13] Seal, A.J., Creeke, P.I., Dibari, F., et al. Low and deficient niacin status and pellagra are endemic in postwar Angola. *Am J Clin Nutr* 85:218–242, 2007.

[14] Heart and Stroke Foundation. *Niacin*, 2011. Available online at http://www.heartandstroke.com/site/c.ikIQLcMWJtE/b.3484125/k.4937/Heart_disease__Niacin.htm. Accessed March 17, 2011.

[15] Genest, J., McPherson, R., Frohlich, J., et al. Canadian Cardiovascular Society/Canadian guidelines for the diagnosis and treatment of dyslipidemia and prevention of cardiovascular disease in the adult–2009. *Can J Cardiol* 25:567–579, 2009.

[16] Aufiero, E., Stitik, T.P., Foye, P.M., et al. Pyridoxine hydrochloride treatment of carpal tunnel syndrome: a review. *Nutr Rev* 62:96–104, 2004.

[17] Bendich, A. The potential for dietary supplements to reduce premenstrual syndrome (PMS) symptoms. *J Am Coll Nutr* 19:3–12, 2000.

[18] Hubner, R.A., and Houlston, R.S. Folate and colorectal cancer prevention. *Br J Cancer* 100:233–239, 2009.

[19] Larsson, S.C., Bergkvist, L., and Wolk, A. Folate intake and risk of breast cancer by estrogen and progesterone receptor status in a Swedish cohort. *Cancer Epidemiol Biomarkers Prev* 17:3444–3449, 2008.

[20] Larsson, S.C., Håkansson, N., Giovannucci, E., et al. Folate intake and pancreatic cancer incidence: a prospective study of Swedish women and men. *J Natl Cancer Inst* 98:407–413, 2006.

[21] Health Canada. *Eating Well with Canada's Food Guide*. Available online at http://www.hc-sc.gc.ca/fn-an/alt_formats/hpfb-dgpsa/pdf/food-guide-aliment/view_eatwell_vue_bienmang-eng.pdf. Accessed December 27, 2010.

[22] American Dietetic Association. Position of the American Dietetic Association: vegetarian diets. *J Am Diet Assoc* 103:748–765, 2003.

[23] Statistics Canada. The effect of supplement use on vitamin C intake: facts and figures, 2010. Available online at http://www.statcan.gc.ca/pub/82-003-x/2010001/article/11128/tbls/tbl3-eng.htm. Accessed March 19, 2011.

[24] Douglas, R.M., Hemilä, H., Chalker, E., et al. Vitamin C for preventing and treating the common cold. *Cochrane Database Syst Rev* 4:CD000980, 2004.

[25] Fischer, L.M., daCasta, K.A., Kwock, L., et al. Sex and menopausal status influence human dietary requirements for the nutrient choline. *Am J Clin Nutr* 85:1275–1285, 2007.

[26] Food and Nutrition Board, Institute of Medicine. *Dietary Reference Intakes: Vitamin A, Vitamin K, Arsenic, Boron, Chromium, Copper, Iodine, Iron, Manganese, Molybdenum, Nickel, Silicon, Vanadium, and Zinc*. Washington, DC: National Academies Press, 2001.

[27] World Health Organization. *Micronutrient Deficiencies. Vitamin A Deficiency: The Challenge*. Available online at www.who.int/nutrition/topics/vad/en/index.html. Accessed April 23, 2008.

[28] Michaelsson, K., Lithell, H., Vessby, B., et al. Serum retinol levels and the risk of fracture. *N Engl J Med* 348:287–294, 2003.

[29] Pryor, W.A., Stahl, W., and Rock, C.L. Beta-carotene: from biochemistry to clinical trials. *Nutr Rev* 58(2 Pt. I):39–53, 2000.

[30] Holick, M.F. Vitamin D: extracellular health. *Endocrinol Metab Clin Nor Am* 39:381–400, 2010.

[31] Institute of Medicine, Food and Nutrition Board. *Dietary Reference Intakes for Calcium and Vitamin D*. Washington, DC: National Academics Press, 2011.

[32] Holick, M.F. Resurrection of vitamin D deficiency and rickets. *J Clin Invest* 116:2062–2072, 2006.

[33] Health Canada. Vitamin D and calcium: updated dietary reference intakes. Available online at http://www.hc-sc.gc.ca/fn-an/nutrition/vitamin/vita-d-eng.php. Accessed September 20, 2012.

[34] Holick, M.F. Vitamin D deficiency: what a pain it is. *Mayo Clin Proc* 78:1457–1459, 2003.

[35] Holick, M.F., and Chen, T.C. Vitamin D deficiency: a worldwide problem with health consequences. *Am J Clin Nutr* 87(Suppl.):1080S–1086S, 2008.

36 Sabat, R., Guthmann, F., and Rüstow, B. Formation of reactive oxygen species in lung alveolar cells: effect of vitamin E deficiency. *Lung* 186:115–122, 2008.

37 Cordero, Z., Drogan, D., Weikart, C., et al. Vitamin E and risk of cardiovascular diseases: a review of epidemiological and clinical trial studies. *Crit Rev Food Sci Nutr* 50:420–440, 2010.

38 Galli, F., and Azzi, A. Present trends in vitamin E research. *Biofactors* 36:33–42, 2010.

39 Bügel, S. Vitamin K and bone health in adult humans. *Vitam Horm* 78:393–416, 2008.

40 Cashman, K.D. Diet, nutrition, and bone health. *J Nutr* 137:2507S–2512S, 2007.

41 The Heart and Stroke Foundation. *Statistics*, 2011. Available online at http://www.heartandstroke.com/site/c.ikIQLcMWJtE/b.3483991/k.34A8/Statistics.htm. Accessed March 4, 2011.

42 Guo, X., Willows, N., Kuhle, S., et al. Use of vitamin and mineral supplements among Canadian adults. *Can J Public Health* 100: 357–360, 2004.

43 Sarubin, A. *The Health Professional's Guide to Popular Dietary Supplements*. Chicago: American Dietetic Association, 2000.

44 American Dietetic Association. Position of the American Dietetic Association: nutrient Supplementation. *J Am Diet Assoc* 109:2073–2085, 2009.

45 Bruno, R.S., and Traber, M.G. Cigarette smoke alters human vitamin E requirements. *J Nutr* 135:671–674, 2005.

46 Ernst, E. The risk–benefit profile of commonly used herbal therapies: Ginkgo, St. John's Wort, ginseng, echinacea, Saw Palmetto, and Kava. *Ann Intern Med* 136:42–53, 2002.

47 Smith, J.V., and Luo, Y. Studies on molecular mechanisms of Ginkgo biloba extract. *Appl Microbiol Biotechnol* 64:465–472, 2004.

48 Solomon, P.R., Adams, F., Silver, A., et al. Ginkgo for memory enhancement: a randomized controlled trial. *JAMA* 288:835–840, 2002.

49 Hu, Z., Yang, X., Ho, P.C., et al. Herb–drug interactions: a literature review. *Drugs* 65:1239–1282, 2005.

50 National Center for Complementary and Alternative Medicine. *Herbs at a Glance: St. John's Wort*. Available online at http://nccam.nih.gov/health/stjohnswort/ataglance.htm. Accessed January 12, 2008.

51 Mills, E., Montori, V., Perri, D., et al. Natural health product–HIV drug interactions: a systematic review. *Int J STD AIDS* 16:181–186, 2005.

52 Zhou, W., Chai, H., Lin, P.H., et al. Molecular mechanisms and clinical applications of ginseng root for cardiovascular disease. *Med Sci Monit* 10:RA 187–192, 2004.

53 Helms, S. Cancer prevention and therapeutics: panax ginseng. *Altern Med Rev* 9:259–274, 2004.

54 Hermansen, K., Dinesen, B., Hoie, L.H., et al. Effects of soy and other natural products on LDL: HDL ratio and other lipid parameters: a literature review. *Adv Ther* 20:50–78, 2003.

55 Caruso, T.J., and Gwaltney, J.M., Treatment of the common cold with echinacea: a structured review. *Clin Infect Dis* 40:807–810, 2005.

56 Health Canada. About natural health product regulation in Canada, 2011. Available online at http://www.hc-sc.gc.ca/dhp-mps/prodnatur/about-apropos/index-eng.php. Accessed March 19, 2011.

Chapter 8

1 Environment Canada. *Water*, 2011. Available online at https://www.ec.gc.ca/eau-water/default.asp?lang=En&n=65EAA3F5-1. Accessed October 10, 2012.

2 World Health Organization and United Nations Children's Fund Joint Monitoring Programme for Water Supply and Sanitation (JMP). *Progress on Drinking Water and Sanitation: Special Focus on Sanitation*. Available online at http://www.who.int/water_sanitation_health/monitoring/jmp2008.pdf. Accessed October 5, 2012.

3 Shen, H.-P. Body fluids and water balance. In Stipanuk, M.H. (ed.) *Biochemical, Physiological, and Molecular Aspects of Human Nutrition*, 2nd ed. St. Louis: Saunders Elsevier, 2006, pp. 973–1000.

4 Murray, B. Hydration and physical performance. *J Am Coll Nutr* 26:542S–548S, 2007.

5 Coyle, E.F. Fluid and fuel intake during exercise. *J Sports Sci* 22:39–55, 2004.

6 Institute of Medicine, Food and Nutrition Board. *Dietary Reference Intakes for Water, Potassium, Sodium, Chloride, and Sulfate*. Washington, DC: National Academies Press, 2004.

7 Gleick, P.H., Wolff, G.H., and Cooley, H. Table 13: Per Capita Bottled Water Consumption, by Country, 1999 to 2004. In: *The World's Water, the Biennial Report on Freshwater Resources: 2006–2007*. Washington, DC: Island Press, 2006, pp. 284–286. Available online at www.worldwater.org/data20062007/Table13.pdf. Accessed October 10, 2012.

8 Health Canada. *Drinking Water*, 2012. Available online at http://www.hc-sc.gc.ca/ewh-semt/water-eau/drink-potab/index-eng.php. Accessed October 12, 2012.

9 Public Health Agency of Canada. *Report from the Canadian Chronic Disease Surveillance System: Hypertension in Canada, 2010*, 2010. Available online at http://www.phac-aspc.gc.ca/cd-mc/cvd-mcv/ccdss-snsmc-2010/2-2-eng.php. Accessed March 18, 2011.

10 Chobanian, A.V., Bakris, G.L., Black, H.R., et al. Seventh report of the Joint National Committee on Prevention, Detection, Evaluation, and Treatment of High Blood Pressure. *Hypertension* 42:1206–1252, 2003.

11 Leenen, F.H., Dumais, J., McInnis, N.H., et al. Results of the Ontario survey on the prevalence and control of hypertension. *CMAJ* 178:1441–1449, 2008.

12 American Heart Association. *Am I at Risk? Factors That Contribute to High Blood Pressure*. Available online at www.americanheart.org/presenter.jhtml?identifier=2142. Accessed August 25, 2008.

13 Carvalho, J.J., Baruzzi, R.G., Howard, P.F., et al. Blood pressure in four remote populations in the Intersalt study. *Hypertension* 14:238–246, 1989.

14 Houston, M.C., and Harper, K.J. Potassium, magnesium, and calcium: their role in both the cause and treatment of hypertension. *J Clin Hypertens (Greenwich)* 10(7 Suppl 2): 3–11, 2008.

15 Health Canada. *Sodium, It's Your Health*. Available online at http://www.hc-sc.gc.ca/hl-vs/alt_formats/pdf/iyh-vsv/food-aliment/sodium-eng.pdf. Accessed March 30, 2013.

16 Sacks, F.M., Svetkey, L.P., Vollmer, W.M., et al. Effects on blood pressure of reduced dietary sodium and the Dietary Approaches to Stop Hypertension (DASH) diet. DASH-Sodium Collaborative Research Group. *N Engl J Med* 344:3–10, 2001.

17 Appel, L.J., Moore, T.J., Obarzanek, E., et al. A clinical trial of the effects of dietary patterns on blood pressure. *N Engl J Med* 336:1117–1124, 1997.

18 Health Canada. *Sodium*, 2012. Available online at http://www.hc-sc.gc.ca/hl-vs/iyh-vsv/food-aliment/sodium-eng.php. Accessed October 12, 2012.

19 Health Canada. *Sodium Reduction Strategy for Canada: Recommendations of the Sodium Working Group*, 2010. Available online at http://cspinet.org/canada/pdf/sodumreductionstrategyforcanada.july2010.pdf. Accessed January 25, 2013.

20 Bügel, S. Vitamin K and bone health in adult humans. *Vitam Horm* 78:393–416, 2008.

21 Tarride, J.E., Hopkins, R.B., Leslie, W.D., et al. The burden of illness of osteoporosis in Canada. *Osteoporosis Int.* Published online March 8, 2012. Available at http://www.springerlink.com/content/1383648644m0k7g2/fulltext.pdf. Accessed January 30, 2012.

22 Osteoporosis Canada. *Facts and Statistics.* Available online at http://www.osteoporosis.ca/index.php/ci_id/8867/la_id/1.htm. Accessed March 19, 2011.

23 Reid, I.R. Relationships between fat and bone. *Osteoporos Int* 19:595–606, 2008.

24 New, S.A., Robins, S.P., Campbell, M.K., et al. Dietary influences on bone mass and bone metabolism: further evidence of a positive link between fruit and vegetable consumption and bone health. *Am J Clin Nutr* 71:142–151, 2000.

25 Teucher, B., and Fairweather-Tait, S. Dietary sodium as a risk factor for osteoporosis: where is the evidence? *Proc Nutr Soc* 62:859–866, 2003.

26 Kerstetter, J.E., O'Brien, K.O., Caseria, D.M., et al. The impact of dietary protein on calcium absorption and kinetic measures of bone turnover in women. *J Clin Endocrinol Metab* 90:26–31, 2005.

27 Institute of Medicine, Food and Nutrition Board. *Dietary Reference Intakes for Calcium, Phosphorus, Magnesium, Vitamin D, and Fluoride.* Washington, DC: National Academies Press, 1997.

28 Nordin, B.E.C., Need, A.G., Morris, H.A., et al. Effect of age on calcium absorption in post-menopausal women. *Am J Clin Nutr* 80:998–1002, 2004.

29 Health Canada. *Dietary Reference Intakes: Reference Intakes for Elements*, 2005. Available online at http://www.hc-sc.gc.ca/fn-an/nutrition/reference/table/ref_elements_tbl-eng.php. Accessed October 11, 2012.

30 Heaney, R.P., Weaver, C.M., and Recker, R.R. Calcium absorption from spinach. *Am J Clin Nutr* 47:707–709, 1988.

31 Tucker, K.L., Morita, K., Qiao, N., et al. Colas, but not other carbonated beverages, are associated with low bone mineral density in older women: The Framingham Osteoporosis Study. *Am J Clin Nutr* 84: 936–942, 2006.

32 Rude, R.K., and Gruber, H.E. Magnesium deficiency and osteoporosis: animal and human observations. *J Nutr Biochem* 12: 710–716, 2004.

33 Al-Delaimy, W.K., Rimm, E.B., Willett, W.C., et al. Magnesium intake and risk of coronary heart disease among men. *J Am Coll Nutr* 23:63–70, 2004.

34 Food and Nutrition Board, Institute of Medicine. *Dietary Reference Intakes: Vitamin A, Vitamin K, Arsenic, Boron, Chromium, Copper, Iodine, Iron, Manganese, Molybdenum, Nickel, Silicon, Vanadium, and Zinc.* Washington, DC: National Academies Press, 2001.

35 Canadian Paediatric Society, Dietitians of Canada, Health Canada. *Nutrition for Healthy Term Infants: Recommendations from Birth to Six Months.* Ottawa: Minister of Public Works and Government Services, 1998.

36 Christofides, A., Schauer. C., and Zlotkin, S.H. Iron deficiency and anemia prevalence and associated etiologic risk factors in First Nations and Inuit communities in northern Ontario and Nunavut. *Can J Public Health* 96:304–307, 2005.

37 Harfield, D. Iron deficiency is a public health problem in Canadian infants and children. *Paediatr Child Health* 15:347–350, 2010.

38 Iron Deficiency Project Advisory Service. *Multi-micronutrient Powders for Children Aged 6–24 months–Sprinkles.* Available online at http://www.idpas.org/InfantIronDef/SprinklesWebpage.html. Accessed October 11, 2012.

39 World Health Organization. *Micronutrient Deficiencies: Iron Deficiency Anemia.* Available online at www.who.int/nutrition/topics/ida/en/index.html. Accessed January 21, 2009.

40 Siah, C.W., Trinder, D., and Olynyk, J.K. Iron overload. *Clin Chim Acta* 358:24–36, 2005.

41 Canadian Hemochromatosis Society. *Hemochromatosis: How Common Is It?* Available online at http://www.cdnhemochromatosis.ca/disorder/how_common.php. Accessed January 28, 2013.

42 Tapiero, H., and Tew, K.D. Trace elements in human physiology and pathology: zinc and metallothioneins. *Biomed Pharmacother* 57:399–411, 2003.

43 Caruso, T.J., Prober, C.G., and Gwaltney, J.M., Jr. Treatment of naturally acquired common colds with zinc: a structured review. *Clin Infect Dis* 45:569–574, 2007.

44 Haase, H., Mocchegiani, E., and Rink, L. Correlation between zinc status and immune function in the elderly. *Biogerontology* 7:421–428, 2006.

45 Beck, M.A., Levander, O., and Handy, J. Selenium deficiency and viral infection. *J Nutr* 133:1463S–1467S, 2003.

46 Food and Nutrition Board, Institute of Medicine. *Dietary Reference Intakes for Vitamin C, Vitamin E, Selenium, and Carotenoids.* Washington, DC: National Academies Press, 2000.

47 Clark, L.C., Combs, G.F., Jr., Turnbull, B.W., et al. Effect of selenium supplementation for cancer prevention in patients with carcinoma of the skin. *JAMA* 276:1957–1968, 1996.

48 Greenwald, P., Anderson, D., Nelson, S.A., et al. Clinical trials of vitamin and mineral supplements for cancer prevention. *Am J Clin Nutr* 85(Suppl):314S–317S, 2007.

49 World Health Organization. *Micronutrient Deficiencies: Iodine Deficiency Disorders.* Available online at www.who.int/nutrition/topics/idd/en/index.html. Accessed May 20, 2008.

50 Vincent, J.B. Recent advances in the nutritional biochemistry of trivalent chromium. *Proc Nutr Soc* 63:41–47, 2004.

51 Di Luigi, L. Supplements and the endocrine system in athletes. *Clin Sports Med* 27:131–151, 2008.

52 Rubin, C.D., Pak, C.Y., Adams-Huet, B., et al. Sustained-release sodium fluoride in the treatment of the elderly with established osteoporosis. *Arch Intern Med* 161:2325–2333, 2001.

53 Palmer, C., and Wolfe, S.H. Position of the American Dietetic Association: The impact of fluoride on health. *J Am Diet Assoc* 105:1620–1628, 2005.

Chapter 9

1 Tjepkema, M. Adult obesity in Canada: measured height and weight. Statistics Canada Cat. No. 82-620-MWE, 2005.

2 Shields, M., and Tjepkema, M. Trends in adult obesity. *Health Rep* 17:53–59, 2006.

3 Tremblay, M.S., Pérez, C.E, Ardem, C.I., et al. Obesity, overweight and ethnicity. *Health Rep* 16:23–34, 2005.

4 Public Health Agency of Canada. *Chronic Diseases in Canada*, December 2009. Available online at http://www.phac-aspc.gc.ca/publicat/cdic-mcbc/30-1/ar_01-eng.php. Accessed April 4, 2012.

5 Setia, M.S., Quesnel-Vallee, A., Abrahamowicz, M., et al. Convergence of body mass index of immigrants to the Canadian-born population: evidence for the National Population Health Survey. *Eur J Epidemiol* 24:611–623, 2009.

6 Finucan, M.M., Stevens, G.A., Cowan, M.J., et al. National, regional, and global trends in body mass index since 1980: systematic analysis of health examination surveys and epidemiological studies with 960 country-years and 9.1 million participants. *Lancet* 377:527, 2011.

7 Stevens, G.A., Singh, G.M., Lu, Y., et al. National, regional and global trends in adult overweight and obesity prevalences. *Pop Health Metrics* 10:22 [Epub], 2012. Available online at http://www.pophealthmetrics.com/content/pdf/1478-7954-10-22.pdf. doi:10.1186/1478-7954-10-22.

8 World Health Organization. *Obesity and Over-weight*, September 2006. Fact sheet no. 311. Available online at www.who.int/mediacentre/factsheets/fs311/en/print.html. Accessed July 2, 2008.

9 Onyike, C.U., Crum, R.M., Lee, H.B., et al. Is obesity associated with major depression? Results from the third NHANES. *Am J Epidemiol* 158:1139–1147, 2003.

10 Anis, A.H., Zhang, W., Bansback, N., et al. Obesity and overweight in Canada: an updated cost-of-illness study. *Obes Rev* 11:31–41, 2010.

11 World Health Organization. *WHO Global Database on Body Mass Index (BMI)*, 2011. Available online at http://apps.who.int/bmi/index.jsp?introPage=intro_3.html. Accessed March 15, 2011.

12 Flegal, K.M., Graubard, B.I., Williamson, D.F., et al. Excess deaths associated with underweight, overweight, and obesity. *JAMA* 293:1861–1867, 2005.

13 Gallagher, D., Heymsfield, S., Heo, M., et al. Healthy percentage body fat ranges: an approach for developing guidelines based on body mass index. *Am J Clin Nutr* 72:694–701, 2000.

14 Redinger, R.N. The physiology of adiposity. *J Ky Med Assoc* 106:53–62, 2008.

15 Bouchard, C., Tremblay, A., Després, J.-P., et al. The response to long term feeding in identical twins. *N Engl J Med* 322:1477–1482, 1990.

16 Albu, J., Allison, D., Boozer, C.N., et al. Obesity solutions: report of a meeting. *Nutr Rev* 55:150–156, 1997.

17 Young, L.R., and Nestle, M. The contribution of expanding portion size to the obesity epidemic. *Am J Public Health* 92:246–249, 2002.

18 Rolls, B.J., Morris, E.L., and Roe, L.S. Portion size of food affects energy intake in normal-weight and overweight men and women. *Am J Clin Nutr* 76:1207–1213, 2002.

19 Statistics Canada. *Canadian Health Measures Survey: Physical Activity of Youth and Adults*, 2011. Available online at http://www.statcan.gc.ca/daily-quotidien/110119/dq110119b-eng.htm. Accessed March 15, 2011.

20 Weinsier, R.L., Nagy, T.R., Hunter, G.R., et al. Do adaptive changes in metabolic rate favor weight regain in weight-reduced individuals? An examination of the set-point theory. *Am J Clin Nutr* 72:1088–1094, 2000.

21 McDonald's Canada. Nutrition facts, 2012. Available online at http://www1.mcdonalds.ca/NutritionCalculator/NutritionFactsEN.pdf. Accessed November 22, 2012.

22 Burger King Canada. Nutritional information, 2008. Available online at http://www.burgerking.ca/RTEContent//Document/nutritionalGuide_webFormat.pdf. Accessed March 22, 2011.

23 Wendy's Canada. Nutrition facts, 2011. Available online at http://www.wendys.ca/food/Nutrition.jsp. Accessed March 22, 2011.

24 Starbucks. Explore our menu, 2011. Available online at http://www.starbucks.com/menu/catalog/nutrition?drink=all#view_control=nutrition. Accessed March 22, 2011.

25 Subway Canada. Canada nutrition information, 2011. Available online at http://world.subway.com/countries/nutrition-files/cannutritionvalues.pdf. Accessed March 22, 2011.

26 Dairy Queen. Nutritional information, 2012. Available online at http://www.dairyqueen.com/us-en/eats-and-treats/nutrition-facts/. Accessed April 2, 2012.

27 Tim Hortons. Canadian nutrition calculator, 2011. Available online at http://www.timhortons.com/ca/en/menu/nutrition-calculator.html. Accessed March 22, 2011.

28 Institute of Medicine, Food and Nutrition Board. *Dietary Reference Intakes for Energy, Carbohydrate, Fiber, Fat, Protein and Amino Acids*. Washington, DC: National Academies Press, 2002.

29 Levine, J.A., Donahoo, W.T., and Melanson, E.L. Cellular and whole-animal energetics. In Stipanuk, M.H. (ed.) *Biochemical, Physiological and Molecular Aspects of Human Nutrition*, 2nd ed. St. Louis: Saunders Elsevier, 2006, pp. 593–617.

30 Rankinen, T., Zuberi, A., Chagnon, Y.C., et al. The human obesity gene map: the 2005 update. *Obesity* 14:529–644, 2006.

31 Wardle, J., Carnell, S., Haworth, C.M., et al. Evidence for a strong genetic influence on childhood adiposity despite the force of the obesogenic environment. *Am J Clin Nutr* 87:398–404, 2008.

32 Stunkard, A.J., Harris, J.R., Pedersen, N.L., et al. The body-mass index of twins who have been reared apart. *N Engl J Med* 322:1483–1487, 1990.

33 Ravussin, E., Valencia, M.E., Esparza, J., et al. Effects of a traditional lifestyle on obesity in Pima Indians. *Diabetes Care* 17:1067–1074, 1994.

34 Norman, R.A., Thompson, D.B., Foroud, T., et al. Genomewide search for genes influencing percent body fat in Pima Indians: suggestive linkage at chromosome 11q21-q22. *Am J Human Genet* 60:166–173, 1997.

35 Esparza, J., Fox, C., Harper, I.T., et al. Daily energy expenditure in Mexican and USA Pima Indians: low physical activity as a possible cause of obesity. *Int J Obes Relat Metab Disord* 24:55–59, 2000.

36 Wynne, K., Stanley, S., McGowan, B., et al. Appetite control. *J Endocrinol* 184:291–318, 2005.

37 Knuston, K.L., and Van Cauter, E. Associations between sleep loss and increased risk of obesity and diabetes. *Ann N Y Acad Sci* 1129:287–304.

38 Batterham, R.L., Cowley, M.A., Small, C.J., et al. Gut hormone PYY(3-36) physiologically inhibits food intake. *Nature* 418:650–654, 2002.

39 Enriori, P.J., Evans, A.E., Sinnayah, P., et al. Leptin resistance and obesity. *Obesity* 14:254S–258S, 2006.

40 Peters, J.C. Control of energy balance. In Stipanuk, M.H. (ed.). *Biochemical and Physiological Aspects of Human Nutrition*, 2nd ed. Philadelphia: W.B. Saunders, 2006, pp. 618–639.

41 Corsica, J.A., and Pelchat, M.L. Food addiction: true or false? *Current Opinion in Gastroenterology* 26:165–169, 2010.

42 Vandenbroeck, I.P., Goossens, J., and Clemens, M. *Foresight Tackling Obesities: Future Choice—Obesity System Atlas*. Government Office for Science, UK Government's Foresight Programme. Available online at http://www.bis.gov.uk/assets/bispartners/foresight/docs/obesity/11.pdf. Accessed March 22, 2011.

43 Christakis, N. A., and Fowler, J. H. The spread of obesity in a large social network over 32 years. *New Eng J Med* 357:370–379, 2007.

44 Kroke, A., Liese, A.D., Schulz, M., et al. Recent weight changes and weight cycling as predictors of subsequent two year weight change in a middle-aged cohort. *Int J Obes Relat Metab Disord* 26:403–409, 2002.

45 National Institutes of Health, National Heart, Lung, and Blood Institute. *The Practical Guide: Identification, Evaluation and Treatment of Over-weight and Obesity in Adults*. NIH publication no. 02-4084. Bethesda, MD: National Institutes of Health, 2000.

46 Wing, R., and Phelan, S. Long-term weight loss maintenance. *Am J Clin Nutr* 82(suppl):222S–225S, 2005.

47 Teixeira, P.J., Silva, M.N., Coutinho, S.R., et al. Mediators of weight loss and weight loss maintenance in middle-aged women. *Obesity*, 18:725–735, 2010.

48 Bundy, C. Changing behaviour: using motivational interviewing techniques. *J R Soc Med* 97:S43–47, 2004.

49 Rodin, R.L., Alexander, M.H., Guillory, V.J., et al. Physician counseling to prevent overweight in children and adolescents: American College of Preventative Medicine position statement. *J Public Health Manag Pract* 13:655–661, 2007.

50 Yale Rudd Center. *Motivational Interviewing for Diet/Exercise and Obesity.* Available online at http://www.yaleruddcenter.org/resources/bias_toolkit/toolkit/Module-2/2-07-MotivationalStrategies.pdf. Accessed November 24, 2012.

51 Acheson, K.J. Carbohydrates for weight and metabolic control: where do we stand? *Nutrition* 26:141–145, 2010.

52 Glandt, M., and Raz, I. Present and future: pharmacological treatment of obesity. *J Obes*, vol. 2011, Article ID 636181, doi:10.1155/2011/636181, 2011.

53 Bent, S., Tiedt, T.N., Odden, M.C., et al. The relative safety of ephedra compared with other herbal products. *Ann Intern Med* 138:468–471, 2003.

54 U.S. Food and Drug Administration. *Sales of Supplements Containing Ephedrine Alkaloids (Ephedra) Prohibited.* Available online at www.fda.gov/oc/initiatives/ephedra/february2004/. Accessed January 11, 2009.

55 Pittler, M.H., and Ernst, E. Dietary supplements for body-weight reduction: a systematic review. *Am J Clin Nutr* 79:529–536, 2004.

56 Li, J.J., Huang, C.J., and Xie, D. Anti-obesity effects of conjugated linoleic acid, docosahexaenoic acid, and eicosapentaenoic acid. *Mol Nutr Food Res* 52:631–645, 2008.

57 Saper, R.B., Eisenberg, D.M., and Phillips, R.S. Common dietary supplements for weight loss. *Am Fam Physician* 70:1731–1738, 2004.

58 Yazaki, Y., Faridi, Z., Ma, Y., et al. A pilot study of chromium picolinate for weight loss. *J Altern Complement Med* 16:291–299, 2010.

59 Hess, A.M., and Sullivan, D.L. Potential for toxicity with use of bitter orange extract and guarana for weight loss. *Ann Pharmacother* 39:574–575, 2005.

60 Sarma, D.N., Barrett, M.L., Chavez, M.L., et al. Safety of green tea extracts: a systematic review by the U.S. Pharmacopeia. *Drug Saf* 31:469–484, 2008.

61 Hsu, C.H., Tsai, T.H., Kao, Y.H., et al. Effect of green tea extract on obese women: a randomized, double-blind, placebo-controlled clinical trial. *Clin Nutr* 27:363–370, 2008.

62 Kurtzweil, P. Dieter's brews make tea time a dangerous affair. *FDA Consumer* July–August 1997. Available online at www.fda.gov/fdac/features/1997/597_tea.html/. Accessed February 18, 2001.

63 Lautz, D., Goebel-Fabbri, A., Halperin, F., et al. The great debate: medicine or surgery. What is best for the patient with type-2 diabetes? *Diabetes Care* 34:763–770, 2011.

64 Pontiroli, A.E., and Morabito, A. Long-term prevention of mortality in morbid obesity through bariatric surgery: a systematic review and meta-analysis of trials performed with gastric banding and gastric bypass. *Ann Surg* 253:484–487, 2011.

65 Maggard, M.A., Shugarman, L.R., Suttorp, M., et al. Meta-analysis: surgical treatment of obesity. *Ann Intern Med* 142:547–559, 2005.

66 Online Surgery. *Advantages and Disadvantages of Bariatric Surgery.* Available online at http://www.onlinesurgery.com/article/advantages-and-disadvantages-of-bariatric-surgery.html. Accessed April 4, 2012.

67 Martin, A.R., Klemensber, J., Klein, L.V. Comparison of public and private bariatric surgery services in Canada. *Can J Surg* 54:154–169, 2011.

68 Klarenback, S., Padwal, R., Wiebe, N., et al. *Bariatric Surgery for Severe Obesity: Systematic Review and Economic Evaluation* [Internet]. Ottawa: Canadian Agency for Drugs and Technologies in Health; 2010 (Technology report no. 129). Available online at http://www.cadth.ca/index.php/en/hta/reportspublications/search?&type=16. Accessed March 11, 2011.

69 Puhl, R. M., and Heuer, C.A. The stigma of obesity: a review and update. *Obesity* 17:941–964, 2009.

70 Kraha, A., and Boals, A. Parents and vehicle purchases for their children: a surprising source of weight bias. *Obesity* 19:541–545, 2011.

71 McClure, K.J., Puhl, R.M., and Heuer, C.C. Obesity in the news: do photographic images of obese persons influence antifat attitudes? *J Health Commun* 20:1–13, 2010.

72 American Dietetic Association. Position of the American Dietetic Association: nutrition intervention in the treatment of anorexia nervosa, bulimia nervosa, and other eating disorders. *J Am Diet Assoc* 106:2073–2082, 2006.

73 Stice, E. Sociocultural influences on body weight and eating disturbance. In Fairburn, C.G., and Brownell, K.D. (eds.). *Eating Disorders and Obesity: A Comprehensive Handbook*, 2nd ed. New York: The Guilford Press, 2002, pp. 103–107.

74 Spann, N., and Pritchard, M. Disordered eating in men: a look at perceived stress and excessive exercise. *Eating and Weight Disorders* 13:e25–e27, 2008.

75 BBC News. Body image worries hit Zulu women. April 16, 2004. Available online at http://news.bbc.co.uk/2/hi/health/3631359.stm. Accessed April 2, 2009.

76 Mediascope. *Body Image and Advertising.* Available online at www.mediascope.org/pubs/ibriefs/bia.htm. Accessed April 20, 2005.

77 Tozzi, F., Thornton, L.M., Klump, K.L., et al. Symptom fluctuation in eating disorders: correlates of diagnostic crossover. *Am J Psychiatry* 162:732–740, 2005.

78 Sullivan, P. Course and outcome of anorexia nervosa and bulimia nervosa. In Fairburn, C.G., and Brownell, K.D. (eds.). *Eating Disorders and Obesity: A Comprehensive Handbook*, 2nd ed. New York: The Guilford Press, 2002, pp. 226–232.

79 Vandereycken, W. History of anorexia nervosa and bulimia nervosa. In Fairburn, C.G., and Brownell, K.D. (eds.). *Eating Disorders and Obesity: A Comprehensive Handbook*, 2nd ed. New York: The Guilford Press, 2002, pp.151–154.

80 Ebeling, H., Tapanainen, P., and Joutsenoja, A. A practice guideline for treatment of eating disorders in children and adolescents. *Ann Med* 35:488–501, 2003.

81 Healthier You. Binge eating disorder. Available online at www.healthieryou.com/binge.html. Accessed April 20, 2005.

82 Sundgot-Borgen, J., and Torstveit, M.K. Prevalence of eating disorders in elite athletes is higher than in the general population. *Clin J Sport Med* 14:25–32, 2004.

83 Goebel-Fabbri, A.E., Fikkan, J., Connell, A., et al. Identification and treatment of eating disorders in women with type 1 diabetes mellitus. *Treat Endocrinol* 1:155–162, 2002.

Chapter 10

1 Gallagher, D., Heymsfield, S., Heo, M., et al. Healthy percentage body fat ranges: an approach for developing guidelines based on body mass index. *Am J Clin Nutr* 72:694–701, 2000.

2 The President's Council on Physical Fitness and Sports. *Physical Activity Protects Against the Health Risks of Obesity.* Available online at www.fitness.gov/digest_dec2000.htm. Accessed June 12, 2008.

3 Fontaine, K.R. *Physical Activity Improves Mental Health.* Available online at www.physsportsmed.com/index.php?art=psm_10_2000?article=1256. Accessed April 7, 2009.

[4] Antunes, H.K., Stella, S.G., Santos, R.F., et al. Depression, anxiety and quality of life scores in seniors after an endurance exercise program. *Rev Bras Psiquiatr* 27:266–271, 2005.

[5] Institute of Medicine, Food and Nutrition Board. *Dietary Reference Intakes for Energy, Carbohydrates, Fiber, Fat, Protein and Amino Acids.* Washington, DC: National Academies Press, 2002.

[6] Statistics Canada. *Canadian Health Measures Survey: Physical Activity of Youth and Adults.* Available online at http://www. statcan.gc.ca/daily-quotidien/110119/ dq110119b-eng.htm. Accessed March 15, 2011.

[7] The Canadian Society for Exercise Physiology. *Canadian Physical Activity Guidelines.* Available online at www.csep.ca/guidelines. Accessed April 1, 2011.

[8] Haskell, W.L., Lee, I.-M., Pate, R.R., et al. Physical activity and public health: updated recommendations for adults from the American College of Sports Medicine and the American Heart Association. *Circulation* 116:1081–1093, 2007.

[9] Manore, M., and Thompson, J. *Sport Nutrition for Health and Performance.* Champaign, IL: Human Kinetics, 2000.

[10] Cairns, S.P. Lactic acid and exercise performance: culprit or friend? *Sports Med* 36:279–291, 2006.

[11] Sundgot-Borgen, J., and Torstveit, M.K. Prevalence of eating disorders in elite athletes is higher than in the general population. *Clin J Sport Med* 14:25–32, 2004.

[12] Kazis, K., and Iglesias, E. The female athlete triad. *Adolescent Medicine* 14: 87–95, 2003.

[13] Remick, D., Chancellor, K., Pederson, J., et al. Hyperthermia and dehydration-related deaths associated with intentional rapid weight loss in three collegiate wrestlers—North Carolina, Wisconsin, and Michigan, November–December, 1997. *MMWR Morb Mortal Wkly Rep* 47:105–108, 1998. Available online at www.cdc.gov/mmwr/preview/mmwrhtml/00051388. htm. Accessed March 25, 2009.

[14] American Dietetic Association. Position of the American Dietetic Association, Dietitians of Canada, and American College of Sports Medicine: nutrition and athletic performance. *J Am Diet Assoc* 109:509–527, 2009.

[15] Tipton, K.D., and Wolfe, R.R. Protein and amino acids for athletes. *J Sports Sci* 22:65–79, 2004.

[16] Jackson, M.J., Khassaf, M., Vasilaki, F., et al. Vitamin E and the oxidative stress of exercise. *Ann N Y Acad Sci* 1031:158–168, 2004.

[17] Finaud, J., Lac, G., and Filaire, E. Oxidative stress: relationship with exercise and training. *Sports Med* 36:327–358, 2006.

[18] Margaritis, I., and Rousseau, A.S. Does physical exercise modify antioxidant requirements? *Nutr Res Rev* 21:3–12, 2008.

[19] Suedekum, N.A., and Dimeff, R.J. Iron and the athlete. *Curr Sports Med Rep* 4:199–202, 2005.

[20] Di Santolo, M., Stel, G., Banfi, G., et al. Anemia and iron status in young fertile non-professional female athletes. *Eur J Appl Physiol* 102:703–709, 2008.

[21] Food and Nutrition Board, Institute of Medicine. *Dietary Reference Intakes: Vitamin A, Vitamin K, Arsenic, Boron, Chromium, Copper, Iodine, Iron, Manganese, Molybdenum, Nickel, Silicon, Vanadium, and Zinc.* Washington, DC: National Academies Press, 2001.

[22] Almond, C.S.D., Shin, A.Y., Fortescue, E.B., et al. Hyponatremia among runners in the Boston Marathon. *N Engl J Med* 352:1550–1556, 2005.

[23] Senay, L.C. Water and electrolytes during physical activity. In Wolinski, I. (ed.). *Nutrition in Exercise and Sport*, 3rd ed. Boca Raton, FL: CRC Press, 1998, pp. 257–276.

[24] Bergstrom, J., Hermansen, L., Hultman, E., et al. Diet, muscle glycogen and physical performance. *Acta Physiologica Scandinavica* 71:140–150, 1967.

[25] Burke, L.M. Nutrition strategies for the marathon: fuel for training and racing. *Sports Med* 37:344–347, 2007.

[26] Bussau, V.A., Fairchild, T.J., Rao, A., et al. Carbohydrate loading in human muscle: an improved 1-day protocol. *Eur J Appl Physiol* 87:290–295, 2002.

[27] Karp, J.R., Johnston, J.D., Tecklenburg, T.D., et al. Chocolate milk as a post-exercise recovery aid. *Int J Sport Nutr Exerc Metab* 16:78–91, 2006.

[28] Berardi, J.M., Price, T.B., Noreen, E.E., et al. Postexercise muscle glycogen recovery enhanced with a carbohydrate-protein supplement. *Med Sci Sports Exerc* 38:1106–1113, 2006.

[29] Di Luigi, L. Supplements and the endocrine system in athletes. *Clin Sports Med* 27:131–151, 2008.

[30] Nissen, S.L., and Sharp, R.L. Effect of dietary supplements on lean mass and strength gains with resistance exercise: a meta-analysis. *J Appl Physiol* 94:651–659, 2003.

[31] Birzniece, V., Nelson, A.E., and Ho, K.K. Growth hormone and physical performance. *Trends Endocrinol Metab* 22: 171–178, 2011.

[32] Kanaley, J.A. Growth hormone, arginine and exercise. *Curr Opin Clin Nutr Metab Care* 11:50–54, 2008.

[33] Chromiak, J.A., and Antonio, J. Use of amino acids as growth hormone-releasing agents by athletes. *Nutrition* 18:657–661, 2002.

[34] Brown, G.A., Vukovich, M., and King, D.S. Testosterone prohormone supplements. *Med Sci Sports Exerc* 38:1451–1461, 2006.

[35] van Amsterdam, J., Opperhuizen, A., and Hartgens, F. Adverse health effects of anabolic-androgenic steroids. *Regul Toxicol Pharmacol* 57:117–123, 2010.

[36] Tokish, J.M., Kocher, M.S., and Hawkins, R.J. Ergogenic aids: a review of basic science, performance, side effects, and status in sports. *Am J Sports Med* 32: 1543–1553, 2004.

[37] NutraBio.com. Congress Passes Steroid Control Act. Available online at www. nutrabio.com/News/news.steroid_control_act_2.htm. Accessed June 25, 2008.

[38] Rowlands, D.S., and Thomson, J.S. Effects of beta-hydroxy-beta-methylbutyrate supplementation during resistance training on strength, body composition, and muscle damage in trained and untrained young men: a meta-analysis. *J Strength Cond Res* 23:836–846, 2009.

[39] McNaughton, L.R., Siegler, J., and Midgley, A. Ergogenic effects of sodium bicarbonate. *Curr Sports Med Rep* 7: 230–236, 2008.

[40] Tarnopolsky, M.A. Caffeine and creatine use in sport. *Ann Nutr Metab* 57(Suppl. 2):1–8, 2011.

[41] Volek, J.S., and Rawson, E.S. Scientific basis and practical aspects of creatine supplementation for athletes. *Nutrition* 20:609–614, 2004.

[42] Shao, A., and Hathcock, J.N. Risk assessment for creatine monohydrate. *Regul Toxicol Pharmacol* 45:242–251, 2006.

[43] Smith, W.A., Fry, A.C., Tschume, L.C., et al. Effect of glycine propionyl-L-carnitine on aerobic and anaerobic exercise performance. *Int J Sport Nutr Exerc Metab* 18:19–36, 2008.

[44] Clegg, M.E. Medium-chain triglycerides are advantageous in promoting weight loss although not beneficial to exercise performance. *Int J Food Sci Nutr* 61:653–679, 2010.

[45] Sökmen, B., Armstrong, L.E., Kraemer, W.J., et al. Caffeine use in sports: considerations for the athlete. *J Strength Cond Res* 22:978–986, 2008.

[46] Ganio, M.S., Klau, J.F., Casa, D.J., et al. Effect of caffeine on sport-specific endurance performance: a systematic review. *J Strength Cond Res* 23:315–324, 2009.

[47] Berger, A.J., and Alford, K. Cardiac arrest in a young man following excess consumption of caffeinated "energy drinks." *Med J Aust* 190:41–43, 2009.

[48] Clauson, K.A., Sheilds, K.M, McQueen, C.E., and Persad, N. Safety issues associated with commercially available energy drinks. *J Am Pharm Assoc* 48:e55–e63, 2008.

[49] Ballard, S.L., Wellborn-Kim, J.J., and Clauson, K.A. Effects of commercial energy drink consumption on athletic performance and body composition. *Phys Sportsmen* 38:107–117, 2010.

[50] Consumer Reports. The buzz on energy-drink caffeine, 2012. Available online at http://www.consumerreports.org/cro/magazine/2012/12/the-buzz-on-energy-drink-caffeine/index.htm. Accessed November, 2, 2012

[51] Health Canada. (2011). Health Canada's proposed approach to managing caffeinated energy drinks. Available online at http://www.hc-sc.gc.ca/fn-an/legislation/pol/energy-drinks-boissons-energisantes-eng.php. Accessed December 19, 2012.

[52] Rath, M. Energy drinks: what is all the hype? The dangers of energy drink consumption. *J Am Acad Nurse Prac* 24:70–76, 2012.

[53] Birkeland, K.I., Stray-Gundersen, J., Hemmersbach, P., et al. Effect of rhEPO administration on serum levels of sTfR and cycling performance. *Med Sci Sports Exerc* 32:1238–1243, 2000.

Chapter 11

[1] Committee to Reexamine IOM Pregnancy Weight Guidelines, Institute of Medicine, National Research Council. *Weight Gain During Pregnancy: Reexamining the Guidelines*. Washington, DC: National Academies Press, 2009.

[2] Bryson, S.R., Theriot, L., Ryan, N.J., et al. Primary follow-up care in a multidisciplinary setting enhances catch-up growth of very-low-birth-weight infants. *J Am Diet Assoc* 97:386–390, 1997.

[3] Health Canada. *Eating Well with Canada's Food Guide*. Available online at http://www.health.gov.nl.ca/health/publications/eatingwellwithcanadasfoodguide.pdf. Accessed November 24, 2012.

[4] Public Health Agency of Canada. *The Sensible Guide to a Healthy Pregnancy*. Available online at http://www.phac-aspc.gc.ca/hp-gs/pdf/hpguide-eng.pdf. Accessed November 24, 2012.

[5] National Women's Health Information Center, U.S. Department of Health and Human Services. *Healthy Pregnancy*. Available online at www.womenshealth.gov/pregnancy/you-are-pregnant/staying-healthy-safe.cfm#a. Accessed November 24, 2012.

[6] Kaiser, L., and Allen, L.A. Position of the American Dietetic Association: Nutrition and lifestyle for a healthy pregnancy outcome. *J Am Diet Assoc* 108:553–561, 2008.

[7] American College of Obstetricians and Gynecologists. ACOG Committee Opinion number 315, September 2005. Obesity in pregnancy. *Obstet Gynecol* 106:671–675, 2005.

[8] Linne, Y., Dye, L., Barkeling, B., and Rossner, S. Long-term weight development in women: A 15-year follow-up of the effects of pregnancy. *Obes Res* 12:1166–1178, 2004.

[9] Oken, E., Taveras, E.M., Kleinman, K.P., et al. Gestational weight gain and child adiposity at age 3 years. *Am J Obstet Gynecol* 196:322.e1–322.e8, 2007.

[10] Poston, L. Gestational weight gain: influences on the long-term health of the child. *Curr Opin Clin Nutr Metab Care* 15:252–257, 2012.

[11] United States Department of Health and Human Services. *2008 Physical Activity Guidelines for Americans*. Available online at www.health.gov/paguidelines. Accessed June 19, 2009.

[12] Koletzko, B., Lien, E., Agostoni, C., et al. The roles of long-chain polyunsaturated fatty acids in pregnancy, lactation and infancy: review of current knowledge and consensus recommendations. *J Perinat Med* 36:5–14, 2008.

[13] Food and Nutrition Board, Institute of Medicine. *Dietary Reference Intakes for Water, Potassium, Sodium, Chloride, and Sulfate*. Washington, DC: National Academies Press, 2004.

[14] Food and Nutrition Board, Institute of Medicine. *Dietary Reference Intakes for Calcium and Vitamin D*. Washington, DC: National Academies Press, 2011.

[15] Kumar, A., Devi, S.G., Batra, S., et al. Calcium supplementation for the prevention of preeclampsia. *Int J Gynaecol Obstet* 104:32–36, 2009.

[16] Holick, M.F. Vitamin D deficiency: what a pain it is. *Mayo Clin Proc* 78:1457–1459, 2003.

[17] Centers for Disease Control and Prevention. Spina bifida and anencephaly before and after folic acid mandate—United States, 1995–1996 and 1999–2000, *MMWR Morb Mortal Wkly Rep* 17:362–365, 2004. Available online at www.cdc.gov/MMWR/preview/mmwrhtml/mm5317a3.htm. Accessed April 17, 2008.

[18] De Wals, P., Tiarou, F., Van Allen, M.I., et al. Reduction in neural-tube defects after folic acid fortification in Canada. *N Engl J Med* 357:135–142, 2007.

[19] Scholl, T.O., and Johnson, W.G. Folic acid: influence on the outcome of pregnancy. *Am J Clin Nutr* 71(Suppl.):1295S–1303S, 2000.

[20] Food and Nutrition Board, Institute of Medicine. *Dietary Reference Intakes for Thiamin, Riboflavin, Niacin, Vitamin B-6, Folate, Vitamin B-12, Pantothenic Acid, Biotin, and Choline*. Washington, DC: National Academies Press, 1998.

[21] Food and Nutrition Board, Institute of Medicine. *Dietary Reference Intakes for Vitamin A, Vitamin K, Arsenic, Boron, Chromium, Copper, Iodine, Iron, Manganese, Molybdenum, Nickel, Silicon, Vanadium, and Zinc*. Washington, DC: National Academies Press, 2001.

[22] Hess, S.Y., and King, J.C. Effects of maternal zinc supplementation on pregnancy outcomes. *Food Nutr Bull* 30(1 Suppl.):S60–S78, 2009.

[23] Mills, M.E. Craving more than food: the implications of pica in pregnancy. *Nurs Womens Health* 11:266–273, 2007.

[24] Statistics Canada. *Births: Analysis*. Available online at http://www.statcan.gc.ca/pub/84f0210x/2008000/part-partie1-eng.htm. Accessed November 24, 2012.

[25] Health Canada. *Congenital Anomalies in Canada*, 2002. Available online at http://www.phac-aspc.gc.ca/publicat/cac-acc02/pdf/cac2002_e.pdf. Accessed May 24, 2011.

[26] Stein, A.D., Zybert, P.A., van de Bor, M., and Lumey, L.H. Intrauterine famine exposure and body proportions at birth: the Dutch Hunger Winter. *Int J Epidemiol* 33:831–836, 2004.

[27] Gluckman, P.D., Hanson, M.A., Cooper, C., and Thornburg, K.L. Effect of in utero and early-life conditions on adult health and disease. *N Engl J Med* 359:61–73, 2008.

[28] Roseboom, T., de Rooij, S., and Painter, R. The Dutch famine and its long-term consequences for adult health. *Early Hum Dev* 82:485–491, 2006.

[29] Casanueva, E., Roselló-Soberón, M.E., and De-Regil, L.M. Adolescents with adequate birth weight newborns diminish energy expenditure and cease growth. *J Nutr* 136:2498–2501, 2006.

[30] McKay, A., Barrett, M. Trends in teen pregnancy rates from 1996–2006: a comparison of Canada, Sweden, U.S.A., and England/Wales. *Can J Hum Sex* 19:43–52, 2010.

[31] Pediatric and Pregnancy Nutrition Surveillance System, Centers for Disease Control and Prevention. *Maternal Health Indicators*. Available online at www.cdc.

gov/pednss/what_is/pnss_health_indica-tors.htm# Maternal%20Health%20Indi-cators. Accessed November 24, 2012.

[32] Weng, X., Odouli, R., and Li, D.K. Maternal caffeine consumption during pregnancy and the risk of miscarriage: a prospective cohort study. *Am J Obstet Gynecol* 198: 279e1–279e8. Epub 2008.

[33] Public Health Agency of Canada. *Caffeine and Pregnancy*, 2008. Available online at http://www.phac-aspc.gc.ca/hp-gs/know-savoir/caffeine-eng.php. Accessed November 24, 2012.

[34] Health Canada. *Safe Food Handling for Pregnant Women*, 2012. Available online at http://www.hc-sc.gc.ca/fn-an/securit/kitchen-cuisine/pregnant-women-femmes-enceintes-eng.php. Accessed November 24, 2012.

[35] Delgado, A.R. Listeriosis in pregnancy. *J Midwifery Womens Health* 53:255–259, 2008.

[36] Goodlett, C.R., and Horn, K.H. Mechanisms of alcohol-induced damage to the developing nervous system. *Alcohol Res Health* 25:175–184, 2001. Available online at http://pubs.niaaa.nih.gov/publications/arh25-3/175-184.pdf. Accessed November 24, 2012.

[37] Berg, C.J., Callaghan, W.M., Syverson, C., and Henderson, Z. Pregnancy-related mortality in the United States, 1998 to 2005. *Obstet Gynecol* 116:1302–1309, 2010.

[38] Thangaratinam, S., and Langenveld, J., Mol, B.W., and Khan, K.S. Prediction and primary prevention of pre-eclampsia. *Best Pract Res Clin Obstet Gynaecol* 25:419–433, 2011.

[39] Office of Minority Health and Health Disparities, Centers for Disease Control and Prevention. *Eliminate Disparities in Diabetes*. Available online at www.cdc.gov/omhd/AMH/factsheets/diabetes.htm. Accessed November 24, 2012.

[40] Damm, P. Future risk of diabetes in mother and child after gestational diabetes mellitus. *Int J Gynaecol Obstet* 104(Suppl. 1):S25–S26, 2009.

[41] Dieticians of Canada. *WHO Growth Charts Adapted for Canada*. Available online at http://www.dietitians.ca/Secondary-Pages/Public/Who-Growth-Charts.aspx. Accessed November 24, 2012.

[42] Food and Nutrition Board, Institute of Medicine. *Dietary Reference Intakes for Energy, Carbohydrates, Fiber, Fat, Protein and Amino Acids*. Washington, DC: National Academies Press, 2002.

[43] Wagner, C.L., and Greer, F.R. American Academy of Pediatrics Section on Breast-feeding, American Academy of Pediatrics Committee on Nutrition. Prevention of rickets and vitamin D deficiency in infants, children and adolescents. *Pediatrics* 112:1142–1152, 2008.

[44] Canadian Pediatric Society. Routine administration of vitamin K to newborns, a joint position statement of the Fetus and Newborn Committee, Canadian Paediatric Society (CPS), and the Committee on Child and Adolescent Health, College of Family Physicians of Canada. *Paediatr Child Health* 2:429–431, 1997.

[45] Health Canada. *Exclusive Breastfeeding Duration–2004 Health Canada Recommendation*. Available online at http://www.hc-sc.gc.ca/fn-an/nutrition/infant-nourisson/excl_bf_dur-dur_am_excl-eng.php. Accessed May 22, 2011.

[46] American Dietetic Association. Position of the American Dietetic Association: promoting and supporting breastfeeding. *J Am Diet Assoc* 105:810–818, 2005.

[47] World Health Organization, United Nations Children's Fund. *Global Strategy for Infant and Young Child Feeding*. Geneva, Switzerland: World Health Organization, 2003.

[48] Guesnet, P., Alessandri, J.M. Docosahexaenoic acid (DHA) and the developing central nervous system (CNS)—implications for dietary recommendations. *Biochime* 93:7–12, 2011.

[49] Hoffman, D.R., Boettcher, J.A., and Diersen-Schade, D.A. Toward optimizing vision and cognition in term infants by dietary docosahexaenoic and arachidonic acid supplementation: A review of randomized-controlled trials. *Prostaglandins, Leukot Essent Fatty Acids* 81:151–158, 2009.

[50] Birch, E.E., Garfield, S., Castaneda, Y., et al. Visual acuity and cognitive outcomes at 4-years of age in double blind, randomized trial of long-chain polyunsaturated fatty acid-supplemented infant formula. *Early Hum Dev* 83:279–284, 2007.

[51] Beyerlein, A., Hadders-Algra, M., Kennedy, K. et al. Infant formula supplementation with long-chain polyunsaturated fatty acids has no effect on Bayley developmental scores at 18 months of age—IPD meta-analysis of 4 large clinical trials. *J Pediatr Gastroenterol Nutr* 50:79–84, 2010.

[52] Simmer, K., Patole, S.K., and Rao, S.C. Longchain polyunsaturated fatty acid supplementation in infants born at term. *Cochrane Database Sys Rev* 23:CD000376, 2008.

[53] Gale, C.R., Marriott, L.D., Martyn, C.N., et al. Group for Southampton Women's Survey Study. Breastfeeding, the use of docosahexaenoic acid-fortified formulas in infancy and neuropsychological function in childhood. *Arch Dis Child* 95:174–179, 2009.

[54] Makrides, M., Smithers, S.H., and Gibson, R.A. Role of long-chain polyunsaturated fatty acids in neurodevelopment and growth. *Nestle Nutr Workshop Ser Pediatr Program* 65:123–133, 2010.

[55] Lawrence, R.M., and Lawrence, R.A. Breast milk and infection. *Clin Perinatol* 31:501–528, 2004.

[56] Ip, S., Chung, M., Raman, G., et al. Breastfeeding and maternal and infant health outcomes in developed countries. *Evid Rep Technol Assess (Full Rep)* 153: 1–186, 2007.

[57] Hamprecht, K., Maschmann, J., Jahn, G., et al. Cytomegalovirus transmission to preterm infants during lactation. *J Clin Virol* 41:198–205, 2008.

[58] Greer, F.R., Sicherer, S.H., and Burks, A.W. Effects of early nutritional interventions on the development of atopic disease in infants and children: the role of maternal dietary restriction, breastfeeding, timing of introduction of complementary foods, and hydrolyzed formulas. *Pediatrics* 121:183–191, 2008.

[59] Ziegler, E.E. Adverse effects of cow's milk in infants. *Nestle Nutr Workshop Ser Pediatr Program* 60:185–196, 2007.

Chapter 12

[1] Slatter, E. *Secrets of Feeding a Healthy Family*. Madison, WI: Kelsey Press, 1999.

[2] Health Canada. *Eating Well with Canada's Food Guide*. Available online at http://www.hc-sc.gc.ca/fn-an/alt_formats/hpfb-dgpsa/pdf/food-guide-aliment/view_eatwell_vue_bienmang-eng.pdf. Accessed December 27, 2010.

[3] Health Canada. *Canada's Food Guide: Children, 2011*. Available online at http://www.hc-sc.gc.ca/fn-an/food-guide-aliment/choose-choix/advice-conseil/child-enfant-eng.php. Accessed February 9, 2013.

[4] Institute of Medicine, Food and Nutrition Board. *Dietary Reference Intakes for Energy, Carbohydrate, Fiber, Fat, Protein, and Amino Acids*. Washington, DC: National Academies Press, 2002.

[5] Institute of Medicine, Food and Nutrition Board. *Dietary Reference Intakes for Water, Potassium, Sodium, Chloride, and Sulfate*. Washington, DC: National Academies Press, 2004.

[6] Nicklas, T.A., and Hayes, D. Position of the American Dietetic Association: nutrition guidance for healthy children ages 2 to 11 years. *J Am Diet Assoc* 108:1038–1047, 2008.

[7] Institute of Medicine, Food and Nutrition Board. *Dietary Reference Intakes for*

Calcium and Vitamin D. Washington, DC: National Academies Press, 2010.

[8] Institute of Medicine, Food and Nutrition Board. *Dietary Reference Intakes for Vitamin A, Vitamin K, Arsenic, Boron, Chromium, Copper, Iodine, Iron, Manganese, Molybdenum, Nickel, Silicon, Vanadium, and Zinc.* Washington, DC: National Academies Press, 2001.

[9] Haas, J.D., and Brownlie, T. Iron deficiency and reduced work capacity: a critical review of the research to determine a causal relationship. *J Nutr* 131: 676S–690S, 2001.

[10] Grantham-McGregor, S., and Ani, C. A review of studies on the effect of iron deficiency on cognitive development in children. *J Nutr* 131:649S–668S, 2001.

[11] Blissett, J., Haycraft, E., and Farrow, C. Inducing preschool children's emotional eating: relations with parental feeding practices. *Am J Clin Nutr* 92: 359–365, 2010.

[12] American Academy of Pediatrics. The use and misuse of fruit juice in pediatrics. *Pediatrics* 107:1210–1213, 2001.

[13] Gillman, M.W., Rifas-Shiman, S.L., Frazier, A.L., et al. Family dinner and diet quality among older children and adolescents. *Archives of Family Medicine* 9:235–240, 2000.

[14] Patrick, H., and Nicklas, T.A. A review of family and social determinants of children's eating patterns and diet quality. *J Am Coll Nutr* 24:83–92, 2005.

[15] Rampersaud, G.C., Pereira, M.A., Girard, B.L., et al. Breakfast habits, nutritional status, body weight, and academic performance in children and adolescents. *J Am Diet Assoc* 105:743–760, 2005.

[16] Alaimo, K., Olson, C., and Frongillo, E. Food insufficiency and American school-aged children's cognitive, academic, and psychosocial development. *Pediatrics* 108:44–53, 2001.

[17] Kleinman, R.E., Hall, S., Green, H., et al. Diet, breakfast, and academic performance in children. *Ann Nutr Metab* 46(Suppl. 1):24–30, 2002.

[18] Toronto District School Board. *Feeding Our Future: The First- and Second-Year Evaluation.* Available online at http://www.tdsb.on.ca/wwwdocuments/about_us/external_research_application/docs/EvaluationFOFProgram19Mar12.pdf. Accessed December 30, 2012.

[19] Health Canada. *Do Canadian Children Meet their Nutrient Requirements through Food Intake Alone?* 2012. Available online at http://www.hc-sc.gc.ca/fn-an/alt_formats/pdf/surveill/nutrition/commun/art-nutr-child-enf-eng.pdf. Accessed February 9, 2013.

[20] Shields, M. Overweight and obesity among children and youth. *Health Reports* 17:27–42, 2006.

[21] Dieticians of Canada. *WHO Growth Charts for Canada.* Available online at http://www.dietitians.ca/Downloadable-Content/Public/BMI_2-19_BOYS_EN.aspx. Accessed January 8, 2012.

[22] Coon, K.A., and Tucker, K.L. Television and children's consumption patterns: a review of the literature. *Minerva Pediatr* 54:423–436, 2002.

[23] Eisenmann, J.C., Bartee, R.T., and Wang, M.Q. Physical activity, TV viewing, and weight in U.S. youth: 1999 Youth Risk Behavior Survey. *Obes Res* 10:379–385, 2002.

[24] Batada, A., Seitz, M., Wotan, M., et al. Nine out of ten food advertisements shown during Saturday morning children's television programming are for food high in fat, sodium, or added sugars, or low in nutrients. *J Am Diet Assoc* 108:673–678, 2008.

[25] Cormier, E., and Elder, J.H. Diet and child behavior problems: fact or fiction? *Pediatr Nurs* 33:138–143, 2007.

[26] Rojas, N.L., and Chan, E. Old and new controversies in the alternative treatment of attention-deficit hyperactivity disorder. *Ment Retard Dev Disabil Res Rev* 11:116–130, 2005.

[27] Health Canada. *Do Canadian Adolescents Meet Their Nutrient Requirements through Food Intake Alone?* 2009. Available online at http://www.hc-sc.gc.ca/fn-an/alt_formats/pdf/surveill/nutrition/commun/art-nutr-adol-eng.pdf. Accessed February 11, 2013.

[28] Beals, K.A., and Manore, M.M. Nutritional status of female athletes with subclinical eating disorders. *J Am Diet Assoc* 98:419–425, 1998.

[29] Kazis, K., and Iglesiasl, E. The female athlete triad. *Adolescent Medicine* 14: 87–95, 2003.

[30] Health Canada. *Canadian Tobacco Use Monitoring Survey (CTUMS)*, 2011. Available online at http://www.hc-sc.gc.ca/hc-ps/tobac-tabac/research-recherche/stat/ctums-esutc_2011-eng.php#tabc. Accessed January 4, 2012.

[31] Facchini, M., Rozensztejn, R., and Gonzalez, C. Smoking and weight control behaviors. *Eat Weight Disord* 10:1–7, 2005.

[32] Palaniappan, U., Jacobs Starkey, L., O'Loughlin, J., et al. Fruit and vegetable consumption is lower and saturated fat intake is higher among Canadians reporting smoking. *J Nutr* 131:1952–1958, 2001.

[33] Health Canada. *Canadian Alcohol and Drug Use Monitoring Survey*, 2009. Available online at http://www.hc-sc.gc.ca/hc-ps/drugs-drogues/stat/_2009/summary-sommaire-eng.php. Accessed June 12, 2011.

[34] Danby, F. W. Nutrition and acne. *Clin Dermatol* 28, 598–604, 2010.

[35] Melnik, B. Dietary intervention in acne: attenuation of increased mTORC1 signaling promoted by Western diet. *Dermatolendocrinol* 4:20–32, 2012.

[36] Human Resources and Skills Development Canada. *Health-Life Expectancy at Birth.* Available online at http://www4.hrsdc.gc.ca/.3ndic.1t.4r@-eng.jsp?iid=3. Accessed June 11, 2011.

[37] Statistics Canada. Health-adjusted life expectancy, at birth and at age 65, by sex and income group, Canada and provinces, occasional (years) (CANSIM Table 102-0121). Ottawa: Statistics Canada, 2006.

[38] Health Canada. *Canada's Aging Population.* Available online at http://publications.gc.ca/collections/Collection/H39-608-2002E.pdf. Accessed June 18, 2011.

[39] Cohn, S.H., Vartsky, D., Yasumura, A., et al. Compartmental body composition based on total-body nitrogen, potassium, and calcium. *Am J Physiol* 239 (*Endocrinol Metabol* 2): E524–E530, 1980.

[40] Institute of Medicine, Food and Nutrition Board. *Dietary Reference Intakes for Thiamin, Riboflavin, Niacin, Vitamin B$_6$, Folate, Vitamin B$_{12}$, Pantothenic Acid, Biotin, and Choline.* Washington, DC: National Academies Press, 1998.

[41] National Institutes of Health, Office of Dietary Supplements. *Dietary Supplement Fact Sheet: Vitamin B12.* Available online at http://ods.od.nih.gov/factsheets/vitaminb12.asp. Accessed August 21, 2008.

[42] Holick, M.F., and Chen, T.C. Vitamin D deficiency: a worldwide problem with health consequences. *Am J Clin Nutr* 87(Suppl.):1080S–1086S, 2008.

[43] Canadian Cancer Society. *Canadian Cancer Statistics, 2012.* Available online at http://www.cancer.ca/~/media/CCS/Canada%20wide/Files%20List/English%20files%20heading/PDF%20-%20Policy%20-%20Canadian%20Cancer%20Statistics%20-%20English/Canadian%20Cancer%20Statistics%202012%20-%20English.ashx. Accessed January 8, 2012.

[44] Blumberg, J. Nutritional needs of seniors. *J Am Coll Nutr* 16:517–523, 1997.

[45] Proctor, D.N., Balagopal, P., and Nair, K.S. Age-related sarcopenia in humans is associated with reduced synthetic rates of specific muscle proteins. *J Nutr* 128:351S–355S, 1998.

[46] Chandra, R.K. Impact of nutritional status and nutrient supplements on immune responses and incidence of infection in older individuals. *Ageing Res Rev* 3:91–104, 2004.

[47] Statistics Canada. *Arthritis, by sex, and by province and territory, 2009*. Available online at http://www.statcan.gc.ca/tables-tableaux/sum-som/l01/cst01/health52a-eng.htm. Accessed June 12, 2011.

[48] Gregory, P.J., Sperry, M., and Wilson, A.F. Dietary supplements for osteoarthritis. *Am Fam Physician* 77:177–184, 2008.

[49] Christen, W.G. Antioxidant vitamins and age-related eye disease. *Proceedings of the Association of American Physicians* 111: 16–21, 1999.

[50] Hajjar, E.R., Cafiero, A.C., and Hanlon, J.T. Polypharmacy in elderly patients. *Am J Geriatr Pharmacother* 5:314–316, 2007.

[51] Canadian Society of Exercise Physiologists. *Canadian Physical Activity Guidelines for Older Adults 65 Years & Older*. Available online at http://www.csep.ca/CMFiles/Guidelines/CSEP-InfoSheets-older%20adults-ENG.pdf. Accessed January 8, 2012.

[52] American Dietetic Association. Position paper of the American Dietetic Association: nutrition across the spectrum of aging. *J Am Diet Assoc* 105:1203–1210, 2005.

[53] Dorner, B., Niedert, K.C., and Welch, P.K. Position of the American Dietetic Association: liberalized diets for older adults in long-term care. *J Am Diet Assoc* 102:1316–1323, 2002.

[54] American Medical Association. *Harmful Consequences of Alcohol Use on the Brains of Children, Adolescents and College Students*, 2002. Fact Sheet. Available online at www.ama-assn.org/ama1/pub/upload/mm/388/harmful_consequences.pdf. Accessed April 27, 2009.

[55] Canadian Centre on Substance Abuse. *Canada's Low-Risk Alcohol Drinking Guidelines*. Available online at http://www.ccsa.ca/Eng/Priorities/Alcohol/Canada-Low-Risk-Alcohol-Drinking-Guidelines/Pages/default.aspx. Accessed January 8, 2012.

[56] Bode, C., and Bode, J.C. Effect of alcohol consumption on the gut. *Best Pract Res Clin Gastroenterol* 17:575–592, 2003.

[57] Lieber, C.S. Relationships between nutrition, alcohol use, and liver disease. *Alcohol Res and Health* 27:220–231, 2003.

[58] Transport Canada. *Canadian Motor Vehicle Traffic Collision Statistics: 2009*. Available online at http://www.tc.gc.ca/eng/roadsafety/tp-tp3322-2009-1173.htm#fig2. Accessed June 13, 2011.

[59] Whitfield, J.B. Alcohol and gene interactions. *Clin Chem Lab Med* 43:480–487, 2005.

[60] Bagnardi, V., Blangiardo, M., La Vecchia, C., and Corrao, G. A meta-analysis of alcohol drinking and cancer risk. *Br J Cancer* 85:1700–1705, 2001.

[61] Dumitrescu, R.G., and Shields, P.G. The etiology of alcohol-induced breast cancer. *Alcohol* 35:213–225, 2005.

[62] Allen, N.E., Beral, V., and Casabonne, D. Moderate alcohol intake and cancer incidence in women. *J Natl Cancer Inst* 101:296–305, 2009.

[63] Saremi, A., and Arora, R. The cardiovascular implications of alcohol and red wine. *Am J Ther* 15:265–277, 2008.

Chapter 13

[1] Canadian Food Inspection Agency. *Causes of Foodborne Illness*. Available online at http://www.inspection.gc.ca/english/fssa/concen/causee.shtml. Accessed January 10, 2013.

[2] Centers for Disease Control and Prevention. *Foodborne Illness*. Available online at www.cdc.gov/ncidod/dbmd/diseaseinfo/foodborneinfections_g.htm. Accessed March 23, 2009.

[3] Health Canada. *Salmonella Prevention*. Available online at http://www.hc-sc.gc.ca/hl-vs/iyh-vsv/food-aliment/salmonella-eng.php. Accessed January 13, 2013.

[4] Samuel, M.C., Vugia, D.J., Shallow, S., et al. Epidemiology of sporadic *Campylobacter* infection in the United States and declining trend in incidence, FoodNet 1996–1999. *Clin Infect Dis* 38 (Suppl. 3):S165–S174, 2004.

[5] Health Canada. *E. Coli*. Available online at http://www.hc-sc.gc.ca/fn-an/securit/ill-intox/ecoli-eng.php. Accessed January 11, 2013.

[6] Koepke, R., Sobel, J., and Arnon, S.S. Global occurrence of infant botulism, 1976–2006. *Pediatrics* 122:73–82, 2008.

[7] Liu, Y. and Wu, F. Global burden of aflatoxin-induced hepatocellular carcinoma: a risk assessment. *Environ Health Perspect* 118:818–824, 2010.

[8] Health Canada. Giardia and cryoptosporidium in drinking water. Available online at http://www.hc-sc.gc.ca/ewh-semt/pubs/water-eau/giardia_cryptosporidium-eng.php. Accessed January 11, 2013.

[9] World Health Organization. Variant Creutzfeldt-Jakob disease. Available online at http://www.who.int/mediacentre/factsheets/fs180/en/. Accessed January 11, 2013.

[10] Canadian Food Inspection Agency. *Enhanced Animal Health Protection Requirements for Canadian Cattle Producers*. Available online at http://www.inspection.gc.ca/english/anima/disemala/bseesb/enhren/catbete.shtml. Accessed January 12, 2013.

[11] Be Food Safe. *4 Easy Lessons in Safe Food Handling*. Available online at http://befoodsafe.ca/uploads/BFS%20BROCHURE_ENGrev3_10f.pdf. Accessed January 12, 2012.

[12] Health Canada. *The Regulation of Pesticides in Canada*. Available online at http://www.hc-sc.gc.ca/cps-spc/pubs/pest/_fact-fiche/reg-pesticide/index-eng.php. Accessed January 12, 2013.

[13] Health Canada. *Pesticides and Food*. Available online at http://www.hc-sc.gc.ca/cps-spc/pubs/pest/_fact-fiche/pesticide-food-alim/index-eng.php. Accessed June 21, 2011.

[14] Canadian Food Inspection Agency. *Information on the Labelling of Organic Products*. Available online at http://www.inspection.gc.ca/english/fssa/orgbio/questlabele.shtml. Accessed June 21, 2011.

[15] Agriculture and Agri-Food Canada. *The Canadian Organic Sector, Trade Data and Retail Sales in 2008*. Available online at http://www4.agr.gc.ca/AAFC-AAC/display-afficher.do?id=1285870839451&lang=eng. Accessed January 13, 2013.

[16] Agriculture and Agri-Food Canada. *Canada's Organic Industry at a Glance*. Available online at http://www4.agr.gc.ca/AAFC-AAC/display-afficher.do?id=1276292934938&lang=eng. Accessed January 13, 2013.

[17] Crinnion, W.J. Organic foods contain higher levels of certain nutrients, lower levels of pesticides, and may provide health benefits for the consumer. *Altern Med Rev* 1:4-12, 2010.

[18] Mukkerjee, A., Speh, D., Dyck, E., et al. Preharvest evaluation of coliforms, *Escherichia coli, Salmonella, and Escherichia coli* 0157:H7 in organic and conventional produce grown by Minnesota farmers. *J Food Prot* 67:894–900, 2004.

[19] Danjour, A.D., Lock, K., Hayter, A., et al. Nutrition-related health effects of organic foods: a systematic review. *Am J Clin Nutr* 90:680–685, 2009.

[20] Danjour, A.D., Dodhia, S.L., Hayter, A., et al. Nutritional quality of organic foods: a systematic review. *Am J Clin Nutr* 90:680–685, 2009.

[21] Health Canada. Mercury in Fish—Questions and Answers. Available online at http://www.hc-sc.gc.ca/fn-an/securit/chem-chim/environ/mercur/merc_fish_qa-poisson_qr-eng.php. Accessed January 13, 2013.

[22] Lander, T.F., Cohen, B., Wittum, T.E., et al. A review of antibiotic use in food animals: perspectives, policy and potential. *Pub Health Rep* 127: 4–22, 2012.

[23] Vogel, L. CMA urges prescription-only antibiotics for agriculture use. *CMAJ* 183: E1007–E1008, 2011.

24 Exon, J.H. A review of the toxicology of acrylamide. *J Toxicol Environ Health B Crit Rev* 9:397–412, 2006.

25 Friedman, M., and Levin, C.E. Review of methods for the reduction of dietary content and toxicity of acrylamide. *J Agric Food Chem* 56:6113–6140, 2008.

26 Morehouse, K.M. *Food Irradiation: The Treatment of Foods with Ionizing Radiation.* Available online at http://legacy.library.ucsf.edu/documentStore/v/z/y/vzy67c00/Svzy67c00.pdf. Accessed February 21, 2013.

27 Health Canada. *Food Irradiation.* June 2008. Available online at http://www.hc-sc.gc.ca/fn-an/securit/irridation/index-eng.php. Accessed January 13, 2013.

28 Osterholm, M.T., and Norgan, A.P. The role of irradiation in food safety. *N Engl J Med* 350:1898–1901, 2004.

29 Canada Gazette Part II. Vol 144. Available online at http://www.gazette.gc.ca/rp-pr/p2/2010/2010-10-13/pdf/g2-14421.pdf. Accessed January 13, 2013.

30 Eichholzer, M., and Gutzwiller, F. Dietary nitrates, nitrites, and N-nitroso compounds and cancer risk: a review of the epidemiologic evidence. *Nutr Rev* 56:95–105, 1998.

31 Health Canada. *Food Additive Dictionary.* April 2006. Available online at http://www.hc-sc.gc.ca/fn-an/alt_formats/hpfb-dgpsa/pdf/securit/dict_add-eng.pdf. Accessed June 25, 2011.

32 International Food Information Council (IFIC) and U.S. Food and Drug Administration. *Food Ingredients and Colors.* November 2004; Revised April 2010. Available online at http://www.fda.gov/downloads/Food/FoodIngredientsPackaging/ucm094249.pdf. Accessed January 13, 2013.

33 Margawati, E.T. *Transgenic Animals: Their Benefits to Human Welfare.* Available online at www.actionbioscience.org/biotech/margawati.html. Accessed January 13, 2013.

34 International Service for the Acquisition of Agri-Biotech Applications. ISAAA Brief 43-2011: Executive Summary: Global Status of Commercialized Biotech/GM Crops: 2011. Available online at http://www.isaaa.org/resources/publications/briefs/43/executivesummary/default.asp. Accessed January 13, 2013.

35 Paine, J.A., Shipton, C.A., Chaggar, S., et al. Improving the nutritional value of golden rice through increased provitamin A content. *Nat Biotechnol* 23:482–487, 2005.

36 Sautter, C., Poletti, S., Zhang, P., et al. Biofortification of essential nutritional compounds and trace elements in rice and cassava. *Proc Nutr Soc* 65:153–159, 2006.

37 Ye, X., Al-Babili, S., Kloti, A., et al. Engineering the provitamin A (beta-carotene) biosynthetic pathway into (carotenoid-free) rice endosperm. *Science* 287:303–305, 2000.

38 National Academy of Sciences, National Research Council. *Genetically Modified Pest-Protected Plants: Science and Regulation.* Washington, DC: National Academies Press, 2000.

39 Shewry, P.R., Tatham, A.S., and Halford, N.G. Genetic modification and plant food allergens: risks and benefits. *J Chromatogr B Biomed Sci Appl* 756:327–335, 2001.

40 Nordlee, J.A., Taylor, S.L., Townsend, J.A., et al. Identification of a Brazil-nut allergen in transgenic soybeans. *N Engl J Med* 334:688–692, 1996.

41 Health Canada. GM foods and their regulation. Available online at http://www.hc-sc.gc.ca/fn-an/gmf-agm/fs-if/gm-foods-aliments-gm-eng.php. Accessed January 13, 2013.

42 Caporael, L.R. Ergotism: the Satan loosed in Salem? *Science* 192:21–26, 1976.

Chapter 14

1 Food and Agriculture Organization of the United Nations. *The 2007–2008 Food Price Swing: Impact and Policies in Eastern and Southern Africa*, 2009. Available online at ftp://ftp.fao.org/docrep/fao/012/i0984e/i0984e00.pdf. Accessed November 23, 2012.

2 Food and Agriculture Organization of the United Nations. *The State of Food Insecurity in the World, 2012*, 2012. Available online at http://www.fao.org/docrep/016/i3027e/i3027e00.htm. Accessed November 2, 2012.

3 Caulfield, L.E., de Onis, M., Blössner, M., et al. Undernutrition as an underlying cause of child deaths associated with diarrhea, pneumonia, malaria, and measles. *Am J Clin Nutr* 80:193–198, 2004.

4 Black, R.E., Allen, L.H., Bhutta, Z.A., et al. Maternal and child undernutrition: global and regional exposures and health consequences. *Lancet* 371:243–260, 2008.

5 World Health Organization. *The Global Burden of Disease: 2004 Update*, 2008. Available online at www.who.int/healthinfo/global_burden_disease/2004_report_update/en/index.html. Accessed May 4, 2009.

6 The World Bank. Mortality rate, infant (per 1,000 live births). Available online at http://data.worldbank.org/indicator/SP.DYN.IMRT.IN/countries/1W?display=default. Accessed November 2, 2012.

7 World Health Organization. *Low Birth Weight: Country, Regional and Global Estimates, 2005.* Available online at http://www.who.int/reproductivehealth/publications/monitoring/9280638327/en/index.html. Accessed February 27, 2013.

8 UNICEF Progress for Children. *A World Fit for Children. Statistical Review.* Available online at www.unicef.org/progressforchildren/2007n6/index_41401.htm. Accessed November 23, 2012.

9 James, P.T., Leach, R., Kalamara, E., et al. The worldwide obesity epidemic. *Obes Res* 9:228S–233S, 2001.

10 Finucane, A., Stevens, G., Cowan, M., et al. National, regional and global trends in body-mass index since 1980: systematic analysis of health examination surveys and epidemiological studies with 960 country-years and 9.1 million participants. *Lancet* 377:557–567, 2011.

11 Food and Agricultural Organization of the United Nations. *The Nutrition Transition and Obesity.* Available online at www.fao.org/FOCUS/E/obesity/obes2.htm. Accessed March 26, 2009.

12 Kelly, T., Yang, W., Chen, C.-S., et al. Global burden of obesity in 2005 and projections to 2030. *Int J Obes (Lond)* 32:1431–1437, 2008.

13 De Onis, M., Blössner, M., and Borghi, E. Global prevalence and trends of overweight and obesity among preschool children. *Am J Clin Nutr* 92:1257–1264, 2010.

14 Vorster, H.H., Bourne, L.T., Venter, C.S., et al. Contribution of nutrition to the health transition in developing countries: a framework for research and intervention. *Nutr Rev* 57:341–349, 1999.

15 Eberwine, D. Globesity: a crisis of growing proportions. *Perspect Health* 7:12–16, 2002. Available online at www.paho.org/English/DPI/Number15_article2_2.htm. Accessed February 12, 2006.

16 Chen, C.M. Overview of obesity in mainland China. *Obes Rev* 9:14–21, 2008.

17 Subramanian, S.V., and Smith, G.D. Patterns, distribution, and determinants of under- and overnutrition: a population-based study of women in India. *Am J Clin Nutr* 84:633–640, 2006.

18 The World Bank. *Global Purchasing Power Parities and Real Expenditures: 2005 International Comparison Program.* Available online at http://siteresources.worldbank.org/ICPINT/Resources/icp-final.pdf. Accessed April 23, 2009.

19 Food and Agriculture Organization of the United Nations. *The State of Food Insecurity in the World 2006.* Available online at

www.fao.org/docrep/009/a0750e/ a0750e00.htm. Accessed May 4, 2009.

20 Bread for the World Institute. *Are We On Track to End Hunger?* 2004. Available online at www.bread.org/learn/hunger-reports/are-we-on-track-to-end.html. Accessed May 7, 2004.

21 Population Reference Bureau. *2012 World Population Data Sheet*. Available online at http://www.prb.org/pdf12/2012-population-data-sheet_eng.pdf. Accessed November 24, 2012.

22 Brown, L.R. *World Facing Huge New Challenge on Food Front—Business-as-Usual Not a Viable Option*. April 16, 2008. Available online at www.earthpolicy.org/Updates/2008/Update72.htm. Accessed August 30, 2008.

23 Rosen, S., and Shapouri, S. Rising food prices intensify food insecurity in developing countries. *Amber Waves* 6(1):16–21, February 2008. Available online at www.ers.usda.gov/AmberWaves/February08/PDF/RisingFood.pdf. Accessed August 30, 2008.

24 McMichael, A.J., and Lindgren, E. Climate change: present and future risks to health, and necessary responses. *J Int Med* doi: 10.1111/j.1365-2796.2011.02415.x.

25 Solomon, S., Qin, D., Manning, M., et al., eds. Intergovernmental Panel on Climate Change (IPCC). *Climate Change 2007: The Physical Science Basis. Contribution of Working Group I to the Fourth Assessment Report of the Intergovernmental Panel on Climate Change*. Cambridge, UK and New York, NY: Cambridge University Press, 2007.

26 Richardson, K., Steffen, W., and Liverman, D. (eds.). *Climate Change: Global Risks, Challenges and Decisions*. Cambridge: Cambridge University Press, 2011.

27 Reijnders, L., and Soret, S. Quantification of the environmental impact of different dietary protein choices. *Am J Clin Nutr* 78:664S–668S, 2003.

28 Steinfeld, H., Gerber, P., Wassenaar, T., et al. *Livestock's Long Shadow: Environmental Issues and Options*, 2006. Available online at http://meteo.lcd.lu/globalwarming/FAO/livestocks_long_shadow.pdf. Accessed March 17, 2009.

29 World Health Organization. *Micronutrient Deficiencies: Iron Deficiency Anemia*, 2012. Available online at http://www.who.int/nutrition/topics/ida/en/index.html. Accessed November 24, 2012.

30 World Health Organization. *Micronutrient Deficiencies: Iodine Deficiency Disorders*. Available online at http://www.who.int/nutrition/topics/idd/en/. Accessed November 24, 2012.

31 World Health Organization. *Micronutrient Deficiencies: Vitamin A Deficiency*. Available online at http://www.who.int/nutrition/topics/vad/en/. Accessed November, 2012.

32 World Health Organization. *The World Health Report, 1998: Life in the 21st Century—A Vision for All*. Geneva: World Health Organization, 1998. Available online at www.who.int/whr/1998/en/index.html. Accessed April 24, 2009.

33 Lopez, A. Malnutrition and the burden of disease. *Asia Pac J Clin Nutr* 13:S7, 2004.

34 Health Canada. *Household Food Insecurity in Canada in 2007–2008: Key Statistics and Graphics*. Available online at http://www.hc-sc.gc.ca/fn-an/surveill/nutrition/commun/insecurit/key-stats-cles-2007-2008-eng.php#a. Accessed June 21, 2011.

35 Jetter, K.M., and Cassady, D.L. The availability and cost of healthier food items. *Am J Prev Med* 30:38–44, January 2006.

36 Statistics Canada. *Infant Mortality Rates by Province and Territory*. Available online at http://www.statcan.gc.ca/tables-tableaux/sum-som/l01/cst01/health21a-eng.htm. Accessed November 24, 2012.

37 Human Resources and Skills Development Canada. *Special Reports—What Difference Does Learning Make to Financial Security?* Available online at http://www4.hrsdc.gc.ca/.3ndic.1t.4r@-eng.jsp?iid=54#a7. Accessed June 24, 2011.

38 Laird, G. *Shelter: Homelessness in a Growth Economy—Canada's 21st Century Paradox. A Report for the Sheldon Chumir Foundation for Ethics in Leadership*. Calgary: Sheldon Chumir Foundation for Ethics in Leadership, 2007.

39 Health Canada. *Canada's Aging Population*. Available online at http://dsp-psd.pwgsc.gc.ca/Collection/H39-608-2002E.pdf. Accessed June 24, 2011.

40 FAO, WFP and IFAD. *The State of Food Insecurity in the World 2012. Economic growth is necessary but not sufficient to accelerate reduction of hunger and malnutrition*, 2012. Rome, FAO.

41 United Nations. *End Poverty: Millennium Development Goals 2015*. Available online at www.un.org/millenniumgoals/. Accessed May 7, 2009.

42 United Nations. *Population Facts*, August 2010. Available online at www.un.org/esa/population/publications/popfacts/popfacts_2010-5.pdf. Accessed November 24, 2012.

43 Berg, L.R., Hager, M.C., and Hassenzahl, D.M. *Visualizing Environmental Science*, 3rd ed. Hoboken, NJ: John Wiley & Sons, 2011.

44 Association of American Geographers. Population Module: Lesson 3, Page 2—How does education affect fertility rates in different places. Available online at www.aag.org/Education/center/cgge-aag%20site/Population/lesson3_page2.html. Accessed May 5, 2009.

45 Central Intelligence Agency. Côte d'Ivoire. *The World Fact Book*. Available online at https://www.cia.gov/library/publications/the-world-factbook/geos/iv.html. Accessed November 24, 2012.

46 World Health Organization. *Infant and Young Child Nutrition: Global Strategy on Infant and Young Child Feeding*, April 16, 2002. Available online at http://whqlibdoc.who.int/publications/2003/9241562218.pdf. Accessed November 24, 2012.

47 World Health Organization. *Guidelines on Breast Feeding and HIV Infection, 2010*. Available online at http://whqlibdoc.who.int/publications/2010/9789241599535_eng.pdf. Accessed November 24, 2012.

48 Tang, G., Qin, J., Dolnikowski, G.G., et al. Golden rice is an effective source of vitamin A. *Am J Clin Nutr* 89:1776–1783, 2009.

49 Greenpeace International. *Golden Rice's Lack of Luster: Addressing Vitamin A Deficiency Without Genetic Engineering*, November 9, 2010. Available online at http://www.greenpeace.org/austria/Global/austria/dokumente/Reports/gentechnik_the%20truth%20about%20GOLDEN%20RICE_2010.pdf. Accessed November 24, 2012.

50 Bienvenido, O.J. *Rice in Human Nutrition*, 1993. Available online at http://www.fao.org/docrep/t0567e/T0567E00.htm. Accessed November 24, 2012.

51 Potrykus, I. Lessons for the 'Humanitarian Golden Rice' Project: regulation prevents development of public good genetically engineered crop products. *N Biotechnol* 27:466–472, 2010.

52 GMO Compass. Golden rice: First field tests in Philippines. Available online at http://www.gmo-compass.org/eng/news/358.golden_rice_first_field_tests_philippines.html. Accessed November 24, 2012.

53 Qaim, M. Benefits of genetically modified crops for the poor: household income, nutrition, and health. *N Biotechnol* 27: 552–557, 2010.

54 Food Banks of Canada. *Facts and Statistics*. Available online at http://www.cafb-acba.ca/main2.cfm?id=10718648-B6A7-8AA0-6A3C6F3CAC0124E1. Accessed June 21, 2011.

55 World Health Organization. Initiative for vaccine research: hookworm disease. Available online at www.who.int/vaccine_research/diseases/soa_parasitic/en/index2.html. Accessed July 23, 2009.

Table and Line Art Credits

Chapter 1

Figure 1.4b: From *Nutrition: Science and Applications* by Lori A. Smolin and Mary B. Grosvenor, John Wiley & Sons, Inc., Copyright © 2008. Reprinted with permission of John Wiley & Sons, Inc.. Figure 1.11: From *Nutrition: Everyday Choices* by Mary B. Grosvenor and Lori A. Smolin, John Wiley & Sons, Inc., Copyright © 2006. Reprinted with permission of John Wiley & Sons, Inc. Hot Topic (left): From *Nutrition: Everyday Choices* by Mary B. Grosvenor and Lori A. Smolin, John Wiley & Sons, Inc., Copyright © 2006. Reprinted with permission of John Wiley & Sons, Inc.

Chapter 2

Figure 2.1: *Canada's Official Food Rules*. Health Canada, 2007. Reproduced with permission from the Minister of Health, 2013. Figure 2.2 (1): From *Nutrition: Science and Applications*, Fourth Edition by Lori Smolin and Mary Grosvenor, John Wiley & Sons, Inc., Copyright © 1998. Reprinted with permission of John Wiley & Sons, Inc. Figure 2.4: From *Nutrition: Science and Applications*, Fourth Edition by Lori Smolin and Mary Grosvenor, John Wiley & Sons, Inc., Copyright © 1998. Reprinted with permission of John Wiley & Sons, Inc. Table 2.1: *Dietary Reference Intakes Tables*. Health Canada, 2010. Adapted and reproduced with permission from the Minister of Health, 2013. Figure 2.7 a, b, c, d *Eating Well with Canada's Food Guide*. Health Canada, 2011. Reproduced with permission from the Minister of Health, 2013. Figure 2.9 *Eating Well with Canada's Food Guide*. Health Canada, 2011. Reproduced with permission from the Minister of Health, 2013. Figure 2.10 *My Food Guide*. Health Canada, 2008. Reproduced with permission from the Minister of Health, 2013. Figure 2.11 *Eating Well with Canada's Food Guide, First Nations, Inuit and Métis*. Health Canada, 2007. Reproduced with permission from the Minister of Health, 2013. Figure 2.12 From *Nutrition: Everyday Choices* by Mary B. Grosvenor and Lori A. Smolin, John Wiley & Sons, Inc., Copyright © 2006. Reprinted with permission of John Wiley & Sons, Inc. Table 2.2: U.S. Food and Drug Administration. Table 2.3: *Status of Disease Risk Reduction Claims in Canada*. Health Canada, 2008. Reproduced with permission from the Minister of Health, 2013.

Chapter 3

Figures 3.1, 3.2: From *Nutrition: Everyday Choices* by Mary B. Grosvenor and Lori A. Smolin, John Wiley & Sons, Inc., Copyright © 2006. Reprinted with permission of John Wiley & Sons, Inc. Figure 3.3: From *Nutrition: Science and Applications* by Lori A. Smolin and Mary B. Grosvenor, John Wiley & Sons, Inc., Copyright © 2008. Reprinted with permission of John Wiley & Sons, Inc. Figure 3.4: From *Nutrition: Everyday Choices* by Mary B. Grosvenor and Lori A. Smolin, John Wiley & Sons, Inc., Copyright © 2006. Reprinted with permission of John Wiley & Sons, Inc. Figures 3.5, 3.6: From *Nutrition: Science and Applications* by Lori A. Smolin and Mary B. Grosvenor, John Wiley & Sons, Inc., Copyright © 2008. Reprinted with permission of John Wiley & Sons, Inc. Figure 3.7: From *Nutrition: Everyday Choices* by Mary B. Grosvenor and Lori A. Smolin, John Wiley & Sons, Inc., Copyright © 2006. Figure 3.9: From *Nutrition: Everyday Choices* by Mary B. Grosvenor and Lori A. Smolin, John Wiley & Sons, Inc., Copyright © 2006. Reprinted with permission of John Wiley & Sons, Inc. Figure 3.11, Thinking It Through: From *Nutrition: Science and Applications* by Lori A. Smolin and Mary B. Grosvenor, John Wiley & Sons, Inc., Copyright © 2008. Reprinted with permission of John Wiley & Sons, Inc. Figure 3.14: From *Nutrition: Everyday Choices* by Mary B. Grosvenor and Lori A. Smolin, John Wiley & Sons, Inc., Copyright © 2006. Reprinted with permission of John Wiley & Sons, Inc. Figure 3.16: From *Nutrition: Science and Applications* by Lori A. Smolin and Mary B. Grosvenor, John Wiley & Sons, Inc., Copyright © 2008. Reprinted with permission of John Wiley & Sons, Inc. Figure 3.17 From *Nutrition: Science and Applications* by Lori A. Smolin and Mary B. Grosvenor, John Wiley & Sons, Inc., Copyright © 2008. Reprinted with permission of John Wiley & Sons, Inc.

Chapter 4

Figure 4.3a: From *Nutrition: Everyday Choices* by Mary B. Grosvenor and Lori A. Smolin, John Wiley & Sons, Inc., Copyright © 2006. Reprinted with permission of John Wiley & Sons, Inc. Figure 4.2b: Adapted from Oldways Preservation Trust and Whole Grains Council (wholegrainscouncil.org); http://blog.greatharvest.com/TheBread-Business-Blog/bid/42503/Whole-Wheat-Flour-is-Packed-with-Nutrients. Figures 4.4, 4.5, 4.7a: From *Nutrition: Everyday Choices* by Mary B. Grosvenor and Lori A. Smolin, John Wiley & Sons, Inc., Copyright © 2006. Reprinted with permission of John Wiley & Sons, Inc. Figure 4.7b: *Nutrition: From Science to Life* by Mary Grosvenor, John Wiley & Sons, Inc., Copyright © 2001. Reprinted with permission of John Wiley & Sons, Inc. Figure 4.8a: From *Nutrition: Science and Applications* by Lori A. Smolin and Mary B. Grosvenor, John Wiley & Sons, Inc., Copyright © 2008. Reprinted with permission of John Wiley & Sons, Inc. Figure 4.9: From *Nutrition: Everyday Choices* by Mary B. Grosvenor and Lori A. Smolin, John Wiley & Sons, Inc., Copyright © 2006. Reprinted with permission of John Wiley & Sons, Inc. Figures 4.10, 4.11 (bar graph): From *Nutrition: Science and Applications*, Second Edition by Lori Smolin and Mary Grosvenor, John Wiley & Sons, Inc., Copyright © 2010. Reprinted with permission of John Wiley & Sons, Inc. Figure 4.11: Canadian Diabetes Association 2013 Clinical Practice Guidelines. http://guidelines.diabetes.ca/. Reprinted with permission from the Canadian Diabetes Association. Figure 4.12: Report from the National Diabetes Surveillance System: Diabetes in Canada, 2009, http://www.phac-aspc.gc.ca/publicat/2009/ndssdic-snsddac-09/2-eng.php, Public Health Agency of Canada, 2009. Reproduced with the permission of the Minister of Public Works and Government Services Canada, 2013. Figure 4.14: Reprinted from *The Lancet*, 374 /9702, Diabetes Prevention Program Research Group, "10-year follow-up of diabetes incidence and weight loss in the Diabetes Prevention Program Outcomes Study," 1677–1686, Copyright 2009, with permission from Elsevier. Figure 4.22: From *Nutrition: Everyday Choices* by Mary B. Grosvenor and Lori A. Smolin, John Wiley & Sons, Inc., Copyright © 2006. Reprinted with permission of John Wiley & Sons, Inc.

Chapter 5

Figure 5.2c: Statistics Canada. *Food Statistics, 2009*. Catalogue no. 21-020-x. 2009. Figure 5.3: From *Nutrition: Science and Applications* by Lori A. Smolin and Mary B. Grosvenor, John Wiley & Sons, Inc., Copyright © 2008. Reprinted with permission of John Wiley & Sons, Inc. Figure 5.4: From *Nutrition: Everyday Choices* by Mary B. Grosvenor and Lori A. Smolin, John Wiley & Sons, Inc., Copyright © 2006. Reprinted with permission of John Wiley & Sons, Inc. Figure 5.5: From *Nutrition: Science and Applications* by Lori A. Smolin and Mary B. Grosvenor, John Wiley & Sons, Inc., Copyright © 2008. Reprinted with permission of John Wiley & Sons, Inc. Figure 5.6a: From *Nutrition: Everyday Choices* by Mary B. Grosvenor and Lori A. Smolin, John Wiley & Sons, Inc., Copyright © 2006. Reprinted with permission of John Wiley & Sons, Inc. Figures 5.7a, c, 5.8a: From *Nutrition: Science and Applications* by Lori A. Smolin and Mary B. Grosvenor, John Wiley & Sons, Inc., Copyright © 2008. Figure 5.9: From *Nutrition: Everyday Choices* by Mary B. Grosvenor and Lori A. Smolin, John Wiley & Sons, Inc., Reprinted with permission of John Wiley & Sons, Inc. Figures 5.10, 5.11: From *Nutrition: Science and Applications* by Lori A. Smolin and Mary B. Grosvenor, John Wiley & Sons, Inc., Copyright © 2008. Reprinted with permission of John Wiley & Sons, Inc. Figure 5.14: From *Nutrition: Everyday Choices* by Mary B. Grosvenor and Lori A. Smolin, John Wiley & Sons, Inc. Figure 5.15: From *Nutrition: Science and Applications* by Lori A. Smolin and Mary B. Grosvenor, John Wiley & Sons, Inc., Copyright © 2008. Reprinted with permission of John Wiley & Sons, Inc., and *Visualizing Human Biology*, *Second Edition* by Kathleen Anne Ireland, John Wiley & Sons, Inc., Copyright © 2010. Reprinted with permission of John Wiley & Sons, Inc. Figure 5.16: Oldways Preservation and Exchange Trust. Figure 5.18: *Eating Well with Canada's Food Guide*. Health Canada, 2011. Reproduced with permission from the Minister of Health, 2013.

Chapter 6

Figure 6.2: From *Nutrition: Science and Applications* by Lori A. Smolin and Mary B. Grosvenor, John Wiley & Sons, Inc., Copyright © 2008. Reprinted with permission of John Wiley & Sons, Inc. Figure 6.3 a-d: From *Nutrition: Everyday Choices* by Mary B. Grosvenor and Lori A. Smolin, John Wiley & Sons, Inc., Copyright © 2006. Reprinted with permission of John Wiley & Sons, Inc. Figure 6.5: From *Nutrition: Science and Applications* by Lori A. Smolin and Mary B. Grosvenor, John Wiley & Sons, Inc., Copyright © 2008. Reprinted with permission of John Wiley & Sons, Inc. Figures 6.6, 6.7a-b: From *Nutrition: Everyday Choices* by Mary B. Grosvenor and Lori A. Smolin, John Wiley & Sons, Inc., Copyright © 2006. Reprinted with permission of John Wiley & Sons, Inc. Figure 6.8a: From *Principles of Anatomy and Physiology*, *12th Edition* by Gerard J. Tortora and Bryan H. Derrickson, John Wiley & Sons, Inc., Copyright © 2009. Reprinted with permission of John Wiley & Sons, Inc. Figure 6.8b: From *Nutrition: Science and Applications* by Lori A. Smolin and Mary B. Grosvenor, John Wiley & Sons, Inc., Copyright © 2008. Reprinted with permission of John Wiley & Sons, Inc. Figure 6.9: From *Nutrition: Science and Applications, Second Edition* by Lori Smolin and Mary Grosvenor, John Wiley & Sons, Inc., Copyright © 2010. Reprinted with permission of John Wiley & Sons, Inc. Figure 6.10c: Percentage population undernourished world map. Available online at http://commons.wikimedia.org/wiki/File:Percentage_population_undernourished_world_map.PNG. Figure 6.12: From *Nutrition: Everyday Choices* by Mary B. Grosvenor and Lori A. Smolin, John Wiley & Sons, Inc., Copyright © 2006. Reprinted with permission of John Wiley & Sons, Inc. Figure 6.16a: From *Nutrition: Everyday Choices* by Mary B. Grosvenor and Lori A. Smolin, John Wiley & Sons, Inc., Copyright © 2006. Reprinted with permission of John Wiley & Sons, Inc. Figure 6.17: From *Nutrition: Science and Applications, Canadian Edition* by Lori A. Smolin, Mary B. Grosvenor, and Debbie Gurfinkel, John Wiley & Sons, Canada, Ltd.., Copyright © 2012. Reprinted with permission of John Wiley & Sons, Canada, Ltd.

Chapter 7

Hot Topic (line graph): United Nations University Press: Miller DF. Enrichment programs: helping mother nature along. *Food Prod Dev* 1978; 12(4): 30-8. http://archive.unu.edu/unupress/food/V191e/ch10.htm. Reproduced with permission of United Nations University Press. Figure 7.3 (left): From *Nutrition: Science and Applications* by Lori A. Smolin and Mary B. Grosvenor, John Wiley & Sons, Inc., Copyright © 2008. Reprinted with permission of John Wiley & Sons, Inc. Figure 7.3 (right): From *Nutrition: Everyday Choices* by Mary B. Grosvenor and Lori A. Smolin, John Wiley & Sons, Inc., Copyright © 2006. Reprinted with permission of John Wiley & Sons, Inc. Figures 7.5, 7.6: From *Nutrition: Science and Applications* by Lori A. Smolin and Mary B. Grosvenor, John Wiley & Sons, Inc., Copyright © 2008. Reprinted with permission of John Wiley & Sons, Inc. Figures 7.7, 7.8, 7.10b: From *Nutrition: Science and Applications, Canadian Edition* by Lori A. Smolin, Mary B. Grosvenor, and Debbie Gurfinkel, John Wiley & Sons Canada, Ltd., Copyright © 2012. Reprinted with permission of John Wiley & Sons Canada, Ltd. Figure 7.11: From *Nutrition: Science and Applications* by Lori A. Smolin and Mary B. Grosvenor, John Wiley & Sons, Inc., Copyright © 2008. Reprinted with permission of John Wiley & Sons, Inc. Figure 7.12: From *Nutrition: Science and Applications, Canadian Edition* by Lori A. Smolin, Mary B. Grosvenor, and Debbie Gurfinkel, John Wiley & Sons Canada, Ltd., Copyright © 2012. Reprinted with permission of John Wiley & Sons Canada, Ltd. Figure 7.13a, b: From *Nutrition: Everyday Choices* by Mary B. Grosvenor and Lori A. Smolin, John Wiley & Sons, Inc., Copyright © 2006. Reprinted with permission of John Wiley & Sons, Inc. Figure 7.13d: From *Nutrition: Science and Applications* by Lori A. Smolin and Mary B. Grosvenor, John Wiley & Sons, Inc., Copyright © 2008. Reprinted with permission of John Wiley & Sons, Inc. and *Visualizing Human Biology*, Second Edition by Kathleen Anne Ireland, John Wiley & Sons, Inc., Copyright © 2010. Reprinted with permission of John Wiley & Sons, Inc. Figure 7.14: From *Nutrition: Science and Applications, Canadian Edition* by Lori A. Smolin, Mary B. Grosvenor, and Debbie Gurfinkel, John Wiley & Sons Canada, Ltd., Copyright © 2012. Reprinted with permission of John Wiley & Sons Canada, Ltd. Figures 7.15-7.17: From *Nutrition: Science and Applications* by Lori A. Smolin and Mary B. Grosvenor, John Wiley & Sons, Inc., Copyright © 2008. Reprinted with permission of John Wiley & Sons, Inc. Figure 7.18: From *Nutrition: Science and Applications, Canadian Edition* by Lori A. Smolin, Mary B. Grosvenor, and Debbie Gurfinkel, John Wiley & Sons Canada, Ltd., Copyright © 2012. Reprinted with permission of John Wiley & Sons Canada, Ltd. Figure 7.19: From *Nutrition: Science and Applications* by Lori A. Smolin and Mary B. Grosvenor, John Wiley & Sons, Inc., Copyright © 2008. Reprinted with permission of John Wiley & Sons, Inc. Figure 7.20: From *Nutrition: Science and Applications, Canadian Edition* by Lori A. Smolin, Mary B. Grosvenor, and Debbie Gurfinkel, John Wiley & Sons Canada, Ltd., Copyright © 2012. Reprinted with permission of John Wiley & Sons Canada, Ltd. Figure 7.21: From *Nutrition: Science and Applications* by Lori A. Smolin and Mary B. Grosvenor, John Wiley & Sons, Inc., Copyright © 2008. Reprinted with permission of John Wiley & Sons, Inc. Figures 7.22, 7.23b: From *Nutrition: Science and Applications, Canadian Edition* by Lori A. Smolin, Mary B. Grosvenor, and Debbie Gurfinkel, John Wiley & Sons Canada, Ltd., Copyright © 2012. Reprinted with permission of John Wiley & Sons Canada, Ltd. Figure 7.24: From *Nutrition: Science and Applications* by Lori A. Smolin and Mary B. Grosvenor, John Wiley & Sons, Inc., Copyright © 2008. Reprinted with permission of John Wiley & Sons, Inc. Figure 7.25 (map): World Health Organization, *Countries categorized by degree of public health importance of Vitamin A deficiency*, April 1995. Available online at http://www.

who.int/vmnis/vitamina/prevalence/mn_vitamina_map_1995.pdf. Figure 7.27: From *Nutrition: Everyday Choices* by Mary B. Grosvenor and Lori A. Smolin, John Wiley & Sons, Inc., Copyright © 2006. Reprinted with permission of John Wiley & Sons, Inc. Figure 7.29a: From *Nutrition: Science and Applications, Canadian Edition* by Lori A. Smolin, Mary B. Grosvenor, and Debbie Gurfinkel, John Wiley & Sons Canada, Ltd., Copyright © 2012. Reprinted with permission of John Wiley & Sons Canada, Ltd. Figure 7.30: From *Nutrition: Science and Applications* by Lori A. Smolin and Mary B. Grosvenor, John Wiley & Sons, Inc., Copyright © 2008. Reprinted with permission of John Wiley & Sons, Inc. Figure 7.31: From *Nutrition: Science and Applications, Canadian Edition* by Lori A. Smolin, Mary B. Grosvenor, and Debbie Gurfinkel, John Wiley & Sons Canada, Ltd., Copyright © 2012. Reprinted with permission of John Wiley & Sons Canada, Ltd. Figure 7.32: From *Nutrition: Science and Applications* by Lori A. Smolin and Mary B. Grosvenor, John Wiley & Sons, Inc., Copyright © 2008. Reprinted with permission of John Wiley & Sons, Inc. Figure 7.34: From *Nutrition: Science and Applications, Canadian Edition* by Lori A. Smolin, Mary B. Grosvenor, and Debbie Gurfinkel, John Wiley & Sons Canada, Ltd., Copyright © 2012. Reprinted with permission of John Wiley & Sons Canada, Ltd.

Chapter 8

Figure 8.2: From *Nutrition: Everyday Choices* by Mary B. Grosvenor and Lori A. Smolin, John Wiley & Sons, Inc., Copyright © 2006. Reprinted with permission of John Wiley & Sons, Inc. Figures 8.3–8.4: From *Nutrition: Science and Applications* by Lori A. Smolin and Mary B. Grosvenor, John Wiley & Sons, Inc., Copyright © 2008. Reprinted with permission of John Wiley & Sons, Inc. Figure 8.10: From *Nutrition: Science and Applications* by Lori A. Smolin and Mary B. Grosvenor, John Wiley & Sons, Inc., Copyright © 2008. Reprinted with permission of John Wiley & Sons, Inc. Figure 8.12: From *Nutrition: Science and Applications* by Lori A. Smolin and Mary B. Grosvenor, John Wiley & Sons, Inc., Copyright © 2008. Reprinted with permission of John Wiley & Sons, Inc. Figure 8.13: *It's Your Health: Sodium*. Health Canada, 2009. Updated: June 2012. Reproduced with permission from the Minister of Health, 2013. Figure 8.14: From *Nutrition: Science and Applications, Canadian Edition* by Lori A. Smolin, Mary B. Grosvenor, and Debbie Gurfinkel, John Wiley & Sons Canada, Ltd., Copyright © 2012. Reprinted with permission of John Wiley & Sons Canada, Ltd. Figure 8.16a: From *Nutrition: Science and Applications* by Lori A. Smolin and Mary B. Grosvenor, John Wiley & Sons, Inc., Copyright © 2008. Reprinted with permission of John Wiley & Sons, Inc. Figure 8.17: From *Nutrition: Everyday Choices* by Mary B. Grosvenor and Lori A. Smolin, John Wiley & Sons, Inc., Copyright © 2006. Reprinted with permission of John Wiley & Sons, Inc. Figure 8.18: From *Nutrition: Science and Applications, Canadian Edition* by Lori A. Smolin, Mary B. Grosvenor, and Debbie Gurfinkel, John Wiley & Sons Canada, Ltd., Copyright © 2012. Reprinted with permission of John Wiley & Sons Canada, Ltd. Figure 8.20: From *Nutrition: Everyday Choices* by Mary B. Grosvenor and Lori A. Smolin, John Wiley & Sons, Inc., Copyright © 2006. Reprinted with permission of John Wiley & Sons, Inc. Figures 8.21, 8.24: From *Nutrition: Science and Applications, Canadian Edition* by Lori A. Smolin, Mary B. Grosvenor, and Debbie Gurfinkel, John Wiley & Sons Canada, Ltd., Copyright © 2012. Reprinted with permission of John Wiley & Sons Canada, Ltd. Figures 8.25b-8.27, Thinking It Through: From *Nutrition: Science and Applications* by Lori A. Smolin and Mary B. Grosvenor, John Wiley & Sons, Inc., Copyright © 2008. Reprinted with permission of John Wiley & Sons, Inc. Figure

8.28: From *Nutrition: Science and Applications, Canadian Edition* by Lori A. Smolin, Mary B. Grosvenor, and Debbie Gurfinkel, John Wiley & Sons Canada, Ltd., Copyright © 2012. Reprinted with permission of John Wiley & Sons Canada, Ltd. Figure 8.29: Yang, X.E., W.R. Chen, Y. Feng. Improving human micronutrient nutrition through biofortification in the soil-plant system: China as a case study. *Environmental Geochemistry and Health*. 2007 Oct; 29(5):413–28. Epub 2007 Mar 24 © Springer Science+Business Media B.V. 2007. With kind permission of Springer Science and Business Media. Figure 8.30: From *Nutrition: Science and Applications* by Lori A. Smolin and Mary B. Grosvenor, John Wiley & Sons, Inc., Copyright © 2008. Reprinted with permission of John Wiley & Sons, Inc. Figure 8.31: de Benoist B et al., eds. Iodine status worldwide. WHO Global Database on Iodine Deficiency. Geneva, World Health Organization, 2004. Data was produced by WHO using the best available evidence and do not necessarily correspond to the official statistics of Member States. Figure 8.34: eprinted with permission from Dietary Reference Intakes for Calcium, Phosphorus, Magnesium, Vitamin D and Fluoride. © 1997 by the National Academy of Sciences, Courtesy of the National Academies Press, Washington, D.C.

Chapter 9

Figure 9.1: *Chronic Diseases in Canada*, Volume 30, no. 1, December 2009, Socio-demographic and geographic analysis of overweight and obesity in Canadian adults using the Canadian Community Health Survey (2005) http://www.phac-aspc.gc.ca/publicat/cdic-mcbc/30-1/ar_01-eng.php Public Health Agency of Canada, 2005. Reproduced with the permission of the Minister of Public Works and Government Services Canada, 2012. Figure 9.5b: National Heart, Lung, and Blood Institute as a part of the National Institutes of Health and the U.S. Department of Health and Human Services. Figure 9.6a: From *Nutrition: Science and Applications* by Lori A. Smolin and Mary B. Grosvenor, John Wiley & Sons, Inc., Copyright © 2008. Reprinted with permission of John Wiley & Sons, Inc. Figure 9.7b: From *Nutrition: Science and Applications, Canadian Edition* by Lori A. Smolin, Mary B. Grosvenor, and Debbie Gurfinkel, John Wiley & Sons Canada, Ltd., Copyright © 2012. Reprinted with permission of John Wiley & Sons Canada, Ltd. Figure 9.8: From *Nutrition: Everyday Choices* by Mary B. Grosvenor and Lori A. Smolin, John Wiley & Sons, Inc., Copyright © 2006. Reprinted with permission of John Wiley & Sons, Inc. Table 9.1: World Health Organization. WHO Global Database on Body Mass Index (BMI), 2011. Available online at http://apps.who.int/bmi/index.jsp?introPage=intro_3.html. Accessed March 15, 2011. Figures 9.12a, 13a: From *Nutrition: Everyday Choices* by Mary B. Grosvenor and Lori A. Smolin, John Wiley & Sons, Inc., Copyright © 2006. Reprinted with permission of John Wiley & Sons, Inc. Hot Topic (table): American Psychiatric Association. (2000). *Diagnostic and statistical manual of mental disorders: DSM-IV-TR*. Washington, DC. Figure 9.14: Vandenbroeck, I.P., Goossens, J. and Clemens, M. *Foresight Tackling Obesities Future Choice—Obesity System Atlas*. Government Office for Science, UK Government's Foresight Programme. Figure 9.15: From *Nutrition: Everyday Choices* by Mary B. Grosvenor and Lori A. Smolin, John Wiley & Sons, Inc., Copyright © 2006. Reprinted with permission of John Wiley & Sons, Inc. Figure 9.19a: From *Nutrition: Science and Applications* by Lori A. Smolin and Mary B. Grosvenor, John Wiley & Sons, Inc., Copyright © 2008. Reprinted with permission of John Wiley & Sons, Inc. Figure 9.21: From *Nutrition: Science and Applications* by Lori A. Smolin and Mary B. Grosvenor,

John Wiley & Sons, Inc., Copyright © 2008. Reprinted with permission of John Wiley & Sons, Inc. Figures 9.23-9.25: From *Nutrition: Everyday Choices* by Mary B. Grosvenor and Lori A. Smolin, John Wiley & Sons, Inc., Copyright © 2006. Reprinted with permission of John Wiley & Sons, Inc. and From *Nutrition: Science and Applications, Canadian Edition* by Lori A. Smolin, Mary B. Grosvenor, and Debbie Gurfinkel, John Wiley & Sons Canada, Ltd., Copyright © 2012. Reprinted with permission of John Wiley & Sons Canada, Ltd.

Chapter 10

Figures 10.1d, 10.3: From *Nutrition: Science and Applications* by Lori A. Smolin and Mary B. Grosvenor, John Wiley & Sons, Inc., Copyright © 2008. Reprinted with permission of John Wiley & Sons, Inc. Figures 10.4, 10.5: Canadian Physical Activity Guidelines, © 2011. Used with permission from the Canadian Society for Exercise Physiology, www.csep.ca/guidelines. Figure 10.5a: From *Nutrition: Science and Applications* by Lori A. Smolin and Mary B. Grosvenor, John Wiley & Sons, Inc., Copyright © 2008. Reprinted with permission of John Wiley & Sons, Inc. Figure 10.7: From *Nutrition: Science and Applications*, Second Edition by Lori Smolin and Mary Grosvenor, John Wiley & Sons, Inc., Copyright © 2010. Reprinted with permission of John Wiley & Sons, Inc. Figures 10.8–10.9: From *Nutrition: Science and Applications* by Lori A. Smolin and Mary B. Grosvenor, John Wiley & Sons, Inc., Copyright © 2008. Reprinted with permission of John Wiley & Sons, Inc. Figure 10.11: From *Nutrition: Science and Applications* by Lori A. Smolin and Mary B. Grosvenor, John Wiley & Sons, Inc., Copyright © 2008. Reprinted with permission of John Wiley & Sons, Inc. Figure 10.15: From *Nutrition: Science and Applications* by Lori A. Smolin and Mary B. Grosvenor, John Wiley & Sons, Inc., Copyright © 2008. Reprinted with permission of John Wiley & Sons, Inc. Figure 10.19: Adapted from Saltin, B., and Castill, D. I. Fluid and electrolyte balance during prolonged exercise. In *Exercise, Nutrition, and Energy Metabolism*. E. S. Horton, and R. I. Tergung, eds. New York: Macmillan, 1988. Reprinted by permission of The McGraw-Hill Companies, Inc. Figure 10.21: From Bergstrom, J., L. Hermansen, E. Hultman, and B. Saltin. Diet, muscle glycogen and physical performance. *Acta Physiologica Scandinavica* 71:140–150, 1967. Wiley-Blackwell Publishers. Figure 10.23: From *Nutrition: Science and Applications, Canadian Edition* by Lori A. Smolin, Mary B. Grosvenor, and Debbie Gurfinkel, John Wiley & Sons Canada, Ltd., Copyright © 2012. Reprinted with permission of John Wiley & Sons Canada, Ltd.

Chapter 11

Figures 11.1, 11.3: From *Nutrition: Science and Applications* by Lori A. Smolin and Mary B. Grosvenor, John Wiley & Sons, Inc., Copyright © 2008. Reprinted with permission of John Wiley & Sons, Inc. Figure 11.3: Adapted from Committee on Nutritional Status During Pregnancy and Lactation. *Nutrition during Pregnancy*. Washington, D.C.: National Academy Press, 1990. Figure 11.5: From *Visualizing Human Biology*, Second Edition by Kathleen Anne Ireland, John Wiley & Sons, Inc., Copyright © 2010. Reprinted with permission of John Wiley & Sons, Inc. Figure 11.6: From *Nutrition: Science and Applications* by Lori A. Smolin and Mary B. Grosvenor, John Wiley & Sons, Inc., Copyright © 2008. Reprinted with permission of John Wiley & Sons, Inc. Thinking It Through: Adapted from Committee on Nutritional Status During Pregnancy and Lactation. *Nutrition during Pregnancy*. Washington, D.C.: National Academy Press, 1990. Figures 11.1, 11.3: From *Nutrition: Science and Applications* by Lori A. Smolin and Mary B. Grosvenor, John Wiley & Sons, Inc., Copy-

right © 2008. Reprinted with permission of John Wiley & Sons, Inc. Figure 11.5: From *Visualizing Human Biology*, Second Edition by Kathleen Anne Ireland, John Wiley & Sons, Inc., Copyright © 2010. Reprinted with permission of John Wiley & Sons, Inc. Figure 11.6: From *Nutrition: Science and Applications* by Lori A. Smolin and Mary B. Grosvenor, John Wiley & Sons, Inc., Copyright © 2008. Reprinted with permission of John Wiley & Sons, Inc. Figure 11.7: *The Sensible Guide to a Healthy Pregnancy*. Public Health Agency of Canada, 2008. Revised, 2012. Reproduced with permission from the Minister of Health, 2013. Figure 11.8, Thinking It Through: From *Nutrition: Science and Applications* by Lori A. Smolin and Mary B. Grosvenor, John Wiley & Sons, Inc., Copyright © 2008. Reprinted with permission of John Wiley & Sons, Inc. Figure 11.10: This figure was published in *The Developing Human, 5e*, by K. Moore and T. Persaud, copyright Elsevier (1993). Figure 11.12: From *Nutrition: Science and Applications* by Lori A. Smolin and Mary B. Grosvenor, John Wiley & Sons, Inc., Copyright © 2008. Reprinted with permission of John Wiley & Sons, Inc. Figure 11.14: Based on the World Health Organization (WHO) Child Growth Standards (2006) and adapted for Canada by Dietitians of Canada, Canadian Paediatric Society, the College of Family Physicians of Canada and Community Health Nurses of Canada. © Dietitians of Canada. 2010. May be reproduced in its entirety (i.e. no changes) for educational purposes only. www.dietitians.ca/growthcharts Figure 11.16b: From *Nutrition: Everyday Choices* by Mary B. Grosvenor and Lori A. Smolin, John Wiley & Sons, Inc., Copyright © 2006. Reprinted with permission of John Wiley & Sons, Inc. Figures 11.20, 11.22: From *Nutrition: Science and Applications* by Lori A. Smolin and Mary B. Grosvenor, John Wiley & Sons, Inc., Copyright © 2008. Reprinted with permission of John Wiley & Sons, Inc.

Chapter 12

Figure 12.1: *Eating Well with Canada's Food Guide*. Health Canada, 2011. Reproduced with permission from the Minister of Health, 2013. Figure 12.4a: Based on the World Health Organization (WHO) Child Growth Standards (2006) and adapted for Canada by Dietitians of Canada, Canadian Paediatric Society, the College of Family Physicians of Canada and Community Health Nurses of Canada. © Dietitians of Canada. 2010. May be reproduced in its entirety (i.e. no changes) for educational purposes only. www.dietitians.ca/growthcharts. Figure 12.4b: Shields, M. Overweight and Obesity among children and youth. *Health Reports* 17: 27-42, 2006. Figure 12.5: Reprinted from the *Journal of the American Dietetic Association*, Vol. 4, Issue 6. Ameena Batada, Maia Dock Seitz, Margo G. Wootan, and Mary Story. *Nine out of 10 Food Advertisements Shown During Saturday Morning Children's Television Programming are for Foods High in Fat, Sodium, or Added Sugars, or Low in Nutrients*. Pages 673–678, copyright 2008, with permission from Elsevier. Figure 12.6 (line graph): Tanner, J.M., Whitehouse, R.H., Marubini, E., Resele, L.F. (1976). The adolescent growth spurt of boys and girls of the Harpenden growth study. *Annals of Human Biology* 1976 Mar: 3(2): 109-26. Figure 12.6 (bar graph): Adapted from Forbes, G.B. Body Composition. In *Present Knowledge in Nutrition*, 6th ed. M.L. Brown, ed. Washington, DC: International Life Sciences Institute-Nutrition Foundation, 1990. Figures 12.7, 12.9: *Eating Well with Canada's Food Guide*. Health Canada, 2011. Reproduced with permission from the Minister of Health, 2013. Figure 12.10a: Health Canada. *Canada's Aging Population*. Available online at http://publications.gc.ca/collections/Collection/H39-608-2002E.pdf. Accessed June 18, 2011. Figure 12.11: *Nutrition: Science and Applications* by Lori A. Smolin and Mary

B. Grosvenor, John Wiley & Sons, Inc., Copyright © 2008. Reprinted with permission of John Wiley & Sons, Inc. Figure 12.12: *Eating Well with Canada's Food Guide*. Health Canada, 2011. Reproduced with permission from the Minister of Health, 2013. Figure 12.13: Adapted from Cohen, S.H., et al. Compartmental body composition based on the body nitrogen, potassium, and calcium. *American Journal of Physiology*. 239: 192-200, 1980 and *Nutrition: Science and Applications* by Lori A. Smolin and Mary B. Grosvenor, John Wiley & Sons, Inc., Copyright © 2008. Reprinted with permission of John Wiley & Sons, Inc. Figures 12.14, 12.15a: From *Nutrition: Science and Applications* by Lori A. Smolin and Mary B. Grosvenor, John Wiley & Sons, Inc., Copyright © 2008. Reprinted with permission of John Wiley & Sons, Inc. Figure 12.15c: Canadian Cancer Society. *Canadian Cancer Statistics, 2012*. Figure 12.16: From *Nutrition: Science and Applications* by Lori A. Smolin and Mary B. Grosvenor, John Wiley & Sons, Inc., Copyright © 2008. Reprinted with permission of John Wiley & Sons, Inc. Figure 12.20: From *Canada's Low-Risk Alcohol Drinking Guidelines* Canadian Centre on Substance Abuse 2012. Developed on behalf of the National Strategy Advisory Committee. Figures 12.22a, 12.23: From *Nutrition: Science and Applications* by Lori A. Smolin and Mary B. Grosvenor, John Wiley & Sons, Inc., Copyright © 2008. Reprinted with permission of John Wiley & Sons, Inc.

Chapter 13

Figure 13.6b: Adapted from Liu, Y. and Wu, F. Global burden of aflatoxin-induced hepatocellular carcinoma: A risk assessment. *Environmental Health Perspectives*. 118:818-824, 2010. Figure 13.9 (logo and Safe Cooking Temperatures table): Canadian Partnership For Consumer Food Safety Education, March 2010. Cooking temperatures provided by Health Canada. Figure 13.9 (thermometer): From *Nutrition: Science and Applications* by Lori A. Smolin and Mary B. Grosvenor, John Wiley & Sons, Inc., Copyright © 2008. Reprinted with permission of John Wiley & Sons, Inc. Figure 13.18: From *Nutrition: Everyday Choices* by Mary B. Grosvenor and Lori A. Smolin, John Wiley & Sons, Inc., Copyright © 2006. Reprinted with permission of John Wiley & Sons, Inc. Figure 13.19c: Data from ISAAA Brief 43-2012: Executive Summary, Global Status of Commercialized Biotech/GM Crops: 2012; http://www.isaaa.org/resources/publications/briefs/44/executivesummary/default.asp

Chapter 14

Figure 14.1a: From *Nutrition: Science and Applications* by Lori A. Smolin and Mary B. Grosvenor, John Wiley & Sons, Inc., Copyright © 2008. Reprinted with permission of John Wiley & Sons, Inc. Figure 14.1c: World Health Organization. *The Global Burden of Disease: 2004 update*, Copyright 2008. Available online at http://www.who.int/health-iinfo/global_burden_disease/GBD_report_2004update_full.pdf. Figure 14.2a: Adapted from Vorster, H.H., Bourne, L.T., Venter, C.S., and Oosthuizen, W. Contribution of nutrition to the health transition in developing countries: A framework for research and intervention. *Nutr. Rev*. 57:341–349, 1999. Wiley-Blackwell Publishers. Figure 14.2b: FAO *The nutrition transition and obesity*, http://www.fao.org/FOCUS/E/obesity/obes2.htm. World Health Organization, 2000. Figure 14.4 (map): World Bank, 2009. World poverty map. International Fund for Agricultural Development (IFAD). Available online at http://www.ruralpovertyportal.org/web/guest/region. Figure 14.5: From *Nutrition: Science and Applications* by Lori A. Smo-

lin and Mary B. Grosvenor, John Wiley & Sons, Inc., Copyright © 2008. Reprinted with permission of John Wiley & Sons, Inc. Figure 14.8: *Household Food Insecurity In Canada in 2007-2008: Key Statistics and Graphics*, http://www.hc-sc.gc.ca/fn-an/surveill/nutrition/commun/insecurit/key-stats-cles-2007-2008-eng.php#a, Health Canada, 2012. Reproduced with the permission of the Minister of Public Works and Government Services Canada, 2013. Figure 14.9a: Special Reports - What Difference Does Learning Make to Financial Security, http://www4.hrsdc.gc.ca/.3ndic.1t.4r@-eng.jsp?iid=54#a7, Human Resources and Skills Development Canada, 2008. Reproduced with the permission of the Minister of Public Works and Government Services Canada, 2013. Figure 14.9b: From *Nutrition: Science and Applications* by Lori A. Smolin and Mary B. Grosvenor, John Wiley & Sons, Inc., Copyright © 2008. Reprinted with permission of John Wiley & Sons, Inc. Figure 14.10: Millennium Development Goals, http://www.un.org/millenniumgoals. Courtesy of the UNDP. Figure 14.12 (bar graph): United Nations Population Fund. 2003. *State of World Population*. Available online from http://www.unfpa.org/publicationsd/index.cfm?filterPub_Type=5. Figure 14.14: From *Visualizing Environmental Science*, Third Edition by Linda Berg, Mary Catherine Hager, and Dave Hassenzahl, John Wiley & Sons, Inc., Copyright © 2011. Reprinted with permission of John Wiley & Sons, Inc.

Appendices

Appendix A: Pages 517-519: *Dietary Reference Intakes: The Essential Guide to Nutrient Requirements*. Reprinted with permission from National Academies Press, Copyright 2006, National Academy of Sciences. Page 520: Institute of Medicine, Food and Nutrition Board, "Dietary Reference Intakes for Energy, Carbohydrate, Fiber, Fat, Fatty Acids, Cholesterol, Protein, and Amino Acids," Washington, DC: National Academy Press, 2002, 2005. Appendix B: Based on the World Health Organization (WHO) Child Growth Standards (2006) and adapted for Canada by Dietitians of Canada, Canadian Paediatric Society, the College of Family Physicians of Canada and Community Health Nurses of Canada. © Dietitians of Canada. 2010. May be reproduced in its entirety (i.e. no changes) for educational purposes only. www.dietitians.ca/growthcharts Appendix C: *Handbook of Clinical Dietetics*, American Dietetic Association, © 1981 by Yale University Press (New Haven, Conn.). Appendix D: Figures D.1, D.2: *Canadian Diabetes Association: Beyond the Basics*. Available online at http://www.diabetes.ca/for-professionals/resources/nutrition/beyond-basics/. Accessed April 6, 2013. Appendix E: Questions adapted from Yale Rudd Center for Food Policy and Obesity. *Motivational interviewing for diet/exercise and obesity*. Available online at ttp://www.yaleruddcenter.org/resources/bias_toolkit/toolkit/Module-2/2-07-MotivationalStrategies.pdf. Accessed March 10, 2013. Appendix F: World Health Organization. *Diet, Nutrition, and the Prevention of Chronic Diseases*. WHO Technical Report Series 916, 2003. Available online at http://whqlibdoc.who.int/trs/who_trs_916.pdf. Accessed August 5, 2012. Appendix G: From N-Squared Computing. First Databank Division of the Hearst Corporation.

Inside Covers

Dietary Reference Intakes: The Essential Guide to Nutrient Requirements. Reprinted with permission from National Academies Press, Copyright 2006, National Academy of Sciences.

Index

A

Aboriginal peoples, 44, 45, 227, 502, 503
absorption, 62
  alcohol, 447–448
  carbohydrates, 107, 123–124
  iron, 277
  lipids, 138, 139, 159
  minerals, 258
  of nutrients, 72–73, 91
  proteins, 169–171, 190, 191
  vitamin B_{12}, 217
  vitamins, 201
absorption mechanisms, 73
acceptable daily intakes (ADIs), 115
Acceptable Macronutrient Distribution Ranges
    (AMDRs), 37
  carbohydrates, 119
  fats, 153
  protein, 183
acesulfame K, 116
acetyl CoA, 109, 143
acne, 434
acrylamide, 478
active, 37
active lifestyle, 353–354
active transport, 73
addiction to food, 316
adenosine triphosphate (ATP), 87, 88, 108,
    109, 142, 205, 276, 357, 371
Adequate Intakes (AIs), 35, 119, 204
adipocytes, 142, 308
adipose tissue, 142
adjustable gastric banding, 328
adolescence, 430–434, 451
  acne, 434
  adolescent growth spurt, 430
  alcohol use, 434
  athletics, 434
  eating disorders, 433
  food guide recommendations, 431
  healthy eating habits, 432–433
  puberty, 430
  recommendations, 431–432
  special concerns, 433–434
  teenage pregnancies, 397
  tobacco use, 434
  vegetarian diets, 432–433
adolescent growth spurt, 430
adolescent pregnancies, 397
adult years, 435–436, 451
  see also older adults
advertisements, credibility of, 22
aerobic capacity, 346
aerobic exercise, 346, 360
aerobic metabolism, 109, 307,
    355, 356–358, 360
aerobic zone, 352
aflatoxin, 466
Africa, 496
age, 148
age-related bone loss, 269
age-specific recommendations, 43
aging, 436–437
  see also older adults
agricultural chemicals, 472–475, 476, 487–488
air displacement, 301

albacore tuna, 43
alcohol, 446–450, 452
  absorption, 447–448
  adolescence, 434
  adverse effects, 448–450
  alcoholic liver disease, 449
  alcoholism, 449
  benefits of, 450
  blood alcohol levels, 447
  excretion, 447–448
  health problems, 449–450
  malnutrition, 449–450
  metabolism, 448
  during pregnancy, 398–399
  recommendations, 446
  short-term effects, 449
  transport, 447–448
alcohol dehydrogenase (ADH), 448
alcohol poisoning, 449
alcohol-related birth defects (ARBD), 399
alcohol-related neuro-development disorders
    (ARND), 399
alcoholic hepatitis, 449
alcoholic liver disease, 449
alcoholics, 207
alcoholism, 449
aldosterone, 253, 262
alimentary canal, 64, 67, 76
allergen, 77
alpha-carotene, 222, 223
alpha-linolenic acid (ALA), 134
Alzheimer's disease, 442
amenorrhea, 334
American Academy of Pediatrics, 424
American Food and Nutrition Board, 34
American Red Cross, 505
amino acid pool, 171, 172
amino acids, 8, 70, 90, 166
  animal *vs.* plant proteins, 9
  conditionally essential amino acids, 167
  Eating Well with Canada's Food Guide, 176
  energy, extraction of, 88
  essential amino acids, 167, 173
  limiting amino acid, 172, 173
  nonessential amino acids, 167, 173
  structure of, 167–168, 190
  supplements, 183
  transport system, 171
amylases, 64
anabolic steroids, 372–373
anabolism, 86
anaerobic, 87–89
anaerobic metabolism, 109, 354, 355, 356, 357
Anderson, Harvey, 181
androstenedione, 373
anecdotal evidence, 21
anemia
  children, 423
  and folate deficiency, 214–215
  and iron, 364
  iron-deficiency anemia, 13, 278–280,
    364, 501
  macrocytic anemia, 214–215
  megaloblastic anemia, 214–215, 390
  pernicious anemia, 217
  sickle cell anemia, 193, 219
  sports anemia, 364

anencephaly, 215
angiotensin II, 253
Angola, 499
animal proteins, 9, 166
animal studies, 20
Anisakis simplex, 466, 468
anorexia athletica, 337
anorexia nervosa, 331, 334–335
anti-caking agents, 482
antibiotics, 475–476
antibodies, 77
anticoagulation agents, 235
antidiuretic hormone (ADH), 253
antigen, 76–77
antioxidants, 148, 152, 203–204, 363–364
appetite, 304
arachidonic acid (ARA), 134, 407
Argentina, 496
arginine, 372
Armstrong, Lance, 375
arsenic, 289
arteries, 83
arterioles, 83
arthritis, 442
artificial sweetener, 115–117
ascorbic acid, 218
aseptic processing, 478
Asian diets, 149, 152
aspartame, 115–116
Aspergillus flovus, 466
assessment, 33
astragalus, 239
atherosclerosis, 145–147
atherosclerotic plaque, 146
athletes, 183, 300
  adolescents, 434
  anabolic steroids, 372–373
  energy and nutrient needs, 361–370
  ergogenic aids, 370–375, 378
  female athlete triad, 337, 362, 434
atoms, 60
ATP. *See* adenosine triphosphate (ATP)
atrophic gastritis, 218, 439–440
attention-deficit/hyperactivity disorder
    (ADHD), 428
autoimmune disease, 110
availability of foods, 6

B

B vitamins, 202
  see also specific B vitamins
bacteria, 462–464
bacterial food-borne infection, 462
bacterial food-borne intoxication,
    462–464
balanced diet, 15–16
balancing calories, 17
Banting, Frederick, 113
bariatric surgery, 328–329
basal metabolic rate (BMR), 305, 308, 349
basal metabolism, 305
Basillus thuringlensis (Bt), 485
Be Food Safe, 470
Beauchemin-Nadeau, Marie-Eve, 183
beaver fever, 465
Bechler, Steve, 327